TSRA

Clinical Scenarios in Cardiothoracic Surgery

2nd Edition

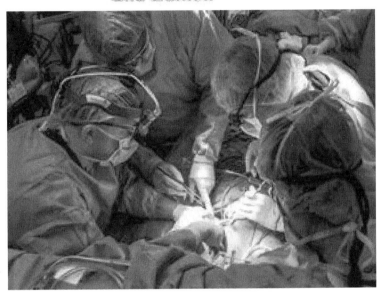

Justin Watson MD
Clauden Louis MD, MS

Edited by:
Justin J.J. Watson MD
Oregon Health & Sciences University
Editor

Clauden Louis MD, MS
University of Rochester Medical Center
Editor

Section Editors:
Alexander A. Brescia, MD, MSc
University of Michigan
Thoracic Section Editor

Jordan P. Bloom, MD, MPH
Massachusetts General Hospital
Adult Cardiac Section Editor

Garrett N. Coyan, MD, MS
University of Pittsburgh Medical Center
Congenital Section Editor

Thoracic Surgery Residents Association
www.tsranet.org

2

Copyright © 2020 by the Thoracic Surgery Residents Association

TSRA/TSDA
633 N. Saint Clair Street
Suite 2100
Chicago, IL 60611
www.tsranet.org

Thanks. We would like to thank the Thoracic Surgery Directors Association (TSDA) for their support with this project and all other initiatives. We would particularly like to thank the TSRA committee members and the multiple contributors that made the creation of this book possible. We would like to thank Xiaoying Lou for her support with this endeavor.

Thank you to my parents Bob & Sara Watson, and my sisters Erika & Kara, for teaching me to be inquisitive, adventurous and fostering my interest in science. This book would not have been possible without the dedicated support and encouragement of my wife, Traci. For understanding my long nights at the hospital and missed bedtime stories, I'd like to thank Bodi. To the section editors and copy editor Jordan, Garrett, Alex & Clauden, thank you for your persistence and tireless pursuit of perfection.

~ JW

To Silvia, Jalen, Sarai for their patience and support. To Jean and Verana for their uplift.

~ CL

To Meghan, Louis, Milo, and all my mentors.

~ AB

To Izabela, Charlotte & Hudson, thanks for your ongoing and unrelenting support of my academic pursuits.

~ JB

To Katie and Jane for their love and support, and my many mentors.

~ GC

4

Forward

How does one learn to make clinical decisions?

Surgeons frequently differentiate between how they learn surgical techniques from how they learn medical techniques. The usual approach is that repetition is the key to learning surgical techniques. Afterall it resembles other mechanical skills say like hitting a golf ball or playing the piano. You must achieve muscle memory allowing you to instinctively adjust the position of your body, the flex of your wrist or perceive a subtle change in anatomy to avoid injuring a hidden vessel. Learning how to make clinical decision on the other hand is something you mostly read about and practice when the opportunity arises. The truth however is that how one learns clinical decision making is no different than how one learns surgical technique. It is a skill that can only be mastered through practice.

Ideally that practice should be deliberate practice, a conceptual framework in education central to the development of expertise in any skill. Pivotal to this framework is the need to break the skill down into manageable components, repeatedly practice those components at the limit of one's current level of mastery, and, most importantly, to receive immediate feedback to correct errors and reinforce correct responses. Ideally this was obtained in the clinic or on the wards. When we saw a patient, we would practice making a clinical decision. We might break it down into components of diagnosis, the evaluation of the extent of the disease (i.e. staging) or treatment allocation. Our faculty would then provide feedback and we would move on.

Unfortunately, these opportunities have been dwindling. The greater need to master an expanding volume of surgical skills is limiting the time available to see patients when the decisions are being made. Time constraints on faculty limits that one-on-one opportunity for feedback. A rapidly expanding body of knowledge means there are more tests, more treatment options etc. that need to be understood and woven into the decision-making process. Finally, one is always at the mercy of whatever patient happens to walk through the door. One may go through an entire fellowship or residency and never see relatively common presentations of various diseases. Without the opportunities to practice or to do so without the availability of immediate feedback limits the development of this vital skill.

Here the TSRA has provided a vital resource to address this very need. *Clinical Scenarios in Cardiothoracic Surgery* provides a basic resource to fill in the gaps that now exist. The first edition was already a boon to trainees as it covered a multitude of topics including some that many residents may not see frequently or even at all. Now one had the ability to practice elements of the decision making on areas where gaps exist. The new second edition has updated the information on the existing chapters and added 19 new chapters in General Thoracic/Adult Cardiac/Congenital Cardiothoracic sections as well as 36-chapter revisions.

I encourage the readers of this book not to simply memorize the content. To truly learn how to make clinical decisions, just like how one learns to operate, one must practice on all sorts of different presentations. The authors do their best to cover the various ways a disease may present but practicing how one makes decisions, while reflecting on how those subtle variations in presentation may impact the decisions, are essential to mastering this skill.

Use this book to initiate discussions with fellow trainees and faculty. Consider nuances in management that may become necessary if a patient presented in a slightly different way. Keep pushing yourself to look at each decision from every angle possible. The more variation you see and practice the more effortless the decisions will become. Use the book to provide some of that expert feedback so crucial for deliberate practice. Get more of it from fellow trainees and your faculty. Most importantly, make notes and add additional details. This book should be well thumbed through by the time you sit for your boards.

Ara. A. Vaporciyan, MD., FACS., MHPE
Professor of Surgery and Chairman of the Department of Thoracic and Cardiovascular Surgery at the University of Texas MD Anderson Cancer Center

TSDA President

Preface

The Thoracic Surgery Residents Association (TSRA) was established in 1997 under the guidance of the Thoracic Surgery Directors Association (TSDA) with the goal of representing residents in cardiothoracic surgery training. Over the last 23 years our identity and mission have expanded to meet the needs of our members by providing peer-based resources and support for cardiothoracic surgery residents to succeed throughout training and launch successful careers.

The prior edition of this book, *TSRA Clinical Scenarios in Cardiothoracic Surgery*, published in 2013 was tremendously successful. The first edition of this book aimed to augment available resident educational resources. It focused on knowledge application in a dynamic decision-making capacity highlighting surgical technique, practical knowledge and clinical acumen based on a variety of different clinical case scenarios. This edition aims to update this review resource while simultaneously expanding the scope of clinical scenarios to keep pace with the ever-changing clinical cardiothoracic training environment.

The aim of this book is to review common, high-yield clinical scenarios that may surface during a cardiothoracic surgeon's practice in congenital, thoracic, or adult cardiac surgery. It was written by residents for residents. We meticulously reviewed and edited all previous clinical case scenario chapters focusing on updated clinical and scientific evidence. The first edition contained 72 chapters authored by over 50 residents and faculty from across the country. The new edition contains 19 new chapters (36-chapter revisions) with 91 chapters authored by 159 residents and faculty nationwide! We have maintained the structure and flow of the book utilizing the three major sections of cardiothoracic surgery: General Thoracic Surgery, Adult Cardiac while expanding the congenital section to be Congenital Cardiothoracic Surgery. While we acknowledge there is some overlap between these fields, i.e. Heart or lung transplant, ECMO etc., we felt this allowed the reader the optimal organization of the material.

Despite the rigorous review process, it should be evident to the reader that there continues to be differences in institutional and/or regional practice patterns especially regarding certain technical aspects or management preferences. The scenarios and their responses reflect the safest practice as determined by the author and reviewers. Due to this variation the reader may choose to utilize algorithms or management pathways not highlighted in this text as long as they are safe, efficacious and supported by current guidelines and literature. TSRA resources are provided as a basic guideline for the study of cardiothoracic surgery and should be used in conjunction with a variety of other educational references and resources and should not used for in training or high stakes examination. We welcome feedback and submission of additional scenarios to Justin Watson (exploringtheworld2@gmail.com) and/or Clauden Louis (claudenlouis@gmail.com).

We would again like to express our gratitude to all the residents and faculty who have contributed to this project. Without each of you this project would not have been possible. We would also like to thank the TSDA and the Joint Council for Thoracic Surgery Education (JCTSE) for their continued support. We sincerely hope you find this book helpful and enjoy reading it. As we continue our busy clinical practices, I want each of you to remember the words of Margaret Mead, "Never underestimate the power of a small group of thoughtful, committed citizens can change the world. In fact, it is the only thing that ever has." I trust that future generations of cardiothoracic surgery trainees will continue to change the world one patient at a time.

Justin Watson, MD
TSRA Vice President 2019

Clauden Louis, MD MS
TSRA Secretary and Communications Chair 2020

August 2020

Contributors

10

11

Table of Contents

I. General Thoracic Surgery

1. EARLY STAGE LUNG CANCER (IA-IIB)

Anthony B. Mozer MD, MBA and David D. Odell MD, MSc

Adapted from 1st edition chapter written by David D. Odell, MD, and Matthew J. Schuchert, MD

Concept

- Indications for lung cancer screening
- Evaluation of the patient with a newly discovered lung nodule
- Indications for surgical resection of isolated pulmonary nodules
- Operative and non-operative treatment approaches for early stage NSCLC

Chief Complaint

"A 57-year-old man is referred to your office after a 1.1 cm irregular nodule is discovered in the right upper lobe of the lung on a CT chest performed to evaluate for pulmonary embolism following a knee replacement."

Differential

Lung cancer (Non-small cell, small cell, carcinoma in situ), neuroendocrine tumor (carcinoid), hamartoma, granuloma, (sarcoid, histoplasmosis, coccidiomycosis, fungal, tuberculosis), infection (viral or bacterial pneumonia), metastasis, infarction, atelectasis

History and physical

The history should focus on the identification of cancer risk factors: tobacco exposure history, occupational exposures (asbestos or other chemical inhalation), and a thorough personal and family cancer history. While primary symptoms related to pulmonary malignancy are absent in > 80% of patients, careful questioning can still elicit findings in some patients. These may be separated into 2 groups: symptoms related to the primary tumor and symptoms indicative of metastatic disease. Primary tumor symptoms include cough, hemoptysis, recurrent respiratory infections, dyspnea, and chest pain. Symptoms that may be attributable to metastatic disease include bone pain, myalgias, headaches, visual changes, anorexia, weight loss, and fatigue.

Tests

Imaging evaluation

CXR

- Low cost and readily available
- Useful for tracking a process over time or for the assessment of advanced disease such as effusion
- Limited utility for TNM staging

Chest CT scan

- Valuable for accurate assessment of the primary tumor
- Valuable for hilar and mediastinal lymph node evaluation (sensitivity and specificity ranging from 65-80%)
- Generally, should have a current CT chest (within 6 weeks) for any patient undergoing resection

PET scan

- Most useful for evaluation of the mediastinal compartment and assessment of metastatic disease.
- Superior to CT alone for lymph node assessment
- Good NPV, poor PPV due to a high rate of false positive results

19

PET-CT scan
- Excellent sensitivity but limited specificity due to false positives
  - 43% false positive rate in the ACOSOG Z0050 trial
- Superior to either CT or PET individually

Bone scan
- Low cost and widely available
- Less specific than PET and largely falling out of clinical favor

Chest MRI
- Useful for characterization of chest wall involvement
- Test of choice if concern for spinal column or brachial plexus involvement
- Poor characterization of primary lung tumor

Bronchoscopy
- Used to assess for presence and location of endobronchial disease
- Washing and brushings may be used for diagnosis in cases where biopsy of a parenchymal lesion is not possible or present
- Should be performed preoperatively in all settings of potential pulmonary resection

Physiologic evaluation
Pulmonary function tests
- *FEV1*. The volume of air expelled in 1 second. This is the single test with the best correlation to postoperative functional outcome. A minimum of 40% predicted postoperative function is needed for a patient to remain free of oxygen dependency after resection. That typically correlates to the following spirometric values prior to resection:
  - 2 L for pneumonectomy
  - 1 L for lobectomy
  - 0.6 L for segmentectomy
- *DLCO*. Diffusing capacity for carbon monoxide. This test is a measure of capillary permeability and the efficiency of gas exchange across the alveolar membrane. Patients need a minimum 40% predicted postoperative function to tolerate resection.
- Predicted postoperative pulmonary (Ppo) function (either FEV-1 or DLCO) can be determined by assessing the proportion of lung to be resected using the formula:
  Ppo-FEV1 = FEV1 x [(19 segments - number of segments to be resected)/19 segments]

Ventilation/perfusion studies
Patients with significant airflow obstruction, central tumors, areas of atelectasis, pleural disease, or prior lung resection may have alterations in ventilation and/or pulmonary blood flow which invalidate the assumptions made with simple spirometric pulmonary function testing. In this circumstance, a quantitative radionuclide ventilation/perfusion scan can better indicate the contribution to ventilation of the region of lung tissue that you intend to resect. For borderline cases, exercise capability may be assessed if there is concern for poor preoperative lung function. A patient who can walk up two flights of stairs likely has adequate reserve to tolerate a procedure. Also, VO2 max less than 15 mL/kg/min is associated with high risk of postoperative adverse events.

Cardiac evaluation
The cornerstone of preoperative cardiac evaluation is obtaining a thorough history from the patient. All patients should have an EKG performed as a baseline prior to surgery. Patients with risk factors or physical exam findings concerning for cardiac disease should be referred

20

to a cardiologist for preoperative evaluation and consideration of a stress test before proceeding with pulmonary surgery.

Index scenario (additional information)

"Following a complete evaluation, the primary nodule is FDG-avid with an SUV of 7.1. There is no evidence of mediastinal adenopathy on CT and no activity beyond the primary nodule on PET. The patient is otherwise healthy and has an FEV1 of 97% predicted and a DLCO 110% predicted."

Treatment/management

In general, the surgeon's primary task is identifying those patients with a disease state amenable to primary surgical resection who are physiologically able to tolerate the operation. Keeping these tenets in mind will help to clearly frame the preoperative evaluation. A detailed understanding of the TNM staging system put forth by the AJCC is important for any practitioner providing care for patients with non-small cell lung cancer (NSCLC).

Early stage cancers are those in which the primary tumor is confined within the lobar lung parenchyma and there is no evidence of mediastinal lymph node involvement or distant disease. The above imaging and diagnostic studies are valuable tools in helping to make this determination preoperatively.

Some preoperative measures that may decrease risk include: smoking cessation, optimizing nutrition and use of epidural anesthesia.

Surgical resection is the therapy of choice for patients with early stage (stage I and II) NSCLC. Surgery also has an important role in the treatment of selected patients with locally advanced disease (stage IIIa), as will be discussed elsewhere. Lobectomy with mediastinal lymph node sampling or dissection remains the surgical standard of care for early stage NSCLC. This approach is based on the findings of a randomized, controlled trial conducted by the Lung Cancer Study Group (LCSG) which compared lobar and sub-lobar approaches to tumor resection. This trial showed a threefold reduction in local recurrence (6.4% vs. 17.2%) and a 30% overall survival advantage (p = 0.088), establishing lobectomy as the 'gold standard' surgical resection. Sublobar approaches to lung cancer resection (wedge and/or anatomic segmentectomy) continue to gain support based on several retrospective series and recent meta-analyses, particularly for patients who would not otherwise tolerate lobectomy. While the term "sublobar" is often used generically, there are two distinct forms of sublobar resection. Segmentectomy involves the resection of an anatomic ventilatory unit, with identification and individual control of the segmental arterial and venous circulation as well as the segmental bronchus. By contrast, wedge resection is a non-anatomic extirpation of a lesion and surrounding tissue. While there are few direct comparisons, the available literature indicates that anatomic segmentectomy is oncologically superior to wedge resection.

Appropriate patient selection and adherence to oncologic principles of resection are paramount if sublobar resection with curative intent is to be offered. The primary factors involved are: a) tumor size b) the ability to obtain an adequate resection margin and c) performance of a careful lymph node assessment at the time of the operation. Achieving an adequate surgical margin is essential regardless of the resection technique chosen. In patients treated with sublobar resection, a margin distance greater than the diameter of the tumor has been shown to significantly decrease rates of local recurrence; however, a true survival advantage has not been shown. A careful analysis of the N1 (lobar and hilar) nodal stations is important for patients considered for sublobar resection. If N1 disease is encountered intraoperatively, a lobectomy should be performed for full evaluation of the intralobar nodes and clearance of regional lymph node metastasis. While there remains great interest in sublobar resection, these operations should be reserved for patients in whom a lobectomy could not otherwise be safely performed and for carefully selected patients with small (< 2cm), peripheral lesions and favorable, low-grade histopathology.

After multi-disciplinary evaluation, stereotactic body radiation therapy/ablative radiotherapy (SBRT/SABR) should be recommended with curative intent to patients who choose not to have surgery or who are deemed medically inoperable due advanced age or comorbidities. When adjusted for patient profile differences, some series demonstrate that SBRT/SABR confers outcomes in overall and disease-free survival comparable to surgical resection for appropriately selected patients. Ablation is of limited utility in many central tumors due to proximity to major airways or vascular structures. Further, the ability to pathologically assess nodal involvement is lost and the potential for local recurrence is higher than that seen with surgical resection in some series.

Operative steps

Lobectomy with *en bloc* resection of N1 lymph nodes combined with mediastinal lymph node sampling or dissection remains the standard surgical procedure in patients with NSCLC. While nuances exist with the approach to each of the lobectomies, certain general principles are applied regardless of the lobe to be resected.

Positioning and incisions

- A double lumen endotracheal tube is placed, and the position verified bronchoscopically both before and after turning the patient (the three segmental bronchi to the right upper lobe should be clearly visible through the tracheal lumen and the blue balloon cuff should be visible). For most cases a left endobronchial tube is sufficient, but make sure to pull it back prior to any left proximal bronchial resections. If you have issues with ventilation on the side you are working on, stop and have anesthesia perform a bronchoscopy and reposition the tube. Alternatively, a bronchial blocker may be used for lung isolation.
- The patient is placed in the lateral decubitus position with the operative side up. An axillary roll is placed, and the arms are brought forward and positioned at a 90° angle from the anterior chest.
- The patient is secured to the operating table and the bed is then flexed to accentuate the interspaces.
- For open lobectomy, the typical incision is a posterolateral thoracotomy through the 5th interspace. VATS lobectomy typically is approached via a 3-4 cm utility incision in the axilla at the 4th interspace along with 2-3 additional working ports in the 7th interspace, anterior axillary line and 9th interspace, posterior mid-clavicular line. The typical port placement for lobectomy using the da Vinci Xi robot (Intuitive Surgical, Inc.) uses 3-4 ports for the robotic arms including two 8mm and two 12mm ports, with one hand's breadth (approximately 6 cm) between each site across the 8th or 9th intercostal space, lower than for a VATS approach. A 12mm thoracoscopic port is placed for the bedside assistant. This port is triangulated between the camera and right robotic arm and just above the diaphragm and commonly serves as the extraction site of the resected specimen.

Mobilization and hilar dissection

- On entry to the chest, a thorough inspection of the pleural surface is performed, and any suspicious lesions are biopsied.
- If there is concern for mediastinal lymph node involvement, mediastinal lymph node dissection and frozen section evaluation may be performed prior to proceeding with lobectomy.
- The inferior pulmonary ligament is identified and mobilized to the level of the inferior pulmonary vein.
- The pleural reflection is incised posteriorly to the level of the azygos vein on the right or the aortic arch on the left. This will allow for good access to and visualization of the bronchus.

- The pleural reflection overlying the anterior mediastinum is incised, taking care to identify and avoid the phrenic nerve. Once the pleura is opened, both the superior and inferior pulmonary veins are identified.

Vascular dissection and division

- The pulmonary vein to the lobe of interest is circumferentially dissected using a blunt technique. For the upper and lower lobes, this dissection is done anteriorly at the hilum. For the right middle lobe, this dissection is performed within the fissure itself. Once identified and dissected free, the vein may be divided with a linear stapler. If performing a right upper or middle lobectomy, ensure visualization of the bifurcation of the upper and middle veins to avoid unplanned conversion of a single lobectomy to a bilobectomy.

- Following division of the vein, the pulmonary artery comes into view. Careful blunt dissection is used to skeletonize the artery and branches. These are individually divided with a vascular stapling device after assuring that the pulmonary artery branches to the other lobe(s) are identified and preserved. For the right upper lobe, the truncus (apical-anterior branch) and ascending or recurrent (posterior ascending) artery to the posterior upper lobe segment are divided. For right middle lobectomy, the middle lobe artery branching anteriorly off the ongoing pulmonary artery is taken. Right lower lobectomy requires division of the ongoing pulmonary artery distal to the middle artery. Note that the superior segmental artery arises near the artery to the middle lobe and may need to be ligated separately; In left lung resections, the apical-anterior branch, anterior, and typically 1-2 lingular branches are encountered for left upper lobe resections. Left lower lobe resections require division of the superior segmental artery and common basilar trunk.

- The vessels may be approached and divided in either order (vein or artery first) depending upon what is anatomically most accessible and safe.

Bronchial division

- After vascular division, the bronchus and perhaps some remaining parenchymal tissue, as in cases of incomplete interlobar fissure, are all that remain. Parenchymal division can be accomplished at this time using an endovascular stapler with a thick tissue staple load. Several firings are typically necessary. The staple line is oriented to follow the direction of the native fissure, with the ongoing pulmonary artery used as a guide for the deep margin in upper lobe resections.

- The peribronchial lymph nodes from the diseased lobe are cleared to expose the bronchial resection margin.

- The bronchus is divided with a linear stapler. The stapler is closed on the bronchus and initially not fired. The anesthesiologist is asked to remove any suction catheters and ventilate the lung on operative side to ensure the remaining lobes aerate normally. If there are questions regarding airway patency, a pediatric bronchoscope may be passed through the operative side of the double lumen tube to visually assess the proposed bronchial stump to assure the airways to remaining lung parenchyma are not compromised. The stapler is then fired, and bronchus divided.

- After completion of the lobectomy, the specimen is removed directly if a thoracotomy was performed or placed in a specimen bag and withdrawn through the access incision if a thoracoscopic or robotic approach was used.

- The bronchial stump closure may be tested for leak intraoperatively by filling the chest with water and ventilating the operative side to assess for bubbling through the staple line. In patients who underwent induction chemoradiotherapy or in whom poor wound healing might be expected, the bronchial stump may be buttressed using a tissue flap (pleura, pericardial fat, divided and mobilize azygos vein, intercostal muscle, etc.).

- Chest tubes are then placed under direct vision to completely drain the post-lobectomy space and the chest wall closed in the typical manner.

23

Technical considerations with specific lobectomies

Right upper lobe

- The pulmonary artery is easily injured while developing the plane between the upper lobe bronchus and the artery itself, as well as during division of the recurrent posterior (posterior ascending) artery as the artery is under some tension in both cases.
- The phrenic nerve is closely related to the apex of the hilum and can be injured when dividing the mediastinal pleura or when taking down adhesions in this region.

Right middle lobe

- The ongoing pulmonary artery runs through the fissure and branches to the lower lobe can sometimes be mistaken for the middle lobe branch. Develop this dissection thoroughly before dividing any arterial branches.
- The arterial branch to the middle lobe is also easily injured by traction once the bronchus to the middle lobe is divided.
- Division of the middle lobe bronchus can easily compromise aeration to the lower lobe. This should be checked carefully prior to stapling.

Right lower lobe

- The middle lobe pulmonary artery is easily injured due to excessive traction while dissecting the lower lobe pulmonary artery branches.
- The middle lobe bronchus can be narrowed or twisted when stapling the basilar branches of the lower lobe bronchus.
- The phrenic nerve is close to the anterior hilum and should be carefully identified.

Left upper lobe

- The aorta and aortic arch are immediately behind the pleural dissection plane used to expose the posterior aspect of the left upper lobe. Small aortic side branches may be encountered, especially if there is an inflammatory component to the tumor process.
- The left recurrent laryngeal nerve loops around the aortic arch before ascending back to the neck. This structure may be injured during mobilization of the apex of the lobe or during aorticopulmonary window lymph node dissection.
- The most common anatomic arrangement of vessels of the main pulmonary artery to the left upper lobe includes apico-anterior, lingular, and posterior branches; however, there is significant variability. Care must be taken to develop a dissection plane travelling immediately along the vessel in order to avoid injury/avulsion to smaller branches that may not be immediately well-visualized.

Left lower lobe

- The ongoing pulmonary artery is typically identified within the fissure. However, the lingular branch often originates at the level of the fissure and may be inadvertently divided if care is not taken to identify this vessel.

Potential questions/alternative scenarios

"As part of a workup for blunt trauma sustained in a motor vehicle crash, a 50-year-old female is referred to you with a chest CT showing an incidental mixed-density nodule in the periphery of the right upper lobe. How do you counsel this patient?

Incidental pulmonary nodules are an increasingly common finding in an era in which CT scanning is commonly used in the diagnosis and workup of disease processes. Ground-glass opacities (GGO) are abnormal findings of uncertain clinical significance which should be followed with q6-12-month CT scans if greater than 6 mm in size to evaluate for growth which may indicate malignant progression. A growing lesion should prompt biopsy, either image-guided needle or surgical, as appropriate. In lower risk patients, incidentally, discovered solid nodules <6mm require no routine follow up, intermediate sized nodules 6-8mm should be serially surveilled, and nodules >8mm should be sampled or assessed with PET/CT. In patients with risk factors for primary lung cancer, solid nodules are considered to carry greater malignant potential than a GGO. A lesion <6mm should be followed for at least

24

1 year to assure no change. Intermediate-sized lesions should be followed with imaging every 12-24 months. Lesions >8mm should prompt PET/CT or biopsy.

"Who should be recommended for low-dose CT for lung cancer screening and what are the risks and benefits?"

The National Lung Cancer Screening Trial (NSLT) showed that screening low-dose CT is indicated for patients 55-74 years old current smokers with smoking history of 30+ pack-years or former smokers who have quit within the preceding 15 years. The major risk is false positive findings and overdiagnosis that require subsequent CT surveillance. The major benefit is a reduction in lung cancer deaths by 20% for individuals in this group.

"Do all patients need neuroimaging prior to resection?"

Routine use of neuroimaging has fallen out of favor in the preoperative evaluation of patients with early-stage lung cancer due to the extremely low rate of occult intracranial metastasis. The current standard of care is a thorough history and physical exam. Neuroimaging (preferentially

MRI) is then pursued for those patients with neurologic symptoms or for patients with clinical stage II or higher NSCLC.

"How do you select patients for mediastinoscopy?"

While some surgeons practice routine mediastinoscopy for all patients with either known or suspected lung cancer, a selective approach is now considered the standard of care. Indications for mediastinoscopy or other forms of surgical mediastinal evaluation in early-stage NSCLC are predicated on the pre-test probability for occult mediastinal disease. These risk factors include: T2 (>3 cm) or larger lesions, pathologically enlarged lymph nodes >1 cm in short axis diameter on CT, increased FDG avidity on PET (SUV >2.5-4.0), and centrally located tumors, even in the absence suspicious imaging. Adenocarcinoma and large cell primary tumor histology are also felt by some to be indications for upfront mediastinal evaluation. Surgical mediastinoscopy remains a valuable tool when clinical suspicion remains high for mediastinal disease despite negative or non-diagnostic mediastinal assessment by endobronchial ultrasound-guided biopsy (EBUS).

"You are evaluating a patient with a left upper lobe NSCLC who has increased FDG uptake on PET in the AP window lymph nodes. The patient is otherwise fit for surgery. How will you
proceed operatively?"

There are two potential options for the evaluation of the AP window lymph nodes in this patient. Traditionally, the level 5 and 6 nodes could be accessed via a Chamberlain procedure. However, in this patient who is a reasonable surgical candidate, a thoracoscopic or robotic approach would offer the benefit of being able to proceed to definitive resection in the same operative setting. The patient would be intubated with a double lumen endotracheal tube and positioned in the right lateral decubitus position as for a lobectomy. A thoracoscopic exploration of the chest would be quickly performed to rule out intrapleural disease and the AP widow lymph nodes excised and sent for frozen section evaluation. If positive, the patient could be treated with neoadjuvant chemotherapy and brought back for surgical resection at a later time. A more conservative approach would be to treat the patient with definitive CRT in the setting of level 5 or 6 N2 disease, although this approach is less favored for single station N2 disease, particularly in the setting of a left upper lobe cancer with level 5 or 6 nodal involvement. If negative, one may safely proceed with lobectomy. Many surgeons perform left upper lobectomy regardless of a positive level 5 or 6 lymph node, as the survival for LUL NSCLC with N2 disease is similar to patients with N1 disease. In this setting, some argue that preoperative sampling of level 5 or 6 nodes is not needed, as the results will not change the treatment plan. Mediastinal lymph node sampling, including level 5 and 6, should still be performed, as patients with positive nodes should be treated with adjuvant therapy.

"You are operating on a patient with a suspected central lung cancer, but there is no biopsy-proven malignancy. What is your intraoperative approach to diagnosis?"

The answer to this question is largely dependent upon the location of the lesion of interest. Careful review of the preoperative CT is helpful in planning the operative approach. Peripheral nodules are typically amenable to wedge resection, allowing for a frozen section diagnosis to be made prior to proceeding with lobectomy. While waiting for frozen section results, mediastinal lymph node sampling can be performed so that the operation continues to progress. In the case of more central lesions, a core needle biopsy can be taken under direct visualization/palpation in most cases. Rarely, an abnormality is centrally located and intimately associated with the pulmonary vasculature, precluding biopsy. In this circumstance, lobectomy is the most minimal resection which can be accomplished safely. It is never acceptable to perform a pneumonectomy without confirm diagnosis of malignancy (e.g., a "diagnostic pneumonectomy").

"While you are preparing to divide the upper lobe pulmonary artery for a right upper lobectomy, the pathology lab calls with results on a previously sampled 4R lymph node. You learn that this is positive for malignancy. How does this change the operative plan?"

This circumstance is really one of the surgeon's own creation. While there is an 8-15% incidence of occult mediastinal lymph node metastasis reported in the literature, this situation is not typically encountered mid-operation. If there is concern preoperatively for mediastinal disease, a mediastinal node dissection and frozen section evaluation should be performed prior to any pulmonary dissection. This will preserve the ability to treat the patient with neoadjuvant therapy and revisit operative resection post-induction with undisturbed tissue planes within the lobe. However, unexpected finding of nodal disease once dissection has begun prompts most surgeons to proceed with lobectomy and complete mediastinal lymph node dissection, with subsequent referral for adjuvant chemotherapy.

"While dissecting the anterior hilum, a rent is made in the pulmonary artery. What is your strategy for managing this complication?"
Pulmonary artery injury is the most feared complication of lobectomy. However, good preparation can minimize the chances for an adverse outcome. During lobectomy, a sponge stick should always be immediately available on the field in case of vascular injury. Whether the approach is open, thoracoscopic, or robotic, this can be used to quickly apply direct pressure to the injured vessel, compressing it against the vertebral bodies and the mediastinum and providing temporary control of the situation. Once this maneuver has been successfully performed and the acute blood loss is under control, plans for repair can be made. In robotic operations, a robotic arm with a rolled sponge (cigar roll) can be positioned to hold pressure over the injury until thoracotomy can be undertaken, or a thoracoscopic instrument with a sponge can be utilized by a bedside assistant.

The most important step at this point is to organize the resources to help care for the patient, including asking for intraoperative assessment or assistance from a partner or senior surgeon, if available. Instruct anesthesia to prepare for the possibility of significant blood loss and expeditiously arrange for appropriate blood products in the room. For proximal injuries, cardiopulmonary bypass may be required for repair and perfusion should be notified to bring a bypass circuit to the OR. All suture materials, instruments, vascular clamps, and other supplies that might be needed for repair should be made immediately available. During this time a wide thoracotomy is performed to provide full exposure to the area of injury.

The first operative step in repair is to achieve proximal and distal control of the vessel. The strategy depends on the location of injury; however, one safe approach to proximal control is to enter the pericardium and encircle the pulmonary artery with an umbilical tape and snare it with a tourniquet at this level. This will provide a free dissection plane proximal to the injury. In many cases, this may be all that is required, and division of the injured artery can be completed with a stapler if it is an injury to a branch that needed to
be resected anyway, with a suture closure on the specimen side to prevent ongoing bleeding as the operation is completed. If the main PA or ongoing PA is injured, a direct suture repair is often possible for smaller injuries. Hemostasis is temporarily achieved by snaring the

26

proximal PA and any major branches feeding the vessel beyond the snare. Vessel loops or small atraumatic vascular clamps may be used for distal and side branch control. Larger injuries may be repaired using a patch technique after vascular control has been gained. Note that obtaining control of the extra-pericardial proximal PA is never a bad idea for right-sided resections, especially if there is concern for a difficult dissection.

"You perform an uncomplicated resection for a 2.5 cm RLL tumor. Final pathology revealed an adenocarcinoma with 2 of 7 hilar lymph nodes positive for malignancy. How will you counsel this patient?"

This patient has T1cN1M0 disease (Stage IIb, AJCC 8th edition). Adjuvant cisplatin or carboplatin-based chemotherapy should be discussed with the patient, and in a multi-disciplinary tumor board setting if possible. Other pathologic factors that are considered high risk in early stage NSCLC include poorly differentiated tumor histopathology, vascular invasion, visceral pleural involvement, and size >4 cm. While the number of clinical trials addressing this question remains small, a meta-analysis of several trials including patients who underwent surgical resection and were then randomized to either cisplatin-based chemotherapy or observation was published in 1995 and remains the most widely accepted data available. This study showed a 13% reduction in the hazard ratio for death and an overall 5% increase in survival in the chemotherapy arm.

Pearls/pitfalls

- Appropriate treatment for lung cancer, especially early stage cancers amenable to surgery, is dependent upon accurate preoperative staging.
- Remember to assess the post-resection pathology report in order to advise patients regarding adjuvant therapy.
- If there is concern about the ability to attain an adequate surgical margin, remember to verify using intraoperative frozen section.
- Consider sleeve resection in the case of a proximal tumor which is not otherwise advanced.
- Thoroughly assess the patient's functional status preoperatively.
- Have a systematic approach to pulmonary resections with good knowledge of arterial and venous control as it applies to individual lobes.
- Have a firm understanding of staging and preoperative physiologic testing.

Suggested readings

- Detterbeck F, Boffa D, Kim A, et al; The Eight Edition Lung Cancer Stage Classification. *Chest* 151:1; 193-203,2017.
- Chemotherapy in Non-Small Cell Lung Cancer; A meta-analysis using updated data on individual patients from 52 randomized clinical trials. Non-Small Cell Lung Cancer Collaborative Group. *British Medical Journal* 311:899-909, 1995.
- NCCN Clinical Practice Guidelines in Oncology: Non-Small Cell Lung Cancer ver. 5.2019 epub @ nccn.org.
- LoCicero J.: Surgical treatment of non-small cell lung cancer. Shields TW et al. (eds) *General Thoracic Surgery* (8th edition) ed. Lippincott, Williams & Wilkins, Philadelphia PA 2019.
- Ginsberg and Rubinstein. Randomized trial of lobectomy versus limited resection for T1 N0 non-small cell lung cancer. Lung Cancer Study Group. *Ann Thorac Surg.* 1995;60[3]: 615.
- Xiangpeng Z, Schipper M, Kidwell K, et al. Survival Outcome After Stereotactic Body Radiation Therapy and Surgery for Stage I Non-Small Cell Lung Cancer: A Meta Analysis. *Int J Radiation Oncol Biol Phys*, Vol. 90(3):603-611, 2014.
- The National Screening Trial Research Team. Reduced Lung-Cancer Mortality with Low-Dose Computed Tomographic Screening. *N Engl J Med* 2011;365:395-409.

2. ADVANCED NON-SMALL CELL LUNG CANCER

Miguel M. Leiva-Juarez, MD and Frank D'Ovidio, MD, PhD

Adapted from 1st edition chapter written by Benjamin Wei, MD, and Betty Tong, MD

Concept

- Preoperative work-up and staging of patients with advanced lung cancer
- TNM staging system and how this is used to guide management
- Indications for induction (neoadjuvant) therapy, surgery, and adjuvant therapies
- Multimodal therapy of advanced lung cancer, including Pancoast/superior sulcus tumors and tumors with chest wall involvement
- Contraindications for surgical resection
- Palliative options for advanced lung cancer

Chief complaint

"You have been referred a patient, previously a heavy smoker, with a 6 cm solid mass at the apex of the right lung. He complains of right shoulder pain radiating down the arm and paresthesias. How do you evaluate this patient?"

Differential

Small cell lung cancer, Non-small cell lung cancer (Adenocarcinoma, squamous cell carcinoma, large cell NSCLC, carcinoid tumor - typical and atypical), pulmonary metastasis, infectious process (i.e., aspergilloma, mycobacterial infection, abscess).

History and physical

History should focus on symptoms suggestive of 1) chest wall invasion, 2) neurologic and/or vascular involvement of a tumor, and 3) metastatic disease. These include: 1) chest wall pain, 2) paresthesias, pain, numbness, swelling, coolness, or weakness of the ipsilateral extremity, and 3) fever, night sweats, weight loss, supraclavicular lymphadenopathy. The patient's overall functional and cardiopulmonary status should also be assessed to determine if he/she would be a potential candidate for operative intervention in case further evaluation reveals this to be indicated. The medical history should include specific questions about other significant comorbidities, prior chest surgery or radiation, smoking history, family and personal history of prior malignancies.

Remember to assess the patient's neurologic and vascular status. Superior sulcus tumors may result in Horner's syndrome, which consists of miosis, ptosis, and anhidrosis of the affected side of the face. When ipsilateral shoulder and arm pain, paresthesias, paresis and atrophy of the hand muscles, and Horner's syndrome are present, this constellation is collectively referred to as Pancoast syndrome. Delineate any neurologic deficits, whether sensory or motor, of the extremity on the side of the mass. Similarly, evaluation of the upper extremities for pulse strength and edema should be done.

Tests

- *PET-CT scan from skull base to knees*: to assess for mediastinal and distant metastatic disease.
- *Brain MRI with IV contrast or head CT with contrast*: to evaluate for intracranial metastases, for which PET-CT is not useful. MRI is preferable. For all suspected cancers stage II and above.
- *Pulmonary function tests*: to evaluate the patient's surgical candidacy based on predicted pulmonary function remaining after resection.

Index scenario (additional information)

"Physical exam reveals diminished sensation on the ulnar aspect of the arm but no weakness. Pulses are intact and there is no arm swelling or Horner's syndrome. PET-CT

28

reveals a 6 cm right upper lobe FDG-avid mass with an SUVmax of 15. The mass appears to invade the chest wall, including the first and second ribs on the right. The mediastinal lymph nodes are enlarged (> 1 cm in diameter) but demonstrate minimal FDG activity (SUV < 2.5). Pulmonary function testing demonstrates FEV1 and DLCO of 65% and 70% predicted, respectively. Brain MRI is unremarkable. What is the next step?"

Treatment/management

The neurologic complaints and findings on physical exam, as well as the location of the mass, suggest that further evaluation for brachial plexus involvement should be performed. MRI is generally the best diagnostic modality for determining whether the brachial plexus and/or spinal cord are involved. MRI, or CT scan with IV contrast, can also help if invasion of the subclavian vessels is a possibility.

"MRI/MRA of the chest shows that the mass is impinging on the T1 nerve root. There is no evidence of invasion into the vertebral foramen or involvement of the vasculature. How would you like to proceed?"
The evidence in this case suggests a superior sulcus tumor. T1 nerve root involvement does not preclude surgery but is associated with paresthesia of the medial upper extremity if resected. Involvement above C8 or the spinal cord is a contraindication to surgery. Resection of C8 may cause Klumpke paralysis (affects the forearm and intrinsic muscles of the hand giving a *claw-like* contracture), which may be an unacceptable outcome to the patient. Based on the PFTs obtained, the patient's predicted postoperative FEV1 and DLCO would be > 40% predicted and he would therefore be a candidate for right upper lobectomy. Invasion of ribs 1-2 necessitates an *en bloc* chest wall resection. Induction chemoradiation followed by surgery has been shown to provide the best chance for cure in this patient population based on the Intergroup 1060 trial (Rusch et al, 2007). However, those with mediastinal disease (N2 or N3) do not have additional benefit from surgery over chemoradiation alone. In addition, oncologists and radiation oncologists generally will not initiate treatment without a tissue diagnosis. Therefore, this patient needs additional studies:

- *Percutaneous CT-guided needle biopsy*: to establish diagnosis.
- *Bronchoscopy*: to evaluate for possible synchronous lesions, mainstem bronchus involvement, and/or abnormal anatomy (endobronchial involvement is another poor prognostic factor).
- *Mediastinoscopy*: to determine if the patient has N2 or N3 disease, in which case he would no longer be a candidate for surgical resection. Mediastinoscopy remains the gold standard for assessment of mediastinal lymph nodes, as there is a significant false positive and false negative rate for PET-CT. Other options include endobronchial ultrasound (EBUS) or navigational bronchoscopy; however, in the setting of negative sampling and high clinical suspicion, a surgical mediastinoscopy would still subsequent need to be performed. If there is a high suspicion of positive aortopulmonary nodes, a Chamberlain's procedure (anterior parasternal thoracotomy) may be necessary to assess these levels (5-6).

"Percutaneous CT-guided biopsy reveals squamous cell carcinoma. Bronchoscopy is unremarkable.   Mediastinoscopy with biopsies of stations 2R, 4R, 4L, and 7 shows no evidence of cancer. What is this patient's clinical stage? What is your treatment plan?"
This patient has clinical stage IIB cancer. It is T3N0, T3 because of chest wall invasion and 6cm size. It remains N0 because mediastinoscopy demonstrated no N2 or N3 involvement. There was no FDG-avid hilar lymphadenopathy on PET-CT therefore the patient is staged at N0. Here it is useful to briefly review the relevant staging of lung cancer (AJCC 8th Edition):
Stage IIB: consists of T1-2N1 and T3N0
Stage IIIA: consists of T1-2N2, T3N1, and T4N0-1

For this patient with a superior sulcus tumor involving or impinging on the T1 nerve, the best strategy is to proceed with neoadjuvant concurrent chemoradiation followed by planned surgical resection. Induction chemoradiation in this situation comprises a platinum-based doublet (ideally cisplatin + etoposide, but cisplatin + vinblastine or carboplatin + pemetrexed (if adenocarcinoma) are also acceptable) administered concurrently with 45-50 Gy of radiation. A repeat PET-CT scan should be performed after induction therapy to determine if the patient has responded to the treatment, or on the other hand, if interval disease progression or development of metastases has occurred.

"The patient undergoes neoadjuvant concurrent chemoradiation with cisplatin and etoposide, as well as 50 Gy of radiation therapy. Aside from some fatigue, he tolerates chemoradiation well and has no significant side effects. Repeat PET-CT scan shows that the mass appears slightly smaller, 4.5 cm in diameter, suggesting a treatment response. There is no evidence of new distant disease."
Our plan is to proceed with surgical resection.

Operative steps

- Consider diagnostic thoracoscopy to evaluate for metastatic pleural disease prior to performing thoracotomy.
- Posterior approach (Shaw-Paulson incision): posterolateral thoracotomy with medial extension between the spine and edge of scapula. This incision is better for access caudal to the thoracic inlet and the chest wall defect can usually be confined under the scapula, avoiding need for chest wall reconstruction.
- Consider harvesting an intercostal muscle flap for bronchial stump coverage in this patient who has undergone preoperative radiotherapy.
- En bloc right upper lobectomy with chest wall resection.
  - Resect 1 rib above and 1 rib below those involved by the tumor – in this case ribs 1-3
  - At least a 2 cm margin laterally/medially
  - Can separate lung from chest wall with a wedge resection if needed with later completion of lobectomy
  - Isolate and divide hilar vessels to the upper lobe individually
  - Send specimen for frozen section to obtain negative soft tissue margins on the chest wall and the bronchus
  - Remember to perform a mediastinal lymph node dissection or sampling
- Perform a chest wall reconstruction if the defect is anterior, large (> 5 cm), or potential for scapular entrapment exists. If the defect is small or is covered by the scapula (but unlikely to be entrapped by it), you can leave the defect unreconstructed. Options include:
  - Biological acellular dermal substitute (e.g., Strattice, AlloDerm)
  - PTFE (2 mm thickness, easy to handle)
  - Prolene mesh alone
  - Prolene with methylmethacrylate sandwich (rigid, but harder to handle/implant)
  - Soft tissue flap with the help of plastic surgery (latissimus – for posterior/anterior locations, pectoralis/transverse rectus abdominis (TRAM) – for anterior locations only) may be necessary if the defect is very large or if there is local radionecrosis from neoadjuvant or prior radiotherapy.

"This patient recovers from surgery. Final pathological staging is ypT3N0. All margins are negative. What additional therapy does he need?"
This patient will need adjuvant chemotherapy, most likely with a cisplatin-based doublet (options include cisplatin + etoposide, cisplatin + vinorelbine, cisplatin + vinblastine; 2nd line for those who cannot take cisplatin = carboplatin + paclitaxel/gemcitabine/pemetrexed). If the patient has mediastinal lymph node metastases

identified on final pathology (missed by preoperative mediastinoscopy), a boost of mediastinal irradiation should be considered (if no prior RT; otherwise chemotherapy only).

Potential questions/alternative scenarios

"You have the same original scenario as above, but it appears that there is invasion of the subclavian vessels on preoperative imaging. What would you do now?"

Again, induction chemoradiation followed by surgery is the ideal strategy, but now the involved portion of the vessel will need to be resected. The anterior (Dartevelle) approach provides excellent exposure in this situation. This incision starts superiorly near the ear and follows the anterior border of the sternocleidomastoid inferiorly, then crosses horizontally towards to the shoulder parallel to and below the clavicle. This horizontal part of the incision can be made lower (and accompanied by a partial sternotomy with anterior thoracotomy in the 2nd or 3rd intercostal space), as needed. The sternal head of the sternocleidomastoid muscle and the inferior belly of the omohyoid are divided to expose the thoracic inlet. Once it is determined that the tumor is resectable, the medial portion of the clavicle is removed. The clavicle, sternocleidomastoid and omohyoid muscles can also be spared using the modified Grunenwald approach, which consists of a transmanubrial incision. The subclavian vein can be ligated and resected without reconstruction. Elevation of the extremity postoperatively minimizes edema as collateral venous networks develop to compensate for venous resection. If there is invasion of the subclavian artery, the section involved should be resected and reconstructed, either with a primary end-to-end reanastomosis or PTFE interposition graft. Branches of the subclavian artery should be ligated with the exception of the vertebral artery unless absolutely necessary to obtain negative margins and in the absence of carotid disease. Carotid-to-subclavian bypass can also be considered. With vascular reconstruction, postoperative anticoagulation is recommended for a period of 6 months. On the left side, the thoracic duct may need to be ligated. Chest wall resection and lobectomy then proceeds after vessels have been resected and anastomosed.

"You have the same original scenario as above, but it appears that there is invasion of the T2 vertebral body. How would you approach this situation?"

Invasion of a vertebral body upstages the patient to a T4 cancer. Typically, this would be suggested by preoperative cross-sectional imaging. An MRI should be obtained to evaluate for spinal cord involvement. Assuming that the cord is not involved, resection of part of the vertebral body can be performed along with the lobectomy. The invasion of more than 2 vertebral bodies is a contraindication to resection. Induction chemotherapy or chemoradiotherapy should be part of the treatment strategy in these patients. Involvement of a spinal surgeon is critical for dealing with this uncommon scenario.

"What if this was not a superior sulcus tumor, but a mass that demonstrated chest wall invasion of ribs 4-5? Would you treat this patient differently? This patient would have a T3N0 with chest wall invasion, but NOT a superior sulcus tumor."

If the patient's mediastinal lymph node staging is negative and the lesion appears technically resectable, you would preferably forgo induction chemoradiation and proceed with chest wall resection and lobectomy with mediastinal lymph node dissection. Induction chemoradiation or chemotherapy with subsequent resection are also options. Principles for chest wall reconstruction, described above, also apply here. This patient would then undergo at minimum adjuvant chemotherapy, regardless of nodal status. Adjuvant radiation would be considered if the patient has either N2 or greater staging on final pathology or positive margins (R1-2).

"How about if this patient had preoperative mediastinoscopy that demonstrated N2 disease? What would you do?"

This patient has stage T3N2 (IIIB) disease with chest wall invasion and should receive definitive chemoradiation + consolidation therapy with durvalumab (PD-L1 inhibitor) (Antonia et al, 2017). Patients who are T3 because of chest wall invasion and N2 do not have any survival benefit from surgery.

31

"You have a patient with a 1.7 cm peripheral left lower lobe tumor, clinical stage I. Surprisingly, however, mediastinoscopy shows that station 4L is positive. What stage is he and how do you treat him?"

This patient is T1b by tumor size (1-2 cm) and N2 (cancer in ipsilateral mediastinal nodes), which is Stage IIIA. Remember that T1-2N2 patients are stage IIIA, while T3-4N2 are stage IIIB. Treatment for N2 patients depends on the patient's clinical condition and which mediastinal lymph nodes are positive. So far, two randomized controlled trials have investigated the role of surgery after chemoradiotherapy (Albain et al, 2009 [North American Intergroup Trial 0139]; vanMeerbeck et al, 2007) without significant survival benefits. However, some patients may benefit from surgical resection after neoadjuvant chemoradiotherapy as long as there is a response to treatment, including those who underwent lobectomy rather than pneumonectomy in Intergroup 0139. Given that patients with persistent N2 disease after chemoradiation do not benefit from resection (Bueno et al, 2000), mediastinal restaging should be performed. In general, stage IIIA patients with high performance status, young, with a single station, microscopic or "non-bulky" (>3 cm, encasing structures, not individually identifiable) N2 disease, and T3-4N1 may be candidates for neoadjuvant therapy with resection. Otherwise, consider proceeding with concurrent chemoradiation and consolidation with durvalumab. The role of immunotherapy as induction is currently under clinical trials and may expand the available treatments to downstage these tumors.

"You have the same patient — 1.7 cm left lower lobe tumor, but 4R is positive. What stage are you dealing with now and how would you treat him?"

This patient is T1bN3 (N3 = cancer in contralateral mediastinal nodes), and stage IIIB. Any N3 disease (and T3-4N2) is classified as stage IIIB. These patients should be treated with definitive chemoradiation and durvalumab.

"Again, same patient—1.7 cm tumor, but mediastinoscopy is negative—however postoperatively you discover that the patient actually has N2 disease. What do you do now?"

This patient was a clinical stage I who has been upstaged postoperatively to pathological stage IIIA. He did not receive preoperative chemotherapy. He should now receive both adjuvant chemotherapy (if a patient is anything beyond N0, he should be considered for chemotherapy) and radiation (N2 or N3 disease discovered postoperatively, as well as positive margins, are an indication for radiation, assuming that the patient has not been irradiated before).

"A patient with a left lower lobe 1.7 cm tumor with negative clinical mediastinal lymphadenopathy and intraoperative frozen biopsies of level 4L nodes come back positive. Would you proceed with surgery?

This is an example of a patient with an occult N2 disease. Recommendations are to continue with the lobectomy and mediastinal lymph node dissection, ensuring to harvest subcarinal and contralateral stations, if you believe that an R0 resection can be achieved. The patient will require adjuvant chemoradiation.

"Your patient has a 6 cm RUL tumor, resected by lobectomy. Final pathology report demonstrates that the hilar nodes are negative for malignancy. Lymph nodes at stations 2R, 4R, 4L, and 7 are negative from mediastinoscopy and mediastinal lymph node dissection at the time of thoracotomy. What stage are we dealing with and would you recommend that this patient receive adjuvant therapy?"

This patient is Stage IIB (T3N0). He is T3 because of size (tumor between 5-7 cm in diameter), and N0 because his ipsilateral hilar nodes are negative. This patient should undergo adjuvant chemotherapy without radiation (unless positive margins).

"You are in the OR with a patient for seemingly straightforward left lower lobectomy for a 3 cm cancer, however upon exploring the chest you determine that the pericardium is involved. How do you proceed?"

If you can determine that the contents *inside* the pericardium (e.g., heart and great vessels) are not involved, proceed with en bloc resection of the lobectomy with involved pericardium. Factors that result in T3 staging, besides chest wall invasion, are size 5-7 cm, that involve the parietal pleura, phrenic nerve, parietal pericardium or separate tumor nodules within the same lobe. Patients with main stem bronchus involvement may be candidates for sleeve lobectomy (see separate section), or pneumonectomy if a parenchymal-sparing lung resection is not possible. Patients with atelectasis of the entire lung may benefit from preoperative laser ablation or debridement of tumor, followed by consideration for a bronchoplastic procedure or pneumonectomy depending on location of the tumor and ability to achieve negative surgical margins. The diaphragm, phrenic nerve, mediastinal pleura, and/or pericardium may be taken *en bloc* with the pulmonary resection if invaded by tumor. These patients do not generally need induction therapy but do benefit from adjuvant chemotherapy. While tumors invading the chest wall, pericardium, or phrenic nerve are staged T3, those invading the mediastinum, diaphragm, heart, great vessels, recurrent laryngeal nerve, carina, trachea, esophagus, or spine are staged T4.

"You are in the OR for that same left lower lobectomy for cancer, however palpating the upper lobe reveals an additional roughly 1 cm nodule. What do you do now?"

In this situation, performing a wedge resection or segmentectomy of the smaller nodule in addition to the left lower lobectomy would be warranted.

"Frozen section reveals non-small lung cancer. What do you do now?"

Proceeding with the lower lobectomy, even if cancer is present in the second nodule, would be reasonable for most patients. Mediastinal lymph node dissection should also be done. Performing an unanticipated pneumonectomy would not be appropriate since this patient has T4 cancer. Depending on location, additional pulmonary tumor nodules with the same histology as the primary site may upstage a cancer to anywhere from stage IIB (T3N0) to stage IV (if contralateral). Assume that patients are N0 or N1 by mediastinal staging for the following:

- *Same lobe (T3)*: lobectomy, followed by adjuvant chemotherapy.
- *Different lobes, same lung (T4)*: lobectomy (for larger nodule) + sublobar resection (for smaller nodule), as lung function permits.
- *Contralateral lung, single nodule (synchronous lesion vs M1a)*: this may represent synchronous primaries or a lung cancer with contralateral metastasis. One strategy to manage these patients is to perform mediastinoscopy followed by resection of the smaller nodule in if the mediastinoscopy is negative. If the mediastinoscopy is positive, assume M1 disease (the mediastinal nodal disease means the disease is in transit and the contralateral lung nodule is more likely to be a metastasis rather than a primary) and treat with chemotherapy. If mediastinoscopy is negative, treat as two synchronous primaries and resect the smaller nodule. A second stage operation involves resection of the larger nodule. The amount of lung resected will depend on the patient's lung function and which lobes are involved.
- *Contralateral lung, multiple nodules*: treat as M1c disease with chemoradiation and consolidation durvalumab.
- *Additional tumor nodule, different histology as primary*: treat as synchronous primaries.

"Invasion of what other structures would also make this patient's cancer T4?"

Involvement of the heart, diaphragm, mediastinum, great vessels, esophagus, recurrent laryngeal nerve, vertebral body, trachea or carina defines T4 staging. T4 disease has historically been considered unresectable and is treated with palliation in most cases. If a patient has a T4N0 or T4N1 cancer, he is stage IIIA, and one can consider resection in certain special circumstances as delineated below:

- *Vertebral body invasion*: obtain MRI to confirm absence of spinal cord involvement, then can consider induction therapy (chemotherapy or chemoradiation) followed by pulmonary resection with vertebral body resection.
- *Carinal invasion*: may be candidate for carinal pneumonectomy if T4N0. If a patient is T4N2, he is stage IIIB and should receive definitive chemoradiation. Patients that require neoadjuvant therapy tend to do poorly after pneumonectomy.
- *Mediastinal invasion:* this would include esophagus, heart, or great vessels. If patient is N0-1 and resection is feasible, should proceed with *en-bloc* resection vs neoadjuvant therapy followed by resection.
- *T4 based on size only (>7 cm)*: if resectable and negative mediastinoscopy, resection with adjuvant chemotherapy.

"You are sent a patient for consideration of lobectomy for biopsy-proven NSCLC, however your imaging reveals numerous liver and bony metastases. What now?"
Metastatic disease is staged and treated in the following manner:

- *M1a*: metastatic pulmonary nodules to contralateral lung, pleural nodules, malignant pleural or pericardial effusion – palliation with pericardiocentesis or thoracentesis.
- *M1b*: single extrathoracic metastasis – palliation with chemotherapy and/or local radiation (if symptomatic), unless:
    - *Synchronous solitary brain met*: may consider pulmonary resection for T1-2 N0 M1 disease after brain met is treated with radiation or surgery in a patient with good performance status. Patients with nodal disease and brain metastases are not surgical candidates (Billing et al, 2001).
    - *Synchronous solitary adrenal met*: FNA to confirm adrenal met, then may consider pulmonary resection and adrenalectomy. Best outcomes with ipsilateral, synchronous, N0-1 lesions (Raz et al, 2011).
    - *M1c*: Multiple extrathoracic metastases including one or more than one organ – palliation

"You perform a left upper lobectomy for clinical stage I cancer. Pathological analysis is consistent with stage I, so he does not receive adjuvant therapy. Surveillance CT scan reveals an LLL nodule consistent with recurrence 2 years later. How would you deal with the following scenarios of locoregional recurrence?"

- *In all cases*: PET/CT (skull base to knee) to evaluate for distant metastatic disease.
- *Isolated parenchymal recurrence*: re-resection if possible, SBRT or RT if not technically feasible; consideration of adjuvant chemotherapy
- *Endobronchial obstruction*: laser ablation, stent, photodynamic therapy, brachytherapy, or radiotherapy for palliation
- *Mediastinal lymph node recurrence*: chemoradiation (if no radiation previously)
- *SVC obstruction*: chemoradiation or radiotherapy ± stenting
- *Oligometastatic disease*: chemotherapy
- *Severe hemoptysis*: endobronchial laser or photodynamic therapy vs embolization

Palliation options

- *Localized symptoms due to primary cancer deemed unresectable*: RT vs endobronchial therapy (laser ablation, stenting, brachytherapy)
- *Limited brain mets:* stereotatic radiosurgery vs surgical resection or whole brain RT (if symptomatic)
- *Disseminated disease*: chemotherapy

34

- *Pleural or pericardial effusion*: thoracentesis or pericardiocentesis ± pericardial window.

Genetic mutation targeted **chemotherapy regimens** for palliation
- *NSCLC*: test for ALK (tyrosine kinase), EGFR, ROS1, BRAF V600E, KRAS mutations and PD-L1 positivity.
  - *If ALK rearrangement+*: alectinib, brigatinib, ceritinib, crizotinib
  - *If EGFR+*: osimertinib, erlotinib, afatinib, gefitinib, dacomitinib
  - *If both ALK/EGFR negative, unknown, or treatment failure with above regimens*: cisplatin-based doublet +/- bevacizumab ("Avastin")
  - *ROS1 rearrangement +*: crizotinib, ceritinib
  - *BRAF V600E+*: dabrafenib + trametinib
  - *KRAS+ cancers*: generally poor response to EGFR inhibitors and chemotherapy
  - *PD-L1+: pembrolizumab, atezolizumab*

Pearls/pitfalls
- Do not operate on N3 disease (this includes patients with involved supraclavicular lymph nodes).
- Do not forget induction chemoradiation in patients with superior sulcus tumors, if you are planning on bringing them to the OR.
- Do not operate on patients with superior sulcus tumors *and* N2 disease.
- Superior sulcus tumors should ideally be treated with induction chemoradiation followed by lobectomy with chest wall resection and mediastinal lymph node dissection.
- Remember to perform head CT or brain MRI with contrast on patients with NSCLC stage II and above.
- Send intraoperative margins on pulmonary resections (bronchial always, chest wall as needed).
- Develop an individualized strategy to deal with N2 disease or bilateral lung masses, based on the patient's pulmonary function, specific characteristics of lesions and mediastinal lymph node, clinical status, and overall performance status.
- Complete evaluation of locally advanced lung cancer includes skull base-knee PET-CT, brain MRI or head CT with IV contrast, pulmonary function testing, bronchoscopy, and mediastinoscopy. CT should include IV contrast if the tumor may invade major blood vessels. MRI is indicated if brachial plexus or spinal cord invasion is possible. If induction or definitive non-surgical therapy is indicated, obtaining a tissue diagnosis is generally required.
- Reconstruct chest wall defects to prevent infection and flail chest unless small or covered by scapula: options include PTFE, prolene, prolene with methylmethacrylate. For larger defects use myocutaneous flaps.
- Any patient with a stage IIA or less with high-risk features (tumor > 4 cm in diameter, with visceral pleural involvement, vascular invasion, poorly differentiated tumors, wedge resected, or N1 on pathology) should receive adjuvant chemotherapy after surgery.
- Stage IIB patients (T1-2N1, T3N0) should generally be treated with surgery followed by adjuvant chemotherapy.
- Stage IIIA patients that are N2 should generally be treated with induction chemotherapy followed by mediastinal restaging, and lobectomy if downstaged. Patients with N2 disease should also eventually receive mediastinal RT as well, whether they undergo surgery or not.

35

- Stage IIIA patients with bulky mediastinal lymphadenopathy and stage IIIB-C patients (T1-4N3, T3-4N2) should be treated with definitive chemoradiation + durvalumab consolidation therapy.
- Nearly all stage IV patients should be treated with chemotherapy, and palliative RT as needed.
- Certain patients with T4 or M1 disease (vertebral body invasion, carinal invasion, solitary metastases to adrenal or brain) may be candidates for surgical resection.

Suggested readings

- National Comprehensive Cancer Network Clinical Guidelines for NSCLC Version 5.2019 (www.NCCN.org). Neoadjuvant treatment for superior sulcus tumors
- Rusch VW, Giroux DJ, Kraut MJ, et al. Induction chemoradiation and surgical resection for superior sulcus non-small-cell lung carcinomas: Long-term results of Southwest Oncology Group Trial 9416. (Intergroup Trial 0160). *J Clin Oncol.* 2007; 25:313-8.
- Rusch VW, Parekh KR, Leon L, et al. Factors determining outcome after surgical resection of T3 and T4 lung cancers of the superior sulcus. *J Thorac Cardiovasc Surg.* 2000, 119:1147-53.

Surgery for N2 disease

- Albain K, Swann RS, Rusch VW, et al. Radiotherapy plus chemotherapy with or without surgical resection for stage III non-small-cell lung cancer: a phase III randomised controlled trial. *Lancet.* 2009;374:379-386. (INT0139)

- Van Meerbeeck JP, Kramer GW, Van Schil PE, et al. Randomized controlled trial of resection versus radiotherapy after induction chemotherapy in stage IIIA-N2 non-small-cell lung cancer. *J Natl Cancer Inst.* 2007; 99(6):442-50.

- Bueno R, Richards WG, Swanson SJ, et al. Nodal stage after induction therapy for stage IIIA lung cancer determines patient survival. *Ann Thorac Surg.* 2000;70:1826–31.

PD-L1 inibition after adjuvant CRT

- Antionia SJ, Villegas A, Daneil D, et al; PACIFIC Investigators. Durvalumab after Chemoradiotherapy in Stage III Non-Small Cell Lung Cancer. *N Engl J Med.* 2017; 377:1919-1929.

Surgery for stage IV lung cancer

- Billing PS, Miller DL, Allen MS, et al. Surgical treatment of primary lung cancer with synchronous brain metastases. *J Thorac Cardiovasc Surg.* 2001;122: 548–53.
- Raz DJ, Lanuti M, Gaissert HC, et al. Outcomes of patients with isolated adrenal metastasis from non-small cell lung carcinoma. *Ann Thorac Surg.* 2011; 92(5):1788–92.

3. SMALL CELL LUNG CANCER
Shair Ahmed, MD, and Allan Pickens, MD

Concept
- Staging small cell lung cancer
- Workup for SCLC
- Appropriate surgical management in SCLC
- Non-surgical management of SCLC

Chief complaint

"A 65-year-old woman presents to your office for a second opinion 3 weeks after a right lower lobe wedge resection for a 9 mm right lower lobe lesion that had been previously biopsied via percutaneous CT guidance, which was non-diagnostic. A VATS wedge biopsy was then performed, with the final pathology revealing SCLC. Her surgeon immediately referred her for chemotherapy and radiation. However, she wants a second opinion. Her comorbidities include hypertension and coronary artery disease. She has a 40 pack-year smoking history."

Differential

Non-small cell lung cancer, small cell lung cancer, carcinoid

History and physical

The symptoms of small cell lung cancer and non-small cell lung cancer are very similar, especially when small cell lung cancer presents at an early stage. Smoking tends to be the most common etiology of SCLC but is also associated with radon and uranium mining. Be aware of the association of small cell lung cancer and paraneoplastic syndromes, which include Cushing syndrome, SIADH, and Lambert-Eaton myasthenic syndrome (LEMS). As SCLC frequently metastasizes to the brain, it is important to ascertain neurological symptoms.

Tests

- *Imaging.* It is extremely important to stage the patient as accurately as possible. Imaging includes whole body PET-CT looking for regional and distant metastases. MRI or CT of the brain should be ordered. The mediastinum should be assessed via cervical mediastinoscopy.
- *Labs.* If paraneoplastic syndromes are suspected, then the appropriate workup should be done.
- *Pulmonary function tests (PFTs).* Lung function needs to be assessed to determine the patient tolerance for pulmonary resection.
- *Bronchoscopy.* It is important to assess for endobronchial lesions that can potentially change management (for example whether to consider a sleeve resection).

Index scenario (additional information)

"The patient's history reveals no evidence of paraneoplastic syndromes and physical exam is benign. On imaging, there is slight uptake along the staple line from the prior wedge resection; however, there is no evidence of regional or distant metastatic spread. There are several sub-centimeter mediastinal lymph nodes that are not PET avid. MRI of the brain reveals no metastases."

Treatment/management

The scenario describes an early-stage SCLC in a functional patient with non-limiting comorbidities. While the bulk of the literature dictates the patient receive platinum-based chemotherapy and radiation, there is a role for surgical resection and adjuvant chemotherapy/radiation for clinical stage I SCLC (T1-2a N0 lesions). The patient should undergo a cervical mediastinoscopy (refer to chapter on Mediastinal Staging), and if there is no mediastinal disease, a completion lobectomy with lymphadenectomy is indicated. Postoperatively, the patient should receive platinum-based adjuvant chemotherapy and radiation.

Potential questions/alternative scenarios

"The patient in the above scenario during mediastinoscopy was found to have mediastinal disease (positive N2 lymph nodes) – how would you proceed?"
The mediastinoscopy should be discontinued and the patient should undergo definitive platinum-based chemotherapy and radiation therapy.

"A similar patient with minimal comorbidities presents with a diagnosis of SCLC by needle biopsy – how would you proceed?"
The pathology should be re-reviewed. If SCLC is confirmed by a second review from a different pathologist, the workup should proceed. If there are no metastases, resection is indicated followed by adjuvant chemotherapy and radiation. On occasion, final histology can reveal a mixed histology that includes non-small cell lung cancer, which is best treated with resection to reduce local recurrence (treat like NSCLC, not SCLC when mixed). In addition, carcinoid tumors can be frequently misdiagnosed as SCLC, so a patient with a suspicious non-metastatic early malignant lesion should be given the chance at surgical resection.

"A similar patient presents with unresectable small cell lung cancer (3 cm right lower lobe lesion, N2 disease, no brain metastases). How would you manage this patient?"
The patient should undergo chemotherapy with platinum-based agents (cisplatin or carboplatin) along with radiation therapy (45-50 Gy). Whereas the literature supports pulmonary resection followed by adjuvant therapy in early stage NSCLC (defined as T1-2N0 or T1N1) with favorable 5-year survival, the ACCP guidelines state that chemotherapy and radiation is first-line treatment for SCLC. The ACCP guidelines do support pulmonary resection for clinical stage I SCLC that are node negative, as metastases is less likely in this subgroup. There is also a growing body of literature that suggests prophylactic cranial irradiation confers increased median survival and lower rate of symptomatic brain metastases for patients with both limited and extensive stage SCLC who achieve a complete or partial response to initial therapy.

Pearls/pitfalls

- Check for paraneoplastic syndromes, such as SIADH, Cushings and Lambert-Eaton myasthenic syndrome.
- Medical treatment includes platinum-based chemotherapy and radiation.
- Histology can provide misdiagnoses, especially percutaneous or endobronchial biopsies. Have pathology re-read. If early stage disease is present, always consider resection.
- For the purposes of pulmonary resection in early stage SCLC, the ACCP guidelines support pulmonary resection followed by adjuvant chemoradiation for patients with clinical stage I SCLC (T1-2a N0).

Suggested readings

- Goldstein SD, Yang SC. Role of surgery in small cell lung cancer. *Surg Oncol Clin N Am.* 2011 Oct;20(4):769-77.
- Jett JR, Schild SE, Kesler KA, Kalemkerian GP. Treatment of small cell lung cancer: Diagnosis and management of lung cancer, 3rd ed: American College of Chest Physicians evidence-based clinical practice guidelines. *Chest.* 2013;143(5 Suppl):e400S-e419S.

4. Pneumonectomy and Sleeve Resection

Ian C. Bostock, MD and Mara B. Antonoff, MD

Adapted from 1ˢᵗ edition chapter written by Michael P. Robich, MD, and Daniel Raymond, MD

Concept

- Preoperative evaluation of patient
- Indications for advanced resections
- Conduct of the operation and pitfalls
- Managing complications

Chief complaint

"A 60-year-old man, 60 pack-year smoker is referred to you are following evaluation for a cough which culminated in the identification of a 4 cm left hilar mass. A whole-body PET-CT has been performed and shows the mass with involvement of the distal left main pulmonary artery and FDG uptake of the mass, with an SUV_{max} of 11, without evidence of distant metastases."

Differential

Primary lung cancer (small cell v. non-small cell), metastatic cancer to the lung, lymphoma, hilar adenopathy.

History and physical

Evaluate for evidence of pre-existing cardiopulmonary disease or prior history of malignancy. Look for evidence of local invasion or metastatic disease. A systematic approach to determine clinical stage and fitness for surgery is of the utmost importance for selecting the appropriate therapy. Hoarseness or chest pain can signify mediastinal/chest wall invasion and thus a locally advanced process. Palpable cervical adenopathy, new bone pain, or new neurologic symptoms would suggest metastatic disease. Evidence of pleural effusion or elevated hemidiaphragm may also suggest an advanced stage process.

Tests

- *Establish diagnosis*: with large, central lesions, preoperative biopsy is necessary prior to attempts at resection in order to exclude diagnoses that would be treated non-operatively, such as small cell lung cancer, lymphoma, and certain metastatic processes. Given the central, hilar nature of the described lesion, endobronchial or ultrasound-guided transbronchial biopsy can be quite helpful. Alternatives such as CT-guided biopsies and navigational bronchoscopy may also be considered. Small, peripheral lesions with a high probability of cancer can be treated with wedge resection with confirmation of malignancy on frozen section, followed by anatomical resection. However, central lesions cannot be wedged for diagnosis and diagnostic pneumonectomy should be avoided.
- *Establish stage.* The current gold standard for clinical staging includes a PET-CT scan and brain imaging (MRI or CT with IV contrast). Mediastinal staging through endobronchial ultrasound (EBUS) and/or cervical mediastinoscopy is necessary to confirm clinical staging prior to proceeding with pneumonectomy or other extensive resection.
- *Pulmonary function assessment.* Assessment for tolerance for pulmonary resection is essential. This is based on history of exercise tolerance and pulmonary function tests. For patients undergoing pneumonectomy, quantitative V/Q scanning is necessary to accurately determine postoperative predicted pulmonary function. Historical indicators of a patient's ability to tolerate a pneumonectomy have included a preoperative forced expiratory volume in one second (FEV1) >2 liters or predicted postoperative FEV1

>800 mL. However, most importantly, one must consider the number of expected functional pulmonary segments postoperatively and calculate the anticipated post-resection FEV1 and DLCO, recognizing that if either of these numbers is expected to fall below 40% of the predicted value for that individual (based on age, race, sex, and height), their pulmonary reserve is inadequate to tolerate the planned resection. Additional testing for borderline candidates may include arterial blood gas, 6-minute walk test, and cardiopulmonary exercise testing.

- *Cardiac evaluation.* Echocardiogram is advisable prior to pneumonectomy to evaluate right heart function and assess for evidence of pulmonary hypertension. Cardiac stress testing or evaluation by a cardiologist is recommended prior to considering a major resection, but dependent as well on the patient's past medical history.

Index scenario (additional information)

"PFTs reveal an FEV1 of 2.6 L (73% of predicted) and DLCO of 71% of predicted. Quantitative lung function tests demonstrate 58% of total perfusion to right lung and 42% to left lung. Stress echo showed no reversible defects. Bronchoscopy reveals a tumor involving the secondary carina on the left without extension along the main stem bronchus. Biopsy reveals a squamous cell carcinoma. There is no radiographic evidence of metastatic disease, including a brain MRI that does not reveal any intracranial abnormalities. PET-CT demonstrates increased uptake in the left hilar lymph nodes, and EBUS evaluation of the mediastinal nodes shows no malignant cells. How would you like to proceed?"

Treatment/management

This patient has clinical T2bN1M0, stage IIB squamous cell carcinoma and pneumonectomy would be indicated in this patient's anatomy and disease. While this patient has already had an endobronchial ultrasound, given the extent of resection, further EBUS sampling or mediastinoscopy to thoroughly ensure lack of N2 or N3 disease may be employed, as well as consideration of VATS lymph node sampling of stations 5/6 if there are suspicious appearing AP window nodes on imaging.

Preoperative discussion should be undertaken with the anesthesia and nursing team to address needs for appropriate IV access, arterial line, Foley catheter, intraoperative fluid management, perioperative antibiotic prophylaxis, DVT prophylaxis, and airway management. For a left pneumonectomy, the patient can be managed with a right-sided double-lumen endotracheal tube, a left-sided double-lumen tube, or a single-lumen tube with a bronchial blocker. Any tube or blocker in the left side will need to be withdrawn prior to division of the left mainstem bronchus. A right-sided double lumen tube is helpful for left-sided resections but can be tricky to place as one must keep an orifice open to the right upper lobe. One must also discuss pain management strategies with the anesthesia team. The authors prefer use of liposomal bupivacaine for posterior intercostal nerve blocks, but non-liposomal bupivacaine for intercostal nerve block or an epidural may alternatively be used.

After appropriate access has been obtained, obtain single-lung ventilation and position the patient in the lateral decubitus position. A posterolateral thoracotomy at the level of the 5th rib provides optimal exposure to the hilum. A muscle-sparing approach can be utilized. The 5th rib may be resected or the 6th rib notched for improved exposure, but this is not mandatory. VATS approach should only be used by those with extensive experience. VATS may be useful prior to thoracotomy to assure that there is no evidence of pleural dissemination.

It is important to examine for evidence of disease spread and biopsy any suspicious lesions/nodes. Pleural disease, pericardial dissemination, or invasion of the aorta, esophagus, or heart are all contraindications to proceeding with pneumonectomy. Bulky, multi-station mediastinal adenopathy is a relative contraindication although unlikely with thorough preoperative evaluation. Chest wall, pericardial, diaphragm, or limited vena cava involvement can be resected *en bloc*. Prior to embarking on pneumonectomy, a final attempt should be made to determine if a lesser resection, including sleeve resection, is possible.

Left pneumonectomy

- Incise the mediastinal pleura circumferentially around the hilum, reflect the phrenic nerve anteriorly with minimal manipulation, and take down the inferior pulmonary ligament.
- Begin with circumferential dissection and isolation of the superior and inferior pulmonary veins.
- Continue dissection cephalad from the superior pulmonary vein and circumferentially isolate the main pulmonary artery. Avoid injury to the recurrent laryngeal nerve (avoid cautery under the aortic arch).
- Following isolation of the main pulmonary artery, place an umbilical tape or clamp.
- Temporary (~1 minute) occlusion of the PA can simulate how the patient will tolerate shunting of all blood flow to a single lung. Look for signs of intolerance, i.e., tachycardia and/or hypotension. If hypotension occurs, assure appropriate location of clamp (make sure not too proximal, obstructing the main PA) and consider TEE evaluation. If clamp reposition does not remedy the situation and RV dysfunction is identified, abort the procedure.
- If extra length of PA is needed, one can divide the ligamentum arteriosum (watch for the recurrent laryngeal nerve) or open the pericardium (from below the inferior PV to above the PA) to expose the origin of the PA.
- Divide the PA. If adequate length, a vascular stapler can be used. If inadequate length, divide the PA between 2 vascular clamps and oversew with 5-0 prolene. Place anchoring sutures on the ends of the PA prior to division of the vessel to prevent the divided vessel from slipping through the proximal clamp.
- Divide the pulmonary veins with a vascular stapler. This step may be done before division of the PA, but dissection and control of the PA is recommended prior to dividing any structures if feasible.
- Expose the left main bronchus to the level of the carina and remove level 4L and 7 lymph nodes. Avoid injury to the recurrent laryngeal nerve.
- Traction applied to the distal airway can facilitate dissection of the proximal main stem to allow for division just distal to the carina. In the setting of endobronchial disease, it is always wise to perform bronchoscopy prior to dividing the airway to ensure that the margin is not too close.
- Once the stapler is applied check airway pressures to look for impingement of remaining airway.
- After removing the specimen, obtain hemostasis and check for leak from the bronchial stump.
- Reinforce the bronchial stump to prevent BPF, which is more important on the right, as the left bronchus will often retract into the mediastinum. Options for bronchial reinforcement include pericardial fat, pericardium, pleura, or azygos vein flaps. Alternatively, consider intercostal muscle, latissiumus dorsi, or serratus anterior flaps in cases of gross infection or previous radiation.
- Complete mediastinal lymphadenectomy.

Right pneumonectomy

- More physiologically taxing and prone to complications.
- Approach is similar to left side, with a few differences:
  - Azygos vein needs to be reflected superiorly to expose the proximal right mainstem bronchus.
  - The superior pulmonary vein may be divided first to provide better exposure to the right PA as long as the surgeon has assured tolerance for resection.

41

- Buttressing of the bronchial stump is mandatory to minimize the risk of postoperative bronchopleural or bronchoarterial fistulae.

Management of the pneumonectomy space

Options include:

- Chest tube attached to pneumonectomy balanced drainage system (not a pleurovac).

- Intrapleural catheter (usually a 8-12 Fr soft tube with a 3-way stopcock).

- No drain. If no drain is placed, consider aspiration of air from the pleural space after the chest is closed.

- Postoperative CXR is examined for mediastinal shift. Air can be added or removed to balance the mediastinum if utilizing a catheter or with angiocath inserted through lateral chest wall if no drain utilized.

- Tubes are usually removed on POD 1 or 2 if mediastinum remains stable and there are no concerns for bleeding. If a chest tube was utilized, the tube tract should be closed carefully to prevent pleurocutaneous fistula and retrograde infection. Tube removal should be performed under sterile conditions.

Potential questions/alternative scenarios

"The morning after a left pneumonectomy, the patient develops progressive hypotension. What is your management?"

The differential for postoperative hypotension is broad, and a systematic approach should be utilized. The physician assessing the patient should consider bleeding, hypovolemia secondary to volume restriction, myocardial ischemia, arrhythmia, epidural-related pressure changes (if applicable), hypoxia, and mediastinal shift. If a chest tube is being utilized, output serves as an indicator of bleeding, unless clotted/clogged. If no chest tube, a stat CXR may reveal a rapidly filling pneumonectomy space, implying bleeding, or significant mediastinal shift that may be impairing cardiac preload (treated by instilling air into the pneumonectomy space to shift the mediastinum back towards the midline). Laboratory hemoglobin/hematocrit values may be helpful, but acute bleeding may not result in an immediate hemoglobin drop. EKG and cardiac enzymes should be utilized to rule out cardiac events. Epidural-related hypotension can be addressed acutely with a volume challenge and temporary cessation of the epidural. Volume challenges may be used judiciously due to concerns regarding post-pneumonectomy pulmonary edema. Hypoxia should be excluded with pulse oximetry, and supplemental oxygen should be titrated.

"Three days after a right pneumonectomy a patient is noted to have a new left lower lobe infiltrate, cough, frothy sputum, and respiratory failure. How will you proceed?"

The mortality rate for pneumonectomy is reported to be 3-12% with a 15-75% rate of complications. The most common complications are respiratory failure, pulmonary edema, pneumonia, empyema, arrhythmias, MI, PE, and BPF. This scenario is describing a BPF in the perioperative setting. Early BPFs occur within one month postoperatively and are usually due to technical errors involving closure of the bronchial stump. Late BPFs occur later than one month and are typically attributed to inadequate healing of the bronchial stump. Incidence of BPF after pneumonectomy is reported to be from 1-10% with a mortality of 30-50%. Immediate management includes positioning the patient **operative side down** and head elevated to avoid contamination of the remaining lung, tube thoracostomy to drain the pleural space, and broad-spectrum antibiotics. Emergent reoperation with repair, coverage of the bronchial stump with a well-vascularized flap, and washout of the pleural space is required. The patient should be treated aggressively for postoperative pneumonia and observed carefully for development of empyema.

"A patient 6 weeks after left pneumonectomy presents to clinic with fever and new onset cough productive of blood-tinged sputum. CXR reveals a declining air-fluid level in the left hemithorax. What's your management?"

This patient is presenting with a delayed or late BPF. A chest tube should be placed to drain the pleural space, administration of broad-spectrum antibiotics, and medical stabilization of the patient. Bronchoscopy and surgical exploration should then be undertaken to evaluate the bronchial stump and the post-pneumonectomy space once the patient has been hemodynamically stabilized. If no obvious BPF is identified, the pleural space should be washed out, debrided, and drained if there is gross contamination. A Clagett window procedure is the next step and should be undertaken after 3-4 week of closed drainage to allow the mediastinum to stabilize. If the BPF presents late, the mediastinum may already be stabilized and the interval to operation may be shorter. In rare circumstances, no contamination is identified, and the chest may be washed out and closed. If there is a visible BPF, the acute management is the same with closed drainage to allow the mediastinum to stabilize. If the fistula closes, a Clagett window closure can be attempted. If the BPF persists, attempts at closure can be made with muscle flaps or omentum once the patient has recovered totally from their initial surgical intervention and subsequent evaluation reveals no evidence of recurrent cancer.

"On preoperative imaging, it appears that control of the PA will be difficult. What are alternative ways to approach this tumor?"
Intrapericardial control of the pulmonary artery can be obtained through a posterolateral thoracotomy. Alternatively, median sternotomy can be performed to gain control of the intrapericardial PA. Both right and left pneumonectomy can be performed via sternotomy.

"The tumor invades the chest wall, pericardium, adventitia of the aorta, superficial muscle of the esophagus, or focal area of SVC. How will you proceed?"
Tumor involving the chest wall, pericardium, focal vertebral body involvement and focal SVC involvement may be resected *en bloc* by surgeons with appropriate experience. Most surgeons would consider aortic or esophageal invasion a contraindication to proceeding. Clips should be placed to guide future radiotherapy if margins are close.

"The tumor involves the proximal vagus nerve on the left. How will you manage this?"
The nerve should be resected en bloc with the specimen. The patient should then be considered for vocal cord medialization in the immediate postoperative period. Strict aspiration precautions should be considered for the immediate postoperative period.

"An active 57-year-old woman is referred to you with a 19 mm carcinoid tumor in the origin of the right upper lobe bronchus. How would you approach the resection?"
After complete history and physical, radiographic staging, and cardiopulmonary testing as for all pulmonary resection candidates, you must decide on a resection strategy. A bronchoplastic resection, such as sleeve resection, is a reasonable consideration in this case to spare the right middle and lower lobes. This type of operation was originally developed for patients who could not tolerate pneumonectomy, but the indications have expanded, and many patients can benefit from a limited resection if anatomically feasible and oncologically appropriate.

Common indications for sleeve resection include:
- Lesions involving main bronchi or lobar bronchi close to the main bronchi
- Benign or low-grade tumors (carcinoid being the most common)
- Bulky peribronchial lymph node involvement
- Tumors in the lateral aspect of the lower trachea or carina

Contraindications:
- Locally advanced T4 tumors
- Patients with N2 or N3 disease *(Note: the exception is in cases of carcinoid tumor, given that chemotherapy and radiation tend to be ineffective. The authors advocate proceeding with carcinoid resections despite advanced nodal disease for greatest*

chance of cure and for optimal management of existing and/or expected airway obstruction symptoms)

- Inability to achieve negative margins

It is important to fully assess the extent of the tumor on bronchoscopy to determine if a sleeve resection will be feasible. The lesion can be biopsied and mucosa proximal and distal to the lesion can be sampled to assess for local spread. Decreased bronchial motion with respiration has been described as a sign of tumor extension.

Operative steps
Right upper lobe bronchial sleeve resection

- Formulate a plan with anesthesiology to ensure a successful ventilation strategy. For sleeve resections on the right, a left-sided double lumen tube should ideally be utilized and *vice versa*. Preoperative bronchoscopy is mandatory.
- Perform a posterolateral thoracotomy in the 5th interspace; harvest the 5th intercostal muscle during entry and carefully preserve the vascular pedicle. (Alternatives to intercostal muscle include pericardial fat or azygos vein)
- Posterior mediastinal pleura is opened to expose the right mainstem, trachea, and esophagus.
- Divide the azygos vein if it helps with exposure.
- Assess for local invasion and resectability. Excessive lymph node dissection should be avoided.
- Dissect and divide the pulmonary veins, arteries, and fissures as usual.
- Sharply divide the **distal mainstem bronchus** and proximal bronchus intermedius perpendicular to the long axis. Get frozen section to assure negative margins (minimum: 5 mm negative margin for high-grade carcinomas and 3 mm for low grade).
- Release inferior pulmonary ligament to decrease tension. Infrahilar pericardial release can provide more length if needed. A mediastinoscopy can also be used to release tension.
- Create an end-to-end anastomosis. Interrupted absorbable suture with knots outside the airway to decrease granuloma formation are preferable in the cartilaginous portion of the airway. Interrupted or running sutures may be used in the membranous portion. Common suture choices include PDS or oiled vicryl. Check for leak by submersion and ventilation to 25 cm water pressure, and then cover the anastomosis with vascularized tissue. Intercostal flaps should be placed primarily between the anastomosis and the pulmonary artery. Complete encirclement of the anastomosis could result in later stenosis if the muscle flap calcifies. Azygos vein, pericardial fat pad, and parietal pleura can provide alternative sources for coverage.

Potential questions/alternative scenarios
"Postoperative day 8 after a right upper lobe sleeve lobectomy, a patient develops fever and respiratory failure. Bronchoscopy shows necrosis and focal dehiscence of the anastomosis. CXR shows increase in the airspace on the operative side. How will you manage?"
Complications after sleeve lobectomy include sputum retention and secondary atelectasis, bronchovascular and bronchopulmonary fistula, and anastomotic failure (stricture and breakdown). Anastomotic breakdown is reported to occur in about 1% of patients. If there is a large air leak, intubation of the left mainstem bronchus will prevent significant ongoing tidal volume loss. If the leak is moderate to small, both lungs can be ventilated, assuming there is adequate drainage of the right pleural space. Therefore, tube thoracostomy and administration of broad-spectrum antibiotics should be the next step after intubation. Further management depends on the timing and size of the dehiscence. Early dehiscence (not clearly defined but occurring in the early postoperative period) may be treated with debridement, additional mobilization of the remaining lung/hilum, and re-anastomosis with tissue coverage in select cases. For dehiscence of 5 mm or less, simple chest tube drainage may be all that is

needed, particularly if there was tissue coverage of the anastomosis and minimal air leakage. For larger segments of dehiscence and those with smaller defects but ongoing significant air leak or pleural contamination, completion pneumonectomy should be considered. Anastomotic strictures may occur late and can typically be treated with balloon dilation. In rare cases, debridement of the stricture may be required with techniques such as laser therapy.

"Postoperative day 14, the previous patient develops hemoptysis. How will you manage them?"
Anastomotic failure can ultimately lead to development of bronchovascular fistula. This patient should be emergently brought to the operating room with preparation for large-volume bleeding. The patient should be carefully intubated with a left sided double lumen ETT, which is bronchoscopically guided into position to avoid anastomotic disruption. If blood or clot is identified at the anastomosis and a bronchovascular fistula is suspected, emergent completion pneumonectomy utilizing sternotomy for proximal pulmonary arterial control should be performed. There is typically no role for angiography and embolization in this potentially fatal setting.

"How do you handle a bronchial size mismatch during the end-to-end bronchial anastomosis?"
Traveling a further distance between bites on the larger sized bronchus should fix small size mismatches. Alternatively, a longitudinal wedge can be cut from the larger bronchus to allow tapering and better size match. Telescoping is an advanced technique that can be considered by those with experience.

"How do outcomes for sleeve lobectomy compare to pneumonectomy for NSCLC?"
Thirty-day mortality has been shown to be approximately 3-5% and 10% for sleeve lobectomy vs. pneumonectomy, respectively. Five- and 10-year survival after sleeve lobectomy have been reported to be 40% and 30-50%, respectively. Several large series have shown a 5-year survival rate of approximately 30-40% for pneumonectomy as well. Sleeve lobectomy is associated with superior 5-year survival rates in some series, decreased operative mortality, and comparable complication rates when compared to pneumonectomy. Pulmonary complications in the initial postoperative period tend to be more frequent with sleeve lobectomy. Factors decreasing long-term survival following a sleeve lobectomy include incomplete resection and increased nodal involvement. Locoregional recurrences with sleeve lobectomy occurred in approximately 30% of patients versus 8-17% in pneumonectomy patients.

Pearls/pitfalls

- Careful preoperative assessment is vital to select appropriate patients for pneumonectomy.
- Always attempt lesser resection when possible especially in patients that are not candidates for pneumonectomy.
- Occlude the PA prior to division to ensure pneumonectomy will be tolerated. Do not divide pulmonary veins prior to this occlusion test.

Suggested readings

- Shields TW, LoCicero, Ponn RJ (eds). Sleeve Lobectomy. Pneumonectomy and its Modifications. *General Thoracic Surgery*. Pennsylvania: Lippincott, Williams & Wilkins. (5th edition).
- Predina JD, Kunkala M, Aliperti LA, et al. Sleeve lobectomy: current indications and future directions. *Ann Thorac Cardiovasc Surg.* 2010 Oct;16(5):310-8.
- Groth SS, Burt BM, Sugarbaker DJ. Management of complications after pneumonectomy. *Thoracic surgery clinics.* 2015 Aug 1;25(3):335-48.
- Beauchamp G. Fundamentals of Standard Sleeve Resection. *Thoracic surgery clinics.* 2018 Aug 1;28(3):285-9.

5. PULMONARY CARCINOID

Ian C. Bostock, MD, and Mara B. Antonoff, MD

Adapted from 1st edition chapter written by Shair Ahmed, MD, and Allan Pickens, MD

Concept

- Classification and presentation of carcinoid tumors (typical vs. atypical)
- Diagnostic options
- Management of typical vs. atypical carcinoid, peripheral vs. central, N0-N2 mediastinal disease
- Special circumstances

Chief complaint

"A 38-year-old woman is referred to your office for evaluation of an incidental lung lesion seen on chest CT during a recent workup for trauma. She denies cough, shortness of breath, or pleuritic chest pain. On chest CT, the lesion is located centrally in the right lower lobe, measures 1.2 cm, and has a smooth homogenous appearance with well-demarcated borders."

Differential

Carcinoid tumor, mucoepidermoid tumors, large cell neuroendocrine tumor, non-small cell lung cancer, small cell lung cancer, pulmonary metastatic disease

History and physical

The symptoms of carcinoid tumors depend on location, whether peripheral or central. Peripheral lesions tend to be asymptomatic and found incidentally. Central lesions present with symptoms such as cough, positional wheezing, recurrent pneumonia, and hemoptysis. Rarely, patients may present with carcinoid syndrome, which consists of diarrhea and episodic flushing. The vast majority of patients presenting with carcinoid syndrome will have advanced disease due to liver metastases. Bronchial carcinoids can present with other paraneoplastic syndromes as well, most notably Cushing's syndrome. The most common source of ectopic adrenocorticotropic hormone (ACTH) is bronchial carcinoid tumors. Patients who present with pulmonary carcinoid tumors are typically younger than patients with NSCLC (median presentation in 40's, ~20 years earlier than NSCLC. Also, there are bimodal peaks in age distribution, at 35 and 55 years).

Tests

- *Imaging.* Chest CT with IV contrast is needed to evaluate the location of the tumor, the characteristics of the lesion (typically homogeneous and well-demarcated), its association with vascular structures, as well as to assess the mediastinum for lymphadenopathy. Carcinoids are metabolically inactive and on PET-CT have very little uptake. However, if PET-CT is performed before a biopsy is obtained, it can be diagnostically useful, as lesions that have low uptake are more likely to be carcinoid as opposed to lesions with high uptake, which tend to be small cell or non-small cell lung cancer. Octreotide scans have been used by some institutions in settings of substantial concern for distant metastatic disease (more likely with central tumors, N2 disease, or carcinoid syndrome). In addition, some institutions perform Gallium DOTATATE PET/CT scans which have been found to be more sensitive than octreotide scans for neuroendocrine tumors.
- *Labs.* If carcinoid syndrome is suspected, proceed with measuring urine 5-hydroxyindoleacteic acid (5-HIAA) with a 24-hour collection (in addition to imaging, which will reveal liver metastasis in most cases). If Cushing's syndrome symptoms exist, then measure serum ACTH. Note that the majority of patients will not have these symptoms, and laboratory workup for carcinoid tumors will typically include standard

preoperative labs such as chemistry panel, complete blood count, and type and screen/cross.

- *Pulmonary function tests (PFTs).* Lung function needs to be assessed to determine tolerance of a pulmonary resection depending on the clinical scenario. This is crucial for central tumors that may require a pneumonectomy or sleeve lobectomy. (See Chapter 4: Pneumonectomy and Sleeve Resection)
- *Bronchoscopy.* Patients with central lesions may have visible disease that can be seen endobronchially. The central tumors are smooth and round; they are often red to reddish brown and covered with bronchial mucosa. Adequate sampling can yield the diagnosis of carcinoid. Endobronchial carcinoids tend to be hypervascular, leading previous authors to historically discourage biopsy. However, this has since been shown to be less of a concern than previously thought, with carcinoid tumors frequently safely biopsied via several approaches: endobronchially, transbronchially (with EBUS), or with transthoracic access (CT-guided percutaneous biopsy). Nonetheless, anyone undertaking biopsy should be prepared to manage potential bleeding.
- *Endobronchial ultrasound with biopsy (EBUS).* If there is suspicious lymphadenopathy, preoperative biopsy via EBUS can be helpful to identify nodes requiring resection. However, preoperative diagnosis of nodal disease should not impact decision to operate, as surgery remains the mainstay of therapy for carcinoid disease, with minimal effectiveness of chemotherapy and radiation.

Index scenario (additional information)

"The patient's history and physical reveal no symptoms and no comorbidities. The mass on CT is 1.2 cm, homogenous, well-demarcated, and centrally located in the right lower lobe with no hilar or mediastinal lymphadenopathy. Bronchoscopy showed no endobronchial lesion. The patient's PFTs revealed an FEV1 of 82% of the predicted value and DLCO of 60% of predicted. How would you proceed?"

Treatment/management

Diagnosis for this situation is based on clinical suspicion while considering patient age and imaging findings. Needle biopsy is feasible, but not mandatory, if high suspicion of carcinoid is present, and treatment may be offered based on clinical presentation in healthy individuals who are low risk for surgery. In the provided scenario, the patient is young, without comorbidities, and has good pulmonary reserve; the patient will likely tolerate a pulmonary resection for diagnostic and therapeutic purposes. Of course, the patient should be appropriately consented with clear discussion of differential diagnosis and possible pathologic findings if surgery is planned without a preoperative tissue diagnosis. It should be noted that intraoperative frozen section cannot differentiate between typical and atypical carcinoid.

Operative steps

Goals – resection to negative margins, perform lobectomy, adequately sample lymph nodes and/or perform complete lymphadenectomy.

- Double lumen ETT, adequate IV access, arterial line, Foley catheter.
- Thoracoscopic approach (VATS)/versus open depending on comfort, tumor location, and potential need for sleeve resection or bronchoplasty
- Take down the inferior pulmonary ligament, send station 9R lymph nodes for permanent.
- Identify and dissect inferior pulmonary vein, locate and preserve the right middle lobe vein; once clearly identified, transect the inferior pulmonary vein.
- Dissect right lower lobe pulmonary artery; transect the right lower lobe branches of pulmonary artery.
- Dissect the right lower lobe bronchus, careful to be distal from the bronchus to the right middle lobe. For endobronchial tumors, bronchoscopic visualization is necessary

at the beginning of the case as well as at the time of airway resection to ensure that margins will be adequate and that sleeve resection or bronchoplasty is not needed. Ensure the preserved lung reinflates prior to transecting the right lower lobe bronchus.

- Complete the fissure between the right middle and right lower lobe.
- Ensure complete lung expansion and leave chest tube posteriorly and to the apex.

Potential questions/alternative scenarios

"The patient in the above scenario presented with a central lesion; however, the patient was found to have hilar lymphadenopathy. How would you proceed?"

Patients with a central carcinoid and hilar adenopathy are more likely to have an atypical carcinoid and should undergo an endobronchial ultrasound with biopsies to stage the mediastinum before resection. This is also consistent with the ACCP guidelines for central lesions and N1 nodal disease. If the patient does have N2 disease, then they should undergo further imaging to work up for distant metastases including brain MRI, CT abdomen/pelvis, +/- PET CT, and/or octreotide scan. Neoadjuvant treatment with re-assessment for resection can be considered, although the modalities available for restaging are suboptimal, and chemotherapy and radiation are of minimal benefit in this disease. Even for advanced nodal disease, as long as there is not distant metastasis, surgical resection remains the most effective strategy for curative treatment.

"A 70-year-old patient presents with a central pulmonary lesion with characteristics suggesting carcinoid and mediastinal lymphadenopathy by imaging. How would you proceed?"

Patients age > 50 with a central pulmonary lesion are more likely to have atypical carcinoid. In this situation, endobronchial ultrasound with biopsies is indicated, which can yield the diagnosis of atypical carcinoid on final path (not frozen) if there is indeed lymph node involvement. Further imaging for distant metastases is warranted. Although the literature is not definitive, preoperative chemotherapy and radiation may also be considered (using regimen for small cell lung cancer, platinum-based chemotherapy) before proceeding to resection. However, many would advocate for proceeding with upfront resection despite N2 disease, followed by consideration of adjuvant chemotherapy given the benefit of resection on long-term outcomes.

"A 65-year-old man presented with a pedunculated endobronchial lesion on diagnostic bronchoscopy, CT chest reveals no extra-bronchial extension of the mass and no hilar or mediastinal disease. How would you manage this patient?"

Endobronchial resection is an option in this select group of patients who have isolated endobronchial pedunculated typical carcinoid. Endobronchial resection is not an option for atypical carcinoid, as these lesions are likely to have further extension. However, if this method is utilized, the patient requires extensive long-term follow-up including bronchoscopy, CT, and EBUS. The procedure may cause significant stricturing from scar tissue, requiring further intervention. Endobronchial resection can also be used to manage symptomatic patients in a palliative manner for whom surgical resection is contraindicated. Adjuncts of management such spray cryotherapy or laser ablation may be helpful. Alternatively, one may also consider sleeve bronchial resection with preservation of all lung parenchyma for a long-term curative resection that will achieve negative margins.

Pearls/pitfalls

- Typical carcinoid defined as tumor with neuroendocrine features, <2 mitotic figures per 10 high power fields (HPFs), and no evidence of necrosis. Typical carcinoid is less aggressive and could be treated with a sub-lobar resection.
- Atypical carcinoid has 2 to 10 mitotic figures per 10 HPFs with evidence of necrosis or architectural disruption. These are more aggressive and should be treated with anatomic lung resection and lymph node dissection, when possible.
- Indolent, well-demarcated homogenous lesions are characteristic of carcinoid.

- Carcinoid has a bi-modal age distribution, with peaks at ages 30-39 and 50-59.
- Carcinoid tumors tend to be metabolically inactive, and will usually not light up on PET.
- Bronchial carcinoids do not present with carcinoid syndrome unless metastatic.
- Endobronchial ultrasound is helpful for hilar or mediastinal disease; if mediastinal disease is present, pursue metastatic workup before resection.
- Resection for typical carcinoid is mainstay of treatment, even if N2 disease present given good long-term survival.
- If chemotherapy needed, use regimen for small cell lung cancer (platinum-based). Radiation is typically not indicated due to poor response rates.
- Recent data have shown excellent long-term outcomes following surgical resection of carcinoid tumors. Interestingly, some authors have found that the presence of nodal metastases and tumor size were not associated with decreased long-term survival.

Suggested readings

- Detterbeck FC. Management of carcinoid tumors. *Ann Thorac Surg*. 2010 Mar;89(3):998-1005.
- Simon GR, Turrisi A; American College of Chest Physicians. Management of small cell lung cancer: ACCP evidence-based clinical practice guidelines (2nd edition).*Chest*. 2007 Sep;132(3 Suppl):324S-339S.
- Wirth LJ, Carter MR, Jänne PA, Johnson BE Outcome of patients with pulmonary carcinoid tumors receiving chemotherapy or chemoradiotherapy. *Lung Cancer*. 2004 May;44(2):213-20.
- Wolin EM. Advances in the diagnosis and management of well-differentiated and intermediate-differentiated neuroendocrine tumors of the lung. *Chest*. 2017 May 1;151(5):1141-6.
- Hendifar AE, Marchevsky AM, Tuli R. Neuroendocrine tumors of the lung: current challenges and advances in the diagnosis and management of well-differentiated disease. *Journal of Thoracic Oncology*. 2017 Mar 1;12(3):425-36.

6. Primary Chest Wall Tumors
Christian C. Shults, MD, and Seth Force, MD

Concept
- Differential for chest wall tumors
- Indicated testing and therapy for the different etiologies
- Techniques for reconstruction
- Adjuvant therapy

Chief complaint

"A 30-year-old man presents with a painless right chest mass that has been slowly growing over the last 5 years."

Differential

Primary chest wall tumor, adjacent tumors with local invasion, metastatic lesions, or non-neoplastic disease. It is helpful to classify lesions in terms of origin (soft tissue vs. bone/cartilage) and then to sub-classify as benign vs. malignant (** indicates most common with % of total, where available).

- *Benign bony and cartilaginous*: fibrous dysplasia ** (30% of all benign chest wall tumors), osteochondroma ** (50% of all benign rib tumors), chondroma ** (15% of all benign rib tumors), plasmacytoma.
- *Malignant bony and cartilaginous*: chondrosarcoma ** (30% of all primary malignant bone tumors), Ewing sarcoma, osteogenic sarcoma, Askin tumor.
- *Benign soft tissue*: desmoid tumor ** (sometimes classified as low grade sarcoma), lipoma, hemangioma, lymphangioma, fibroma, rhabdomyoma, neurofibroma.
- *Malignant soft tissue*: malignant fibrous histiocytoma (MFH) ** (most common primary chest wall tumor), rhabdomyosarcoma ** (second most common primary chest wall tumor), liposarcoma, neurofibrosarcoma, leiomyosarcoma.
- *Adjacent tumors (24% of all chest wall tumors)*: lung, breast, pleura, mediastinum, skin (including melanoma).
- *Metastatic tumors (32% of all chest wall tumors)*: sarcoma and carcinoma.
- *Non-neoplastic conditions*: inflammatory and cystic lesions.

History and physical

The majority of chest wall lesions are the result of metastases (sarcoma most common) or invasion of adjacent malignancies. Primary chest wall tumors are typically slow-growing masses and 75% are painless. Malignant lesions or those arising from bone tend to be painful due to expansion into the cortex or periosteum, destruction of the cortex, or resulting fractures. Important information obtained in the history includes: age (there is an age distribution associated with most masses), symptoms (pain usually indicates malignancy or invasion into bone), history of trauma, and any history of associated disease, weight loss, or previous mass/cancer. The physical exam should focus on whether the mass is soft or firm, fixed or mobile, and tender or painless. A rapid increase in size suggests a malignant lesion. Evidence of previous incisions or trauma should also be assessed.

Tests

- *CXR*: first step, many tumors have a classic radiographic appearance.
- *CT*: highest yield (site, size, bony involvement, screen lungs for metastasis).
- *MRI*: most sensitive, differentiate tumor as well as relationship to critical structures (vascular, neural).
- *PET*: differentiate benign from malignant, delineate tumor grade.
- Diagnosis is ultimately made with biopsy (unless resection planned regardless of diagnosis) and can be performed by core needle biopsy, excisional biopsy (lesions < 5 cm), or incisional biopsy (lesions > 5 cm). It is crucial that the biopsy be performed

along the plane of potential surgical resection. Frozen section is usually of little use for diagnostic purposes given frequent bone and cartilage involvement.

- *Labs*: baseline parameters, coags.

Treatment/management

Chest wall tumors are a heterogenous group of lesions. However, the general strategy remains the same for most lesions. History and imaging may be enough to make the diagnosis or lead one to have a suspicion of the likely diagnosis. Tissue should be obtained when the diagnosis remains in question, although in many circumstances the diagnosis will be made when the lesion is resected. Core needle, incisional, or excisional biopsies are options that must be considered based on the tumor characteristics and suspected diagnosis. Biopsies should not compromise future treatment and care should be taken to perform biopsies oriented within the potential plane of resection. Most benign lesions can be observed, unless they are symptomatic. Malignant lesions must be resected. Treatment involves appropriate excisional margins (2-4 cm) for malignant lesions to minimize the chance of local recurrence. Reconstruction may be required and if so, soft tissue coverage of the reconstruction material may also be required.

Index scenario (additional information)

"Let's say the lesion in question is slow growing, as mentioned, and the appearance on the CT scan is consistent with lipoma."

Slow growing lesions with benign characteristics on CT scan are likely benign. Treatment includes biopsy to rule out a malignant tumor and confirm the suspected histologic diagnosis. Use of core needle, incisional, or excisional biopsy is based primarily on size. Core needle biopsy is a reasonable first step in larger lesions. However, if a diagnosis cannot be made, then incisional biopsy is needed. Excisional biopsy for smaller lesions (2-4 cm) would also be appropriate.

"Describe your approach to an excisional biopsy (benign or malignant)?"

Excisional biopsy may be appropriate for small lesions or lesions that are thought to be benign, but tissue confirmation is needed. Margins typically only need to be grossly negative in these circumstances. Benign lesions that tend to recur (as noted in other scenarios above and below), chondromas (benign lesion with significant risk of harboring occult areas of malignant sarcoma), or other specific lesions may require "wide" local excision, typically with 2-4 cm margins. Excisional biopsies do not require resection of the overlying skin; however, the incisions should be oriented so that if final pathology does demonstrate malignant disease, then the area can be re-resected, including the previous incisions, overlying skin, and surrounding structures. Wide local excision may be accomplished with light monitored sedation versus GETA depending on the size and extent of resection. Oblique incision parallel to the ribs about 2-4 cm on each side of the lesion. Incise through the skin, dermis, and subcutaneous tissue and raise a flap around the tumor leaving fascia on the muscle. Bovie out a circle around the tumor down to the bone with at least 2-4 cm margin of tissue. Ensure that the tumor is freely mobile within the soft tissue and not involving the bone (if the lesion is a primary bone tumor then the rib or bone would be resected with the appropriate margin). Undermine the undersurface of the tumor and hand off the specimen with properly oriented marking sutures. If the suspicion for malignancy is low, send for permanent pathology, as frozen sections are not likely to change management. If there is any question about margins, then send the specimen for frozen and/or send a specimen of free margin in the area of concern. Get hemostasis and re-approximate the remaining muscle, subcutaneous tissue, and dermis. You may need to mobilize the muscle laterally to release tension.

"Let's say instead of a 30-year-old man it is a 3-year-old boy with what appears to be a hemangioma on the chest wall."

Treatment for hemangiomas in children is non-operative except for cosmetic reasons or complications such as bleeding or ulceration. If there is any question as to the diagnosis, a T2

MRI will show a high signal intensity in the case of hemangioma. Given its benign nature, excision with grossly negative margins is all that is needed. Biopsy in this instance is unnecessary and may cause bleeding.

"What if this lesion were a lymphangioma?"
Lymphangiomas are benign chest wall lesions that are most commonly found in children. Surgical resection is required to prevent recurrence. OK-432 and acetic acid sclerotherapy may also be used.

"Let's say the patient is a 24-year-old woman with a history of trauma to the area and Gardner's Syndrome?"
With a history of Gardner's Syndrome, the desmoid tumor alarm should be going off in your head. 50% of these tumors occur in the abdomen; however, the chest wall is the most common extra-abdominal site. They originate from fibroblasts of the deep muscle and connective tissue and most commonly present in the teens – 30's. 62% are painful and associated with a history of trauma, thoracotomy, and Gardner's Syndrome. They are slow growing and have a very high recurrence rate. Wide local excision with 4 cm margins is optimal. Adjuvant radiation is commonly used to decrease local recurrence rates with both negative and positive margins. There is an 89% 5-year probability of local recurrence with positive margins and 18% if the margins are negative.

"Let's say the patient is a 25-year-old man with a chest wall tumor on the posterolateral aspect of the 6th rib. The mass is slow growing, asymptomatic, and was incidentally found. The x-ray shows a ground glass appearance of the central area of the rib with thinning of the cortex and irregular calcification in the medulla. How would you manage this patient?"
These are all characteristics of a benign lesion, the most common of which (30%) is fibrous dysplasia. These typically present in the age range of 20-30s, on the posterior or lateral aspect of the ribs and are asymptomatic, slow-growing, and usually found incidentally. They are associated with Albright Syndrome (skin lesions and precocious puberty in girls). Imaging shows the classic ground-glass appearance in the central area of the rib, thinning of the cortex, and irregular calcifications in the medulla. Treatment is local excision for painful lesions. Asymptomatic lesions can be left alone (unless the diagnosis is in doubt). In general biopsies of these lesions are low yield.

"Let's say the patient is a 20-year-old man with growths arising from the cortical bone anteriorly at the costochondral junction along the sternum with caps that feel cartilaginous. X-ray/CT Scan shows a pedunculated protuberance with intact cortex and stippled calcification in the area of the tumor. How would you treat this lesion?"
This is the classic presentation of an osteochondroma. These are cartilage capped growths that arise from the cortical bone of the sternum anteriorly at the costochondral junction along the sternum. These chest wall tumors most commonly present in the patients 20's with a 3:1 M:F predominance. Imaging findings are as described with a pedunculated protuberance, intact cortex, and stippled calcification in the area of the tumor. Malignant degeneration is rare in these lesions and wide local excision with margins of 2-4 cm is warranted for lesions that are symptomatic, enlarging, or if the diagnosis is in doubt and the patient is an adult.

"You are referred a 30-year-old woman with an asymptomatic, slow-growing mass with X-ray/CT findings showing a periosteal lytic mass with a thinning cortex and sclerotic borders. How would you manage this patient?"
This is most likely a chondroma (benign chest wall tumor), however it is hard to distinguish chondroma from a malignant, degenerative chondrosarcoma. Therefore, the treatment is excision with wide margins of 2 cm in all cases. These masses are asymptomatic, slow-growing, most commonly ages 20-40 with M = F. If the lesion proves to be malignant of final pathology (frozen will not help in determining this), then re-resection with 4 cm margins is necessary.

"You are seeing another patient, a 60-year-old man with pain and no palpable mass in the lateral chest wall. He is also hypercalcemic with a urinalysis positive for Bence-Jones protein. What is the suspected diagnosis and how would you treat this patient?"

Pain with no mass, hypercalcemia, and Bence-Jones proteinuria are key here. This is a plasmacytoma, which is highly associated with multiple myeloma. These chest wall tumors most commonly occur in men, 60-70 yo, and present with pain and no palpable mass. These patients will have Bence-Jones protein in the urine with abnormal protein electrophoresis and hypercalcemia. A bone marrow biopsy will confirm the diagnosis. These patients are treated with surgery for the purposes of tissue diagnosis only (core needle or incisional biopsy), followed by high-dose radiation. 35% to 55% of patients progress to multiple myeloma, with an overall 5-year survival 25% to 35%.

"You are referred a 60-year-old man with a painless slow-growing mass that on CT scan appears to originate from the muscle and grows along the fascial planes between muscle fibers. How would you treat?"

This is a malignant soft tissue malignant fibrous histiocytoma (MFH). This is the most common chest wall sarcoma. It has a male > female predominance and most commonly occurs in the 50's to 70's. These lesions are painless, and slow growing, originate in the muscle, and grow along the fascial planes between the muscle fibers. Treatment is wide local resection. There is a high local recurrence rate with metastasis 30-50% of the time. 5-year survival is 38%. Adjuvant radiation is given for inadequate margins or high histologic grade. You may also perform re-resection of low-grade tumors.

"A 15-year-old boy with a rhabdomyosarcoma is now referred to you. How would you treat this patient?"

Most common in children and adolescents. Treatment is wide local excision and multi-drug chemotherapy. Neoadjuvant therapy followed by surgical excision has a 75% survival rate versus 25% for surgery alone.

"You are seeing a 50-year-old man with a large encapsulated tumor. Previous biopsy of the mass shows a liposarcoma. How would you treat this malignant lesion?"

Liposarcomas occur most commonly in men ages 40-60. They present as large encapsulated tumors. Treatment consists of wide excision to prevent local recurrence. 5-year survival rates are 60%. Other soft tissue malignancies include neurofibrosarcoma and leiomyosarcoma.

"A 40-year-old woman presents with a painful, hard, fixed mass at the costochondral angle and with a history of trauma to the region several years ago. The CT scan shows a mixed lytic and sclerotic pattern with an ovulated mass originating from the medulla with cortical lesions as well as some areas of thickened cortex."

This is a chondrosarcoma. This is the most common primary malignancy of the anterior chest wall. It occurs most commonly in 30-60-year olds M = F. It is associated with prior trauma and presents as a painful hard, fixed mass. 80% arise from the costochondral angle and 20% from the sternum. CT scan will show a mixed lytic and sclerotic pattern with a mass originating from the medulla with cortical lytic lesions as well as some areas of thickened cortex. Treatment consists of resection of localized lesions with wide local excision (2-4 cm, or one uninvolved rib above and below). This tumor is radio-resistant, and radiation is reserved for positive margins only. Outcome is highly dependent upon the grade of the tumor: Low-grade (mild hypercellularity) has a 96% 10-year survival with few metastases. High-grade (marked hypercellularity) have metastases 75% of the time and a 5-year survival of only 20-30%. Poor prognostic factors include high tumor grade, large tumor size, incomplete resection, local recurrence, metastasis and patient age over 50 years.

"Walk me through how you would resect this tumor or any primary bone tumor on the anterolateral chest wall."

Operative steps

Chest wall resection for an anterolateral chest wall tumor

- Based upon preoperative imaging you would first identify the superior and inferior margins of resection.
- The patient would receive a double lumen tube and an epidural.
- The patient would be positioned in lateral decubitus with the involved side up. (If lateral chest wall lesion.)
- Complete resection is the best chance for cure. Objectives for resection would be a 2-4 cm margin including the rib above and the rib below the tumor as well as involved skin (including biopsy site) and parietal pleura if involved.
- Make an oblique incision parallel to the ribs about 4 cm on each side of the lesion down through the skin.
- Dissect through the dermis and subcutaneous tissue, raise a flap around the tumor leaving fascia on the muscle.
- Get enough exposure to palpate a rib above and a rib below easily.
- Bovie out a circle around the tumor down to the bone with at least 2-4 cm margin of tissue. Score the ribs anteriorly and posteriorly.
- Drop the lung and enter the pleura at the intercostal space below, above, or anterior to the tumor. Note that it is not always necessary to explore the chest at this time if the CT shows no evidence of intrapleural involvement. If there is any doubt, then plan on placing a retractor of choice and exploring the pleural space prior to proceeding.
- Free the intercostal musculature and neurovascular bundles surrounding the upper and the lower ribs. Clear the periosteum 1.5 cm from each border and separate the rib from the underlying pleura. Cut the ribs. An additional 1 cm posterior and anterior margins of the ribs are sent separately and marked appropriately to ensure free margins. Note that in the case of a costochondral tumor, this may require ligation of the mammary artery and resection of the cartilaginous ribs near the sternum. If it abuts the sternum it may require partial resection of the sternum as described below.
- Ligate and divide the neurovascular bundles accompanying the upper and lower ribs that were resected.
- Any soft tissue margin with questionable involvement should be sent for pathologic frozen section to assess whether wider margins are required.

In all patients with a malignant primary chest wall tumor the 5-year freedom from recurrence rate is 56% in patients resected with 4 cm margins and 25% with 2 cm margins.

Potential questions/alternative scenarios

"What if the tumor was not palpable and the patient is obese?"

Multiple options exist. The lesion can be marked by radiology using the CT scanner in an orientation that is perpendicular to the epicenter of the lesion. Alternatively, intraoperative ultrasound could be used to aid with localization. If the lesion involves the rib, a quick VATS procedure could be performing placing a camera away from the tumor to identify the its boundaries and mark with a long spinal needle if needed.

"What if the tumor is adherent to the lung, sternum, or the pericardium?"

Tissue adherent to the tumor—including superficial chest wall muscles, lung, thymus, pericardium, or diaphragm—should be resected en bloc. If the sternum is involved, it may require partial or total sternectomy along with excision of the contiguous bilateral costal margins. Try to maintain the circumferential integrity of the chest wall for pulmonary function. If the lower sternum is involved, preserve the manubrium. If the sternal body is involved, a subtotal sternectomy is performed, preserving the upper 2 cm of manubrium and clavicles. If the manubrium is involved, spare the lower half of the sternum. Rigid reconstruction of the sternum is required. Note that advanced primary lung cancers are discussed in a separate chapter. However, if the lung is adherent to the rib in the setting of a primary lung cancer, then the resection proceeds very much as

54

described above with a few important caveats. It is critical in this scenario to explore the chest before starting your resection. If the tumor is high, then this is easily done through an anterolateral or posterolateral thoracotomy in the 4th or 5th intercostal space. Place your retractor, palpate the lung and assess the degree of chest wall invasion from within the chest. At this point you can either perform the chest wall resection through a separate incision exactly as described above and then perform the lobectomy or perform the lobectomy first followed by the chest wall resection. What if the mass is in the 5th rib in the middle of the thoracotomy exposure that you intended to use for the lobectomy? Enter the intercostal space anterior or posterior to the tumor (depending on location) and proceed as just described. You will obviously not need a separate incision for the chest wall resection in this case as it will be a part your thoracotomy incision. The thoracotomy incision will be closed primarily as usual, but the posterior or anterior chest wall defect will require reconstruction as described below.

"How would you reconstruct the defect?"
A subsequent reconstruction may use simple prosthetic placement or more complex tissue transposition techniques. Technique is dependent upon the location and size of the defect.

"Let's say you have a high posterior defect above the 5th rib and < 10 cm?"
All high posterior defects above the 5th rib and < 10 cm do not need reconstruction since the defect will be covered by scapula. Resection that involves the 5th rib can lead to entrapment of the scapula in the defect if it is not reconstructed.

"What if it is an anterior defect?"
All anterior defects < 5 cm do not require reconstruction. Resection of three or more ribs, or removal of two or more ribs with baseline pulmonary compromise needs reconstruction.

"What if you've resected bilateral sternoclavicular joints?"
Resection of bilateral sternoclavicular joints, the entire sternum, or upper part of the manubrium needs reconstruction (unilateral sternoclavicular joint not typically reconstructed)

General reconstruction techniques
Materials
- *Rigid reconstruction*: Marlex-methylmethacrylate sandwich, titanium bars, bio-absorbable bars (biobridge)
- *Non-rigid reconstruction*: Gortex, marlex, bovine pericardium

Technique
Suture prosthetic mesh to the chest wall under tension. Infected/irradiated fields: bovine pericardium or processed cellular matrix (Alloderm). A Marlex "sandwich" used when more rigid support is needed: sternal or anterolateral resections. Mesh is measured to 2x the size of the defect. A 2 to 3 mm layer of methyl methacrylate is then poured on one half of the mesh and then the other half of the mesh is folded over. The mesh edges are then sutured to the edge of the wound defect with permanent suture. One technique that is commonly used: drill holes in the exposed rib edges anteriorly and then posteriorly. Bring in the measured material and use thick non-absorbable sutures (i.e., 1-0 prolene) in an interrupted fashion through the ribs and then the material of choice. Along the top and bottom the suture goes around the staying rib and then through the material. Tie all sutures at the end. Muscle and soft tissue will then be mobilized above this material as needed to achieve complete coverage.

"What if the field is infected?"
Prosthetic reconstruction is contraindicated in infected wounds, in which case skeletal reconstruction should be delayed or biologic material should be used (Biobridge). In these cases, autologous tissue such as muscle and omentum can be used. Soft tissue reconstruction

55

can be used when skeletal stability is not required. Soft tissue options include: split-thickness skin grafts, muscle grafts, or musculocutaneous grafts (latissimus dorsi, pectoralis major, serratus, rectus abdominus, external oblique).

"A 50-year-old man with prior radiation to the chest presents with a rapidly expanding painful mass and elevated alkaline phosphatase levels. The CT scan shows a sunburst pattern and shows the tumor lifting the periosteum. What is the most likely diagnosis based on the imaging findings? How would you manage this patient?"

This is an osteogenic sarcoma. These chest wall tumors are most commonly seen in the long bones. Osteogenic sarcomas represent approximately 6% of all primary chest wall malignancies. These masses are rapidly expanding, painful, and cause elevated alkaline phosphatase levels. CT will show the classic sunburst pattern (sometimes seen on radiograph – representing calcifications at the right angles to the cortex) and Codman's triangle wherein the tumor lifts the periosteum and creates a shadow between the cortex and the raised periosteum. This tumor most commonly occurs in teenagers or adults. It is seen in patients with Paget disease, prior radiation, or prior bone infarction. It is associated with mutations in the RB gene p53. Biopsy can be performed as a core needle, incisional, or excisional. Treatment is neoadjuvant chemotherapy and wide local excision. Outcome is poor with metastasis with a 20% survival rate – lung is the primary site of metastasis. Overall survival is 14-20%.

"A 15-year-old boy presents with a rapidly enlarging painful mass. The CT scan shows an onion-peel appearance. What is the most likely diagnosis based on the imaging findings? How would you manage this patient?"

This is Ewing sarcoma with the classic radiographic appearance of the onion-peel that occurs from the bony destruction and the reactive multiple layers of new periosteal formation. This tumor occurs most commonly in 10-15 year-old males (M:F 2:1). With this presentation you must first get a core biopsy to confirm the diagnosis. This is done with reverse-transcription polymerase chain reaction analysis of the gene locations. Treatment is neoadjuvant chemotherapy followed by wide local excision. Radiation is added for additional cortical control and for positive margins. Survival is 56-65% at 5 years and 43% at 10 years.

"A 17-year-old boy presents with a large soft tissue mass that involves the chest wall with pleural thickening. Core biopsy shows small round cells on light microscopy and the cells stained positive for neuron-specific enolase (NSE) and electron microscopy showed dense core granules in the cytoplasm. What is the diagnosis and how would you treat?"

This is an Askin tumor, which is a primitive neuroectodermal tumor (PNET) from the Ewing sarcoma family of tumors. The radiographic findings will be non-specific. This tumor is difficult to differentiate from other small cell tumors of childhood and young adulthood (Ewing's) especially if only using light microscopy. Positive staining for neuron-specific enolase and dense core granules in the cytoplasm help to differentiate Askin tumors. Workup and treatment are the same as for Ewing's tumor. The presence of a posterior and pleural-based mass in the chest or the presence of a retroperitoneal mass in the abdomen should alert you to the possibility of spread along the sympathetic chain. Presence of these metastatic foci would have significant treatment implications. These tumors are more aggressive than Ewing's with a 5-year survival of 16%.

"A 30-year-old man presents with a right chest wall soft tissue mass. An incisional biopsy showed plasmacytoma. Do you proceed with resection alone?"

No. Plasmacytoma of the chest wall, even if solitary, should be considered a systemic disease. Resection is reasonable but systemic therapy with radiation and/or chemotherapy is key.

Pearls/pitfalls

- Heterogeneous group of tumors (diagnosis is key)
- Needle aspiration not adequate, need tissue for diagnosis, ideally open biopsy

- Plan biopsy to lie within resection margins along the long axis of the tumor
- Most benign lesions can be observed unless symptomatic or otherwise complicated; malignant lesions must be excised
- Complete resection is the most important prognostic factor
- Most chest wall tumors are resistant to chemo/radiation
- If there is any doubt as to diagnosis, tissue diagnosis by histologic examination is required
- If suspicion for malignancy you want 4 cm margin, check margins with frozen
- Do not place mesh in an infected field; reconstruct with biologics or native tissue, or plan to return when the infection is cleared for reconstruction
- Must reconstruct:
  - Posterior defects below 4th rib
  - All anterior defects > 5 cm
  - Resection of three or more ribs
  - Removal of two or more ribs with baseline pulmonary compromise
  - Resection of the manubrium
  - Resection of the entire sternum

Suggested readings

- Garner M, Fackche NT, Brock MV. Management of Primary Chest Wall Tumors. Cameron JL and Cameron AM (ed). *Current Surgical Therapy*. Philadelphia: Elsevier 2020: 873-879.
- Allen TC, Cagle PT. Pathology of chest wall tumors. Franco KL, Thourani VH (eds). *Cardiothoracic Surgery Review*. Philadelphia: Lippincott Williams & Wilkins 2012:1169.
- Fabre D, Missenard G, Fadel E, Kolb P, Besse B, Darteville P. Surgical treatment of chest wall tumors. Franco KL, Thourani VH (eds). *Cardiothoracic Surgery Review*. Philadelphia: Lippincott Williams & Wilkins 2012:1178.
- Nicastri DG, Swati GN, Williams EE, Flores RM, Jones DR. Chest wall tumors. LoCicero J III, Feins RH, Colson YL, Rocco G. *Shields' General Thoracic Surgery*. Philadelphia: Lippincott Williams & Wilkins, 2018: 636.

7. MEDIASTINAL STAGING

Sarah Yousef, MD, and Matthew Schuchert, MD

Adapted from 1st edition chapter written by David D. Odell, MD, and Jonathan D'Cuhna, MD

Concept

- Indications for mediastinal evaluation
- Approaches to mediastinal staging
- Potential complications of mediastinoscopy and management

Chief complaint

"A 54-year-old man with a 30 pack-year smoking history is referred to you by his primary care physician after a 4.3 cm right upper lobe mass was discovered on chest CT that was obtained to evaluate a 'persistent pneumonia'. A subsequent CT-guided biopsy of this lesion was pathologically consistent with adenocarcinoma. CT scan shows evidence of mediastinal lymphadenopathy."

History and physical

A focused history should be taken including a smoking history, history of exposures and recent illnesses, and an evaluation of the patient's surgical candidacy. History of recent upper respiratory tract infection or pneumonia may increase the likelihood of reactive mediastinal adenopathy. Any prior history of surgical intervention in the neck or chest as well as prior chest radiation should be carefully reviewed as these issues may increase the difficulty of surgical staging. Current smokers should be strongly encouraged to quit smoking 2-3 weeks prior to any surgical intervention, if possible. A thorough physical exam should be performed with special attention paid to palpation of the cervical and supraclavicular lymph nodes. Neck extension should be evaluated to enhance understanding of the ability to position the patient for mediastinoscopy.

Differential for mediastinal lymphadenopathy:

Mediastinal lymph node metastasis (N2 or N3 disease), reactive lymphadenopathy (due to a concomitant congestive heart failure or pulmonary infectious process), prior granulomatous disease (especially in patients with exposure history for tuberculosis, histoplasmosis, coccidiomycosis or other caseating infections), sarcoidosis, secondary lymphatic malignancy (lymphoma). It is important to remember that mediastinal adenopathy may be seen in several clinical scenarios and that occult nodal metastasis may be present in a radiographically normal mediastinum. In fact, the rate of unsuspected pathologic mediastinal nodal disease in central and cN1 tumors with a radiographically normal mediastinum range from 20 to 42%.

Preoperative workup for NSCLC:

- PET/CT
- **Mediastinal staging (if indicated)**
- MRI brain (if indicated)
- Risk assessment with PFTs, stress test

"You counsel the patient that prior to surgical resection, a complete staging evaluation is necessary. He undergoes a PET-CT which demonstrates increased FDG avidity in the 4R and 7 nodal stations. The nodes are 1.4 cm in size at each of these stations, but normal on the contralateral side."

The current American and European guidelines for preoperative mediastinal nodal staging in NSCLC recommend *tissue confirmation of regional nodal spread in all cases except those with small (3 cm or less) peripheral carcinomas with no evidence of nodal involvement on CT and PET.*

The following scenarios warrant mediastinoscopy:

- Hilar or mediastinal LNs > 1 cm in short axis diameter

- PET positive hilar or mediastinal LNs
- Bilateral pulmonary nodules
- Higher order resection (bronchoplasty, pneumonectomy)
- Pancoast tumor
- Solitary metastasis
- Central tumors
- Small cell carcinoma

Cervical mediastinoscopy allows for access to level 2, 4, and 7 lymph node stations and remains the gold standard approach for preoperative mediastinal assessment. At least 3 stations should be sampled (4L, 4R, and 7). Though mediastinoscopy remains the gold standard, EBUS is often utilized as the initial staging modality, with confirmatory mediastinoscopy if EBUS is negative. EBUS allows for access to nodal stations 2, 3, 4, 7, 10, and 11 and is less invasive than mediastinoscopy. Many studies have shown that EBUS has similar yields without significant differences in nodal staging accuracy when compared to mediastinoscopy, but EBUS has lower complication rates. Endoscopic ultrasound has also been used as an adjunct in mediastinal staging and offers access to the level 5, 7, 8 and 9 lymph node stations.

Tumors of the left upper lobe commonly have initial lymph node metastases to the aorticopulmonary window lymph node (levels 5 and 6). These stations are not accessible by mediastinoscopy or by EBUS. This is one of the few scenarios in which resection can be considered in the setting of N2 disease (level 5 and 6 are level 2 nodes). Studies have shown similar survival for patients who undergo resection with N1 disease and those who undergo resection for a left upper lobe tumor and positive level 5 or 6 lymph nodes. One option would be to confirm N2 involvement of the level 5 or 6 lymph nodes by biopsy and if positive, refer the patient for induction CRT. Another would be to give induction therapy without the biopsy, restage with PET-CT, and proceed with resection if there is no evidence of disease outside the primary and level 5 or 6 nodes. Finally, one may choose to proceed with resection and mediastinal lymph node dissection, followed by adjuvant CRT. On the other hand, if 5 and 6 appear abnormal in the setting of a right-sided tumor, sampling would be mandatory as this would indicate potential N3 disease.

Thoracoscopy is the preferred approach for sampling this nodal station and would also allow for an excellent evaluation of the ipsilateral nodes (including hilar lymph nodes) as well as evaluation of the primary tumor. Most often, frozen section staging is performed before proceeding to resection in the same operative setting. Thoracoscopic mediastinal lymph node evaluation is typically aimed at levels 4R and 7 from the right chest and levels 5, 6, and 7 from the left chest. The Chamberlain procedure (anterior mediastinotomy) is also an option for sampling levels 5 and 6, though this approach is becoming infrequently performed.

Mediastinoscopy: Operative steps
- General anesthesia in hospital-based setting.
- Supine positioning with a transverse scapular roll to elevate the chest and allow extension of the neck. The patient should be positioned with the head as high as possible on the operating room table to maximize extension. The surgical field should be prepped to include both the neck and entire anterior chest/upper abdomen in case emergent conversion to sternotomy is required.
- Incision is made transversely 1-2 cm above the sternal notch. The platysma is divided transversely. The strap muscles are separated vertically in the midline. The dissection is carried in the midline down to the pretracheal fascia.
- Incise the fascia with sharp scissors and enter the avascular pretracheal space.
- Blunt finger dissection along the anterior trachea into the mediastinum. One should be able to reach the carina, as well as the R and L mainstem bronchi.
- Establish vascular landmarks (innominate artery, arch of the aorta, R main PA) by digital palpation.

- Insert the mediastinoscope and follow the dissected pretracheal plane.
- Keeping the trachea and bronchi in view with the mediastinoscope is important to maintain orientation.
- Complete the dissection to the level of the carina by advancing the scope and performing blunt dissection with a suction device. Bluntly dissect along the right and left main stem bronchi, which will also help to maintain orientation.
- Lymph nodes are identified and individually dissected free from surrounding tissues using the suction device. Samples of nodal tissue are taken with a large cup laryngeal biopsy forceps. The upper paratracheal stations are typically sampled first, followed by the lower paratracheal stations. The subcarinal space is sampled last as this is most prone to bleeding.
- Level 2 nodes are above the innominate vein, level 4 are below the innominate vein and level 7 are within the subcarinal space.
- After sampling is complete, the scope is withdrawn as the region is inspected for bleeding. The skin incision is then closed in layers.

Evaluation of the nodal status by mediastinal staging along with evaluation for distant metastasis by PET CT allow for complete staging of lung cancer. The AJCC 8th edition represents the most recent TNM classification and clinical staging system.

Potential questions/alternative scenarios
"Will you plan to proceed to resection if there are no nodal metastasis demonstrated on frozen section?"
Either immediate or delayed resection is a reasonable choice. Some surgeons advocate a staged approach, with mediastinoscopy performed in a separate setting from the definitive resection for patients who present a higher operative risk due to medical comorbidities. In this setting, the staging procedure affords the opportunity to evaluate the patient's response to general anesthesia. Confidence in your pathology team is important when making decisions based on frozen section. Delaying surgery following mediastinoscopy has the potential to make the mediastinal lymph node sampling/dissection more complicated when one returns during the formal resection.

"In assessing the 4R lymph node station on mediastinoscopy, a dark structure is seen but you are unsure if this is a lymph node."
Do not biopsy any structure that is not clearly identified as a lymph node. The azygos vein and R pulmonary artery are both potentially mistaken for lymph nodes in the 4R position. Proceed with further gentle dissection around the node. If you are still unable to determine that the structure is not vascular, a long 21-gauge spinal needle may be used to aspirate the structure through the mediastinoscope.

"During mediastinoscopy, biopsy of a clearly defined lymph node in the subcarinal space results in significant bleeding, obscuring vision."
When the source of bleeding is clearly known to be a node or a small vessel within a nodal packet, the situation is best managed by passing a one-inch gauze packing strip into the mediastinum via the mediastinoscope. Alternatively, or additionally, one may pack operating room sponge(s) into the mediastinum for additional counter-pressure. The packing is allowed to remain in place for 2-10 minutes and then withdrawn. Selective use of electrocautery under direct vision may also be helpful in controlling bleeding from nodal vasculature. Use of electrocautery should be avoided when taking lymph node biopsies from the 4L station to avoid injury to the left recurrent laryngeal nerve.

"While attempting to biopsy the 4R lymph node station, a copious amount of blood fills the mediastinoscope, immediately obscuring vision. Simultaneously, the patient becomes hypotensive."
In this scenario, a major vascular injury has occurred. Immediate recognition of the situation and mobilization of the appropriate resources is necessary to achieve a favorable outcome. To

achieve temporary vascular control, one should pack the mediastinum with gauze via the mediastinoscope (as described above). The operating room team, anesthesia, and perfusion should be alerted regarding your concerns. Blood for transfusion should be brought to the operating room. Intravenous access should be optimized. The surgeon should also call for additional surgical support as having additional sets of hands is key. In this biopsy location, the two structures most likely to be injured are the azygos vein and the right main pulmonary artery. Either of these vascular injuries will require immediate open operative intervention. When uncertain, a median sternotomy offers the most flexibility in dealing with vascular injuries given the ability to initiate cardiopulmonary bypass. Median sternotomy is preferred for injuries to the aortic arch, innominate artery, main pulmonary artery, and the superior vena cava. Even the azygos vein can be repaired via sternotomy. Consideration may also be given to proceeding to lobectomy rather than repair, especially if the tumor itself involves the right upper lobe. Selection of the appropriate operative approach for repair will depend upon the surgeon's assessment of the most likely area of injury.

Regardless of the incision, the primary operative goal is to quickly achieve vascular control. For proximal injuries, this may require cardiopulmonary bypass. Generally, assume the injury is worse than you think, as this is often the case. Further, you must be prepared as sometimes the injury may extend as you try to repair it. Once the incision is made, the injury is visually assessed and a plan for control and repair is formulated. Hilar injuries often require intrapericardial access for adequate proximal control (refer to Early Stage Lung Cancer chapter). Vascular clamps are placed proximally and distally to the injury and repair/resection is then performed in a controlled manner.

"The bleeding source is localized to the right main pulmonary artery. After entering the pericardium, you are unable to get control of the injury proximally."

While many pulmonary vascular injuries can be adequately controlled and exposed for repair with local dissection, proximal injuries will typically require support with cardiopulmonary bypass for repair. Local control is established with direct pressure until a cardiopulmonary bypass circuit is available. Give full dose heparin and then place a proximal aortic cannula and two-stage venous cannula via the right atrium. Once ACT is within reasonable range (ideally > 480), initiate CPB. This will afford good decompression for repair. It is not necessary to arrest the heart in most circumstances to repair injuries to venous structures or the pulmonary arteries.

"An injury to the aortic arch is suspected, what will be your approach to assessment of the injury and repair?"

The initial goal is to attain control of bleeding in this situation. This may be accomplished by aggressively packing the mediastinum with gauze as described above. Rarely, this maneuver is not effective and either digital compression via the mediastinoscopy incision or emergent sternotomy may be required. If the injury is to the innominate artery, then perform a median sternotomy, give 10,000 units of heparin, obtain proximal and distal control, and repair directly or with a graft interposition.

Any injury to the aortic arch should be repaired with the assistance of cardiopulmonary bypass and may require circulatory arrest depending upon the extent of the injury. Once the bleeding is controlled, a careful assessment of the injury is necessary in order to plan the operation. The typical location of injury is along the undersurface of the aortic arch. Median sternotomy allows for direct visualization. TEE evaluation is invaluable to assess for the presence of aortic dissection and in some cases to localize the injury itself and guide cannulation. If the injury is focal, repair with pledgeted suture may be appropriate. However, care must be taken to rule out the presence of a dissection if a limited local repair is performed. If the injury is too extensive or your suture does not stop the bleeding, then give heparin and initiate CPB. Hopefully the injury is proximal to where you can safely cannulate and clamp. It this is true, then there should not be a need for circulatory arrest. If you can't clamp and cannulate distal to the injury then cannulate wherever you can on the ascending or arch, keep digital pressure on the injury, get venous access (2 stage RA vs. bicaval) and start cooling. Once you get to 20°, circ arrest and repair with or without graft material as needed.

61

Recannulate the graft/ascending aorta and start warming. If there is a dissection this gets more complicated as a formal dissection repair will be required (refer to Aortic Dissection and Iatrogenic Dissection chapters).

Pearls/pitfalls

- Mediastinal metastasis may be found in as high as 10% of patients with a negative PET CT.
- Radiographic definition of pathological adenopathy is > 1 cm in short axis diameter.
- Recurrent laryngeal nerve injuries occur most commonly on the left and are usually a result of traction during dissection, not direct biopsy. 5-10% of patients may have hoarseness following mediastinoscopy.
- In addition to the complications highlighted above, mediastinoscopy has the following additional complications: tracheobronchial tree tear, esophageal tear, recurrent nerve injury, pneumothorax, thoracic duct injury, mediastinitis, venous air embolism, stroke, and tumor implantation.
- Contraindications (relative) to mediastinoscopy are as follows: Tracheostomies or laryngectomy, large goiter with calcifications, aneurysm or heavy calcification of the aortic arch or innominate artery, previous violation of the pretracheal plane by process such as mediastinitis, superior vena cava syndrome.

Suggested readings

- Call S, Obiols C, Rami-Porta R. Present indications of surgical exploration of the mediastinum. *J Thorac Dis*. 2018;10(Suppl 22):S2601-S2610.
- Krantz SB, Howington JA, Wood DE, et al. Invasive Mediastinal Staging for Lung Cancer by The Society of Thoracic Surgeons Database Participants. *Ann Thorac Surg*. 2018;106(4):1055-1062.
- Detterbeck FC. The eighth edition TNM stage classification for lung cancer: What does it mean on main street? *J Thorac Cardiovasc Surg*. 2018;155(1):356-359.
- Nasir BS, Tasufuku K, Liberman M. When Should Negative Endobronchial Ultrasonography Findings be Confirmed by a More Invasive Procedure? *Ann Surg Oncol*. 2018;25(1):68-75.

8. PULMONARY METASTASECTOMY
Fatuma Kromah, MD, and Dennis Wigle, MD

Concept
- Knowledge of primary tumors that metastasize to the lung
- Presentation of a patient with pulmonary metastasis
- Diagnostic evaluation
- Criteria for surgical intervention
- Contraindications and limitations to pulmonary metastasectomy
- Technical aspects of metastasectomy
- Pitfalls in pulmonary metastasectomy
- Non-surgical management

Chief complaint
"A 41-year-old female former smoker is referred to you with a history of surgical resection and adjuvant chemotherapy 3 years prior for locoregionally-advanced colon cancer. She is now referred to you after a CT scan revealed bilateral pulmonary nodules, an enlarged subcarinal lymph node, and a mass in the posterior right hepatic lobe. What are your differential diagnoses and how would you proceed?"

Differential
- Metastatic colon cancer to the liver and lung
  - Colorectal cancer pulmonary metastasis fast facts
    - 5-15% metastases at the time of initial diagnosis.
    - 5-year survival in untreated metastatic disease: 5-10%.
    - 3-year survival after pulmonary metastasectomy: 78%.
    - 5-year survival after pulmonary metastasectomy: 30-50%.
- Primary lung cancer with metastasis to the liver
- Synchronous primary lung and liver cancers
- Primary liver cancer with metastasis to the lung
- Metastatic colon cancer and primary lung cancer
- Benign lesions

NOTE: Other primary tumors that metastasize to the lung with some published pulmonary metastasectomy survival rates
- Sarcomas
  - Soft tissue sarcoma
    - 3-year survival without metastasectomy: 2%.
    - 3-year survival with metastasectomy: 23%
  - Osteogenic sarcoma
    - Favorable diagnostic factors: less than two metastases and disease-free interval (DFI) > 24 months.
- Breast carcinoma
  - 5-, 10-, 15-year survival with pulmonary metastasectomy: 38%, 22%, and 20% respectively.
- Head and neck cancer
  - 5-year survival rates after metastasectomy: 29% to 59%
- Renal cell carcinoma
  - 5-year survival with pulmonary metastasectomy:
    - 42-45% after complete resection

- o   8-22% after incomplete resection
- Germ cell cancer
    - 5-year survival with pulmonary metastasectomy for testicular germ cell cancer: 68%.
- Melanoma
    - 5-year survival with incomplete resection: 13%
    - 5-year survival with pulmonary metastasectomy: 21%
- Gastric
    - 5-year survival with chemotherapy: 2%
    - 5-year survival with pulmonary metastasectomy: 33%.
- Endocrine tumors
    - 5-year survival with pulmonary metastasectomy: 61%
- Gynecologic tumor
    - Uterine cancer 5-year survival rate with metastasectomy: 53%.
    - Cervical cancer 5-year survival rate with metastasectomy: 0-52%.
- Hepatocellular carcinoma
    - 5-year overall survival (OS): 40.9%.

History and physical

Patients presenting with pulmonary metastases are asymptomatic 75% to 90% of the time with lesions found incidentally during staging and follow-up of the primary malignancy. In obtaining a history, one should inquire about symptoms like hemoptysis that may be caused by centrally located lesions, cough suggesting endobronchial involvement, pain as a result of pleural involvement or chest wall invasion, and dyspnea which may be suggestive of airway obstruction or pleural effusion. Assessing the patient's cardiac and pulmonary functional status is vital in determining candidacy for surgical intervention. Inquiry of cancer risk factors like tobacco usage should be made with smoking cessation counseling as needed. Additionally, a thorough history to include the patient's comorbidities, prior surgeries (especially any prior thoracic surgeries), and family history of cancer should be obtained. It is also important to ensure that there are no symptoms related to recurrent colon cancer.

"This patient's history and physical exam is otherwise unremarkable except for a prior smoking history (20 pack-years) and the abdominal surgical scars. Her performance status is ECOG score zero (good functional status). What tests or studies should be obtained?"

Tests

- *CXR*: may be initial imaging identifying the suspicious lesion(s).
- *Computed tomography scan*: Gold standard for pulmonary metastases. 4-5 mm helical CT scans detect 20% more nodules than conventional CT scan and result in 12% increase in the number of definite nodules detected. Suggested timing for obtaining CT scan is within 4 weeks of metastasectomy.
- *PET-CT scan.* PET may be positive in only 67.5% of metastatic pulmonary nodules and is not sensitive for evaluation of lung nodules in the metastatic setting. PET mediastinal staging has a sensitivity, accuracy, and negative predictive value of 100%, 96%, and 100%, respectively, versus 71%, 92%, and 95% for CT scan alone.
- *Bronchoscopy*: important for central lesions with possible endobronchial invasion.
- *Endobronchial ultrasound (EBUS) and mediastinoscopy*: used only if there is suspicious mediastinal lymphadenopathy. If the mediastinum is positive, the survival benefit of metastasectomy decreases significantly and it is arguable whether one should proceed with resection.
- *Pulmonary function testing (PFT)*: is required for assessing performance status and ability to tolerate surgery (see other chapter on lung cancer regarding PFT criteria for resection).

"The CT scan characteristics of the lesions were highly suspicious for metastasis, so a biopsy was not performed. The patient undergoes chemotherapy. Follow-up CT scan shows stable pulmonary nodules and decrease in the size of the liver metastasis with internal necrosis. What would you do next?"

Treatment/management

Since the pulmonary lesions are stable, it is decided the patient will undergo abdominal surgery first and subsequently the pulmonary metastasectomy. The patient undergoes a right hepatectomy. The hepatic lesion is consistent with colon metastasis. One month postoperatively, a repeat CT scan showed no new intra-abdominal metastases. There is a new 1.5 cm lymph node adjacent to the SVC and pulmonary vein in addition to the bilateral pulmonary nodules. You decide on simultaneous bilateral pulmonary metastasectomies with video assisted thorascopic surgery (VATS) for wedge resections and mediastinal lymphadenectomy.

Operative steps

- General anesthesia with double-lumen endotracheal tube
- Lateral decubitus position with flexion of bed
- VATS incisions and examination of the lung and chest cavity
- Identification of the pulmonary nodules by visualization and digital palpation
- Wedge resections with 1 cm margins using endoscopic stapler and ensuring that excessive lung parenchymal tissue is not resected
- Placement of wedged lung into a protective bag and removal from the chest cavity to prevent droplet spread or contamination
- Specimen should be sent for frozen section to make sure that the lesion is not a primary lung cancer (particularly since the patient has a smoking history)
- Mediastinal lymph node dissection
- Obtain hemostasis, place chest tube, and re-expand the lung under direct visualization
- Close incisions
- Reposition patient in lateral decubitus position on opposite side and repeat as above

"The final pathology report comes back and further examination of the dissected lymph nodes shows one lymph node positive for metastatic cancer. Is there a role for lymph node dissection during pulmonary metastasectomy?"

The reported incidence of mediastinal nodal metastases: 5%-28.6% for all cell types. Lymph node metastases at the time of pulmonary metastasectomy have an adverse effect on prognosis. Three-year survival with negative lymph nodes has been shown to be 69%, compared with 38% for patients with positive lymph nodes. Complete mediastinal lymph node dissection improves staging and can guide treatment. This area is somewhat controversial, as many surgeons do not routinely perform a mediastinal lymph node sampling or dissection at the time of metastasectomy. However, if there are FDG-avid mediastinal lymph nodes or enlarged lymph nodes (> 1 cm in the short axis), then mediastinal lymph dissection is certainly warranted, if surgical resection is still pursued.

Potential questions/alternative scenarios
"What are the selection criteria for pulmonary metastasectomy?"
Patients may be considered for pulmonary metastasectomy if there is proven control of the primary tumor (no recurrence or residual disease at the primary site) with complete R0 resection, ability to resect all metastatic disease, and sufficient cardiopulmonary reserve for the planned resection. Re-resection can be considered in selected patients. Ablative techniques (SBRT, RFA) can be considered when the patient is not a surgical candidate (inadequate physiologic reserve, refuses surgery) and the lesion(s) is amenable to complete

ablation. Patients with resectable synchronous metastases can be resected synchronously or using a staged approach.

"What surgical options and approaches are there for bilateral pulmonary metastases?"

The surgical approach used for metastasectomy is based on the principle of performing a complete resection with preservation of lung tissue (in case of future metastasectomy). Standard therapy is wedge resection with a 1 cm negative margin. Deep or centrally located lesions may require anatomic resection: segmentectomy, lobectomy, or, rarely, pneumonectomy. Approaches include:

- *Sternotomy.* Allows for simultaneous exposure, visualization, examination, and palpation of bilateral lungs. Issues with sternal wound healing after radiation. Difficult access to the posterolateral left lung.
- *Sequential thoracotomies.* Allow healing and recovery from the first surgery before performing the next. Optimal time for contralateral resection is unclear, however most recommend a repeat chest CT for surgical planning prior to the subsequent resection.
- *Bilateral thoracotomies (clamshell).* Allows access to both hemithorax during the same operation. Internal mammary arteries are sacrificed. Increased morbidity versus unilateral approach.
- *Video-assisted thoracic surgery (VATS).* Less pain and shorter hospital stay. Studies have shown comparable 5-year overall survival rates and median survival for thoracotomy and VATS. Lose bimanual tactile ability, potentially resulting in higher rate of missed metastases.

"The patient presents to you one year after her pulmonary metastasectomy with a CT scan of the chest that now shows new right-sided pulmonary nodules suspicious for colon metastases. Is there any evidence to support performing multiple metastasectomies for recurrent pulmonary metastases? How is survival affected?"

Multiple attempts to re-establish intrathoracic control of metastatic disease can be justified in carefully selected patients, but the magnitude of benefit decreases with each subsequent attempt. 5-year survival for patients undergoing 2 metastasectomies is 60%, 3 metastasectomies is 33%, and 4 or more metastasectomies is 38% (all-comers, not just colon metastases). From the time a recurrence is declared unresectable, 2-year survival is 19% (median 8 months).

"What if the patient has insufficient cardiopulmonary reserve to tolerate surgery or has had multiple prior surgeries? Alternatively, what if the patient is a surgical candidate but declines surgery? What alternative treatments are available?"

- *Stereotatic body radiation therapy (SBRT).* Safe, tolerable, and effective local treatment option in select patients.
- *Radiofrequency ablation (RFA).* Inclusion criteria are: lesions < 5 cm in diameter, inoperable non–small cell lung cancer, and no more than four secondary lesions bilaterally. The feasibility depends on factors including the presence of an "access window" and proximity to hilar structures. Uncorrectable coagulopathy is an absolute contraindication for RFA. Complications of RFA include pneumothorax, pleural effusion, hyperpyrexia, infection, and hemorrhage.
- *Neodymium:yttrium-aluminum garnet laser (Nd:YAG).* Treatment with Nd:YAG laser may facilitate complete resection of multiple bilateral centrally located metastases, is lobe sparing, and can improve long-term survival.
- *Isolated lung perfusion.* An alternative chemotherapeutic delivery method that allows high local doses with reduced incidence of systemic toxicities.

Pearls/pitfalls

- Metastasectomy should not be performed unless there is sufficient evidence supporting local control of the primary tumor site.

- Pulmonary metastatic lesions should be amenable to complete resection to consider metastasectomy.
- Good prognostic indicators for pulmonary metastasectomies are resectability, disease-free interval greater than 36 months, and solitary metastases in select patients.
- A VATS approach for pulmonary metastasectomy in select patients offers comparable survival benefit compared to open procedures.
- Mediastinal staging is essential in identifying patients who are not disease-free and who may require additional treatment, as the presence of lymph node metastasis has an adverse effect on prognosis.
- Pulmonary metastasectomy can be performed concomitantly, sequentially, or staged without a change in survival.
- Local ablative therapy is a safe and effective modality. These techniques are proving to be a satisfactory alternative to surgery with an increasing role in non-surgical candidates and those who do not want surgery. The alternatives should be addressed from a multidisciplinary approach.

Suggested readings

- Pastorino U, Buyse M, Friedel G, et al. Long-term results of lung metastasectomy: Prognostic analyses based on 5206 cases. *J Thorac Cardiovasc Surg* 1997;113:37-049.
- Ercan S. Nichols FC. Trastek VF. Deschamps C. et al. Prognostic significance of lymph node metastasis found during pulmonary metastasectomy for extrapulmonary carcinoma. *Ann Thorac Surg.* 2004 May;77(5):1786-91.
- Jaklitsch MT, Mery CM, Lukanich JM, et al. Sequential thoracic metastasectomy prolong survival by re-establishing local control within the chest. *J Thorac Cardiovasc Surg* 2001;121:657-67.
- National Cancer Comprehensive Network Clinical Practice Guidelines in Oncology – Colon Cancer Version 1.2018. https://oncolife.com.ua/doc/nccn/Colon_Cancer.pdf.
- Erhunmwunsee L, D'Amico TA. Surgical Management of Pulmonary Metastases. *Ann Thorac Surg.* 2009;88:2052-2060.
- Onaitis MW, Petersen RP, Haney JC, et al. Prognostic factors for recurrence after pulmonary resection of colorectal cancer metastases. *Ann Thorac Surg.* 2009;87(6):1684-8.
- Gonzalez M and Gervaz P. Risk factors for survival after lung metastasectomy in colorectal ancer patients: systematic review and meta-analysis. *Future Oncol.* 2015;11(2 Suppl):31-3.

9. PLEURAL EFFUSIONS AND EMPYEMA
Nakul Vakil, MD, and Daniel Raymond, MD

Concept
- Diagnosis of pleural effusions
- Initial management
- Fluid analysis
- Operative management
- Pitfalls and alternative solutions

Chief complaint

"A 70-year-old man on the medical service is referred to you because of an increasing right-sided pleural effusion and shortness of breath."

Differential

The differential for shortness of breath is broad. However, a history and physical as well as review of imaging will suggest if the SOB is most likely caused by the effusion or another etiology (cardiac, pulmonary embolism, etc). The differential for an effusion includes cardiogenic, infectious, malignant or hepatic (hepatic hydrothorax) causes.

History and physical

Dyspnea is the most common complaint associated with an effusion. Chest auscultation (decreased breath sounds, dullness to percussion, etc.) can help establish a diagnosis. Presence of systemic signs of infection (fevers, WBC elevation) can lead one to suspect an empyema/parapneumonic effusion. Heart sound auscultation and assessment of JVD/lower extremity edema could suggest a cardiac etiology. Abdominal exam revealing caput medusa or ascites may suggest hepatic pathology (hepatic hydrothorax). A known, prior, or suspected neoplasm, chest pain, and prior smoking/asbestos exposure may suggest a malignant etiology.

Tests

- *CXR*. Plain AP or PA/lateral will identify the effusion. Traditional teaching is to obtain a decubitus film to rule out loculations. This may not be needed with the availability of ultrasound/CT scanning. Typically, there will need to be at about 200 cc of fluid to see blunting of the costophrenic angle on a plain film.
- *Ultrasound (U/S)*. U/S can provide information regarding loculations, the distance between the effusion and chest wall, and depth of the effusion itself.
- *Chest CT*. CT scan provides additional information on the lung tissue, mediastinal lymph nodes, and upper abdominal pathology which may differentiate pleural versus non-pleural processes. CT scanning will also provide information on thickness of pleura, pleural nodularity, anatomy of loculated fluid, and entrapment. Contrasted CT scans are superior at identification of adenopathy and differentiating atelectatic lung from pleural masses.

Index scenario (additional information)

"The patient has been hospitalized over the past several days for urosepsis. His unilateral right effusion has recently increased and is accompanied by low grade fevers and an increasing oxygen requirement. He is already on antibiotics for the resolving urosepsis. CXR shows a moderate right-sided effusion."

Treatment/management

Thoracentesis is typically the first step after radiographic evaluation of an effusion. Thoracentesis often confirms a suspicion based on H&P and imaging. It is both diagnostic (exudative versus transudative, cytology, gram stain and culture) and can be therapeutic in cases of certain effusions. Thoracentesis can be done: 1.) using real time ultrasound, 2.) with ultrasound marking of the chest wall for guidance of subsequent thoracentesis, 3.) one to two rib spaces below the area of dullness to percussion, or 4.) with CT guidance. The traditional teaching is to drain less than 1500 cc initially or to stop drainage when the patient has chest discomfort or coughing in order to avoid re-expansion pulmonary edema. Thoracentesis should generally be avoided in patients on mechanical ventilatory support because of a higher risk of pneumothorax and difficult positioning – these patients are better candidates for tube thoracostomy. The gross appearance of aspirated fluid may suggest the process at work. Bloody aspirates are associated with trauma or malignancy; purulence suggests an empyema, and milky appearance suggests a chylothorax. Less obvious distinctions can be made based on the pleural fluid analysis.

Fluid is typically sent for culture, cytology, cell count with differential, LDH, glucose, protein, and pH. Additional tests can be ordered when esophageal or pancreatic etiologies are suspected such as amylase. Although there are others, Light's criteria is the classic way of making this determination based on pleural fluid characteristics. It has a very high sensitivity but is less specific. Exudates are defined as: pleural to serum protein ratio > 0.5, pleural to serum LDH ratio > 0.6, and a pleural LDH > 2/3 the upper limits of the laboratory's normal serum LDH value. Different strategies are employed for benign versus malignant effusions.

Benign effusions

Transudative

Most benign transudative effusions are caused by congestive heart failure and/or renal failure and tend to be bilateral. These should be medically managed with treatment of the underlying cause. Nephrotic syndrome and hepatic hydrothorax are with fewer common causes. These too should be managed with attention to the underlying process. Recurrent symptomatic effusions can be ameliorated with thoracentesis. Tube thoracostomy is not recommended in hepatic hydrothorax.

Exudative

Management of exudative effusions is more complex. Parapneumonic effusions are those exudative effusions associated with a pneumonia or other lung infections. The evolution of an exudative effusion is from an exudative phase with negative bacterial studies and free-flowing fluid, to a fibropurulent phase (positive bacterial studies) and frequently with loculation, and finally to a chronic, organized phase with a pleural rind.

- Uncomplicated parapneumonic effusions generally do not need drainage (other than what was achieved already by thoracentesis). These can be managed with appropriate antibiotics. Most of these resolve on their own, but a small percentage progress to empyema. If the patient is symptomatic (i.e., dyspneic), the effusion should be drained.

- The presence of purulence or positive bacterial studies necessitates drainage. This can be done with tube thoracostomy or image-guided (US or CT) placement of small-bore drains. If this fails, one can consider fibrinolysis through an existing tube (i.e., intrapleural administration of tPA). Failure is defined as incomplete drainage of the empyema or incomplete expansion of the lung. Failure of tube thoracostomy, presence of a trapped lung, or a persistent effusion (greater than two to three weeks where there is likely to be a significant inflammatory process) necessitates either thoracoscopic or open decortication.

- Uncomplicated post-cardiotomy exudative effusions can almost always be managed medically or with thoracentesis. Surgery is for the few who develop lung entrapment.

- Patients who fail surgical treatment of the empyema or those with bronchopleural fistulae may need open pleural drainage by a cavernostomy (Eloesser flap or Clagett window).

Malignant effusions

Metastatic disease to the pleura affects pleural fluid reabsorption and/or production. Moderate to large symptomatic effusions can be managed initially with thoracentesis (also diagnostic) and with pleurodesis or an indwelling pleural catheter, as malignant effusions tend to recur.

- *Pleurodesis*: only possible when there already is pleural apposition (i.e., cannot work in cases of lung entrapment). This can be done either through an existing catheter or thoracostomy tube, or during a VATS procedure.
- *Indwelling pleural catheter.* This is an option for patients who lack pleural apposition and in those whom the risks of an operative intervention (decortication) outweigh the benefits (e.g., PleurX Catheter).

Potential questions/alternative scenarios

"Thoracentesis reveals purulence and an exudative effusion by Light's criteria. The empyema is only partially drained on post-procedure imaging. Records indicate he has had this effusion for three weeks."

First, the fluid should be sent for culture and IV antibiotics should be tailored appropriately. The patient's effusion has likely progressed to the fibropurulent or chronic, organized phase. If the patient is not septic and is hemodynamically stable, taking a more conservative approach (non-operative) is reasonable. A non-contrast CT of the chest will be helpful to determine if there are extensive loculations or the presence of a thick rind. If there are minimal loculations and no rind, placement of one or two chest tubes may allow for complete drainage of the pleural space. If there are significant loculations, then the surgeon has a couple of options. One or two chest tubes can be placed, and fibrinolysis attempted with tPA administration through the tubes. If only one or two pockets of undrained fluid remain, image-guided (either CT or US) thoracentesis or placement of smaller pleural catheters may provide adequate drainage. If this fails, proceed to the OR for VATS or open drainage. Alternatively, since the chance of complete drainage is lower in the presence of significant loculations, it is reasonable to proceed to the OR for drainage and disruption of loculations at the first encounter rather than prolonging the course with multiple chest tubes. Rarely is a complete decortication needed at this stage but be prepared for the possibility of finding a thicker rind than anticipated. Moreover, if the patient has persistent fevers or starts becoming septic, then earlier operative intervention is required. Success may be higher with an open then VATS procedure, although it is very reasonable to start with VATS.

"You are referred another patient who has recovered from a left-sided pneumonia. He was noted to have a parapneumonic effusion at the time of infection, which was drained by thoracentesis once. His repeat CXR 2 weeks later shows clear lungs, but a persistent left-sided effusion. This is again drained by thoracentesis and pleural fluid cultures are negative. After drainage of the effusion, the lung does not re-expand fully. A non-contrast CT does not show any loculations. The patient gets progressively shorter of breath over the next 3 days and the effusion has re-accumulated. How would you manage this patient?"

The patient likely has a fibrothorax. First, a bronchoscopy should be performed to make sure there is no mucus plugging that is preventing ventilation of the atelectatic lung. Assuming the airways are clear, then it can be assumed the lung is not expanding due to an entrapped lung. Treatment is decortication. Thoracoscopic treatment may not be successful as this is likely a long-standing process; it can be attempted with a low threshold to convert to open thoracotomy.

Operative steps

Decortication

Thoracoscopic or open approaches are reasonable; however, success with thoracoscopic approaches decreases with increased duration of effusion and presence of a chronic empyema. Objectives of decortication are 1.) Wide drainage - break up loculations, drain residual fluid, leave well-placed drainage tubes 2.) Lung expansion - separate the pleural peel from the visceral pleura along the entire pleural surface (including the diaphragmatic pleural surface) in order to establish complete lung expansion.

- Double lumen intubation, 2 large bore IV's, Foley.
- Position the patient in the right decubitus position with the left side up and isolate the lung.

70

- A posterolateral thoracotomy in the fifth intercostal space will provide adequate exposure. If a VATS approach is to be taken, care must be taken to avoid placing the initial port too low in the chest, as there will be volume loss from the atelectatic lung, and the diaphragm will be higher than usual. The remaining ports are placed under direct thoracoscopic vision.
- Care must be taken when entering the chest, as the lung may be adherent to the parietal pleura.
- Once in the chest, residual fluid should be drained and sent for gram stain and culture.
- The pleural peel, or rind, must then be meticulously dissected away from the visceral pleura of the lung; avoid tearing into the parenchyma. Doing so will result in air leaks postoperatively, necessitating prolonged chest tube drainage.
- Decorticating the lung may result in significant bleeding from the lung surface due to the extensive inflammation. Blood transfusion may be needed if this is excessive.
- The lung must be freed up circumferentially, including the diaphragmatic surface of the lung.
- Once the lung has been freed up, the chest is irrigated and the atelectatic lung is then ventilated. Areas that do not expand fully may need additional decortication. Full lung re-expansion is crucial for a successful decortication.
- Multiple chest tubes are placed to assure adequate drainage and the chest is closed.
- Bleeding from the lung surface typically subsides with full lung re-expansion and pleural apposition, but it is not uncommon for there to be some persistent oozing for a few hours postoperatively. Make sure clotting factors are replaced as needed. Get as much hemostasis as possible prior to leaving the OR
- The patient should be extubated as soon as possible to reduce air leaks. At times some positive pressure may be warranted for adequate lung expansion of residual segments.
- Chest tubes remain until all air leaks have resolved and drainage is minimal.

"A 67-year-old man with recent STEMI treated with multiple drug eluting stents, EF of 30%, on Plavix, and renal failure now presents one month after a pneumonia that was complicated by a parapneumonic effusion treated with thoracostomy tube drainage. His chest CT shows an effusion with multiple locules of gas and a thick pleural peel, consistent with an empyema. There are also multiple pockets of fluid that are not easily accessible by percutaneous drainage. He is septic, but blood pressures are stable on minimal pressor support. He has been on broad spectrum antibiotics for 2 days. You feel that he needs drainage and decortication but are concerned that he is too high risk to tolerate this. What are some alternative options?"

An Eloesser flap represents a quicker and safer operation for a very ill and debilitated patient who may not tolerate a full decortication. One needs to ensure that the lung is in fact trapped and will not collapse based on timing (>3 weeks), imaging alone (thick rind), or imaging pre- and post-drainage (lung stays entrapped). Resect a segment of 2 to 3 ribs in the dependent portion of the chest. Suture the skin to the thickened pleural rind or the ribs to keep the site open. The cavity can be irrigated daily and the chest packed with wet to dry gauze. Once the patient is medically stable, nutritionally replete, the cavity begins to granulate in, and significant air leaks have resolved, then a VAC dressing may be applied. Alternatively, the space can be filled with tissue (muscle or omental flap) to obliterate the space once the empyema cavity has been cleared of infection.

"You are consulted on a patient with metastatic breast cancer who is severely debilitated. She was admitted with complaints of dyspnea and was found to have a moderate left pleural effusion, which was drained by thoracentesis. Cytology was positive. Her post-drainage CXR shows full lung re-expansion and her symptoms are significantly improved. She wants to know if you can do anything to prevent this from happening again."

This patient is a good candidate for pleurodesis given that the lung has fully expanded and the high likelihood of recurrence. Chemical irritants (sclerosants) cause pleural inflammation, eventually causing fusion of the visceral and parietal pleura if there is good pleural apposition. Adequate pleural drainage is needed for at least 48-72 hours after the sclerosing agent is administered to prevent re-accumulation of fluid and separation of the pleural surfaces. Options include sterile talc, doxycycline, or bleomycin. These agents can cause significant discomfort due to the inflammation they cause, and adequate analgesia is required. Talc can be administered through a chest tube (but not smaller pleural catheters) at the bedside or through small incisions (VATS or open) in the operating room. Doxycycline or bleomycin can be administered via chest tube or smaller pleural catheters. If pleurodesis is unsuccessful in this debilitated patient with metastatic disease, then placement of a permanent indwelling pleural catheter (e.g., PleurX Catheter) is another option.

"You are referred a patient with metastatic esophageal cancer who is severely debilitated. The patient has a right-sided malignant effusion that has been drained by thoracentesis multiple times in the past. The most recent post-drainage CXR is read as a right hydropneumothorax. How would you manage this patient?"
This patient has an entrapped lung with a space that will re-accumulate. In other words, there is no pneumothorax. These patients cannot be successfully managed with pleurodesis, as pleural apposition is needed for pleurodesis to be successful. Severely debilitated patients may not tolerate a thoracotomy for palliation of symptoms and survival in this type of metastatic cancer may be limited. In this case, the patient may be best served by a long term indwelling, tunneled pleural catheter that can be placed with or without VATS (Pleurex).

"You are consulted on a patient with a history of Child's class B cirrhosis and ascites. He has had multiple prior thoracenteses for a recurrent, transudative, right pleural effusion. The patient now has severe shortness of breath and opacification of the right chest on portable CXR despite drainage only 2 days ago. How would you proceed?"
This is likely a hepatic hydrothorax. Treatment is continued serial thoracenteses for relief of symptoms and aggressive treatment of portal hypertension, including diuresis, and consideration for TIPS. Chest tubes should be avoided in cirrhotic patients with hepatic hydrothorax due to concerns for development of pleurocutaneous fistulae, as chest tube output will remain significant until the underlying disease process has been treated.

Pearls/pitfalls

- *Light's criteria for exudative process*: pleural to serum protein ratio > 0.5, pleural to serum LDH ratio > 0.6; highly sensitive, less specific.
- Pleurodesis is an option only when there is pleural apposition, consider decortication or indwelling catheter drainage in cases of lung entrapment. Pleurodesis (versus repeated tapping) should be considered for malignant pleural effusions in patients with pleural apposition and life expectancy greater than 1-2 months.
- Most parapneumonic effusions do not require tube thoracostomy drainage. Tube thoracostomy is indicated for effusions that cause dyspnea or for those with purulence or positive cultures.
- In cases of benign effusion, the goals of tube thoracostomy are drainage of fluid and full lung expansion; if this fails, then one should consider VATS or open decortication. VATS or open decortication should be first-line treatment in well-established effusions which are unlikely to benefit from local therapy.
- Avoid chest tubes in patients with hepatic hydrothorax.

Suggested readings

- British thoracic society pleural disease guideline 2010 – a quick reference guide. *Thoracic Society Reports.* 2(3): 20.

10. Bronchopleural Fistula

Yogesh Patel, DO, and DuyKhanh P. Ceppa, MD

Concept

- Diagnosis of bronchopleural fistula (BPF)
- Initial management
- Operative management

Chief complaint

"A 65-year-old male with history of COPD and recent history of R sided pneumonectomy 2 weeks ago presents to the ED with fevers, nausea, anorexia, shortness of breath, and copious secretions. Patient describes the secretions are clear/salmon colored. He also elicits symptoms of failure to thrive since discharge from the hospital. You are called by the ED physician to come evaluate this patient."

Differential

Bronchopleural fistula, pleural effusion, pneumonia

History and physical

Bronchopleural fistula (BFP) is one of the most feared complications following pulmonary resection. It can occur with any anatomic pulmonary resection surgery (segmentectomy, lobectomy, or pneumonectomy). While the incidence of BPF overall is low, it is higher following pneumonectomy (4.5% to 20%) than after lobectomy (0.5% to 1%). Risk factors for developing a BPF are preoperative or postoperative chemotherapy or radiation therapy, a long bronchial stump, poor nutritional status, prolonged ventilation, residual tumor at a bronchial margin, heavy smoking, chronic obstructive pulmonary disease, chronic steroid therapy, and surgical technique. Symptoms of BPF vary widely and are dependent on the timing of presentation. Patients present most commonly with a history of fever, coughing up copious secretions (due to drainage directly from communication with the pleural space), and general malaise. If there is spillage of secretions into unresected lung, patients may have shortness of breath and/or symptoms similar to pneumonia. Occasionally, patients also report having chest pain. In patients who still have a chest tube in place, a new or persistent, large volume air leak may be the only presenting symptom. Late or missed cases may present with direct fistulas that drain via the skin of the chest wall.

Tests

- *Chest x-ray.* Usually reveals presence of increased air on the affected side. In cases of pneumonectomy, it can take a few weeks for the post-pneumonectomy space to fill with fluid. Therefore, it is best to compare compare the CXRs with the one at discharge.
- *Chest CT.* Similar to CXR, CT can show changing air-fluid levels on the affected side and failure of the space to fill with fluid. It may show presence of air bubbles around bronchial stump or even actual identification of the fistula itself.
- *Labs.* Since the patient is presenting with signs of sepsis, it is important to send routine labs such as a complete blood count and a basic metabolic panel. Blood and sputum cultures should all be sent as there is concern for sepsis from an infected pleural space. Type and screen along with a coagulation panel should be ordered if there is possibility of surgery. Pleural fluid should be sent for cytology and culture when a chest tube has been placed.
- *Bronchoscopy.* Bronchoscopy is diagnostic of a BPF. It allows direct visualization of anatomy and appropriate evaluation of the bronchial stump. For smaller/subtle BPFs, injection of fluid can elicit bubbling at the site of fistula.

Index scenario (additional information)

"By the time you get to the ED, a CXR and CT scan of the chest may have already been completed. Review the CXR and compare it to the patient's CXR at discharge. The patient's right sided post-pneumonectomy space has a significantly increased air. In addition, on the CT, subcutaneous air is noted throughout the chest wall. The patient states that he has not had an appetite since discharge and has been spiking consistent fevers >101.5F for the past 3 days. His sputum production was initially thin earlier in the week and became foul smelling and thick about 2 days ago. His WBC is elevated at 25,000, and his metabolic panel is suggestive of dehydration with an elevated BUN/Cr and pre-renal pattern. Blood and sputum cultures have been sent. The patient now asks what is going on?"

Treatment/management

Initial management of suspected BPF in a post-lung resection patient is to position the patient with affected side down. This will minimize communication of the infected pleural space with the tracheobronchial tree and attempt to prevent aspiration of infected material into non-operative/preserved lung. At the same time, appropriate resuscitation of the patient and initiation of broad-spectrum antibiotics should be completed. Following this, a chest tube should be placed on the side of suspected BPF. This will drain the infected pleural space and minimize further pulmonary decompensation of the patient. Drainage of purulent fluid and a persistent air leak from pleural space will again confirm diagnosis of BPF. In some cases, patients may not have an air-leak following chest tube placement; absence of an air leak does not rule out a BPF.

After initial drainage, depending on timing of presentation of BPF, surgery is usually indicated in the post lung resection patient. Surgical management can be divided into three important principles: 1) debridement and washout of necrotic/infected tissue, 2) revision of affected bronchial stump, and 3) obliteration of the previously infected pleural space. Patients who have developed BPF in the early postoperative period (<14 days) are candidates for early surgical repair if the patient is able to tolerate surgery. If patients present in the late postoperative period (>14 days), surgery is usually delayed treating and improve poor nutritional status and physical strength. During time to delay, it is important to make sure the patient continues to have adequate chest tube drainage of infected pleural space.

Operative steps
Debridement/Washout and Drainage

If surgery is pursued, a thoracoscopic approach can initially be utilized. Thoracoscopy usually plays a role in washing out the hemithorax and drainage in the setting of a smaller BPF that can be controlled endoscopically. However, in most cases (particularly if a revision of the bronchial stump is required), a thoracotomy may be needed. Following operative washout and debridement, adequate drainage of the infected pleural space can be accomplished with well-placed chest tubes, continuous irrigation via chest tubes, or open packing of the infected pleural space. The chest tubes or separate irrigation catheters can be used for continuous irrigation or for irrigation multiple times a day with antibiotic solution. When there is sufficient evidence of minimal contamination or complete sterilization, revision of bronchial stump, obliteration of the space, and closure can be performed. Culture of irrigation fluid or Gram stain of pleural tissue can be used to determine sterilization of pleural cavity.

In patients who have extremely poor nutritional status and would not be able to tolerate major thoracic surgery or who are unlikely to heal a closure, an open window thoracostomy (Eloesser flap) can be used as a last resort option. An open window thoracostomy allows for adequate drainage, source control, and packing of thoracic cavity until it is cleared of infection. Augmentation of the thoracostomy window with vacuum assisted closure device can decrease the duration of dressing changes and further improve drainage. Once the patient's nutritional/physical status has improved and the thoracic cavity has been sterilized, bronchial stump revision and closure of chest wall can be performed. It is essential to minimize tension with chest wall closure and sometimes resection of ribs and mobilization of chest wall musculature must be performed in order to gain a tension-free closure.

Revision of Bronchial Stump

Revision of bronchial stump can include re-resection of the stump along with closure and reinforcement of the stump with well-vascularized tissue. Attempts should be made to leave a final stump that is less than 1cm in length measured from the carina (in cases of pneumonectomy). The first choice for well-vascularized tissue is muscle due to its rich blood supply. Latissimus dorsi, intercostal, serratus anterior, pectoralis major, trapezius, and rectus abdominis can all be mobilized for a flap. In many cases, the latissimus dorsi is unable to be used as it has previously been transected during the initial or subsequent thoracotomies. Involving a consultant from plastic surgery may be helpful at this stage. In cases of poor nutritional status where muscles are severely atrophied, vascularized pericardial fat pad or omentum remains an option.

Obliteration of the Cavity/Space

Three procedures have been described to help obliterate the pleural space:

- *Claggett Maneuver*: This entails filling the sterilized pleural cavity with antibiotic solution. Early on, if chest wall closure had been accomplished in addition to appropriate placement of chest tubes, antibiotic solution is infused via the tubes to fill the cavity. After infusion of antibiotic solution, the chest tubes are removed, and the skin is sutured closed. If an open thoracostomy window was performed, when ready for closure, antibiotic solution is filled into the chest cavity followed by chest closure in multiple layer to prevent leakage.

- *Muscle Flap Transposition (described above)*: The ability of various muscle flaps to reach most regions of the pleural space make them a great option for obliteration of the space.

- *Thoracoplasty*: This involves resection of multiple adjacent rib segments to allow the chest wall to collapse inwards to fill the space. Thoracoplasty can be morbid and physically disfiguring and, hence, is not commonly used in today's era. It may also have a negative physiologic impact on the preserved lung due to the impaired respiratory mechanics related to multiple rib resections.

Potential questions/alternative scenarios

"When placing the initial chest tube, does location matter?"

In a post pulmonary resection pleural space, the diaphragm can be elevated to accommodate for the volume loss from the resected lung tissue. Therefore, during chest tube placement, it is important to consider a higher rib interspace for chest tube placement to prevent inadvertent placement of the chest tube into the abdominal cavity.

"How is an open window thoracostomy performed?"

- Patient is positioned, prepped, and draped identical to a thoracotomy.
- A U-Shaped incision is performed over the most dependent portion of the space, making sure to span over a few ribs
- A skin flap is created and dissected down to the level of the chest wall. Segments of 2-3 adjacent ribs within the U-shaped skin flap are resected to create a "window."
- The skin flap is then inverted, folded into the chest cavity and sutured directly to the parietal pleura. With time, this creates an epithelized tract.
- The pleural cavity can be packed with saline/antibiotic soaked bandages or even a wound vac at this point.

"When is bronchoscopic closure or treatment indicated?"

Bronchoscopic closure of a BPF can be effective with smaller BPFs. Size is the most important aspect for endoscopic options. BPFs larger than 8mm are generally unable to be treated with bronchoscopic interventions. Options for closure include stents, glues, sealants, coils, tissue expanders, or even Amplatzer devices. Results for bronchoscopic interventions are variable and differ between treatment centers. In high risk surgical patients, bronchoscopic closure can be used as a bridge until surgical options can be pursued. In cases of malignancy, attempted bronchoscopic closure may be the only palliative option.

"You are considering operating on a patient who previously underwent a left-sided pneumonectomy. Based on imaging and bronchoscopy, the left mainstem tracheal stump has retracted and may no longer be accessible via the left chest. What options or approaches can be used?"
In some cases, especially with left sided surgery, the bronchial stump can retract underneath the aorta. A common approach for carinal exposure is via a right posterolateral thoracotomy. The right lung can be mobilized and retracted allowing access to the mediastinal pleura. The mediastinal pleura can then be incised inferior to the carina, providing access. An alternative approach is through a median sternotomy. The benefit of a median sternotomy is that it provides a virgin field which makes for easier exposure. Following median sternotomy, the pericardium is opened and the space between the SVC and aorta is dissected out. The posterior pericardium is incised at the level of the carina to provide adequate exposure. In some cases, central ECMO may be necessary if exposure is difficult or the patient is unstable.

Pearls/pitfalls
- BPF is a challenging and often fatal complication following pulmonary resection and strategies to prevent BPF should be undertaken during the initial surgery (i.e., coverage of post-pneumonectomy stump with vascularized tissue).
- Other causes of BPF can include malignancy, infection (e.g., tuberculosis, abscess), and trauma.
- Initial management of BPF includes draining the affected side to minimize contamination of remainder of the tracheobronchial tree and preserved lung.
- The major principles of BPF treatment are drainage of pleural space, control of infection (includes revision of bronchial stump if applicable), and pleural cavity obliteration.
- Open window thoracostomy is not preferred and should be used in cases where source control cannot not be achieved after initial washout and debridement.
- Nutritional and physical conditions of the patient play an extremely important role in deciding the timing of surgery (if indicated).

Suggested readings
- Berry MF and Harpole DH. Bronchopleural Fistula After Pneumonectomy. *Adult Chest Surgery, Second Edition.* Eds. David J. Sugarbaker, et al. New York, NY: McGraw-Hill, 2014.
- Liberman M and Cassivi SD. Bronchial Stump Dehiscence: Update on Prevention and Management. *Semin Thorac Cardiovasc Surg.* 2007;19(4):366-373.
- Lois M and Noppen M. Bronchopleural fistulas: an overview of the problem with special focus on endoscopic management. *Chest* 2005;128(6):3955-65.
- Sarkar P, Chandak T, Shah R, Talwar A. Diagnosis and management bronchopleural fistula. *Indian J Chest Dis Allied Sci.* 2010;52(2):97-104.
- Shen KR, Bribriesco A, Crabtree T, et al. The American Association for Thoracic Surgery consensus guidelines for the management of empyema. *J Thorac Cardiovasc Surg.* 2017;153(6):e129-e146.

11. INFECTIOUS LUNG DISEASE

David Mauchley, MD, and Scott Mitchell, MD

Concept
- General work-up for a patient with a pulmonary infection
- Bacterial pulmonary abscess
- Aspergilloma
- Zygomycosis
- Multidrug-resistant tuberculosis

Chief complaint
"You are called by one of your internal medicine colleagues to evaluate a 75-year-old woman admitted for presumed community acquired pneumonia. Since admission 24 hours ago, she has had persistent fevers and productive sputum despite IV antibiotic therapy. You have been consulted because she has additionally developed hemoptysis in the last few hours."

Differential
Community-acquired pneumonia, tuberculosis, invasive fungal infection, pulmonary abscess, bronchiectasis, malignancy (post-obstructive infection)

History and physical
Typical symptoms of the majority of pulmonary infections include cough, dyspnea, sputum production, and pleuritic chest pain. Timing and duration of these symptoms is important to determine whether this is an acute or chronic problem. A patient with a bacterial pulmonary abscess would likely have had symptoms for a shorter period than a patient with recurrent infections in the setting of bronchiectasis. The immunologic status of the patient is also very important when evaluating a patient with complicated lung infection. Immunosuppressed patients (previous transplant, chemotherapy, long term steroid use) are more likely to suffer from invasive *Aspergillus* infection. A history of structural lung disease (bullous emphysema, fibrotic lung disease, cavitary tuberculosis, sarcoidosis with bullae) makes the diagnosis of mycetoma (*aspergillus, histoplasma, blastomyces, coccidioides*) more likely.

Typical physical exam findings in patients with lung infections include fever, tachycardia, and tachypnea. Crackles on auscultation are also common. In the setting of a parapneumonic effusion, breath sounds may be diminished or absent on the affected side. Evaluation of dentition can be of some use in patients with suspected bacterial pulmonary abscess, as aspiration of anaerobic organisms from oral infections can lead to abscess formation.

Tests
- *Imaging.* PA/lateral CXR can identify the location of consolidation in the event of pneumonia. There might also be evidence of a pulmonary abscess or parapneumonic effusion on plain film. Chest CT will give more detailed anatomic information and should be ordered in the event that the plain films do not offer a definitive diagnosis.
- *Labs.* Any patient hospitalized with a pulmonary infectious problem that requires surgical consultation should have a complete blood count, basic electrolytes, renal and hepatic function tests, and a coagulation panel sent. In febrile patients, blood cultures, urinalysis, and urine culture should be obtained. All patients with a suspected pulmonary infection should have a sputum culture sent. If a pulmonary resection is being entertained, preoperative spirometry and diffusion capacity can be used to estimate perioperative risk. If surgery is indicated, a type and screen or crossmatch should be ordered depending on the complexity of operation and likelihood of major blood loss.

77

- *Identification of organisms.* In order to successfully treat a pulmonary infection, it is helpful to accurately identify the precipitating pathogen. Sputum should be collected in any patient suspected of having a pulmonary infection, but these samples are negative 50% of the time in cases where the presence of infection has been proven in other ways. Furthermore, many sputum samples come back contaminated with normal respiratory flora, making them useless. There are a number of other more invasive means of obtaining an accurate diagnosis.
  - *Fiberoptic bronchoscopy.* This method allows direct sampling of the infected part of the lung. Collection of bronchoalveolar lavage samples from this area helps eliminate contamination with normal respiratory flora.
  - *Endobronchial ultrasound.* In rare cases where samples of pulmonary parenchyma are needed for definitive sampling. Fine needle aspirates can be taken under ultrasound guidance.
  - *Transthoracic needle aspiration.* Performing an aspiration or biopsy of a suspected area of infection eliminates the possibility of contamination with respiratory flora considerably. This technique is particularly helpful when obtaining samples from an abscess cavity or pleural effusion/empyema.

Index scenario (additional information)
"The patient's history and physical reveal that her symptoms of cough, malaise, and fever have been going on for approximately one week. Her hemoptysis started yesterday and is ultimately what brought her to the hospital. Over the last month she has noticed that she has developed some difficulty swallowing and frequently chokes when eating. She is previously healthy and is on no medications. Her WBC is elevated at 25,000 and the rest of her labs are normal. Sputum, blood and urine cultures are pending. CT scan shows a 5 x 6 cm cavity in the superior segment of her right lower lobe with an air-fluid level and surrounding parenchymal consolidation."

Treatment/management
Given her history, there is high suspicion for a bacterial pulmonary abscess, particularly with the recent aspiration symptoms. Furthermore, pulmonary abscesses frequently will develop in the superior segments of either lower lobe because of their dependent locations. The posterior segments of the upper lobes are also frequently involved for the same reason. Treatment of a bacterial pulmonary abscess is medical initially and involves antibacterial therapy, chest physiotherapy/postural drainage, and nutritional support. Antibiotic coverage should start broad and be narrowed based on culture results. If aspiration is suspected or the patient recently has significant dental work, anaerobic coverage should be initiated. The most commonly involved organisms are: Peptostreptococcus, Bacteroides, Staph aureus, Strep pneumo, Haemophilus, Klebsiella, Mycobacteria. Antibiotics are generally continued for 6-8 weeks.

Differentiating a simple bacterial pulmonary abscess from an infected cavitary lung carcinoma can be challenging. If there is any question of malignancy, flexible bronchoscopy can be performed to rule out an obstructing tumor or other foreign body and as a way to obtain a tissue sample if possible. Additional culture specimens can be obtained at the same time to help target the offending organism. If the bronchoscopy is unrevealing and there is still high suspicion for malignancy, transthoracic biopsy of the thickest part of the cavity's wall may lead to a diagnosis.

For those abscesses that show no signs of draining internally on bronchoscopy, external catheter drainage may be required. This is typically performed by interventional radiology and is necessary in the minority of bacterial pulmonary abscess cases (i.e., persisting fevers, abscess is not receding or is getting bigger despite appropriate antibiotics). Catheter drainage has greatly decreased the need for surgical intervention in these cases. Catheter placement through areas of suspected pleural symphysis is optimal to minimize leakage into the pleural space.

Surgical intervention is only required in approximately 10% or less of lung abscesses. The indications for surgery are:

- Persistent infection secondary to bronchial obstruction from foreign body or tumor
- A multidrug-resistant pathogen
- Large abscess greater than 6 cm
- Massive hemoptysis
- Rupture of abscess cavity with resultant empyema/bronchopleural fistula
- Cavitary malignancy, or inability to rule out malignancy

Typically, surgical management is limited to excision of the involved parenchyma. Most commonly, this requires a lobectomy or segmentectomy depending on the size of the cavity. These cases may be attempted with a video-assisted thoracoscopic (VATS) approach, but the adhesions associated with the abscess cavity may make the resection difficult. A double lumen endotracheal tube should be utilized to prevent potential spilling of purulent debris into the contralateral lung. Use of autologous tissue buttressing of the bronchial stump is suggested only in difficult to treat (i.e., multidrug resistant) infections. In cases where there is concern for residual pleural space, rotation of latissimus or omental flaps can be used to fill the thoracic cavity. If rupture of the abscess cavity has occurred prior to surgical intervention, decortication in addition to resection may be required.

Cavernostomy is reserved for patients in whom antibiotic therapy and percutaneous drainage have failed and are too unstable to tolerate a resection. After drainage and debridement of the cavity, the space should be filled with a vascularized soft tissue flap and closed. The alternative to this is to marsupialize the cavity to the atmosphere via limited rib resection. This should be reserved for the most critically ill patients as the morbidity from the resultant wound is not trivial. One last situation where cavernostomy may be the best approach is in the patient who would require a pneumonectomy to adequately resect their cavity. Pneumonectomy in the setting of lung abscess carries very high morbidity and mortality rates. The rate of both bronchopleural fistula (BPF) formation as well as empyema without BPF are much higher in this situation.

Potential questions/alternative scenarios

"You are asked to see a 35-year-old man who is one-year status post kidney transplant who has fevers, cough, and a 4 cm by 4 cm cavitary lesion in his right upper lobe."

The immunosuppression that is required for the kidney transplant makes a fungal infection much more likely. Abscess cavities secondary to histoplasma or blastomycosis are possible, but aspergilloma is more likely. An aspergilloma is a conglomeration of Aspergillus hyphae, fibrin, mucus, and cellular debris. They may occur in immunocompetent patients with structural lung disease such as bullous emphysema, fibrotic lung disease, cavitary tuberculosis, or sarcoidosis with bullae. In immunocompromised patients, the aspergillus will rapidly destroy lung parenchyma and create a cavity. Often, they are asymptomatic until they cause hemoptysis, but can cause pulmonary symptoms such as cough and pleuritic chest pain. The classic CT scan finding is a ball of tissue within a cavity that does not entirely fill the space, leading to the radiologic description of an "air crescent sign." Diagnosis can be verified with sputum culture or serum antibodies specific to aspergillus.

Surgical therapy is indicated in any patient with aspergilloma and hemoptysis and is also indicated in the following circumstances due to poor prognosis: Increasing size of aspergilloma on imaging, immunosuppression, increasing aspergillus-specific IgG, and HIV infection. In those with hemoptysis, preoperative embolization of feeding bronchial arteries can temporize the bleeding, but surgical resection is recommended at this point because the aspergilloma will invariably recruit new blood supply. Surgical therapy often requires lobectomy, but in cases of small lesions may only require a sublobar resection. These operations tend to be quite difficult due to the dense vascular adhesions associated with the cavity.

"You are asked to see a 55-year-old man who was admitted to the MICU with diabetic ketoacidosis (DKA), fevers, and respiratory failure. Over the course of the last 12 hours, his oxygen requirement has gone up from 40% to 60% and he has a rapidly expanding right sided infiltrate on CXR. CT scan shows a dense infiltrative process localized to the right upper lobe and part of the middle lobe with possible involvement of the chest wall."

The combination of findings above are concerning for a zygomycosis (previously known as mucormycosis) infection. Pulmonary zygomycosis is most commonly seen in poorly controlled diabetics, specifically those who present to the hospital in DKA, and neutropenic patients, such as those undergoing bone marrow transplantation. Patients with pulmonary zygomycosis typically present with fevers and pulmonary infiltrates refractory to antibiotics. The progression of disease is often very rapid, and it will spread across anatomic boundaries. It is not uncommon to see invasion of the chest wall, pericardium, and other surrounding structures.

Treatment of pulmonary zygomycosis involves three key components: reversal of underlying condition (ketoacidosis, neutropenia), antifungal therapy, and surgical debridement. Antifungal treatment consists of high-dose amphotericin B (1-1.5 mg/kg per day) and is continued until all signs of infection have resolved. Operative intervention is indicated in patients who have disease limited to one lung. All involved lung parenchyma should be resected in addition to involved chest wall tissue. Patients with pulmonary zygomycosis who undergo aggressive surgical debridement have a significant survival advantage to those who are treated medically. However, overall prognosis remains poor as many of these patients are marginal surgical candidates due to the rapid progression of infection and their underlying comorbidities.

"A 48-year-old man with known multidrug-resistant tuberculosis (MDR-TB) is referred to your clinic for possible surgical resection of persistent disease. He has been on medical treatment for several months and remains sputum culture positive. On CT scan he has a 9 cm by 13 cm cavity in his right upper lobe that has been slowly increasing in size over this time period."

MDR-TB is defined as a strain of TB that is resistant to at least isoniazid and rifampin. Despite this resistance, most MDR-TB cases will not require surgical intervention, although resection of persistent parenchymal disease in these patients is clearly associated with improved outcomes. Surgery is usually needed to treat the complications of MDR-TB infection. The most common of these complications include:

- Massive hemoptysis
- Bronchopleural fistula
- Empyema
- Bronchiectasis or destroyed lung
- Broncholiths
- Aspergilloma

Preoperative evaluation of these patients should focus on optimizing the patient's baseline physical status to reduce the chances of morbidity and mortality. The nutritional status of a patient with MDR-TB is often compromised and may require enteral tube feeds preoperatively. Routine cardiac and pulmonary function testing should be performed, although in the case of a patient with cavitary disease or destroyed lung, resecting the diseased lung will not often alter overall pulmonary function. To further elucidate this in patients with borderline spirometry and diffusion capacity, a VQ scan can be helpful.

The most common parenchymal resection for MDR-TB is lobectomy, followed by pneumonectomy. In the patient described above, removal of his right upper lobe will greatly increase his chances of obtaining a negative sputum culture as the cavity serves as a reservoir of bacteria that are isolated from circulation and antibacterial medications. Approach to resections for MDR-TB is typically through a posterolateral thoracotomy, although a video-assisted approach can be used for lesions that are surrounded by lung parenchyma. In cases involving the pleura, an extrapleural dissection may be needed to remove the lung without causing soilage of the pleural space. The bronchial stump should be covered with muscle or omentum in patients with a positive preoperative sputum smear, significant drug resistance, or polymicrobial contamination (remember to preserve an intercostal flap at the time of thoracotomy). When adhesive disease involves the hilum, it can be easier to gain intrapericardial control of the pulmonary vessels. In pneumonectomy cases that result in significant contamination of the pleural space, it is advisable to leave an intentional Eloesser flap to prevent postoperative empyema. This space may then be closed several weeks later with instillation of modified antibiotic solution (Clagett procedure).

Pearls/pitfalls

- Surgical resection is rarely required for infectious lung disease.
- When required, surgical resection is limited to involved parenchyma. This often will require a segmentectomy or lobectomy.
- Resection for infectious lung disease can feasibly be performed via VATS; however, vascular adhesions can complicate the dissection and there should be a low threshold for conversion to an open procedure.
- Cavitary malignancy should always be ruled out in the setting of a suspected pulmonary abscess that is not responsive to conventional therapy.
- Aspergilloma, and other fungal infections, are rare in immunocompetent patients without structural lung disease.
- When performing a resection for infection with multidrug-resistant organisms, it is advisable to cover the bronchial stump with a vascular tissue pedicle.

Suggested readings

- Passera, E. et al. Pulmonary Aspergilloma: Clinical Aspects and Surgical Treatment Outcome. *Thorac Surg Clin.* 2012; 22: 345-61.
- Jaroszewski, D. et al. Diagnosis and Management of Lung Infections. *Thorac Surg Clin.* 2012; 22: 301-24.
- Merritt, R. et al. Indications for Surgery in Patients with Localized Pulmonary Infection. *Thorac Surg Clin.* 2012; 22: 325-332.
- Weyant, MJ. et al. Multidrug-Resistant Pulmonary Tuberculosis: Surgical Challenges. *Thorac Surg Clin.* 2012; 22: 271-276.

12. Malignant Pleural Mesothelioma

Shawn S. Groth, MD, Marcelo C. DaSilva, MD, and David J. Sugarbaker, MD

Concept

- Discuss the preoperative testing to determine resectability for patients with malignant pleural mesothelioma (MPM)
- Discuss the indications and critical surgical steps for extrapleural pneumonectomy (EPP) and extended pleurectomy/decortication (EPD)
- Discuss the postoperative management and complications after EPP and EPD

Chief complaint

"A 65-year-old man is referred to you by his primary care physician for evaluation of right pleural thickening and nodularity. As part of a workup for a two-month history of dyspnea, a chest x-ray was obtained four weeks ago which revealed a right pleural effusion. A thoracentesis was performed with 1000 cc of cloudy, serous fluid being drained. Cytology was negative for malignancy. A non-contrast chest CT was obtained that demonstrated diffuse pleural thickening and nodularity of the right hemithorax and resolution of the effusion."

Differential

The differential for pleural thickening and pleural nodules includes benign etiologies, such as mesothelial hyperplasia, benign pleural plaque, benign solitary fibrous tumor of the pleura, lipoma, mesothelial cyst, adenomatous tumor, and schwannoma. Malignant causes include primary pleural tumors such as malignant pleural mesothelioma, malignant solitary fibrous tumor, pleural thymoma, sarcoma (liposarcoma, leiomyosarcoma, rhabdomyosarcoma), pleuropulmonary blastoma, small cell carcinoma of the pleura, and desmoid tumor. Neoplasms with pleural metastases may also present in this fashion with primaries such as primary lung cancer, extrathoracic carcinomas, extrathoracic sarcomas, melanoma, and germ cell tumors being the most common.

History and physical

A focused history should inquire into common presenting symptoms for MPM (i.e., dyspnea, chest pain, fevers, cough, hemoptysis, and anorexia), asbestos exposure, family history of MPM, chest radiation, and an assessment of the patient's functional status. Nutrition is a vital aspect of caring for all cancer patients; inquire about weight loss, anorexia, and dietary intake. A focused physical examination should include a general assessment of the patient's physiological and nutritional status. Auscultate and percuss the chest to assess diminished breath sounds, chest wall excursion (contraction of the hemithorax often suggests chest wall invasion), and palpable chest wall masses (including previous biopsy sites). Assess for cervical, supraclavicular, and axillary adenopathy. Examine the abdomen for masses and/or ascites (signs of peritoneal involvement).

Tests

Tissue diagnosis

- *Approach.* The first step is to obtain tissue for diagnosis. Only 30% to 50% of MPM patients are diagnosed by thoracentesis and cytology. The authors prefer a thoracoscopic biopsy of the pleura, which provides a definitive diagnosis with a high degree of accuracy and minimal risk. In most instances, this can be done as an outpatient procedure.
- *Histological subtypes.* The primary MPM histological subtypes are epithelioid, sarcomatoid, and biphasic (which is composed of at least 10% epithelial and sarcomatoid elements). Pure sarcomatoid and biphasic tumors carry the worse prognosis.

82

- *Pathology review.* The diagnosis of MPM should be confirmed by an experienced pathologist. In addition to hematoxylin and eosin staining, the diagnosis of MPM is based on immunohistochemical features (antibodies to calretinin, keratin antibody AE1/AE3 - a product of Wilm's tumor susceptibility gene 1 (WT1)). Antibodies to CEA, Leu-M1, and TTF1 suggest NSCLC. Antibodies to calretinin and WT1 are consistent with epithelioid MPM, whereas sarcomatoid MPM has nuclear pleomorphism and stains strongly for keratin.

Pretreatment staging

- *CT.* A non-contrast chest CT is the primary imaging modality for diagnosis, staging and post-treatment surveillance of MPM. Common CT findings in MPM include: pleural thickening, involvement of the fissure, pleural effusion, contraction of the involved hemithorax and mediastinal shift. Once the diagnosis is established, it is useful to assess for mediastinal adenopathy, mediastinal invasion, chest wall invasion, transdiaphragmatic involvement, and contralateral disease.

- *PET/CT.* The authors also routinely obtain an integrated PET/CT scan. It increases the sensitivity to detect mediastinal lymph node metastases, subtle chest wall involvement, and occult extrathoracic disease. The baseline SUVmax has prognostic significance and, if neoadjuvant chemotherapy is given, is a useful metric to follow on post-treatment imaging.

- *MRI.* A gadolinium-enhanced chest MRI is a useful adjunct to chest CT to assess for chest wall, transdiaphragmatic, mediastinal, and contralateral invasion. We obtain a chest MRI for all of our patients.

- *Mediastinal lymph node biopsy.* All potential candidates for resection should undergo EBUS-TBNA, EUS-FNA, or cervical mediastinoscopy for histologic assessment of N2 disease. Those with N2 disease should undergo neoadjuvant chemotherapy.

Physiological fitness

- Appropriate candidates for surgery should have a good functional/performance status (i.e., Karnofsky performance status of 70 or greater), normal hepatic function, normal renal function (CrCl > 60 mL/min), and adequate cardiopulmonary reserve.

Assessment of cardiopulmonary status

- *Oximetry.* For all patients, we assess their oxygenation saturation (by pulse oximetry) at rest and with activity (i.e., during a 6-minute walk test). It provides an invaluable and inexpensive assessment of their pulmonary function.

- *Pulmonary function tests (PFTs).* All patients should have formal PFTs. For patients with COPD or pulmonary fibrosis, assess DLCO as well. Patients with poor underlying pulmonary function (postop predicted FEV1 < 40% or DLCO < 40%) are not candidates for resection.

- *Quantitative VQ scan.* All potential candidates for resection should have a quantitative VQ scan. Such an assessment is used to calculate the postoperative predicted (PPO) FEV1 (FEV1 x % perfusion to non-affected lung) to ascertain whether or not the patient could tolerate a pneumonectomy without an undue risk for respiratory complications. Patients with a ppoFEV1 below the following values are not candidates for resection: EPD, < 1.0 L; left EPP, < 1.0 L; right EPP, < 1.2 to 1.4 L. The relative perfusion to each lung is also important for determining candidacy for a resection. For instance, a patient with a ppoFEV1 of 1.2 L and a relative perfusion of 10% to the affected lung is less likely to have complications than a patient with a ppoFEV1 of 1.2 L and a relative perfusion of 50%. In such patients, other parameters should be taken into consideration when determining medical operability.

- *Transthoracic echo (TTE).* All patients should undergo a TTE to assess LV and RV function, underlying valve disease and to estimate PA pressures (from the degree of

TR). Patients with an estimated PA pressure of 30 mmHg and a right atrial pressure roughly 1/3 systemic are not candidates for resection.

- *Cardiac stress test.* All patients with an active cardiac condition should undergo preoperative stress testing. Consider preoperative testing in patients with at least one cardiac risk factor and a functional capacity of 4 metabolic equivalents or less.

"The patient underwent pleuroscopy and biopsy of a parietal pleural nodule; final pathology demonstrated the presence of epithelioid MPM. He then underwent a PET/CT which demonstrated diffuse FDG uptake throughout the right pleural space; there is no abnormal FDG uptake elsewhere. A chest MRI showed no evidence of chest wall, diaphragmatic, contralateral, or mediastinal extension. Mediastinoscopy was negative for N2 disease. The patient has been reading on the internet about various treatment options and is curious about your thoughts on who should get chemotherapy and who should undergo a resection."

Treatment/management
Neoadjuvant chemotherapy
Patients with N2 disease, chest wall invasion, and contralateral disease should be referred for neoadjuvant chemotherapy. The preferred regimens for neoadjuvant and adjuvant therapy are platinum-based agents and pemetrexed or platinum-based agents and gemcitabine.

Definitive chemotherapy
Patients who are deemed medically inoperable and those with advanced disease should be referred for definitive chemotherapy.

Cytoreductive surgery
The best chance for cure is complete removal of macroscopic disease (i.e., an R1 resection). Patients with marginal cardiopulmonary function who are unlikely to tolerate an EPP may still be candidates for EPD. The decision to perform EPD or EPP will be based on the patient's physiologic reserve, age, and the extent of disease (minimal versus bulky disease). With either procedure, the goal is a complete macroscopic resection of all tumor.

Adjuvant chemotherapy
Patients who undergo EPD (especially those with node-positive disease) should undergo postoperative chemotherapy. For patients who undergo EPP, those patients with biphasic histology and those with node-positive disease should also undergo postoperative chemotherapy.

Radiation therapy
Radiation therapy can be given to improve local control after EPP (not EPD), to treat and palliate chest wall disease, and to treat a focus of mediastinal disease.

Operative steps
Pleurectomy/decortication (EPD)
Goals – explore and determine resectability, complete macroscopic removal of all tumor, and mediastinal lymph node dissection. *Note: The incision, exposure, and extrapleural dissection are similar for EPPs and EPDs.*

- Double-lumen endotracheal tube.
- *Tube and lines*: PA catheter on operative side, peripheral IVs, arterial line, Foley catheter, NG tube (to facilitate identification of the esophagus during the extrapleural dissection and to prevent large volume aspiration until resolution of the postoperative ileus).
- Extended posterolateral thoracotomy (divide latissimus dorsi and serratus anterior).
- Excise the 6th rib.

- Begin the extrapleural dissection around the circumference of the thoracotomy, separating the parietal pleura from the endothoracic fascia.
- Continue posterolaterally up to and over the apex of the lung, sweeping the pleura off the subclavian vessels.
- For right-sided tumors, continue along the anterior mediastinum over the SVC to the SVC-azygos recess; avoid injury to the internal mammary vessels.
- Continue extrapleural dissection inferiorly and posteriorly along the azygos for right-sided tumors or along the aorta for left-sided tumors to the retrocrural space and retroperitoneum.
- After completing the extrapleural dissection, the tumor is stripped off the pericardium to the hilar cuff.
- The tumor is incised with a scalpel in-line with the thoracotomy.
- A plane is created between the lung and the visceral pleura. The tumor is bluntly dissected free from the underlying lung to the level of the hilar cuff, where the incision in the tumor is extended down to the hilar reflection. The upper and lower halves of the tumor shell are removed.
- Depending on tumor involvement, the diaphragm and/or the pericardium may need to be resected (and reconstructed).
- Mediastinal lymph node dissection.
- Place chest tubes and close.

Extrapleural pneumonectomy (EPP)

Goals – explore and determine resectability, complete macroscopic removal of all tumor, and mediastinal lymph node dissection. *Note: The incision, exposure, and extrapleural dissection are similar for EPPs and EPDs.*

- Double-lumen endotracheal tube.
- Tube and Lines: PA catheter on operative side, peripheral IVs, arterial line, Foley catheter, NG tube (to facilitate identification of the esophagus during the extrapleural dissection and to prevent large volume aspiration until resolution of the postoperative ileus).
- Extended posterolateral thoracotomy (divide latissimus dorsi and serratus anterior).
- Excise the 6th rib.
- Begin the extrapleural dissection around the circumference of the thoracotomy, separating the parietal pleura from the endothoracic fascia.
- Continue posterolaterally up to and over the apex of the lung, sweeping the pleura off the subclavian vessels.
- For right-sided tumors, continue along the anterior mediastinum over the SVC to the SVC-azygos recess; avoid injury to the internal mammary vessels.
- Continue extrapleural dissection inferiorly and posteriorly along the azygos for right-sided tumors or along the aorta for left-sided tumors to the retrocrural space and retroperitoneum.
- Palpate the pericardial sac for tumor invasion.
- Avulse the diaphragm from the chest wall, and bluntly dissect the diaphragm off the peritoneum.
- Open the pericardium anteromedially.
- Hilar dissection.
- Dissect and divide the PA (intrapericardial division for right EPP and extrapericardial division for left EPP).
- Intrapericardial division of the pulmonary veins.
- Divide the bronchus under bronchoscopic visualization, leaving a < 1 cm stump.
- Complete the pericardiotomy.

- Complete mediastinal lymph node dissection.
- Mobilize a tongue of greater omentum for bronchial stump coverage.
- Reconstruct the diaphragm with a dynamic patch of 2 pieces of 2 mm PTFE mesh.
- Reconstruct the pericardium with a fenestrated PTFE patch (regardless of side).
- Buttress the bronchial stump with the omental flap.
- Place a 14 Fr red rubber catheter and close.
- Remove air via the red rubber catheter to balance the mediastinum (Right EPP: men 1000 cc and women 750 cc, Left EPP: men 750 cc and women 500 cc).

Potential questions/alternative scenarios

"While still in the OR following a right EPP, the patient has a sudden rise in his CVP and PA pressure and a drop in his blood pressure and cardiac output when being turned from lateral to supine."

Turn the patient back in the lateral decubitus position, re-prep and re-open the thoracotomy. The pericardial patch is likely the cause of tamponade and should be replaced with a looser patch.

"On postoperative day number 2 after a right EPP, your patient has a cardiac arrest while in the ICU."

An emergency thoracotomy, removal of the pericardial patch, and open cardiac massage should be performed to address potentially correctable mechanical causes of the arrest (cardiac herniation, a constrictive pericardial patch, kinking of the IVC by the diaphragmatic patch, or a pericardial effusion). Closed chest compressions are ineffective after pneumonectomy. After resuscitation, the patient should be taken back to the OR for a washout and closure.

"A routine CXR on postoperative day number three after a right EPP demonstrates complete filling of the pneumonectomy space and contralateral mediastinal shift."

Place a small drainage catheter in the 2nd intercostal space, midclavicular line to slowly remove fluid to balance the mediastinum. The fluid should be sent for culture and Gram's stain as well as for triglycerides and cell count.

"The culture is negative. The triglyceride level is 900, and the fluid is lymphocyte rich."

These findings are consistent with a chylothorax. (See Chylothorax chapter for details on management.)

"Five weeks after a left EPP, a patient presents with fevers, malaise, and a drop in his air-fluid level. You are concerned about a possible bronchopleural fistula (BPF) and empyema."

If the patient is acutely toxic, place a chest tube in the pneumonectomy space (above the level of the thoracotomy). The patient ultimately needs a bronchoscopy and open surgical drainage (i.e., a Clagett Window or Eloesser Flap). All synthetic material (i.e., the PTFE patches) should be removed.

"You have a patient booked for a left EPP who you referred for induction therapy. He now returns to the office with a PET-CT for post-treatment staging and he is noted to have uptake along the contralateral costophrenic margin. How would you proceed? What if the patient had only left-sided disease with extensive involvement of the left hemidiaphrag? The read on the PET-CT states that there is questionable extension into the peritoneal cavity. How would you manage this patient?"

Contralateral pleural disease would make this patient unresectable. However, this should be confirmed by biopsy, most easily performed via thoracoscopy. Peritoneal involvement would also make this patient unresectable. A staging laparoscopy would be prudent in this case to rule out intra-peritoneal disease prior to proceeding with resection.

86

Preoperative evaluation

- Always assure that you have a recent (within the previous 4 weeks) imaging study (i.e., CT, MRI, or PET/CT).
- Never biopsy the visceral pleura or nodules on the surface of the lung. Such biopsies often lead to chronic BPFs and impair patients from receiving definitive treatment.

Surgery

- Remove all prior biopsy scars due to the risk for tumor seeding.
- During the extrapleural dissection for a left EPP, it is easy to begin dissecting behind the aorta, thereby injuring the intercostals. To avoid this, begin on the arch and stay in the preaortic plane.
- During diaphragmatic resection for a left EPP, leave a 1-2 cm rim of left crus for suturing during patch reconstruction to prevent gastric herniation.

Postoperative management

- After EPP, extubate in the OR to minimize positive pressure on the bronchial stump.
- After EPD, continue with positive pressure ventilation for the next 24 hours to help tamponade bleeding from the surface of the lung and chest wall.
- PA catheters are essential to optimizing postoperative fluid status and cardiac function.
- For patients with diaphragmatic reconstruction who require long-term postoperative enteric nutritional support, place an open jejunostomy tube.
- Pneumoperitoneum for laparoscopy can induce a tension pneumothorax. Be cognizant of this potential adverse sequela.

Suggested readings

- Sugarbaker DJ, RB Bueno, Colson YL, Jaklitsch MT, Krasna M, Mentzer SJ. Pleural Malignancy (Part 20). *Adult Chest Surgery.* McGraw-Hill. New York, 2015.
- Wolf AS, Daniel J, Sugarbaker DJ. Surgical Techniques for Multimodal Treatment of Malignant Pleural Mesothelioma: Extrapleural Pneumonectomy and Pleurectomy/Decortication. *Semin Thorac Cardiovasc Surg.* 2009;21(2): 132-48.
- DaSilva MC and Sugarbaker DJ. Technique of Extrapleural Pneumonectomy. *Oper Tech Thorac Cardiovasc Surg.* 2010;15(4): 282-293.
- Kaufman AJ and RM Flores. Technique of Pleurectomy and Decortication. *Oper Tech Thorac Cardiovasc Surg.* 2010;15(4): 294-306.
- Rusch VW. Pleurectomy and Decortication: How I Teach It. *Ann Thorac Surg.* 2017;103(5):1374-7.
- Maat A, Durko A, Thuijs D, Bogers A, Mahtab E. Extended pleurectomy decortication for the treatment of malignant pleural mesothelioma. *Multimed Man Cardiothoracic Surg.* 2019;2019. doi: 10.1510/mmcts.2019.023.

13. CHYLOTHORAX

Jenalee N. Coster, MD, and Shawn S. Groth, MD, MS

Adapted from 1st edition chapter written by Ryan A. Macke, MD, and Benny Weksler, MD

Concept

- Presentation and diagnostic workup of chylothorax
- Differences in management of traumatic and neoplastic chylothorax
- Options and justification for medical and surgical management
- Describe the anatomy of the thoracic duct and the steps of thoracic duct ligation
- Role of lymphangiographic thoracic duct embolization
- Pitfalls in management of chylothorax

Chief complaint

"You have successfully completed a redo coarctation repair via left thoracotomy on an otherwise healthy 45-year-old man. It is now postoperative day 4. Left chest tube output has been high (> 1 L/day). After starting a regular diet, the chest output changes from serous to milky in appearance."

Differential

Sympathetic effusion, chylothorax, empyema, esophageal perforation

History and physical

Causes of chylothorax are categorized as congenital, traumatic, and neoplastic. Congenital occurs most commonly in neonates and is usually idiopathic in nature likely due to abnormal lymphatic development. Traumatic chylothorax is most common and can complicate any thoracic operation (most commonly esophagectomy, aortic procedures, left pneumonectomy and resection of posterior mediastinal masses) or lower neck operations (such as radical neck dissection or central line placement – particularly in the pediatric population). Blunt trauma resulting in hyperextension of the spine and violent vomiting or coughing can disrupt the thoracic duct at the level of the diaphragm, resulting in a traumatic chylothorax. Neoplastic processes such as lymphoma, primary lung cancer, or metastatic disease can cause obstruction of the thoracic duct resulting in rupture of lymphatic tributaries leading to chylothorax. Infection, filariasis, venous obstruction (SVC, subclavian, or jugular veins), cirrhosis, tuberculosis, and pulmonary lymphangioleiomyomatosis (LAM) are less common etiologies of chylothorax. A history of the above procedures, injuries, or conditions and the presence of a pleural effusion, high output serous chest drainage in patients who are not taking oral intake, or milky chest drainage should prompt additional workup to rule out a chylothorax or to confirm the suspected diagnosis. The following chapter focuses primarily on the more common traumatic and neoplastic causes of chylothorax.

Tests

The presence of a change in the chest tube effluent from serous to non-clotting, milky fluid is a classic presentation for chylothorax. In patients who are NPO with high serous chest tube output and chylothorax is suspected, triggering the characteristic change of appearance is accomplished by feeding high fat content substances (e.g., heavy cream or olive oil). Dyes such as Evan's blue (injected subcutaneously) or methylene blue (added to enteral intake) may also be used. Additionally, fluid analyses can confirm the diagnosis. Lymph is comprised of fat, proteins, and lymphocytes. Sending fluid for triglycerides count with a concentration of > 110 mg/dL is diagnostic of a chyle leak in 99% of cases, whereas a chyle leak is present in less than 5% of cases with a concentration of < 50 mg/dL. In cases where the triglyceride level is equivocal and suspicion remains high, the fluid should be sent for chylomicrons. The presence of any concentration of chylomicrons is diagnostic, as these lipoproteins are not present in serum. Microscopic examination may demonstrate fat globules that stain with Sudan-3 or clear with alkali/ether, with both tests being diagnostic of a chyle leak.

Imaging for chylothorax is usually limited to CXR or CT Chest demonstrating pleural effusion. Lymphangiography is an invasive test that may be useful in difficult cases, such as failed thoracic duct ligation or left-sided chylothoraces. Lymphangiography may be used to localize the site of leak and plan the approach for additional invasive procedures. Furthermore, thoracic duct embolization can be accomplished at the time of lymphangiography via a variety of coils. This may be an option in a patient who will not tolerate an operation or those in whom operative ligation has failed. At some specialized centers, thoracic duct embolization may be attempted prior to operative ligation, though there is a paucity of evidence supporting this approach.

Index scenario (additional information)

"The patient described above is afebrile, hemodynamically stable, and is otherwise doing well on the floor. Chest tube drainage was sent for fluid analysis, showing a triglyceride level of 220 mg/dL and chylomicrons of 50, confirming your suspicion of chylothorax. Discuss your management going forward." How long would you treat medically before deciding to re-operate?"

Treatment/management

The four components of medical management are:
1) Minimize chyle production and flow through the thoracic duct
2) Drainage of the chylous effusion
3) Replacing fluid losses
4) Nutritional support

The main role of the thoracic duct is to transport absorbed lipids from the intestine to the venous system. Chyle is composed of lipids (free fatty acids, cholesterol, cholesterol esters, and phospholipids), proteins (such as albumin and fibrinogen), fat-soluble vitamins, enzymes, lymphocytes (mostly T lymphocytes), and antibodies. The thoracic duct also carries extravasated proteins and excess interstitial fluid along with chyle. The composition and volume of chyle depends primarily on the timing, lipid-content, and amount of enteral intake. It takes approximately 90 minutes for ingested lipids to reach the systemic circulation. Long-chain fatty acids are absorbed by the intestine and are transported by chylomicrons in the thoracic duct giving chyle the characteristic milky appearance. Short and medium chain fatty acids (< 10 carbon atoms) are absorbed directly into the portal system bypassing lymphatic circulation. A reduced fat diet restricting long chained fatty acids and supplementing medium chained fatty acids or complete bowel rest with TPN decreases the volume of chyle and increases the chance of spontaneous healing of the duct leak. It is important to note that intravenous lipids do not increase chyle flow through the lymphatic system.

Adjuncts to dietary management include octreotide, a somatostatin analogue. Though the benefit is unproven, octreotide may reduce gastrointestinal secretions and absorption and, in turn, lymph production.

An undrained chylothorax will eventually lead to a chylous effusion and compressive atelectasis, resulting in dyspnea. Drainage is required typically by tube thoracostomy. Ongoing drainage of a chyle leak leads to loss of important lipids, proteins, vitamins, and lymphocytes resulting in malnutrition and immunosuppression. As such, an uncontrolled chylous effusion can be extremely morbid, leading to other complications, and can be fatal.

Medical management is more effective in lower output chyle leaks (<500mL/day), but compliance may be poor. Spontaneous closure/sealing of thoracic duct leaks are expected in roughly half of patients treated with non-operative/medical therapy. Half of patients will require some form of invasive procedure. Morbidity and mortality increase significantly if the chylothorax has not resolved by one week. High output chylothoraces (> 1 L/day) are less likely to resolve with medical management alone. Cut-offs points for determining failure of medical therapy are controversial. In general, alternative methods to treat the chylothorax should be carried out if the leak fails to seal after 2 weeks of medical therapy or if there is greater than 1 L of output daily. The threshold to abandon non-operative/medical management should be lowered for patients who are immunosuppressed or malnourished.

"You decide to keep treating the patient with bowel rest, octreotide, and TPN. Two weeks have now passed, and the patient continues to have ~500 cc/day of chest tube output. Fluid analysis shows a persistently elevated triglyceride level. What would you do next? Describe your approach to thoracic duct ligation."

Persistent chylothorax has been confirmed with the triglyceride level of > 110 mg/dL and the patient has failed to resolve the leak after two weeks of non-operative management. Output remains considerable. Invasive procedures, such as surgical ligation of the thoracic duct, lymphatic tributary clipping, application of biologic sealant (i.e., fibrin glue), obliteration of the pleural space by surgical or chemical pleurodesis, pleuroperitoneal shunting, or lymphoscintigraphy with thoracic duct embolization or cisterna chyli fenestration, are options for failed medical management.

An understanding of the anatomy of the thoracic duct is a critical component of its management. "Normal" anatomy isn't the norm. Approximately, 40% to 50% of patients have "abnormal" anatomy, including multiple ducts, aberrant termination, and multiple terminal channels. These variations must be taken into consideration when managing chylothoraces.

Suspected location/laterality of the chyle leak plays an important role in surgical approach to thoracic duct ligation. Unilateral chylothoraces can usually be approached on the side of the chylous effusion if direct ligation or tributary clipping is planned. However, the exact location of the thoracic duct injury or leaking lymphatic tributaries may not always be identifiable once in the operating room. In this case, mass ligation of the thoracic duct just above the diaphragm via the right chest is the preferred approach. Therefore, right sided chylothorax should always be approached from the right, permitting direct or mass duct ligation.

Careful planning is required for left-sided chylothoraces. Preoperative lymphoangiography or VATS inspection may be useful to avoid redo or second thoracotomy and allows the surgeon to attempt to localize the leak by direct visualization. Administration of cream through an NG tube can be helpful to stimulate lymphatic flow and identify the location of the leak. If the leak cannot be identified with preoperative lymphangiography or by VATS, the safest approach is to perform a mass ligation via the right chest, which will in effect treat the left chylothorax. Some surgeons always recommend a right-sided mass ligation of the thoracic duct, even in left sided chylothoraces. Bilateral chylothoraces should be treated with mass duct ligation via the right chest.

Operative steps
Direct thoracic duct ligation or tributary clipping
- Direct ligation of the thoracic duct or clipping of the duct tributaries may be performed thoracoscopically or via thoracotomy. If an open approach is preferred, the chest can be entered through the previous thoracotomy if one was performed.
- Provocative measures, such as providing heavy cream down an NG tube during the operation, can be taken to help identify the leak once in the chest.
- Once adhesions have been lysed and the site located, the duct is ligated proximally and distally with non-absorbable suture.
- If there is no injury to the main duct, but rather leakage is noted from disrupted lymphatic tributaries, the tributaries are clipped.

- The addition of a sealant, such as fibrin glue, may be added as a secondary measure following direct ligation or clipping to assist sealing the leak.
- Drains and chest tubes are positioned near the site of repair to monitor output postoperatively.
- If the site of the chylous fistula cannot easily be identified, dissection in the thoracic duct fat to attempt to find the leak should be avoided, as this may result in additional injury to the duct or disruption of lymphatic tributaries. Failure to identify the leak should prompt one to consider mass ligation of the thoracic duct.

Mass thoracic duct ligation
- Mass duct ligation is performed via the **right chest** thoracoscopically or open. If a previous thoracotomy is present, the chest may be re-entered through the same incision. However, a high thoracotomy may not provide adequate access near the hiatus. A thoracotomy in the 6th or 7th intercostal space is ideal.
- For a VATS approach, a camera port is placed in the 7th or 8th intercostal space in the posterior axillary line. Working ports are placed in the 8th or 9th intercostal space in line with the tip of the scapula and just below the tip of the scapula. A lung retraction port is placed in the 5th intercostal space anterior to the latissimus.
- A retraction stitch may be placed in the tendinous portion of the diaphragm to improve exposure of the hiatus.
- Once the diaphragm is retracted inferiorly, the lung is retracted anteriorly.
- The goal of mass ligation of the thoracic duct is to ligate all tissue in the area limited posteriorly by the azygos vein, anteriorly by the esophagus, and medially by the descending aorta, just above the diaphragm to cease all flow of chyle through the thoracic duct.
- A plane is developed just anterior to the azygos vein and dissection is carried down to the aorta. The esophagus is identified anteriorly and all the tissue between the azygos vein and esophagus is doubly ligated with non-absorbable sutures. Large clips may be added proximally and distally for reinforcement. Biologic sealant, such as fibrin glue, may be added as well.
- Drains and chest tubes are then placed to monitor postoperative output.
- Pleurectomy or chemical pleurodesis may be performed as an added measure of security to promote pleural symphysis and sealing of leaking tributaries or accessory ducts not addressed by the mass ligation. A fully expanded lung is necessary for this to be effective.

Potential questions/alternative scenarios
"Describe the anatomy of the thoracic duct. What percentage of patients do you suspect have this 'normal anatomy'? What are some common variants seen in thoracic duct anatomy?"

The thoracic duct is the main channel that drains lymph from the entire body to the venous system, with the exception of the heart, dome of the liver, and right upper body (face, neck, arm, and thorax). The thoracic duct originates at the cisterna chyli, which is located anterior to the spine between vertebral bodies T10 to L3. The duct passes through the aortic hiatus and ascends to the right of the midline, posterior to the esophagus, between the descending thoracic aorta and azygos vein. The duct then passes behind the aorta crossing the midline between T5–T6 and ascends through the thoracic inlet along the left aspect of the esophagus. Once in the neck, the duct arches laterally, traveling anterior to the left subclavian and thyrocervical arteries, phrenic nerve, and anterior scalene muscle before passing posterior to the carotid sheath and jugular vein. The thoracic duct drains into the posterior aspect of the left jugular-subclavian vein confluence.

The right thoracic duct drains the right upper body and typically terminates at the right jugular subclavian vein confluence. This duct is small and rarely seen. It is estimated that this "normal" anatomy is present in only half of patients.

Some of the more common variants include multiple terminating trunks draining into the venous system, multiple trunks passing through the mediastinum, variable points of cross-over from right to left, and variable drainage pathways of the accessory ducts draining the right upper body. Less than 40% of patients will drain directly into the jugular-subclavian venous confluence, with the duct commonly terminating at the jugular, subclavian, or both veins.

"You have a patient who is 3 days out from an Ivor Lewis esophagectomy for esophageal cancer. Right chest tube output has been moderate (~500 cc/day). Following initiation of enteral feeds via a jejunostomy tube, you are called because the chest tube has put out 750 cc's of milky fluid so far today. Of note, the patient had a preoperative weight loss of 20 pounds and has a BMI of 21. Discuss how your management may or may not differ from the previous patient and why. Do you perform routine thoracic duct ligation during esophagectomy?"

Post-esophagectomy chylothorax occurs in approximately 1-5% of patients. A more aggressive approach is advocated for treatment of this patient population due to higher failure rates with medical therapy alone. Also, many patients who undergo esophagectomy are already malnourished and will not tolerate a longer period of medical management due to the nutritional losses that occur. If the chyle leak does not seal after 3-5 days of medical management, surgical intervention is recommended. Drainage of > 1 L/day is the recommended cut-off for failure of non-operative management (others have shown a lower chance of spontaneous duct closure with > 400 mL/day). Some even advocate surgical intervention at the time of diagnosis in this patient population. The advantages of early intervention are avoiding malnutrition and immunosuppression that accompanies a high output chylous fistula and re-entering the chest at a time where adhesions are soft and minimal. The conduit vascular pedicle is at risk with dissection near the hiatus during mass thoracic duct ligation, making late reoperation a high-risk endeavor.

Although adding a prophylactic mass thoracic ligation to an esophagectomy adds minimal time and risk of morbidity to the procedure, there is not overwhelming evidence to support routine ligation at the time of resection. However, should a ductal injury be identified intraoperatively, direct suture ligation should be performed. It should be noted that identification of a thoracic duct leak intraoperatively is rare since most patients are in a fasting state and without the presence of lipids, the draining chyle will be serous in appearance.

"Following mass ligation of the thoracic duct, your patient continues to have a refractory right chylothorax. Beside medical management, what are some other options to manage this patient?"

Refractory chylothorax can be problematic. Failure of medical therapy should be treated surgically with direct or mass ligation of the thoracic duct, with success rates upwards of 90% being expected. Reoperation with mass ligation of the duct may be successful in patients who underwent direct ligation or tributary clipping on the first attempt. In patients who have failed surgical ligation or those in which re-entrance into the chest is problematic, lymphangiography may be useful to identify the location of the chylous fistula. In addition, thoracic duct embolization or cisterna chyli fenestration may be carried out at the time of lymphangiography. Thoracic duct embolization is an invasive procedure that can be separated into two separate phases and can take 4-6 hours. It requires a pedal or pelvic intranodal lymphangiography for visualization of the cisterna chyli. Once the cisterna chyle is visualized, percutaneous access is required through a transabdominal approach. The duct is cannulated via Seldinger technique and contrast is injected to identify the fistula on delayed imaging. The site or sites of the leak may then be embolized with use of a variety of materials. If the duct cannot be cannulated, the cisterna chyli may be fenestrated via multiple needle passes under fluoroscopic guidance to promote drainage of lymph into the peritoneal cavity and decrease flow to the thoracic duct. Chyle is reabsorbed in the peritoneum, minimizing nutritional losses. Percutaneous embolization and fenestration has minimal risk of morbidity and mortality, although this procedure is highly operator-dependent. Up to 60% of attempts to cannulate the cisterna chyli are unsuccessful. If the thoracic duct is able to be cannulated, then success rates of embolization approach 90%. If the thoracic duct is unable to be cannulated percutaneously then cisterna chyli fenestration has a reported success rate of up to 72%; furthermore, performing lymphangiography has also demonstrated success in cessation of chyle leak. Regardless, this technique is a useful alternative for patients unwilling or unable to undergo reoperation or in refractory cases where mass or direct ligation has failed.

If the refractory chylothorax is low output and the lung is fully expanded with drainage, pleurectomy or chemical pleurodesis may be performed to promote pleural symphysis and sealing of the leak.

"You are re-consulted on a patient you did a mediastinoscopy on 2 weeks ago to confirm the diagnosis of lymphoma. She now complains of dyspnea and has a right pleural effusion. You place a chest tube and complete fluid analysis which confirms the diagnosis of chylothorax. What is the cause of chylothorax in this patient? How would you manage this patient going forward?"

Neoplastic processes may lead to lymphatic duct obstruction by direct invasion, mass effect/compression, or tumor embolism. The obstruction eventually leads to rupture of lymphatic tributaries and accumulation of a chylous effusion. Lymphoma accounts for over half the cases of neoplastic chylothorax. Treatment of the primary lesion with radiation and/or chemotherapy will usually resolve the chylothorax due to either shrinkage of the culprit lesion with relief of the obstruction or fibrosis of the lymphatics and closure of the leak. However, in some patients the symptoms of the effusion are not tolerated, thus waiting for the systemic therapy to take effect may not be an option. Given the abnormal lymphatic drainage in these patients, larger or symptomatic effusions should be drained by tube thoracostomy. It is likely that most duct injuries or leaks do not resolve by healing of the duct itself, but rather are sealed by pleural symphysis; therefore, adequate drainage is necessary for pleural apposition to occur. Some advocate chest tube drainage and chemical pleurodesis via the indwelling tube with such irritants as tetracycline, doxycyline, bleomycin, or talc to promote pleural fusion and sealing of the lymphatic leak. High-output or inadequately drained chylous effusions are unlikely to heal with this technique.

Lymphangiography with percutaneous embolization or cisterna chyli fenestration may be a useful alternative. Surgical intervention, such as pleurectomy and/or duct ligation, is not recommended in patients with non-traumatic chylothorax caused by neoplastic disease to avoid delaying initiation of systemic therapy. Pleuroperitoneal shunting is one surgical option that has been used in this patient population with some success. These shunts relieve dyspnea by draining the effusion, while nutrients are reabsorbed as the chyle is drained into the peritoneal cavity. Ascites is an absolute contraindication to pleuroperitoneal shunts.

Pearls/pitfalls

- Chylothorax should be in the differential for post-traumatic or postoperative high, serous chest tube output. Further workup is needed to confirm the diagnosis.
- Understand the basic principles of medical management for treatment of chylothorax and have a threshold for treatment failure.
- The site of the thoracic duct leak may not be easily identified intraoperatively. Anticipate this scenario "curveball" and have a plan for how to manage it.
- Mass ligation via the right chest can be used to treat right, left, or bilateral chylothorax and is probably the safest answer when describing surgical management of chylothorax.
- Variations in thoracic duct anatomy are nearly as common as "normal" anatomy.

- Thoracic duct ligation and pleurectomy should be avoided when possible for management of neoplastic chylothorax.

Suggested readings

- Johnstone DW. Anatomy of the Thoracic Duct and Chylothorax. In: Shields TW, LoCicero J III, Reed CJ, Feins RH (eds.) *General Thoracic Surgery*. 7th ed. Philadelphia, PA: Lippincott Williams & Wilkins; 2009:827-834.

- Merigliano S, Molena D, Ruol A, et al. Chylothorax complicating esophagectomy for cancer: a plea for early thoracic duct ligation. *J Thorac Cardiovasc Surg*. 2000; 199: 453-457.

- Reisenauer, JS, Puig, CA, Reisenauer, CJ, et al. Treatment of postsurgical chylothorax. *Ann Thorac Surg*. 2018;105:254-62.

- Schenker, MP, Baum, RA. Percutaneous Therapy for Traumatic Chylothorax. In; Sugarbaker, DJ, Bueno, R, Colson, YL, Jaklitsch, MT, Krashna, MJ, Mentzer, SJ (eds). *Adult Chest Surgery*. 2nd Ed. New York, NY: McGraw-Hill Education, 2015: 1063-68

- Shah R, Luketich JD, Schuchert MJ, et al. Postesophagectomy chylothorax: incidence, risk factors, and outcomes. *Ann Thorac Surg*. 2012; 93: 897-904.

- Itkin M, Kucharczuk JC, Kwak A, Trerotola SO, Kaiser LR. Non-operative thoracic duct embolization for traumatic thoracic duct leak: experience in 109 patients. *J Thorac Cardiovasc Surg*. 2010 Mar;139(3):584-589; discussion 589-590.

14. Hemoptysis

Jenalee N. Coster, MD, and Shawn S. Groth, MD, MS

Adapted from 1st edition chapter written by Matthew D. Taylor, MD, and Christine L. Lau, MD, MBA

Concept

- Differential for hemoptysis
- Initial patient stabilization
- Indications for OR (Rigid bronchoscopy, endobronchial therapies, surgical resection)
- Role of embolization
- Treatment according to etiology

Chief complaint

"A 67-year-old man is admitted to the medical intensive care unit (MICU) with acute respiratory distress. An urgent thoracic surgery consultation is requested for 'airway bleeding.'"

Differential

The most common cause of hemoptysis is chronic inflammatory disease (bronchiectasis, cystic fibrosis, aspergillosis, and TB). Other causes of hemoptysis include acute infections (e.g., necrotizing pneumonia), tracheoinnominate fistula (usually occurs 1-2 weeks after tracheostomy), neoplasms, autoimmune lung diseases (SLE, Wegener's granulomatosis, polyarteritis nodosa, Takayasu's arteritis), trauma (e.g., penetrating, blunt, or iatrogenic [Swan-Ganz catheters]), pulmonary embolism (can result in infarction, hemorrhage, and subsequent necrosis), arteriovenous fistula (usually congenital in origin, represents 2% of all cases of massive hemoptysis), cardiovascular disease (associated with elevated pulmonary venous pressures such as mitral stenosis or congenital heart disease). The differential should also include oropharyngeal tumors or oropharyngeal trauma, as well as upper GI causes that may be mistaken for hemoptysis. The definition of "massive" hemoptysis varies in the literature varies from 200 to 1000 cc per day. It is uncommon (about 1.5% of all episodes of hemoptysis). Importantly, it only takes about 400 cc of blood to cause significant hindrance of O2 transfer. Because systemic pressures are higher than pulmonary arterial pressures, most (90-95%) of episodes of massive hemoptysis are from the bronchial arteries.

History and physical

The priority is to assess and protect airway, breathing, and circulation. Do not proceed to history and physical nor further testing until the primary survey has been addressed. Once stabilized, obtain a medical history focusing on possible infectious causes, tracheostomy, malignancy, trauma, underlying cardiovascular disease, and chronic inflammatory diseases. Ask about any history of upper GI problems. Also inquire about coagulopathies, history of easy bleeding, and any anticoagulant medications. Physical examination in the unstable patient is outlined below under treatment/management. Once stabilized, proceed with the secondary survey which confirms airway, breathing, and circulation. Verify that vitals and saturations are stable. Assess the patient's mental status, cardiovascular exam, and distal pulses. Examine the oropharynx for evidence of trauma or masses. A nasolaryngoscope may be useful for evaluation of the nares and oropharynx. Look for stigmata of liver disease (caput medusae, ascites). Place an NG tube with lavage to rule out active UGI bleeding.

Tests

Below is a list of tests that will be relevant to the patient's management. They can be ordered during or after the primary survey and patient stabilization. These tests aim to elucidate the etiology of the bleed as well as the patient's overall state of health.

- *Bronchoscopy (diagnostic and therapeutic).* Define the location of the bleeding source. Should be the first step in management and work-up of hemoptysis. Rigid or flexible depending on the scenario (see below). Have dilute epinephrine ready as a lavage, since this may help vasoconstrict smaller, superficial areas of bleeding.

- *CXR*: parenchymal disease, air fluid levels (abscess).
- *Basic labs*: CBC, complete metabolic panel, ABG, and coagulation studies.
- *CT chest with IV contrast (for the stable patient only)*. Rule out lung mass, tracheal lesions, or cavitary lesions. Evaluate for a blush or area of possible target of embolization.
- *PFTs (for the stable patient only)*. Determine ability to tolerate lung resection if needed.
- *Echo, stress testing (for the stable patient only)*. Evaluate cardiovascular fitness in patients at risk of cardiovascular disease prior to any pulmonary resection.

Index scenario (additional information)
"This patient is currently coughing up 2 cups of clotted blood while you are evaluating him. His oxygen saturation is 86% on 10 L of oxygen. Hematocrit is 19. He has no tracheostomy. He is tachypneic. What is your next step in management?"

Treatment/management
Primary survey and initial stabilization:
A - *Airway* - This patient in his current state warrants a definitive airway via a single lumen endotracheal tube (ETT) using rapid sequence intubation (succinylcholine, etomidate, cricoid pressure).
B - *Breathing* – Confirm that the ETT is allowing adequate ventilation (by assessing auscultation, endtidal CO2, and/or pCO2 on ABG) and oxygenation. Bronchoscopy is crucial to clear initially formed clot that may accumulate in the trachea to allow adequate ventilation and localize the source of bleeding; otherwise, asphyxiation and death may ensue. If the bleeding is profuse and inhibiting ventilation, place a bronchial blocker or advance the ETT into the unaffected mainstem bronchus (flexible bronchoscopy will be needed to make this determination), inflate the cuff, and reassess. This should allow you to catch up from a ventilatory and hemodynamic standpoint. It may help to position the patient with the affected lung side down (dependent) to prevent aspiration of blood into the unaffected lung.
C - *Circulation* – Obtain large bore IV access, start resuscitation with blood products, and correct coagulopathy. Note that blood loss of > 600 mL in 4 hours is associated with a 71% mortality. Blood loss of > 1 L in 24 hours is associated with a 58% mortality. Continue with a quick secondary survey as described above with any adjunctive tests that are reasonable to order. In this case CXR, labs, NG tube, and flexible bronchoscopy (if not already done) are reasonable. It is useful to have irrigation, low dose epinephrine as a lavage, and suction available at the time of flexible bronchoscopy. Pull the ETT back to the trachea above the carina. Advance the scope, irrigate, suction, and evaluate the area of interest as well as the other lobes as tolerated.

"You have been able to stabilize the patient from a hemodynamic and ventilatory standpoint. You notice bleeding coming from the RLL bronchus. It is persistent. A CXR showed an air fluid level in the RLL. NG tube lavage was clear. Coagulation factors were corrected. ABG shows an HCT of 26% after transfusion. How do you wish to proceed?"
In a patient who is hemodynamically stable, easily ventilated with a controlled airway, and only minor or moderate hemoptysis, it may be reasonable to take a slightly less aggressive approach. Sedatives and anti-tussive medications will help to minimize coughing and recurrent bleeding. Bronchodilators should be avoided, as they have a vasodilatory effect on the pulmonary vasculature. Hypertension should be controlled. Imaging with a CT angiogram or angiography may provide useful information that will help determine the next subsequent steps in treatment. In this scenario, it is difficult to adequately evaluate and treat the right lower lobe lesion through the flexible bronchoscope at the bedside. There is known identified ongoing hemorrhage. The most prudent and efficient course of action is to proceed to the OR suite for rigid bronchoscopy.

Rigid bronchoscopy

In a patient with uncontrolled bleeding without a controlled airway, rigid bronchoscopy is warranted. A rigid bronchoscope has a larger diameter which facilitates suctioning and instrumentation. The smaller diameter of the flexible bronchoscopes limits interventions, which is why rigid is preferred in emergency cases with large-volume hemoptysis. A jet ventilation circuit will be needed. This patient already has a single lumen ETT in place. Flexible bronchoscopy and large bore catheter suctioning is performed to clear the airway of as much blood as possible. Jet ventilation and rigid bronchoscope are prepared, and the patient is extubated and the rigid scope is passed as follows:

- A teeth guard is placed on the upper teeth. The left hand of the surgeon is placed palm down and grasps the upper teeth. The rigid bronchoscope is slid between the index and thumb and acts as a fulcrum as the scope is passed distally. Anesthesia or an assistant can help to expose the vocal cords with a laryngoscope, sweeping the tongue away and lifting the epiglottis. The beveled tip of the rigid scope should be anterior and will help to lift the epiglottis as well. Once the cords are seen through the rigid scope, it is rotated 90° to allow the tip to pass through the cords.

- A large bore suction catheter is passed through the rigid scope and the airway is cleared of as much clot as possible to visualize the carina/determine right from left.

- The main stem of the unaffected lung is intubated, and jet ventilation is carried out until oxygen saturations are stable and within normal range.

- The rigid scope is then pulled back and the main stem bronchus of the affected lung is intubated with the rigid scope. Additional suctioning is carried out until the source of bleeding is identified or O2 saturations decline. The affected lobar or segmental bronchus is then treated with ice-cold saline lavage (1 liter) with 1 mg of epinephrine (mixed prior to lavage) in the bleeding orifice for 10-15 seconds. This facilitates clot clearance and has the potential to slow or stop the bleeding altogether.

- It is necessary to alternate between intubation (with the rigid scope) of the unaffected lung, followed by ventilation and recovery, then intubation of the affected lung, followed by treatment.

- A flexible bronchoscope may be passed through the rigid scope to better visualize areas of bleeding. This also allows passage of a Fogarty embolectomy balloon into an affected segmental bronchus to prevent ongoing bleeding into the remaining lung if ice-saline lavage is unsuccessful. A bronchial blocker may be used to occlude a lobar or main stem bronchus. Balloon occlusion may be useful as temporizing measures while arrangements are made to proceed with an operation, transfer to the angio suite, optimize hemodynamics, or allow for reversal of coagulopathy.

- If bleeding is from any orifice except the right upper lobe, the rigid bronchoscope may be wedged for selective lavage. The flexible scope allows good access to the upper lobe and can be wedged for lavage. Wedging the rigid scope in the right upper lobe is difficult, but for bleeding from all other lobes, the rigid scope provides optimal access for lavage and other treatments.

Potential questions/alternative scenarios

"After performing saline/epinephrine lavage, the patient continues to bleed uncontrollably. What is the next step in management?"

If there is an identifiable endobronchial mass causing bleeding endobronchial thermal ablation may be useful. It is important to remember when using thermal techniques to decrease the inhaled oxygen to an FiO2 of less than 0.34 to prevent airway fires. Endobronchial thermal ablation devices range from CO_2 to Argon Plasma Coagulation (APC) to Nd:YAG and Nd:YAP lasers. CO_2 was the first laser introduced to medicine; however, it has several disadvantages including a long wavelength (10,600 nm) and shallow depth of penetration (0.23 mm) which may limit its effect on hemostasis. APC uses argon as a conduction of electricity to promote photocoagulation of tissues. It also has limited tissue penetration (1-2mm) which is beneficial on bleeding airway mucosa, but it is of limited use if a large vessel is the source of bleeding. Nd:YAG and Nd:YAP lasers with a shorter wavelength utilize flexible quartz filaments for delivering which allows it to be used through a flexible bronchoscope, a property that increases its popularity for endobronchial therapy. One disadvantage of the Nd:YAG/Nd:YAP lasers are the variable depth of penetration and thus should not be used on the mucosa as can cause perforation but are preferable for bleeding masses. If saline lavage and endobronchial therapies are unable to control bleeding, one option is to place a Fogarty embolectomy balloon catheter into the segmental orifice or a bronchial blocker into the lobar or main stem bronchus to tamponade the bleed. The bronchus of the unaffected lung is then intubated, a tube exchanger in passed through the rigid scope, and a single lumen (or double lumen tube if the unaffected side happens to be the left) is passed over the tube exchanger into the unaffected bronchus after the rigid scope has been removed. The patient should then be transferred to angiography for bronchial artery embolization with single lung ventilation. Bronchial artery embolization is successful in 90% of cases. Bronchial artery embolization is ideal for situations where there are multiple sources of bleeding. Embolization may also play a role for temporizing ongoing hemoptysis until a more definitive surgical plan is devised.

"Attempts at bronchial artery embolization have failed. What is your next plan of action?"
This constitutes failure of non-surgical options. The next step would be pulmonary resection of the bleeding source which in this case is the RLL. Traditional incisions/exposures can be used for this form of pulmonary resection. Operative mortality for lobectomy for hemoptysis is approximately 10%. The procedure follows the steps described under pulmonary resections in the lung cancer chapters with the exception that the tissue will be much more inflamed, friable, and bloody. Lymph node sampling/dissection is not required unless cancer is suspected. In the case of bleeding from the right or left lung and one is not able to locate the lobar or segmental source by bronchoscopy or angiography, a pneumonectomy may be required. This would only be advised if it is truly a life-threatening situation and exsanguination/asphyxiation appears imminent.

"The patient has successful arterial embolization for massive hemoptysis. The etiology of the patient's hemoptysis is an aspergilloma with a cavitary lesion. How do you wish to proceed?"
The patient should be treated with IV antifungal therapy (i.e., Amphotericin) for at least a week followed by reassessment of clinical status, CXR, and CT scan. If the patient has not had a recurrence of bleeding nor evidence of sepsis, and the imaging shows a stable cavitary lesion with or without regression, then continue conservative management. In the meantime, it is not unreasonable to obtain PFTs and cardiovascular workup in the event that a resection is warranted. If the patient has a recurrence or the abscess fails to improve after 2-3 weeks of therapy, then consider percutaneous drainage with infusion of intracavitary Amphotericin B. If the patient's clinical condition fails to improve, then resection may be warranted. Note that any recurrent bleed will be handled just as outlined above in the index scenario. If resection becomes necessary, you will want to do this on an elective or urgent basis rather than an emergently. Also note that prior to any resection a malignancy should be ruled out (refer to chapter on Pulmonary Infections).

"Pulmonary function testing indicates that the patient would not tolerate resection. What is the next plan of action?"
CT-guided intracavitary amphotericin paste has been successful in preventing recurrent hemoptysis and for obliterating the cavitary site.

"A 65-year-old obese man with a history of COPD and colon cancer develops profuse bleeding from a tracheostomy. The tracheostomy was placed 1 week ago for respiratory insufficiency after an open colectomy. What is the next step in the management of this patient?"
You would proceed as outlined above for the index scenario with a few alterations. The first maneuver would be to overinflate the tracheostomy cuff to tamponade bleeding. If this

maneuver is not successful, remove the tracheostomy and obtain endotracheal intubation while a finger is inserted through the tracheostomy stoma providing manual compression of the innominate artery to the posterior table of the sternum. The patient is then taken emergently to the OR where a sternotomy is performed, and the fistula is repaired. TIF carries a high mortality rate. As such the most expeditious, simple method to control bleeding is preferred, rather than a complicated repair or interposition graft (depending on availability of operative consultation at one's hospital). A median sternotomy is the preferred approach. Ligate the innominate at its origin. Distal ligation should be proximal to the bifurcation of the right subclavian and right common carotid arteries. The tracheal injury is debrided, repaired using a buttress of muscle or thymus.

"A 68-year-old man with a known tracheal mass (presumed squamous cell carcinoma from outside reports) presents with hemoptysis. You stabilize the patient in the ICU as outlined above and can pass an ETT with bronchoscopic guidance just beyond the lesion. You clear the airways with the bronchoscope and note no distal bleeding source. Once stable, you pull the tube back to irrigate and visualize the bleeding source and note the presence of an irregular mass occupying 50% of the circumference at the mid trachea and extending about 2 cm in length. The mass is very friable with multiple bleeding points. How do you proceed?"

You approach this patient just as you did the index case above. Here you are lucky that you could get the tube beyond the lesion. If there was any difficulty in doing this, you should not pull the tube back and "peek" at the lesion, but rather go directly to the OR for rigid bronchoscopy. In the current scenario you were able to get a sense of the characteristics of the mass but will not be able to control the bleeding safely with a flexible bronchoscope at the bedside. Proceed to the OR for rigid bronchoscopy. Your primary objective is to obtain hemostasis. Endobronchial therapies with laser or APC may be beneficial here in this scenario. Obtain biopsies before laser ablation with the understanding that a biopsy of the lesion may prompt more bleeding. Once hemostasis is obtained and tracheal mass is debulked, the patient will need a complete workup to determine if resection is feasible. Refer to the chapter on Tracheal Tumors for staging and treatment options for constricting tracheal masses.

Pearls/pitfalls

- *Initial stabilization of patient* – ABCs: airway protection with intubation, IV access, correction of coagulopathy
- Treatment for massive hemoptysis:
    - *Bronchoscopy*: iced-saline/epinephrine lavage, laser coagulation, topical coagulants, endobronchial thermal therapies, endobronchial blockade, and single lung ventilation strategies.
    - Bronchial artery embolization.
    - Surgical resection of bleeding source.

Suggested readings
- Khemasuwan, D., Mehta, AC., Wang, K. Past, present, and future of endobronchial laser photoresection. *J Thorac Dis.* 2015: 7(S4): S380-S388.
- McNamee C, Conlan A. Massive hemoptysis. Lewis MI and McKenna RJ, (eds). *Medical Management of the Thoracic Surgery Patient.* Philadelphia: Saunders 2009:174-80.
- Radchenko, C., Alraiyes, A.H., and Shojaee, S. A systematic approach to management of massive hemoptysis. *J Thorac Dis.* 2017: 9: S1069-S1086.
- Wigle DA, Waddell TK. Investigation and management of massive hemoptysis. Patterson GA, Cooper JD, Deslauriers J, Lerut AEMR, Luketich JD, Rice TW, and Pearson FG (eds). *Pearson's Thoracic and Esophageal Surgery.* Philadelphia: Churchill Livingstone 2008:507-27.

15. COPD, EMPHYSEMA, AND SPONTANEOUS PNEUMOTHORAX

Mara B. Antonoff, MD, and Traves D. Crabtree, MD

Concept

- Differential diagnosis for spontaneous pneumothorax
- Surgical management options for emphysema/bullous disease
- Considerations of candidacy for lung volume reduction surgery
- Conduct of lung volume reduction operative procedures
- End-stage emphysema and basic lung transplant considerations

Chief complaint

"A 51-year-old man presents to the emergency department complaining of sudden onset of shortness of breath and pleuritic chest pain. Chest x-ray demonstrates right-sided hyperlucency with absence of pulmonary markings."

Differential

The diagnosis of pneumothorax is revealed by the X-ray findings. Potential etiologies include: trauma, iatrogenic injury, primary spontaneous pneumothorax, or secondary spontaneous pneumothorax from underlying conditions such as bullous diseases/chronic obstructive pulmonary disease (COPD), connective tissue disorders, malignancy, cystic disease, catamenial disease, or infection.

History and physical

A very limited history and exam should occur after the diagnosis of large pneumothorax, with tube thoracostomy performed early. A focused history should be obtained in order to rule out traumatic/iatrogenic sources and to elucidate any underlying lung disease as potential etiology of a secondary spontaneous pneumothorax. If underlying pulmonary processes are present, questions should focus on severity of disease and overall fitness for operative intervention. A focused exam should be performed, with emphasis on return of breath sounds bilaterally, adequacy of pulmonary excursion, work of breathing, and stigmata of chronic pulmonary disease, such as clubbing.

Tests

- *CXR*: mandatory in all.
- *Chest computed tomography (CT)*: identify blebs and delineate surgical anatomy, particularly in patients with underlying lung disease, prior chest surgery, or possible loculations.
- *Pulmonary function testing*: assess forced expiratory volume in 1 second (FEV1) and diffusion capacity in the lung of carbon monoxide (DLCO).

Index scenario (additional information)

"This patient has a PMH significant for COPD and long-standing smoking history. He describes a similar episode of spontaneous pneumothorax treated with right-sided chest tube 6 months prior. The patient reports periodic DOE and generalized limitations in activity due to SOB. Chest CT reveals re-expansion of the right lung with chest tube in place and several large apical blebs, right greater than left, with fairly normal underlying lung parenchyma. The patient has a continuous, large air leak."

Treatment/management

The pneumothorax was adequately treated/temporized with chest tube placement. Indications for surgical intervention include recurrent pneumothoraces, persistent air leak following tube thoracostomy, failure of lung re-expansion, extensive underlying parenchymal disease that puts the patient at higher risk for recurrence, or patients with limited health care access in the event of recurrence (i.e., pilots). Recurrence rates for primary pneumothoraces range from

16-52%, and, for secondary pneumothoraces, range from 40% to 56%; this risk can be reduced dramatically by operative bleb resection. In conducting bleb resection, it is imperative that one also performs adjunct procedures to enhance lung apposition to the chest wall, including pleurectomy or mechanical/chemical pleurodesis. Bleb resection with pleurectomy results in a recurrence rate of 1-5%. Pleural abrasion mechanical pleurodesis is technically less demanding and has a recurrent pneumothorax rate of approximately 2%. Mechanical pleurodesis and pleurectomy both carry an elevated risk of hemorrhagic complications compared with chemical pleurodesis. Chemical pleurodesis may be performed intraoperatively or via chest tube and is most commonly performed using talc, with doxycycline used alternatively (autologous blood [blood patch] and bleomycin have also been described). Instillation of talc slurry or other sclerosing agents via the chest tube tends to have a pneumothorax recurrence rate of 8-25%, while use of aerosolized talc with video-assisted thoracic surgery (VATS) has a reported recurrence rate of 5% to 9%. It is important that the lung be fully expanded for pleurodesis to be effective, as the pleural surfaces must be in apposition for obliteration of the pleural space to occur. It is also important to note that pleurodesis is often done with reservation in young patients or patients who may require additional surgery given the difficulty of chest re-entry, and in such cases mechanical pleurodesis may be preferred over chemical. It is thus important to consider all variables when deciding pleurodesis.

VATS has served as a favorable option replacing posterolateral thoracotomy as an operative approach for this disease process. With a minimally invasive approach, one can obtain good visualization and carry out the procedure with less pain and shorter length of hospital stay. Bleb resection, pleurectomy, and pleurodesis can be performed in a single setting.

Operative steps

- General endotracheal anesthesia with double-lumen endotracheal tube; large-bore intravenous access, arterial line (as clinically indicated), Foley catheter.
- Lateral decubitus positioning. VATS approach unless contraindicated.
- Take care upon entering chest to avoid injury to underlying lung and perform complete adhesiolysis in order to gain adequate visualization.
- Attempt to identify leaking bulla (which may be challenging in an isolated lung). A brief period of low-volume ventilation on the affected side may facilitate localization.
- Resect leaking bulla, if it can be identified. Use sequential firings of an endoscopic stapler; consider buttressed staple loads, however minimal evidence to support use. If a bleb cannot be clearly identified, some advocate an apical wedge resection regardless.
- Re-inflate underlying lung under direct vision and be prepared to perform a toilet bronchoscopy if unable to re-expand.
- Consider using spray sealant on the staple line to minimize the risk of prolonged postoperative air leak, however minimal evidence to support
- Perform apical pleurectomy, scoring pleura along the rib with electrocautery and peeling downward with grasper. Be sure to avoid aggressive pleurectomy in area of recurrent laryngeal nerve (RLN), phrenic nerve, and sympathetic chain.
- Mechanical pleural abrasion with folded cautery scratch pad. Here, too, be careful to avoid injury to RLN, phrenic nerve, or sympathetic chain.
- Chemical pleurodesis: 1-2 spray bottles (4 grams per bottle) of aerosolized talc, allowing contents to disperse around thoracic cavity.
- Leave a chest tube and place to -20 cm H_2O in operating room to rule out bleeding, then switch to water seal, which has shown to have better results in the immediate postoperative period. Chest tubes are typically left in place for 48 to 72 hours to allow for pleural symphysis to develop. Resolution of any air leaks is also necessary prior to tube removal.

Potential questions/alternative scenarios

101

"What if this same patient were referred to you in an outpatient setting for his chronic symptoms (in the absence of the pneumothorax)? What surgical options might be considered for management of severe, symptomatic emphysema?"

Based on the findings of the National Emphysema Treatment Trial, lung volume reduction surgery (LVRS) has been shown to be efficacious, safe, and durable in the management of *select* patients with disabling emphysema refractory to maximal medical therapy. Patients should be enrolled in preoperative pulmonary rehabilitation, which may improve some patients to the point that they will no longer require surgery, optimize some persistently symptomatic patients preoperatively, and identify patients too unfit to undergo operative intervention. Additional medical optimization should include oxygen and bronchodilators as indicated. Spirometry should be performed, and FEV1 and DLCO used to quantify the extent of airflow obstruction and gas trapping. Radiographic evaluation (non-contrast chest CT) is used to identify patients with characteristics most favorable for lung volume reduction surgery. Patients with severe, heterogeneous, upper-lobe predominant disease tend to have the greatest improvements in exercise tolerance, spirometry, and quality of life postoperatively. In addition, long-term survival is also improved in patients with heterogeneous, upper-lobe predominant disease and a low maximal workload during exercise testing who undergo LVRS compared to medical therapy. Outcomes tend to be more variable and less promising among patients with homogeneous or non-upper-lobe predominant emphysema, for this reason these patients are typically treated with medical therapy alone. Patients should not be considered for LVRS if they are currently smoking (or are < 6 months tobacco-free) or if they have a concurrent malignancy, advanced age, or other medical contraindications to operative intervention. Previous thoracic surgical procedures are relative but not absolute contraindications for LVRS.

"What if this patient had a homogeneous distribution of emphysematous changes? When should patients with end-stage emphysema be considered for lung transplantation?"

Patients with a homogeneous distribution of emphysema on CT have had less successful outcomes with LVRS, such that it is not recommended in individuals with such anatomic disease distribution. For these patients, lung transplantation remains a viable option. Other relative indicators which might suggest that a patient will be better served by lung transplantation than with LVRS include: oxygen dependence > 6 liters/minute at rest, FEV1 or DLCO < 20% of the predicted value, $PaCO_2$ > 55 mmHg, and pulmonary hypertension. Long-term survival following lung transplantation for end-stage emphysema is poorer than that of patients transplanted for cystic fibrosis, alpha-1 antitrypsin deficiency, and primary pulmonary hypertension. *However*, survival following lung transplantation for COPD has been shown to be comparable to survival following LVRS, and transplant remains an appropriate consideration for patients failing maximal medical management and unlikely (based on anatomic considerations) to benefit from LVRS.

Pearls/pitfalls

- Patients with secondary spontaneous pneumothorax are more likely to have prolonged air leaks and to have recurrent pneumothoraces; consideration should be given to operative management of such individuals.

- A VATS approach can be highly effective in the management of emphysema/bullous disease. Greatest efficacy is achieved by performing bleb resection, apical pleurectomy, and mechanical and/or chemical pleurodesis.

- LVRS serves as a potential operative strategy in patients with severe emphysema refractory to medical management. Good outcome is predicted by heterogeneous disease (mostly apical blebs) and symptomatic COPD.

- Patients with homogeneous disease, significant oxygen dependence at rest, FEV1 < 20% of the predicted value, $PaCO_2$ > 55 mmHg, and pulmonary hypertension may not have optimal outcomes with LVRS. In these individuals, careful consideration may be given to lung transplantation.

102

- Chambers A, Scarci M. In patients with first-episode primary spontaneous pneumothorax is video-assisted thoracoscopic surgery superior to tube thoracostomy alone in terms of time to resolution of pneumothorax and incidence of recurrence? *Interact Cardiovasc Thorac Surg.* 2009;9(6):1003-8.

- Criner GJ, Cordova F, Sternberg AL, Martinez FJ. The National Emphysema Treatment Trial (NETT): Part I: Lessons Learned about Emphysema. *Am J Respir Crit Care Med.* 2011;184(7):763-770.

- Criner GJ, Cordova F, Sternberg AL, Martinez FJ. The National Emphysema Treatment Trial (NETT): Part II: Lessons Learned about Lung Volume Reduction Surgery. *Am J Respir Crit Care Med.* 2011;184(8):881-893.

16. THORACIC TRAUMA
Sagar S. Damle, MD, and Michael J. Weyant, MD

Concept
- ATLS resuscitation
- Differential diagnosis for possible injuries
- Diagnostic tests
- Conduct of care with prioritization of injuries
- Specific operative interventions for particular injuries

Chief complaint
"A 35-year-old man is brought into the ED after a gunshot wound to the left chest. His vital signs are reportedly stable with volume resuscitation in the field. He is reportedly awake but dazed and confused."

Differential
Penetrating injuries to lung, heart, esophagus, chest wall. Also, blunt force injuries to lung, esophagus, and heart. Note that hemodynamically significant cardiac injuries are discussed in the Cardiac Trauma chapter.

History and physical
Focus on the critical steps of ATLS resuscitation. Remember that during ATLS protocols, diagnosis and treatment are done simultaneously during primary survey, which serves as your history and physical. Define the pattern of injury (i.e., anterior "box", posterior "box" - refer to Cardiac Trauma chapter). Remember the steps: A-B-C-D-E then secondary survey.
- *Airway*: confirm patient has adequate airway, especially if patient has large degree of subcutaneous emphysema. Intubate early for airway stability.
- *Breathing*: Confirm adequacy of oxygenation/ventilation. Look for chest wall deformities, entry/exit wounds sites, and flail movement of chest wall. Evaluate for extent of crepitus and/or chest wall hemorrhage. Get CXR. Also remember to CONFIRM result of therapy – did repeat CXR demonstrate evacuation of hemothorax? Most lung injuries will not lead to severe inability to ventilate and oxygenate patient. However, if the patient has a central airway injury from trauma, consider mainstem intubation or double-lumen ventilation during your "B" assessment.
- *Cardiovascular*: Examine for pulses and hemodynamic stability. Listen to heart sounds and check for JVD. Remember the penetrating injuries near great vessels or heart, and blunt force, may lead to pseudoaneurysms, cardiac trauma, etc. without direct injury. Perform FAST and rule out tamponade. If equivocal, place central venous catheter and evaluate
- CVP. D and E will not be covered in this topic.

Tests
- *Labs*. Usual trauma labs are useful. Particularly important to obtain ABG and Type & Cross.
- *X-rays*. "BIG 3." Lateral C-spine, CXR and pelvis. Clearly, we will be most concerned with CXR with particular attention to: pneumothorax, hemothorax, mediastinal shifting, apical cap, multiple rib fx, scapula fx, 1st rib fracture, loss of aortic knob/contour, and left effusion without rib fracture. Although a CXR is a quick test, it often lacks sensitivity and specificity.
- *FAST or E-FAST*. Particularly useful will be the subxiphoid view and bilateral hemithoraces, if done. Ideal for evaluating for possible tamponade in ED. Remember that repeat FAST also has a tremendous value as some fluid pockets will develop later.

- *CTA chest.* Especially useful to rule out great vessel injury. Patient should be hemodynamically stable to undergo CT. Do not send tenuous patient to the scanner. CT is of particularly higher yield in patients with high-impact mechanisms or CXR findings suggestive of injury (apical cap, 1st rib fx, scapula fx, multiple rib fx, loss of aortic knob etc.). CT is also useful for transmediastinal GSWs to outline tract and evaluate for possible collateral damage. Echocardiography (TEE) and angiography have limited, if any role, in evaluation of traumatic thoracic injuries with today's CT technology.

Index scenario (additional information)

"The patient is awake but has labored breathing. During his initial primary survey, he is intubated, and 2 large bore IVs are placed, and he is started on NS resuscitation. He is noted to have an entry wound in the left axilla and an exit wound in the right 4th ICS in the anterior axillary line. In addition, he has a large abrasion over the lateral left chest wall, consistent with a sledgehammer blow. While getting trauma X-rays, he is hypotensive with tracheal deviation to the left. A right chest tube is placed with return of a large amount of air and 300 cc of blood. CXR does not demonstrate any retained bullet fragments but does demonstrate multiple fractured ribs on the left and a large amount of subcutaneous air, as well as bilateral hemothoraces and near-complete collapse of the left lung. After placing a left-sided chest tube, there are large air leaks with > 1000 cc of blood return from the left tube upon initial insertion. Although he seems to stabilize somewhat, over the next 30 minutes, the left chest tube output is 600 mL and there is a severe blowing air leak in the right chest tube. How would you proceed?"

Treatment/management

Again, life-saving treatment is done during primary survey. During airway evaluation, if one suspects a high airway injury, consideration can be made for mainstem intubation. However, ideally, rapidly performed bronchoscopy should be done or available, as well to diagnose. Unfortunately, bronchoscopic findings of airway injuries may be subtle and can be easily missed. Also, availability of a bronchoscope in the ED can be variable. During evaluation of adequacy of breathing and oxygenation/ventilation, chest tubes should be placed liberally with suspected thoracic trauma. Evaluate for amount, type, and persistence of drainage. After intervention, make certain to re-evaluate patient for improvements after each therapeutic intervention. During cardiac evaluation, perform FAST initially and REPEAT at intervals to assess for accumulation of fluid, especially in patient who goes from stable to unstable. Have a low threshold to place large IVs and potential central access for CVP evaluation and more rapid resuscitation. If patient is in extremis or loses vital signs in ED, consider ED thoracotomy for stabilization. If hemodynamics is transiently stabilized, but decompensation continues, rapidly transport patient to the OR for operative intervention. If the patient's chest tube output remains low and hemodynamics are stable, consideration should be given for CTA to evaluate the bullet tract and associated injuries.

Operative steps

- Operative approach will vary based on injury.
- *Positioning.* Supine with patient prepped from chin to toes (standard trauma prep/drape). Although a lateral decubitus position would be possible, it limits one's ability to gain access to the abdominal cavity or contralateral hemithorax. Avoid suggesting this positioning.
- *Anesthesia considerations.* Double-lumen intubation, while ideal, is typically not possible due to trauma situation and airway edema. Consider alternatives for lung isolation including main stem intubation and bronchial blockers.
- *Incision.* The most versatile approach will be a thoracotomy with the patient in a supine position. This allows the possibility to extend the incision into the contralateral chest for treatment of contralateral injuries (i.e., clamshell). In addition, the clamshell also allows excellent exposure to the heart and great proximal great vessels. For this

105

scenario, perform clamshell thoracotomy from the beginning as there is significant hemorrhage from the left chest and persistent pneumothorax on the right. The sternum can be quickly divided transversely with either a sternal saw or heavy scissors. Be cognizant of the internal mammary arteries (i.e., ligate).

- After incision, control life-threatening bleeding with pressure, clamps, etc. as needed and available.
- If poor or limited venous access, place right atrial cannula for rapid infusion.
- In this scenario, bronchoscopy should be performed to evaluate for central airway injury, which typically can be addressed with either segmental resection (if extensive damage or tissue loss) or primary closure (if limited damage).
- Also, in this scenario, address source of bleeding in the left chest with appropriate therapy. Bleeding from bullet tract in lung can be addressed with tractotomy and oversewing of bleeding vessels. Tractotomy is performed by placing the anvil of a GIA stapler in the bullet tract and opening the lung parenchyma with stapler to the periphery of lung. Great vessel injuries must be addressed with proximal/distal control and either primary repair (rare) or interposition graft (vein or graft).

"In the operating room, you perform a clamshell thoracotomy to gain access to both chests. You note the bullet tract entering the left lung with profuse bleeding coming from the tract. The bullet appears to have traversed the mediastinum behind the great vessels. You note an injury to the trachea. How would you proceed?"

It appears that at the moment, there is reasonable control of the airway. If the ETT is too high and the tracheal injury is making it difficult to ventilate the patient, advance the ETT gently with a combination of fiber optic bronchoscopy and direct palpation. Once the airway control is established, even temporarily, address the bleeding from the lung with a tractotomy. Next, turn attention back to the tracheal injury. Unroof the mediatinal pleura overlying the trachea for a reasonable distance from the right chest. Identify the injury and freshen the edges. If possible, primary repair should be performed. If a near-circumferential injury, one may need to perform a segmental resection and primary anastomosis (refer to chapters on benign and malignant tracheal disease). Of note, the distal trachea, as well as the right *and* left mainstem bronchi can be relatively easy to reach from the right chest. Since most injuries occur posteriorly, this provides good access for repair. More proximal tracheal injuries must be approached from the neck, typically with a collar incision (discussed in Tracheal Tumor chapter). The distal trachea can also be reached via sternotomy. After opening the anterior pericardium, the SVC is mobilized laterally to the patient's right and the ascending aorta/arch to the patient's left. The posterior pericardium is then opened to gain access to the airway.

"Is there anything else you would do?"

Airway injuries and transmediastinal GSWs are often associated with other injuries. Especially in this case, one MUST evaluate the esophagus. Therefore, prior to closing chest, perform EGD. If any questions, explore area around the esophagus near bullet tract. Repair primarily if there is healthy tissue. Widely drain and buttress with well-vascularized tissue.

Potential questions/alternative scenarios

"After placing the left-sided chest tube, you note greenish fluid coming from the chest tube. Does this change your evaluation and/or operative approach?"

Clearly this should raise the suspicion of a diaphragmatic injury and probably gastric or small bowel injury (either from the trauma or from iatrogenic injury from your chest tube placement since stomach or bowel is in the chest). Acute diaphragmatic ruptures can be approached through the abdomen or through the chest. In this scenario, the chest would be ideal since there is now contamination of the pleural space. A low left thoracotomy (6th or 7th intercostal space, imaging can help to determine the optimal entry site) will be needed. The visceral organ perforation is repaired and then returned to the abdomen. Since there has been minimal scarring, primary repair of the diaphragm is usually feasible. There will typically be a rim of diaphragm that remains along the ribs. Horizontal mattress (+/- pledgets, if infected using felt pledgets is not advised) stitches using non-absorbable suture are placed to bring the free edge of the diaphragm to the costal rim of diaphragm. If the defect is large and some of the diaphragm muscle is destroyed, debridement is required and a patch (i.e., PTFE, Gortex, Alloderm) may be needed. A biologic mesh would be ideal the setting of contamination, such as described here. If there were no contamination in the chest, the herniated viscera can be reduced from the abdomen and the repair performed in similar fashion from below. In this scenario, the chest should be washed out and multiple chest tubes left to avoid the late complication of an empyema.

Diaphragmatic injuries are one of the most commonly missed traumatic injuries. These injuries may be small and not easily seen on initial trauma imaging. Ruptures such as these may become symptomatic with time as the intra-abdominal content eventually find their way into the chest. Chronic diaphragmatic ruptures are typically approached from the chest, as reduction of the herniated viscera may require lysing of adhesions or the contents may become incarcerated. The diaphragm also becomes less pliable in the setting of chronic rupture and primary repair may not be accomplished without tension; in which case a patch is needed.

"Soon after arrival in the ED, the patient becomes suddenly hypotensive and unresponsive. The nurses are unable to palpate a pulse."
Although controversial, this is an indication for an ED thoracotomy. Institutional protocols will vary, the basic steps involve a large anterolateral thoracotomy, typically in the 6th ICS. All dissection is done with a scalpel or scissors. Next, the pericardium is opened widely anterior and longitudinal to the phrenic nerve and the heart is delivered into the left chest. The pleura is incised over the distal aorta and a cross-clamp is applied. At this point, cardiac massage can begin as well as damage control or repair of cardiac trauma or lung trauma (refer to Cardiac Trauma).

"After initial evaluation of the patient, he is noted to have only a tangential gunshot wound without penetration into the thorax. However, on CXR, he is noted to have multiple rib fractures and some 'haziness' in the right lung fields. He states that he feels short of breath, but he is oxygenating well. What is your approach to treat him now?"
Do not fall into the trap of the stable patient and jump into your planned chest tube. He should still undergo ABCDE of ATLS. However, he clearly needs a right-sided chest tube to evacuate potential clot.

"On repeat CXR after chest tube placement, he continues to have some 'haziness' in the right hemithorax. What now?"
Confirm that the patient is stable and that the chest tube is functioning properly with tidaling and drainage. If the patient is stable, consider obtaining a CT scan to evaluate for retained hemothorax vs. diffuse pulmonary contusions. If the CT demonstrates retained blood, there are two options. One is to place a second chest tube and the other is to plan for a VATS cleanout once he is stable, usually within 24-48 hours. Either approach is reasonable; however, a second chest tube is often not enough and may not avoid a trip to the operating room. Some data suggest that early VATS offers early time to discharge and less chest tube days than a second chest tube. Early evacuation of hemothoraces is also easier, as the blood/clot is typically still liquified. Delays in evacuating the hemothorax may result in organization of the clot and formation of a pleural rind, which then would require evacuation of the hemothorax as well as a more time-consuming decortication. Particularly in the setting of trauma, retained hemothoraces may become infected, again arguing for early evacuation and washout of the chest.

If there is in fact no retained hemothorax, which can easily be assessed on CT, one must be concerned about pulmonary contusion. Multiple rib fractures should raise the suspicion of underlying pulmonary contusion. Adequate pain control is of paramount importance in the setting of multiple rib fractures to avoid splinting and promote
adequate ventilation. Pain from multiple rib fracture and underlying pulmonary contusion should be treated aggressively with an epidural, intercostal nerve blocks, or a PCA. Judicious

fluid management may be helpful in the setting of pulmonary contusion but may not be prudent in the setting of polytrauma. There should be a low threshold for intubation and mechanical ventilation in the setting of multiple rib fractures and extensive pulmonary contusion, particularly in the setting of flail chest.

"Instead of being shot, the patient was stabbed with a long ice pick. His vitals are otherwise stable, but his CXR demonstrates a small left hemopneumothorax. What is your approach."
ABC's first. Clearly, you do not want to remove the object in the ED. Urgently prep the patient and OR for operative thoracotomy. Dual-lumen ventilation is ideal. Have blood readily available.

"You note the ice pick enters the left chest in the lower axilla and you make a posterolateral thoracotomy. Upon entering the chest, the lung is deflated, and the ice pick traverses the superior segment of the lower lobe and appears to enter the aorta. What is your operative plan?"
Luckily, the situation is controlled, for the most part. Ideally, we should get proximal and distal control of the aorta before removing the ice pick. However, this is not always possible. Another option is to dissect out the lateral aspect of the aorta where the ice pick enters and place a side biting clamp around it. With the side-biter ready to go, remove the ice pick and side-bite the aorta. Remember to give a little heparin as well, if the patient will tolerate it. Then, dissect the adventitia, identify the hole and repair it. This repair may require a few interrupted sutures or a patch. Be sure to have perfusion and circuit in the room in the event there's a need for cardiopulmonary bypass. Cannulation might include distal descending aortic with left atrial for partial bypass or femoral venous and arterial.

"Your assistant removed the ice pick but inadvertently lacerates the aorta. There is torrential bleeding. After occluding the aorta with your hand, you notice that there is a piece of aortic wall on the ice pick and a nearly circumferential hole in the aorta. Now what?"
Again, plan to get proximal and distal control. Then, resect the damaged portion of the aorta and perform a primary repair. Use of cardiopulmonary bypass, circulatory arrest or partial left heart bypass will depend on the location and severity of the injury as well as any associated dissection flap.

"The ends of the aorta will not come together."
Place an interposition graft of Dacron and wash the chest out thoroughly.

Pearls/pitfalls
- Be wary of the "stable patient." Many intrathoracic injuries (tamponade, tension ptx, ongoing hemothorax) will present with a "stable" picture, but decompensation occurs quickly. All thoracic injuries, especially those to "the anterior box" require complete evaluation before declaring the patient stable for observation.
- Do not deviate from ATLS protocols and get side-tracked.
- Operative planning should be done considering all possible scenarios.

Suggested readings
- Bastos R, Baisden CR, Harker L et al. Penetrating thoracic trauma. *Semin Thorac Cardiovasc Surg.* 2008:20:19-25.
- Bastos R, Calhoon JH, Baisden CE. Flail chest and pulmonary contusion. *Semin Thorac Cardiovasc Surg.* 2008:20: 39-45.
- Carpenter AJ. Diagnostic techniques in thoracic trauma. *Semin Thorac Cardiovasc Surg.* 2008:20: 2-5.

108

17. THORACIC OUTLET SYNDROME

Roman V. Petrov, MD, and Kaj H. Johansen, MD

Concept

- Anatomy of thoracic outlet region
- Variants of thoracic outlet syndrome (TOS): neurogenic, venous, arterial
- Clinical presentation and key physical findings
- Workup of patients with TOS
- Non-operative and operative management of different variants of TOS

Chief complaint

"You are seeing a 29-year-old woman who complains of right shoulder and neck pain, occipital headaches, and weakness/numbness of her right arm over the last several months. She is seeking disability benefits and requesting an oxycontin refill."

Differential

Oftentimes patients referred for evaluation of thoracic outlet syndrome (TOS), especially the neurogenic variant, have a long-standing history of symptoms and an extensive, fruitless work-up. As such, this diagnosis frequently is a diagnosis of exclusion. Conditions to differentiate carpal tunnel syndrome, ulnar nerve compression, cervical spine strain, cervical degenerative disk disease/spinal stenosis, brachial plexus injury, fibromyalgia, syringomyelia, polymyalgia rheumatica, structural shoulder injury, compression from tumor (i.e., superior sulcus tumor).

TOS consists of a constellation of symptoms produced by compression of the subclavian vessels and/or the brachial plexus by the musculoskeletal structures of the thoracic outlet. The exact mechanism of compression is not always clear; however, the first rib is almost always involved. For this reason, resection of the first rib for decompression is the surgical treatment of choice in most cases. Three variants of thoracic outlet exist – neurogenic (brachial plexus compression, nTOS – 95%), venous (effort thrombosis, Paget-Schroetter syndrome, vTOS - 5%), and arterial (aTOS – 1%).

Understanding the anatomy of the thoracic outlet is critical for treatment of this patient population. A key anatomic region involved in TOS is the scalene triangle, which is bordered by 1.) *anterior border:* the anterior scalene muscle (ASM) originating from the transverse processes (TP) of C3-C6 and inserting on the first rib 2.) *posterior border:* middle scalene muscle (MSM) originating from TP of C2-C7 inserting on the superior-lateral surface of the first rib posteriorly 3.) *base:* superior border of the first rib. The brachial plexus and subclavian artery pass between the anterior and middle scalene muscle, while the subclavian vein passes anteromedial to the triangle.

The brachial plexus consists of 3 trunks traversing the scalene triangle. These include the upper trunk (C5-C6 roots), middle trunk (C7 root) and the lower trunk (C8-T1 roots). Several additional nerves pass through the scalene triangle – the phrenic nerve (C3-C5 roots) travels on the anterior surface of the ASM from lateral to medial before diving under the subclavian vein and down through the mediastinum toward the diaphragm. The long thoracic nerve (C5-C7) passes through the belly of the MSM as it travels distally toward the serratus anterior muscle. The sympathetic chain travels along the posterior inner surface of the ribs and consists of multiple ganglia.

The subclavian artery, after rising from the upper mediastinum, gives off vertebral, internal mammary and thyrocervical branches before entering the scalene triangle. It then arches over the first rib, anterior to the brachial plexus and posterior to ASM. The subclavian vein passes over the first rib anterior to the ASM, but outside of the scalene triangle, and is prone to compression between ASM, first rib, subclavius muscle, and the clavicle (costoclavicular space). The thoracic duct can be found on the left side where it enters the junction of the subclavian and internal jugular veins. Compression also may take place between the coracoid process, pectoralis minor (PM) tendon, and the chest wall (PM space).

The "classic" anatomy of thoracic outlet is found in less than half of patients and many

109

variations of thoracic outlet region anatomy have been described with additional fibrous bands, muscle structures and bony abnormalities (i.e., cervical ribs). While such anatomic variants are often believed to be predisposing factors, their contribution to symptoms is unclear.

History and physical

A careful review may elicit a history of hyperextension neck trauma (e.g., whiplash). However due to a variable latent period, up to several years between the inciting episode and the appearance of symptoms, a history of trauma can be overlooked. Other conditions predisposing to TOS include repetitive occupational trauma (leads to fibrosis of scalene muscles), bodybuilding (hypertrophy of scalene muscles), poor posture and aging (lead to narrowing of scalene triangle), obesity, pregnancy and others. Clavicular fractures/deformities or a cervical rib can compress thoracic outlet structures and can predispose to TOS as well.

Pain, paresthesia, and weakness are the primary symptoms of nTOS. These symptoms usually affect the arm and hand, most commonly in the ulnar nerve distribution (lower brachial plexus trunk). Extension of the pain to the shoulder, neck, and occipital region is common. Bilateral TOS is not uncommon, although symptoms on one side are usually more prominent. Late, worrisome findings include hand grip weakness and intrinsic hand muscle atrophy.

Physical examination focuses on eliciting symptoms with active and passive range of motion of the arm, neck and head. Degree of disability, such as muscle atrophy and weakness, are assessed as well as sensory abnormalities. Palpation over the scalene triangle may elicit tenderness. Provocative maneuvers include:

- *Elevated arm stress test (EAST)*: arms elevated (surrender positions) repetitive opening and closing of fists elicits typical symptoms.
- *Brachial plexus tension test of Elvey*: arms out, wrists dorsiflexed, tilting of the head produces symptoms on the contralateral side.
- Adson maneuver and Wright test are not useful in diagnosis of nTOS because of their low sensitivity and specificity.

In patients with aTOS, a pulsatile supraclavicular mass or bruit (subclavian aneurysm) and splinter hemorrhages or finger and hand ischemia (signs of distal embolization) should be sought. Axillo-clavicular venous compression and thrombosis (Paget-Schroetter Syndrome or vTOS) may manifest as upper extremity pain, discoloration, and swelling. A prominent net of collateral subcutaneous veins in cases of chronic thrombosis may be present (Urschel's sign).

Tests

nTOS is typically a clinical diagnosis of exclusion and most of the studies are performed to rule out other conditions.

- *Plain radiography, CT, MRI.* Can help identify bony abnormalities, such as spinal stenosis, cervical ribs, disk disease.
- *Electromyography (EMG).* Usually negative due to the intermittent nature of compression but may help to exclude other neurogenic conditions.
- *Ulnar nerve conduction velocity (UNCV).* Has been shown to be useful in nTOS patients and should be obtained in all patients in whom the diagnosis is suspected. Delayed UNCV across the supraclavicular fossa increases the chances that surgical treatment will be needed. Conduction velocities across the median and ulnar nerves are determined at the supraclavicular fossa, mid-upper arm, distal to the elbow, and at the wrist. Normal ulnar nerve velocities at the supraclavicular fossa are > 85 m/s, lower than 55 m/s is considered to be significantly abnormal. Values more distally along the nerve do not have predictive value in the workup of nTOS, but normally are slower as one moves distally down the nerve.
- *Scalene muscle block.* Relief of symptoms with injection of local anesthetic or botulinum toxin into the belly of ASM is highly sensitive and moderately specific for the diagnosis of nTOS and predicts success of surgical decompression.

110

"The patient admits to having progressive symptoms over several months and now has disabling weakness in her right arm. She is employed as a librarian, but is unable to reach for books on upper shelves and frequently drops objects from her hand. She also admits to frequent tension headaches. On physical examination she has decreased sensation in her medial hand and fingers and internal forearm. Hypothenar atrophy is noted. There is tenderness over the right supraclavicular region. EAST and Elvey tests are positive. Chest and C-spine X-rays do not reveal any abnormalities, MRI is negative. UNCV shows ulnar nerve conduction of 65 m/s and EMG studies were normal."

Treatment/management

Initial management for all patients with a confirmed or suspected diagnosis of nTOS consists of physical therapy. This should focus on stretching the scalene muscles, normalizing posture, and strengthening muscle of the shoulder girdle. NSAIDs, muscle relaxants, and non-narcotic analgesics are adjuncts. Progress is reassessed in 4-6 wks. Two-thirds of the patients with nTOS improve with physical therapy and avoid surgical intervention. Most patients with an UNCV of < 60 m/s will require surgery but should be treated with physical therapy first. Failure of conservative therapy is an indication for surgical decompression. Indications for surgical decompression without a trial of physical therapy includes nTOS with motor deficits (compared to sensory only), mixed symptoms (both neurologic and vascular symptoms), and vascular symptoms (arterial and venous TOS are always immediate surgical indications, addressed in scenarios below).

Two main surgical approaches currently employed – transaxillary (best for nTOS and vTOS) and supraclavicular (best for aTOS). A posterior transthoracic approach and a VATS approach have also been described.

Operative steps

Transaxillary approach for first rib resection

Pros: cosmetically hidden incision, easy exposure of the first rib, no traction on the brachial plexus.

Cons: poor exposure of scalene muscles, incomplete brachial plexus neurolysis, inadequate vascular exposure.

- Single lumen ETT, supine position with arm elevated above the head with cushion under the shoulder.
- Transverse incision at axillary hairline between pectoralis major and latissimus dorsi, blunt dissection over chest wall to the apex of the axilla. Watch for the intercostobrachial cutaneous nerve.
- Identify first rib, neurovascular bundle beneath the rib, and ASM insertion.
- Divide ASM over a right-angle clamp near its insertion on the first rib (protect phrenic).
- Expose the first rib in a subperiosteal plane using a periosteal elevator to strip the intercostal muscle off inferiorly (sweep away pleura to avoid a pneumothorax) and middle scalene muscle off posteriorly-superiorly (watch for long thoracic on its posterior margin).
- A wedge of the first rib is taken out of its mid-portion, including the scalene tubercle (insertion site) to aid with retraction.
- The medial remaining first rib (distal rib) is retracted anteriorly and the subclavian vein is swept off its posterior aspect, the costoclavicular ligament is divided, and the rib is separated from its sternal attachment and removed. Additional bands/adhesions are then removed to completely decompress the vein.
- The posterior remaining first rib (proximal rib) is retracted away from its bed and the subclavian artery and brachial plexus are swept off its posterior aspect. Dissection can be carried in the subperiosteal plane all the way back to its articulation with the

transverse process of the first vertebra and the rib disarticulated and removed. Care must be taken to avoid injuring the first thoracic nerve root immediately deep to the rib (avoided by keeping dissection on the rib).

- If the entire rib is not removed, leaving the most distal and proximal extent of the rib in place, the edges of the cut rib should be blunted with a Rongeur forceps. Some advocate removal of the entire rib to prevent future compression by regenerative fibrocartilage.
- Resect any additional fibrous bands crossing the brachial plexus (neurolysis).
- If a cervical rib is present, it should be resected at this time in similar fashion.
- Asses for pneumothorax – consider chest tube.
- Close over JP.

Supraclavicular approach for first rib resection
Pros: wide exposure of all structures, complete scalene resection, complete plexus neurolysis, resection of accessory ribs, obligatory for arterial reconstructions.
Cons: less cosmetic, traction on the plexus during rib resection.

- Single lumen ETT, supine with neck extended or beach-chair position with arm prepped for range of motion during the case.
- Transverse incision two finger breadth above clavicle. Divide omohyoid, reflect scalene fat pad laterally, exposing ASM (phrenic).
- Circumferentially dissect ASM (watch for vein anteriorly, artery and trunks posteriorly and phrenic) and divide with scissors from scalene tubercle.
- Reflect ASM superior and resect off TPs at origin (watch for nerve roots).
- Perform complete neurolysis of brachial plexus, consider Seprafilm or Surgi-Wrap.
- Retract plexus forward and detach MSM from first rib with periosteal elevator (watch for long thoracic).
- Assess residual compression and need for first rib resection by range of motion of the arm.
- Detach intercostal muscle from inferior aspect of the rib with periosteal elevator and after protecting brachial plexus with the finger divide rib posteriorly (watch for pleura, brachial plexus and long thoracic).
- Depress the rib inferiorly and divide just medial to scalene tubercle, posterior to subclavian vein (watch for the vein).
- Smooth cut edges with a rongeur. The first rib may be removed in its entirety as described above, as well. Re-approximate fat pad and close over JP drain.

High posterior thoracoplasty approach for first rib resection
Pros: excellent exposure of nerve roots and brachial plexus, good vascular exposure, good for reoperations.
Cons: larger incision, less cosmetic, uncommon incision/exposure.

- Single lumen ETT, lateral decubitus position.
- Vertical incision between spine and scapula, divide trapezius, rhomboid and posterior serratus.
- Identify and dissect first rib subperiosteally (watch for T1), divide first rib at the neck, rongeur out the head.
- Resect cervical rib, fibrous bands, perform neurolysis, consider Seprafilm or Surgi-Wrap. Perform sympathectomy of T1-3 ganglia (watch for stellate ganglion).

Potential questions/alternative scenarios
"A 48-year-old mechanic presents to the ED with pain in his right hand and numbness that began acutely this morning. You notice that he has an absent pulse and petechiae in the first and second digits. His hand appears dusky and motor function is slightly diminished.

112

He notes a similar episode that resolved about a month ago. He does not have a history of arrhythmias (i.e., AF), diabetes, nor peripheral vascular disease. He does complain of symptoms consistent with arm claudication with repetitive maneuvers. How do you proceed?"

This scenario gives an example of aTOS – post-stenotic aneurysm with distal embolization. Occasionally acute thrombosis or retrograde thrombosis and cerebral embolization develops. Workup includes vascular lab imaging: CT angiography and/or angiography. In acute arterial thrombosis, endovascular restoration with regional thrombolysis or thrombectomy may be possible and should be attempted first. The patient should be anticoagulated after flow has been reestablished. The primary issue (compression of the subclavian artery) can then be addressed more electively. In elective situations, resection of the aneurysm and bypass or interposition graft is used for reconstruction (proximal and distal control, heparinization prior to clamping) following first rib decompression as described above.

"A 28-year-old pitcher presents with acute right arm swelling. He was diagnosed with a subclavian-axillary vein clot on duplex in the ED. How would you manage this patient?"

This is an example of Paget-Schroetter Syndrome, a variant of vTOS. This syndrome typically affects young athletes with excessive/repetitive use of the arm (i.e., pitchers, basketball players, weightlifters). Compression of the subclavian/axillary vein is caused by compression against the first rib by a congenitally, laterally displaced costoclavicular ligament along with a hypertrophied ASM. Diagnose with venous duplex and venogram. Patients should also be worked up for a hypercoagulable state. Initial treatment is with catheter directed thrombolysis (access through basilic vein, cross thrombus with wire and pulse-spray catheter with tPA infusion). After successful thrombolysis, the patient is treated with a heparin bridge and started on Coumadin. Patients with evidence of venous compression should undergo TOS decompression after 3 months of coumadin therapy. Failed thrombolysis is an indication for open thrombectomy and decompression during the same admission versus long-term coumadin therapy if the patient does not wish to have operative intervention.

"Six months after a transaxillary first rib resection, a 55-year-old man with nTOS presents with recurrence of symptoms. How would you manage this situation?"

Recurrent TOS – distinguish true recurrence (initial improvement followed by recurrence – due to scarring) vs. false (lack of initial improvement – inadequate surgery – either wrong diagnosis or wrong procedure (i.e., 2nd rib resection). Thorough workup and imaging for assessment of performed procedure. Start with PT. If repeat surgical intervention deemed to be necessary, the preferred approach is a high posterior thoracoplasty.

Pearls/pitfalls

- No confirmatory studies, clinical diagnosis.
- Don't rush to OR. Treat nTOS with physical therapy first.
- Supraclavicular approach offers better decompression, resect a segment of ASM rather than simply detach it.
- Do not overlook aTOS and vTOS – these are game changers and will push you to OR early.
- Not all patients are drug seekers. With appropriate diagnosis and management most get better and return to work.

Suggested readings

- Osgood MJ and Lum YW. Thoracic Outlet Syndrome: Pathophysiology and Diagnostic Evaluation. Sidawy AN and Perler BA. *Rutherford's Vascular Surgery and Endovascular Therapy* 9th ed.
- Humphries MD and Freischlag JA. Thoracic Outlet Syndrome: Surgical Decompression of the Thoracic Outlet. Sidawy AN and Perler BA. *Rutherford's Vascular Surgery and Endovascular Therapy* 9th ed.

113

18. THORACIC SYMPATHECTOMY

Eric Krause, MD and Whitney Burrows, MD

Concept

- Evaluation of the patient with focal hyperhidrosis
- Evaluation of the patient with refractory electrical storm

Chief Complaint

"A 20-year-old male sophomore in college presents to your clinic with complaints of profuse palmar sweating during the day requiring that he carry a handkerchief with him to wipe his hands. He has trouble in chemistry lab with frequently smudging his lab notebook. He has avoided dating and social interactions due to embarrassment from shaking hands."

Differential

The patient needs to be evaluated for primary vs secondary hyperhidrosis. Primary hyperhidrosis is idiopathic and generally starts early in childhood and is exacerbated in puberty. In contrast to secondary hyperhidrosis, sweating does not occur while asleep. It is generally confined to the face, palms, axilla, and plantar surfaces. Patients can experience symptoms in any one or a combination of these locations. It is likely due to excessive response to both emotional stressors and heat. It has a familial component in 25-50% of the time.

Secondary hyperhidrosis has more generalized symptoms that present in adulthood and whose sweating does occur while asleep. It can be caused by infections, malignancy (lymphoma, pheochromocytoma, etc), hyperthyroidism, menopause, diabetes, and spinal cord injuries causing autonomic dysreflexia.

Primary Focal Hyperhidrosis

Primary focal hyperhidrosis is defined by secretion of sweat in amounts greater than physiologically needed for thermoregulation. The usual presentation is excessive sweating that interferes with patients' quality of life. The incidence of it ranges between 1-3% of the population. It occurs most frequently is hotter climates but can be found in all races and in all climates. It affects men and women equally. Diagnosis relies on the history and physical.

The human body has between 1.5-4 million sweat glands divided into three types: eccrine, apocrine and apoeccrine. Eccrine glands are the most prevalent and are responsible for the sweating of hyperhidrosis. However, the exact pathway that leads to this hyperactivity has not been defined as of this writing. What is known is that they are innervated by the sympathetic nervous system and controlled by the neurotransmitter acetylcholine. In general, the ganglia that innervate the areas of interest for our discussion are T2 for facial blushing/hyperhidrosis, T3 for palmar hyperhidrosis and T4 for axillary hyperhidrosis. The sweat they produce is serous and generally not odorous, unlike the sweat from apocrine glands. The eccrine glands become active at puberty and are controlled by adrenergic nerve fibers. Apoeccrine glands are present in the axilla and are of little importance to this discussion. Overall, the body's sweat glands are unevenly distributed with much higher concentrations on the palms than the back and forehead. On average only 5% of the glands are functional at a time, but when fully active, up to 10L of sweat can be produced per day.

As stated previously, symptoms are generally confined to the face, axilla, palms and plantar surfaces; either in one location or a combination of them. The classic presentation is excessive sweating without provocation in the palms and plantar surfaces of the feet. Uniformly, patients who present for surgical evaluation have experienced severe social and psychological consequences. They, like the index patient, avoid social situations due to fear of shaking hands and embarrassment from sweating through clothing. These fears and problems routinely also complicate the work environment, causing patients even further distress.

Patients will describe severe symptoms of facial blushing, axillary, palmar and plantar sweating that affects both their social and work lives to the point of severe emotional distress. Many patients avoid social interactions due to embarrassment and can also be debilitating at work. Patients will also describe bringing a change of shirt and socks to work with them so they can change throughout the day. Patients should also be questioned for symptoms related to secondary illness including elevated heart rate, weight loss, numbness and loss of motor function.

Since patients with primary idiopathic hyperhidrosis are generally younger, their physical exam is generally normal. A focused physical exam focused on the head, neck, cardiac, pulmonary and abdominal exams should be performed to ensure that the patient can tolerate surgery.

Tests

The diagnosis of hyperhidrosis is mostly made by the history and physical exam and minimal ancillary testing is needed, unless it is to determine if the patient is a candidate for surgery. Patients can be evaluated using both qualitative and quantitative metrics. In terms of quantitative testing, gravimetry can be performed. This involves weighing filter paper before and after exposure to the affected areas. The minor starch-iodine test involves placing iodine and starch on areas in question and waiting for sweat production. A purple color appears wherever sweat is produced.

Because no quantitative test can determine if a patient has focal hyperhidrosis, qualitative metrics are usually performed. According to the International Hyperhidrosis Society guidelines, patients should first be asked if they have experienced at least six months of focal and visible excess sweat production without cause. If yes, then do they have at least two of the following symptoms: bilateral and symmetrical sweating, sweating that impacts the patient's life, at least one episode per week, symptom onset prior to age 25, sweating stops when the patient is asleep and a family history of similar symptoms. The Hyperhidrosis Impact Questionnaire (HHIQ) is useful for research, but not clinical application due to its length, 41 questions. The Hyperhidrosis Disease Severity Scale (HDSS) is shorter test that has good correlation between it and the quantitative gravimetry assessment. A score of 3 or 4 indicates severe hyperhidrosis. A 1-point reduction correlates to a 50% decrease in symptoms and a two-point decrease equates to an 80% decrease.

Index scenario (additional information)

The patient says that he is considering leaving school if he cannot achieve better control of his symptoms and that he is willing to try anything to get them under control. He wants to know what you recommend.

Treatment/management

Non-surgical management

Non-surgical management of hyperhidrosis is first line therapy and generally should be attempted prior to surgical evaluation, although some would argue that for severe palmar hyperhidrosis thoracoscopic sympathectomy/sympathicotomy should be first line therapy. Non-surgical treatments can be divided into topical agents, iontophoresis, botulism toxin injections, and anticholinergic agents

- *Topical agents* are first line agents and include aluminum chloride hexahydrate ($AlCl_3$-$6H_2O$) and topical anticholinergic agents (discussed later). Aluminum chloride hexahydrate is both the most common and effective topical agent. It works by physically blocking the eccrine glands, preventing sweating. Most over the counter antiperspirants contain this agent up to 12% concentrations; however, prescription preparations are as high as 35%. The compound is most effective

115

when it is applied at bedtime, allowing it to be in contact with the skin for 6-8 hours uninterrupted. At times, patients use occlusive wraps or gloves to aid in absorption. This cycle is repeated, generally three to seven times a week until euhidrosis is reached. Then treatments continue as a maintenance therapy several times a week as needed. If therapy is stopped, symptoms recur quickly, generally within a week. Because of these limitations it is most commonly used for axillary symptoms. The most common side effect is skin irritation that can lead to over 20% of patients to stop therapy. Concerns that the aluminum can be absorbed through the skin and contribute to Alhziemer's have proven unfounded. However, care should be taken in patients with renal failure who take aluminum hydroxide phosphate binders.

- *Iontophoresis* generally involves submersion of the affected area in submerged water (occasionally with anticholinergic agents included), while electrical current is applied. The mechanism of action for the decrease in sweat excretion is unknown, but it is an FDA approved treatment. Treatments are performed at home three to four times a week for 20 to 30 min until euhidrosis is achieved. After that, maintenance therapy continues every one to four weeks. Side effects are uncommon if used on intact skin but relate to irritation and dryness at the site of treatments. Given the need to submerge the affected area, this treatment is mostly limited to palmar and plantar surfaces, although there is a commercially available device for the underarms.
- *Botulinum toxin* is approved by the FDA for hyperhidrosis. Injections inhibit the release of acetylcholine at the neuromuscular junction and sympathetic cholinergic nerve endings. Euhidrosis is generally achieved within 4 days and lasts between 6 and 19 months, depending on the dose used. When used properly it has a very good safety profile with minimal side effects; however, when used for palmar hyperhidrosis, weakness of the intrinsic hand muscles has been reported.
- Anticholinergic agents can be given either orally or topically. Oral agents include glycopyrrolate and oxybutynin and lead to improvement in the majority of patients, but significant side effects (blurred vision, constipation, headaches, dry mouth and urinary retention) limit their usefulness. Systemic symptoms are occasionally reported when used with iontophoresis.

If non-surgical management fails to control their symptoms and the decision is made to proceed with a sympathectomy, all patients must be trialed on a low dose beta blocker prior to surgery. This is to mimic some of the common side effects of surgery. If patients experience intolerable bradycardia, exercise intolerance, or lethargy this would be a relative contraindication to surgery.

Surgical Interventions
The goal of surgery is to interrupt the sympathetic chain at the appropriate level that corresponds to the patient's symptoms. No uniform consensus exists as to the proper level and extent of interruption that should be performed. Nor is there a consensus as to the proper surgical technique, which includes the following:
- Sympathectomy is the removal or ablation of the ganglion itself along with removal of the chain above and below it.
- Sympathicotomy is the transection of the chain at a specific level, general over the rip head.
- Clipping is similar to sympathicotomy but involves the application of a surgical clip at a specific point without removal or ablation of the chain. The theory is that if patients wish to have the procedure reversed it can be accomplished by the removal of the clips. However, this has only been shown to be effective if removed within the first two weeks. After that, the sympathetic chain has atrophied and the new accessory nerve connections that mediate the compensatory sweating have been formed. At that point the process is irreversible.
- Selective sympathectomy or ramicotomy leaves the sympathetic chain itself intact and removes only the rami communicantes.

Surgical sympathectomy/sympathicotomy historically was performed through open incisions, but now the preferred method is through a thoracoscopic approach using either one or two trocars. The patient is brought to the operating room and intubated either with a single or double lumen tube. They are then placed supine with their arms outstretched and secured to arm boards. They are then positioned either in "beach chair" or steep reverse trendelenburg. If a single trocar technique is performed a 10mm incision is made in the axilla at the level of the hair line and the chest is entered at either the 2nd or 3rd interspace. If two trocars are used, the first 5mm incision is generally in the 4th or 5th interspace in the midclavicular line with the second 5mm incision in the axilla at the hairline.

After entering the chest the proper level/rib must be identified. Three landmarks are used to do this. First is palpation of the first rib using a blunt probe. The first rib also has a characteristic contour that can be visualized. Secondly one can identify the supreme intercostal vasculature, with the vein being the most recognizable, that runs in the first intercostal space. Third, there is a characteristic fat pad that usually overlays the first rib head, slightly obscuring it. After identifying the proper level to be addressed based on the patient's symptoms (T2 for facial blushing, T3 for palmar, T4 for axillary) the parietal pleura is incised lateral to the chain. The chain is then carefully isolated and then interrupted using electrocautery or sharp transection. The key being that the chain must be completely disrupted at the proper level. Some surgeons advocate for multi-level interruptions to ensure disruption of the chain; however, this may lead to more compensatory sweating as a side effect. The surgeon must also investigate the area lateral to the sympathetic chain in order to identify and to ablate any accessory fibers, commonly referred to as *Kuntz* nerves or fibers; these are commonly identified at the second rib level. Failure to address these accessory pathways may be the cause of some surgical failures.

After the chain has been interrupted, the lung is re-expanded. It is not necessary to leave a chest tube in place as the air can be fully evacuated either through the trocars or through a small tube held under water at the field while anesthesia completes multiple Valsalva maneuvers. Then the patient is extubated, and a postoperative chest x-ray is performed. Generally, patients are discharged later that same day.

Side effects are almost unavoidable and to be expected. Patients must be counseled that they will invariably suffer from compensatory sweating that could be worse than their original problem. Compensatory sweating is sweating of areas that were previously dry and are commonly the torso, thighs and legs. The pathogenesis of the compensatory sweating is likely due to abnormal thermoregulation and abnormal feedback following sympathectomy. Further, the overall amount of sweat does not change, rather that it changes its location. Most patients, especially patients who experience palmar-plantar hyperhidrosis, generally tolerate the compensatory sweating well. However, a small percentage have symptoms severe enough to make them regret having surgery. Risk factors for intolerable compensatory sweating include multi-level interruptions, resections above T2 and preoperative axillary symptoms.

The most feared complication is if the upper T1 nerve root is disrupted causing the patient to suffer an ipsilateral Horner's syndrome (miosis, ptosis, anhidrosis). Other complications are no different than for any other VATS procedure.

Alternative Indications for Thoracic Sympathectomy/ Sympathicotomy

Other indications for thoracic sympathectomy/sympathicotomy include Raynaud's, complex regional pain disorders (CRPDs), long QT syndrome, and refractory electrical storm. For all these procedures the conduct of the operation is the same; however, the target level on the sympathetic chain changes based on the indication. For Raynaud's and CRPDs the sympathetic chain is interrupted at the T1 to T3 ganglion. Refractory electrical storm is defined as tachyarrhythmias requiring three or more electrical cardioversions in a 24 hour period and that the tachyarrhythmias are not controlled by correcting reversible causes and maximum antiarrhythmic therapy. These patients can be difficult to treat and should be managed by a multidisciplinary team that includes cardiology, electrophysiology, and cardiothoracic surgery. One emerging treatment option is cardiac denervation to decrease sympathetic tone reaching the heart. This can be accomplished by ethanol and radiofrequency ablations, but thoracic sympathectomy/sympathicotomy has gained favor in the appropriately selected patient. This technique has previously been effective in the treatment and prevention of refractory VT in pediatric and young adult patients with long QT syndrome. While the first thoracoscopic cardiac denervation was performed in 2000, few adult experiences have been published, with the largest case series reporting between 10 and 20 patients. Most of the published reports describe at least bilateral interruption of the T1 ganglion, most with more extensive disruption beyond that. However, at the University of Maryland we have had success with single trocar, left sided only procedures targeted at the caudal half of the T1 ganglion that lies at the first rib level. We only perform a sequential right sided procedure if necessary. The reasoning for the staged approach is that the left sympathetic chain maps as more excitatory to cardiac function than the right sympathetic chain, which, is more inhibitory. This staged approach has been successful in both low EF patients and in patients on VA ECMO. Every patient that has been treated had a reduction in the number of shocks, with approximately 70% not receiving any shocks after the procedure. These results are consistent with other published studies.

Indications for thoracic sympathectomy/sympathicotomy include failed endovascular ablations, inability to perform the procedure (mechanical aortic valve, lack of access), a pronounced adrenergic response by the patient that corresponds to tachyarrhythmias and inability to wean from mechanical circulatory support due to the tachyarrhythmias. If there is doubt as to whether the patient will benefit from the procedure a peripheral block of the sympathetic chain can be performed to simulate cardiac denervation. If the tachyarrhythmias cease for the duration of the block, the patient will likely benefit from surgical intervention. Ideally a temporary Horner's Syndrome would be caused by this procedure to ensure that the sympathetic chain has been appropriately blocked.

No matter the amount of resection, the risk of Horner's syndrome is greatly increased for this indication because the T1 ganglion itself is being targeted. Patients and/or their families should be warned of this increased risk. In our experience, by targeting the lower half of the ganglion, we have had clinical success without any instances of Horner's Syndrome.

Pearls/pitfalls

- Side effects and complications must be explicitly delineated when discussing sympathectomy/sympathicotomy. Side effects such as compensatory sweating is unavoidable and will be experienced by all patients. Complications are rare, but still must be discussed.
- Careful identification of the proper rib and ganglion is imperative in this operation both for success and to avoid Horner's Syndrome.

Suggested readings

- LaPar, Damien. TSRA Review of Cardiothoracic Surgery (2nd Edition) (Kindle Locations 4534-4544). Kindle Edition.
- Grondin, S.C. (2008) Hyperhidrosis, *Thoracic Surgery Clinics*, Vol 18, No 2. (May 2008)
- Wehman B, Mazzeffi M, Chow R, et al. Thoracoscopic Sympathectomy for Refractory Electrical Storm After Coronary Artery Bypass Grafting. *Ann Thorac Surg* 2018 Mar;105(3):e99-e101.
- Okajima K, Kiuchi K, Yokoi K, et al. Efficacy of bilateral thoracoscopic sympathectomy in a patient with catecholaminergic polymorphic ventricular tachycardia. *J Arrhythm.* 2016;32(1):62–66.
- Hofferberth SC, Cecchin F, Loberman D, Fynn-Thompson F. Left thoracoscopic sympathectomy for cardiac denervation in patients with life-threatening ventricular arrhythmias. *J Thorac Cardiovasc Surg* 2014 Jan;147(1):404-9.
- Cerfolio RJ, De Campos JRM, Bryant AS, et al. The Society of Thoracic Surgeons Expert Consensus for the Surgical Treatment of Hyperhidrosis. *Ann Thorac Surg.* 2011;91:1642-8.

19. Thoracic Organ Procurement

Rebecca Phillip, MD, Rajasekhar Malyala, MD, and Suresh Keshavamurthy, MD

Concept

- Heart procurement procedure
- Lung procurement procedure
- Donor criteria for heart procurement and lung procurement
- Management of complications during procurement

PART ONE – Heart procurement

Chief complaint

"Patient recipient is a 65-year-old gentleman with end-stage ischemic dilated cardiomyopathy, who had undergone three-vessel coronary artery bypass grafting ten years prior, suffered a myocardial infarction earlier this year, and since that event has had chronic decompensated heart failure. He has been sustained on 0.25 mcg/kg/min of milrinone infusion and was readmitted for volume overload."

Criteria for viable donor graft

- Donor 50-60 years of age, or younger (donors younger than 16 years of age are not generally used for adult recipients)
- Absence of the following:
  - Prolonged cardiac arrest
  - Prolonged severe hypotension
  - Hemodynamic stability without high dose inotropic support (<20 ug/kg/min of dopamine at the time of procurement)
  - Severe chest trauma with evidence or concern for cardiac injury
  - Pre-existing cardiac disease or vascular disease (coronary artery disease, hypertension, diabetes mellitus, cardiomyopathy, history of sudden cardiac death in first degree relative, cardiac channelopathies, mitochondrial diseases, peripheral arterial disease)
  - Extracerebral malignancy and glioblastoma
  - Septicemia
  - Positive serology for HIV, Hepatitis B, Hepatitis C (although Hepatitis C positive serology may be accepted in higher acuity situations)
  - Intracardiac drug injection or extensive history of smoking, alcohol use, and illicit drug use (cocaine or intravenous administration)

Donor history and physical

"The donor is a 38-year-old woman who was found at home by a friend, unresponsive, after a suspected drug overdose. EMS arrived and found the patient to be in PEA arrest. CPR was initiated and continued for 48 minutes, with subsequent return of spontaneous circulation. Norepinephrine and epinephrine were given to maintain blood pressure. Patient was areflexive on arrival to hospital, subarachnoid hemorrhage was suspected, and the patient was placed on hypothermia protocol and cooled to 36 degrees for 24 hours. The patient remained areflexive and was declared brain dead via clinical exam, transcranial doppler, and cerebral blood flow nuclear study. The patient was confirmed as an organ donor and the family was in support.

The donor had a medical history significant for depression, hypertension, drug-related seizures, migraines, and had a fifteen-year smoking history. She had previously had two cesarean sections, an appendectomy, and cholecystectomy. She had traveled once outside of the country to Mexico.

She was 172cm tall and weighed 104kg, giving her a BMI of 35 and her blood type was A."

Tests

- *Electrocardiogram*
- *Chest radiograph*
- *Arterial blood gases*
- *Labs* (ABO, HIV, HBV, HCV)
- *Pulmonary artery catheter evaluation/CVP*
- *Echocardiogram imaging* (transthoracic and transesophageal, if available)
- *Cardiac catheterization* results (if performed)

Index scenario (additional information)

"Upon arrival to the donor medical facility you introduce yourself and your team to the operating room staff as well as the other procurement teams present, which include a lung procurement team. You request to review the electrocardiogram, echocardiography, and catheterization imaging of the donor patient. Evaluate the morphology of the aortic, mitral and tricuspid valves and any valvular abnormalities; the dimensions of the left ventricle and interventricular septum (septal width larger than 1.5cm would be concerning and may warrant declining the heart). You confirm no obstructive coronary artery lesions. You confirm with the anesthesiologist the donor hemodynamics, inotropic and pressor infusion rates, and the most recent arterial blood gas. You request to see the donor history and physical documents, with results from any recent labs or cultures, including the certification of brain death documents from two sources. You confirm the donor and recipient blood typing and compatibility from two sources. You verify and sign that you have reviewed all the above items and that you are there to procure the heart. You report to your home recipient team that there are no discrepancies or abnormalities with the donor organ thus far. You confirm all of the correct equipment is available by reviewing items with the host OR staff as well as the organ procurement organization staff. Make sure to request and keep available internal defibrillator paddles in case these are needed during manipulation of the heart while procurement is underway.

Operative steps

Evaluation of Donor Heart

- Access is gained through a median sternotomy, performed in the standard fashion.
- A pericardial well is created with three silk stay sutures on the surgeon's side and three on the assistant's side. These can be clamped all three together on each side with a single hemostat, allowing for easy access to the pleura by simply transferring the hemostat across the field, and tenting the pericardium away from the pleura.
- The heart and great vessels are examined for any anatomic abnormalities or traumatic injuries. The heart is evaluated for any signs of atherosclerotic coronary artery disease. It is important to palpate the left main coronary to the left of the main pulmonary artery, the left anterior descending artery, and the right coronary artery. This is done gently by using the pulp of the finger.
- Palpable thrills are assessed, and ventricular contractile function is visually examined. It should be noted if the right atrium is turgid, pink, or dark blue.
- The anatomy of systemic and pulmonary venous drainage is confirmed to rule out any abnormal variants.
- Next, the pleura is entered bluntly on each side, without cautery, to avoid any risk of burn injury to the lung parenchyma. This can be done by the lung team.
- The lung team will then perform visual inspection and palpation of both lungs and recruitment of any atelectatic segments.
- The results of the initial donor organ exam, including donor hemodynamics and inotropic/pressor requirements, as well as the anticipated cross clamp time is then communicated to the recipient team.

Donor Heart Dissection

120

- The aorta is separated from the main pulmonary artery and from the right pulmonary artery. This is to facilitate adequate cross clamp application. A wet umbilical tape is passed around the aorta and secured with a hemostat.
- The superior vena cava is separated from the right pulmonary artery. The superior vena cava is dissected free to the level of the innominate vein.
- A heavy silk ligature is passed on a right-angle clamp around the superior vena cava cephalad to the azygos vein and fixed with a Rummel and hemostat.
- A second heavy silk ligature is passed around the azygos vein. Care must be taken not to damage the upper lobe branch of the right pulmonary artery that lies near the azygos vein.
- The azygos vein can then be ligated but it does not need to be divided, as this may risk injury to this vessel and subsequent hemorrhage.
- The inferior vena cava is looped with a heavy silk tie, fixed to a hemostat. If a liver procurement team is present, the level of division should be agreed upon at this time.
- The posterior pericardium between the superior vena cava and the aorta, and cephalad to the right pulmonary artery, can be incised in order to allow palpation and gentle dissection of the trachea above the carina. This will facilitate tracheal access during subsequent lung resection. Care must be taken not to dislodge the endotracheal tube. In a heart that is irritable or tenuous, this step should be omitted to avoid causing arrhythmias.
- A 4-0 polypropylene horizontal mattress suture is placed in the anterior middle portion of the ascending aorta, leaving enough room distally for cross clamp placement, and fixed with a Rummel and hemostat for future cannula placement.
- A second 4-0 polypropylene purse-string suture is placed at the distal main pulmonary artery, near or at the bifurcation of the main pulmonary artery (this should be 1-2 cm from the pulmonary valve to allow for enough pulmonary artery cuff during cardiac implantation).

Donor Heart Preservation

- At this time the heart procurement team will ensure that all donor organ dissection is complete with the accompanying procurement teams.
- Heparin (30,000 units) is administered via a central venous line. Several minutes should elapse prior to placement of cannulas.
- The plegia lines are flushed and de-aired.
- The cardioplegia (standard cannula) and pulmoplegia (6.5mm metal tip high flow) cannulas are placed, each rummel is tightened, and infusion tubing is connected to the respective cannulas.
- The lung team will administer a bolus of prostaglandin E1 into the main pulmonary artery adjacent to the pulmoplegia cannula.
- A partial occluding clamp is placed on the left atrial appendage, well away from the base, to avoid tearing the tissue or injuring the circumflex coronary artery. A one-centimeter incision is made in the tip of the appendage above the level of the clamp.
- The left atrial appendage clamp can remain in place until just prior to aortic cross clamp application.
- The superior vena cava is ligated by tying the silk ligature or cinching the rummel tightly.
- The inferior vena cava is then vented by hemitransection.
- The left atrium is vented via the tip of the left atrial appendage by removing the clamp that was previously placed.
- The left atrial appendage is the preferred left atrial venting incision when there is a lung procurement team working simultaneously; however, there are several other methods of venting the left atrium which may be better options if only the heart is

being procured, such as venting the left atrium via the interatrial groove. A sucker can be placed through this incision into the left heart to facilitate emptying if needed.

- Confirm ligation of the superior vena cava, partial transection of the inferior vena cava, and removal of the clamp from the left atrial appendage.
- Confirm adequate decompression of the left ventricle.
- Apply the aortic cross-clamp. This should be placed cephalad to the cardioplegia catheter, fully around the aorta, but not encompassing the pulmonary artery which lies beneath.
- Start the infusion of cardioplegia solution such that the root pressure is 60-80mmHg; some surgeons prefer to run it by gravity whereas others recommend transducing the root pressure to accurately measure this. The key is to have a firm aorta below the clamp and a soft and decompressed LV.
- Ice saline slush is applied to the heart for topical cooling.
- A volume of 2 liters of cardioplegia solution is administered to the heart (University of Wisconsin/Celsior/HTK [histidine-tryptophan-ketoglutarate]/Del Nido as per our center's preference). An additional 1 liter of cardioplegia solution can be started in order to continue cardioplegia administration while awaiting the completion of the pulmoplegia solution. This will keep the ascending aorta pressurized and prevent any pulmoplegia solution from entering the coronary arteries. This is also performed if the myocardium appears to be thick and additionally cardioplegia is deemed necessary.
- Confirm rapid arrest of the heart by cessation of any contraction or electrical activity.

Donor Heart Excision

- The inferior vena cava is completely transected, taking care not to injure the right inferior pulmonary vein.
- The superior vena cava and azygous vein are transected below the silk ligature.
- The aorta is then transected at the base of the innominate artery. The aorta can be dissected more distally and divided after the left carotid artery if more length of aortic tissue is required for implantation (in the case of a recipient with an LVAD where the outflow graft is inserted high onto the aorta, if the recipient has an aneurysmal aorta, or in some recipients with congenital defects). Avoid injury to the pulmonary artery at the attachment of the ligamentum arteriosum.
- The main pulmonary artery is divided just proximal to the bifurcation, at the pulmoplegia cannulation site taking care to retain the bifurcation of the PA for the lung team.
- The heart is then lifted, and an incision is made in the posterior left atrium, midway between both pulmonary veins, toward the base of the left atrial appendage, taking care to stay halfway between the left inferior pulmonary vein and coronary sinus.
- A 1 cm cuff of tissue is kept on the left atrium to ensure adequate margin for lung implantation.
- The heart is further elevated, and the rest of the left atrial excision is completed from inside the left atrium. All four pulmonary vein orifices should be visualized with adequate cuff margins retained on both the heart and lung blocks.

Donor Heart Transport

- The heart is removed from the field and submerged in a sterile plastic bag or transport container with cold preservation solution. No ice is placed directly in the container.
- The heart is inspected for any undetected pathology, valvular abnormalities, and a patent foramen ovale. If present, a patent foramen ovale is sutured closed.
- Any iatrogenic injuries are promptly communicated to the implant surgeon.
- The initial sterile bag or container is placed in a second sterile bag and this is filled with sterile ice slush to cover the heart.

122

- The package is then placed in a third sterile bag and covered with sterile ice slush. This is then labeled and placed in an ice chest for transport.
- Any donor pericardium or lymph tissue are placed in the ice chest as well.
- Pertinent documents such as electrocardiogram, echocardiogram report, or cardiac catheterization reports are secured in or on the ice chest. The ice chest is closed securely for transport.
- The recipient heart team is notified that the procurement has been successful. Any further abnormalities are reported. An estimated time of donor arrival is communicated.

Alternative Practices
Venting of the heart

- The *left atrial appendage* can be incised to vent the left heart. This is often an attractive option as it allows great visualization of the drainage and it does not require manipulation of the heart. It is easily visualized even if the pericardial well is filled with blood from drainage and ice slush. However, left atrial appendage tissue is very thin and when venting at this site care must be taken not to tear the appendage down to its base which would risk injury to the circumflex coronary artery, whether through manipulation or by using a rigid vascular clamp. In addition, access through the appendage may not provide adequate drainage and an additional vent site may be required at a point in procurement where it is difficult to access the pulmonary veins or the interatrial groove. Furthermore, the left atrial appendage incision must be repaired/oversewn prior to implantation of the donor graft. This is the only form of venting that is performed when doing a combined heart-lung *en bloc*.
- The *interatrial (Sondergaard's or Waterston's) groove* can be used for venting as well (towards the dome of the left atrium). This method has the advantage of not impacting the left atrial appendage, with no need for later repair. This approach is effective whether or not a lung team is present, although it may require confirmation of the atrial cuff by both teams prior to making the venting incision. It also allows for the venting incision to be extended for completion of the left atrial cuff during excision. This can be done from the patient's right on the surgeon's side without lifting the apex of the heart. Venting through the groove will not risk dynamic occlusion of the incision from the heart itself, as one may encounter when venting through the posterior left atrial wall. However, this site requires some dissection of interatrial groove before cross clamp and more manipulation of the heart, carrying the risk of hemodynamic compromise or atrial fibrillation.
- The *posterior left atrial wall* between the pulmonary veins and the coronary sinus can be incised to vent the left heart. This approach also does not necessitate later appendage repair. A left atrial wall approach should be avoided if there is concomitant lung procurement. In addition, drainage may be difficult after the heart is released, since the heart may obstruct adequate drainage. If poor drainage does occur, a suction cannula may be placed into the incision. However, this will require lifting the heart again during cardioplegia infusion, which should be avoided if possible since it may cause aortic valve insufficiency and interrupt administration of cardioplegia.
- An incision into the *right superior pulmonary vein* may be used to vent the left heart. This can be done from the patient's right side (surgeon's side). This approach may work well when the heart alone is being procured but should not be used if the lungs are also being procured.
- Venting the heart into the *right pleural space* may be performed if the lungs are not being procured. The right pleural space may be entered and during excision the heart can be exsanguinated into the right chest, allowing an emptier pericardium and improved visualization during excision.

Sternal incision

- An alternative to the classic single line sternal incision is a Y-shaped incision that allows the surgeon to begin more inferiorly to the sternal notch so as to leave the upper chest and neck free of scar. This may be beneficial for the donor's eventual viewing and funeral arrangements and should be performed if specially requested.

Azygous vein dissection

- The azygos vein does not need to by be encircled during initial dissection and can be later encircled and ligated during excision. This will minimize the chance of tearing this structure and causing hemorrhage during initial dissection or injuring the upper lobe branch of the right pulmonary artery which lies in close proximity.

Excision in isolated heart transplant

- Pulmonary vein transection of each of the pulmonary veins at the level of the pericardium is preferable.
- Pulmonary artery transection at the right and left pulmonary arteries is preferable.

Donation after cardiac death (DCD)

- DCD procurements are donations of organs from a donor after cessation of all cardiopulmonary function. This may be a patient who has suffered devastating and irreversible injury, who is near death and in whom further treatment is futile, but who does not meet formal brain death criteria.
- The procurement will occur at a time the family has decided to withdraw care. When life sustaining support is withdrawn, support is withdrawn, asystole is pronounced, death is declared, then the organs are immediately procured in the operating room.
    - o Withdrawal of life-sustaining support is planned and performed at a time to facilitate procurement of organs.
    - o After circulation has ceased for a period of several minutes (2-5 depending on local and institutional policies), death is declared.
    - o The donor can be declared in the operating room or can be taken rapidly to the operating room, prepped and draped, and the procurement commences.
- The time from withdrawal of life-sustaining support to cardioplegia administration should be less than 30 minutes for donor heart grafts.
- DCD procurement can most easily be performed when the donor and recipient are in a common location, or alternatively through the use of extracorporeal circulatory support devices.

Potential questions/alternative scenarios
Dysrhythmias during procurement

"You are harvesting a heart from an in-hospital donor patient, an ideal situation! This will allow for ease of communication between yourself and the recipient team, optimized timing for both procedures, and minimal ischemic time. As you begin the dissection of the donor heart the atria begin to fibrillate. You stop dissecting but the arrhythmia does not resolve. The ventricular rate is 142 and the blood pressure begins to fall, systolic blood pressure reaches 80. The anesthesia team asks if you would like to treat this with medication. However, you would prefer if the donor heart did not have medication on board during implantation. You ask for the defibrillator paddles and deliver a synchronized shock which restores normal sinus rhythm."

- *Sinus tachycardia* is the most common arrhythmia reported in during heart procurement and may ensue when there are elevated levels of catecholamines present, the donor is hypotensive, or there is significant anemia. This may also be caused by the use of vasoactive medications. In a young and healthy donor heart some degree of tachycardia may be well tolerated. If tachycardia is compromising heart function or causing hypotension, then it should be addressed. The tachycardia may be treated with

124

short acting beta blocker such as esmolol or labetalol. The donor should be monitored closely as beta blockers can cause hypotension or bronchospasm.

- *Atrial fibrillation* occurs in donor patients and will need to be addressed during procurement. It may be due to physiological stress, especially in a young healthy donor, but may also portend concurrent heart disease and warrants a careful evaluation for any pre-existing heart disease that was missed on initial donor evaluation. Atrial fibrillation may cause decreased cardiac output due to decreased diastolic filling time and loss of atrial kick, as well as clot formation and risk of embolization. Medications such as amiodarone, diltiazem, or esmolol may be administered in order to achieve cardioversion or rate control; however, ideally the donor would not be receiving these medications during implantation. Long-acting beta blockers and digoxin should not be used. If the ventricular response rate is greater than 130 bpm, and this is causing hypotension, then synchronous electrical cardioversion is indicated and is the preferred option.
- *Ventricular fibrillation* can also occur during donor heart procurement and this may be due to physiological stress on the donor or excess manipulation of the heart. Prompt defibrillation with internal defibrillator paddles should be performed.

Left ventricular distention after cross-clamp application
"The heart is vented, and the aortic cross clamp is applied. Cardioplegia and pulmoplegia solution begins to run. Ice slush is placed on the heart and lungs. However, the left ventricle begins to distend. You manually decompress while confirming drainage from the left atrial appendage incision is running clear. However, the ventricle begins to distend again. What do you do?"

- The procuring surgeon must be constantly watching and evaluating for left ventricular distention after the heart is vented, arrested, and the cross-clamp is applied. If the heart does not have adequate drainage, and the left ventricle begins to distend, then the surgeon must act expeditiously to remedy this situation. The left sided vent site should be checked for drainage and a sucker should be placed in the left heart or adjusted. If this does not decompress the left ventricle then the cardioplegia should be stopped, the cross-clamp released, the left ventricle manually decompressed. The cross-clamp can subsequently be reapplied and, if necessary, an additional vent site can be made (in the left atrial appendage or interatrial groove).

PART TWO – Bilateral lung procurement (lungs divided on back table for single lung)
Chief complaint
"Patient recipient is a 28-year-old woman with cystic fibrosis and chronic respiratory failure, a history of bronchopulmonary aspergillosis, with home oxygen requirements of 6L NC, who was admitted after suffering seizures at home and having worsening respiratory distress."
Criteria for viable donor graft
- Donor 55 years of age or younger
- ABO compatibility
- Smoking history less than 20 pack years
- Arterial PO2 >300 mmHg on FiO2 of 100% and PEEP 5cm H2O
- Normal chest radiograph
- Sputum free of bacteria, fungus, significant numbers of white blood cells, on gram stain and fungal stain
- Bronchoscopy showing absence of purulent secretions or signs of aspiration
- Absence of the following:
  - Severe chest trauma with evidence or concern for lung injury
  - Sepsis or aspiration
  - Previous cardiopulmonary surgery
  - Prolonged cardiac arrest
  - Prolonged severe hypotension

125

- o Hemodynamic stability without high dose inotropic support (<15 ug/kg/min of dopamine for 24 hours)
- o Extra-cerebral malignancy and glioblastoma (excluding basal cell carcinoma or squamous cell carcinoma of the skin)
- o Positive serology for HIV, Hepatitis B, Hepatitis C (although Hepatitis C positive serology may be accepted in higher acuity situations)

Donor history and physical

"The donor is a 48-year-old woman who was found by her family, twenty minutes after she went to bed, with a noose around her neck and unresponsive. Her family performed ten minutes of CPR before EMS arrived. Initial rhythm was recorded as asystole. Return of spontaneous circulation was obtained after another 6 minutes of CPR by the emergency response team. On arrival to the ED the patient was hypotensive and unresponsive and was intubated for airway protection. The patient progressed to brain death and was pronounced by clinical exam and apnea test. The patient was confirmed as an organ donor and the family was in support. The donor had a medical history significant for depression and menorrhagia from uterine fibroids. She had no history of smoking, alcohol use, or illicit drug use. She was 163cm tall and weighed 153kg, giving her a BMI of 26 and her blood type was A."

Tests

- *Chest radiograph* and *CT imaging* if available (required if >20 pack-year smoking history, donor age greater than 55 years, or concern for pneumonia)
- *Arterial blood gases*
- *Serologic screening*: HIV, HepB sAg, hepatitis serology, HSV, CMV, RPR
- *Ventilator*: Peak inspiratory pressure less than 30 cmH2O

Index scenario (additional information)

"Upon arrival to the donor medical facility you introduce yourself and your team to the operating room staff as well as the other procurement teams present, which happen to include a heart procurement team. You request to review the chest radiographs and any available computed tomography imaging. You confirm with the anesthesiologist the donor hemodynamics, inotropic/pressor requirements, and the most recent arterial blood gas. You request to see the donor history and physical documents, with results from any recent labs or cultures, including the certification of brain death documents from two sources. You confirm the donor and recipient blood typing and compatibility from two sources. You verify and sign that you have reviewed all the above items and that you are there to procure the lungs. You report to your home recipient team that there are no discrepancies or abnormalities with the donor organ thus far."

Operative steps

Evaluation of Donor Lungs

- Access is gained through a standard median sternotomy.
- A bronchoscopy should be performed while the cardiac team continues opening the chest. This can be done simultaneously to opening, if the lung procurement surgeon is assisting in opening, and there is an additional member of the lung procurement team.
- A pericardial well is created with three silk stay sutures on the surgeon's side and three on the assistant side. These can be clamped all three together on each side with a single hemostat, allowing for easy access to the pleura by simply transferring the hemostat across the field, and tenting the pericardium away from the pleura.
- The pleura is then entered bluntly on each side without cautery to avoid any risk of burn injury to the lung parenchyma.
- The lungs are then visually inspected and palpated. The recruitment of any atelectatic segments is performed by gentle massage. The lungs should not be displaced from the

126

pleural cavity or hyperinflated while attempting to resolve atelectatic segments as this risks injuring the lungs causing hemodynamic compromise.

- The anesthesia team is asked to inflate the lungs and sustain 30cm H2O pressure while time is given to confirm adequate inflation.

- With a small gauge needle and syringe, blood samples are taken from each of the pulmonary veins, being careful not to manipulate the heart too during this process. This final set of blood gases are sent for analysis. The ventilator settings while these samples are drawn must be FiO2 100% and PEEP 5.

- The results of the initial donor organ exam, including donor hemodynamics and inotropic/pressor requirements, arterial blood gases, results of the bronchoscopic exam, as well as the anticipated cross clamp time, is now communicated to the recipient team.

Donor Lung Dissection

- The heart procurement team will dissect free the great vessels

- A 4-0 polypropylene horizontal mattress suture is placed at the distal main pulmonary artery for the pulmoplegia catheter, near or at the bifurcation of the main pulmonary artery (this should be 1-2 cm from the pulmonary valve to allow for enough pulmonary artery cuff during cardiac implantation).

- The tip of the pulmoplegia cannula should be pointed back towards the pulmonary valve (not towards the bifurcation of the artery). This will ensure even distribution of pulmoplegia solution to each lung.

- The posterior pericardium between the superior vena cava and the aorta, and superior to the right pulmonary artery, can be incised in order to allow palpation and gentle dissection of the trachea above the carina. Care must be taken not to dislodge the endotracheal tube. Importantly, the posterior membranous trachea must be handled with care as this tissue is fragile and prone to injury.

- The anterior, lateral, and medial portions of the trachea can be dissected to facilitate easier subsequent resection.

- The fascia between the trachea and the esophagus should be left untouched. This does not need to be dissected at this time and doing so may risk injury to the esophagus or dislodgement of the endotracheal tube.

Donor Lung Preservation

- At this time the heart procurement team will ensure that all donor organ dissection is complete with the accompanying procurement teams.

- Heparin dose of 30,000 units is administered via a central venous line. Several minutes should elapse prior to placement of cannulas.

- During this brief period a final recruitment of atelectatic lung segments can be performed by the anesthesia team.

- The cardioplegia (standard cannula) and pulmoplegia (6.5mm metal tip high flow) cannulas are placed, each Rummel is tightened, and infusion tubing is connected to the respective cannulas.

- The lung team will administer a bolus of prostaglandin E1 into the main pulmonary artery adjacent to the pulmoplegia cannula to initiate lung preservation, this should be done several minutes before the cross-clamp is applied, allowing time for it to circulate. The donor will often become hypotensive after administration of PGE1, and thus all participating teams should be notified prior to its administration.

- Ventilation should be with an FiO2 of 40% and a PEEP of 3-5 cm H2O.

- The cardiac team will begin steps to decompress the heart and apply the aortic cross-clamp. The SVC is ligated, the left atrium is vented, and the IVC is partially transected. The aortic cross-clamp is then applied.

- The cardioplegia solution is now infused. The pulmoplegia solution should be initiated after the heart arrests so as not to cause any distention of the heart via pulmonary venous return.

- The pulmoplegia bag is hung from a high IV hook, ideally 1 meter above the patient, and is infused via gravity pressure. The pulmoplegia, Perfadex (Vitrolife Inc., Englewood, CO) is infused from two large bags (2.8 liters each) until one liter remains in the final bag. During infusion the lungs should be ventilated at half of the normal tidal volumes.

- The anesthesia team is asked to decrease the ventilatory pressure to allow for saline ice slush to be placed in both pleural spaces.

- The surgeon may visualize through the left atrial appendage incision that pulmoplegia solution is returning from all pulmonary veins. This confirms equal perfusion of both lungs. Additionally, both lungs should be visually inspected and blanching of the tissue should be noted to confirm adequate pulmoplegia administration.

- Suction should be utilized to prevent leakage of pulmoplegia through the mitral valve causing distention of the left ventricle. The solution returning through the pulmonary veins should eventually be confirmed to be clear in appearance.

- Continued cardioplegia until the completion of pulmoplegia will maintain aortic root distention and prevent leakage of any amount of pulmoplegia into the coronary arteries.

Donor Lung Excision

- The heart excision is begun. The left atrial incision is made in the posterior left atrial wall, parallel to the atrioventricular groove, toward the base of the left atrial appendage. Taking care to stay halfway between the left inferior pulmonary vein and coronary sinus. The left atrial incision is then extended toward the inferior edge of the inferior vena cava on the right.

- A cuff of tissue, one centimeter from the atrioventricular groove, is kept on the left atrium to ensure adequate margin for cardiac implantation.

- The heart is further elevated, and the rest of the left atrial excision is completed from inside the left atrium. All four pulmonary vein orifices should be visualized with adequate cuff margins retained on both the heart and lung blocks. The heart excision is completed, and the heart is removed from the chest.

- To begin the lung excision, the inferior pulmonary ligaments are carefully divided on both sides. Retracting the lung gently anteriorly will allow for better visualization of the ligament and lower risk of damaging lung parenchyma.

- The pericardium is then divided on both sides, taking care to stay above the phrenic nerve, as this will avoid injury to hilar structures.

- On the right side, the azygous vein must be divided in order to free the right lung. On the left side, the lung is freed up to the aortic arch taking care to avoid injury to the left main bronchus.

- To separate the lungs from the esophagus, it is helpful if the NG tube remains in place, to allow easier handling of the esophagus.

- The pericardium is freed from the diaphragm and reflected superiorly, along with the left atrial cuff and the hilar structures, to access the plane along the anterior surface of the esophagus. The lung bloc is then sharply dissected off of the esophagus, maintaining a plane close to the esophagus, and working from inferior to superior. Note: some institutions will harvest the esophagus and aorta with the lung bloc to facilitate bronchial artery revascularization or as per institutional protocol.

- The inner curvature of the aorta may be left attached to the right pulmonary artery to prevent any damage to the pulmonary artery in trying to dissect it free. In addition, some aortic tissue may remain in the area of the ligamentum arteriosum so as not to injure the pulmonary artery.

128

- The lungs should then be freed from any remaining aortic tissue and arch vessels as well as any other mediastinal tissue.
- Recruitment before tracheal stapling should be at 60% tidal volume (this will prevent barotrauma while transporting the lungs at higher altitudes).
- The endotracheal tube is pulled back, high into the trachea, to facilitate stapling.
- The trachea is divided two finger breadths above the carina, or as high as possible. This is performed with two TIA 30 staple firings in succession (Auto Suture Company Division, United States Surgical Corporation, Norwalk, Connecticut). After the first staple line is fired on the distal trachea with the lungs remaining partially inflated, the endotracheal tube is removed completely, and the proximal staple line is applied. Then the trachea is transected between these staple lines with a fresh scalpel.
- The lung block is dissected free from any remaining mediastinal fascia. The double lung block is removed from the chest cavity and brought to the back table. Here it is placed in a sterile plastic bag filled with Perfadex solution and no ice.
- At this time, the remainder of the pulmoplegia solution is given in a retrograde fashion at the back table. A deflated Foley catheter tip may be fixed to the pulmoplegia tubing so that it may be gently positioned in the pulmonary veins. The total remaining liter of Perfadex solution is given in four approximate 250mL infusions directly into each of the four pulmonary veins. The return of clear solution from the pulmonary arteries should be confirmed. While this solution is given, gentle massage of the corresponding lobe can be performed, to flush any clot in the pulmonary arteries. The burden of clot in each lung may be reported to the implant team.
- The lung block is preferably divided so that right and left lungs are stored separately. This allows for the second lung to remain cold and protected during implantation of the first lung.
- The left atrial cuff and the pulmonary artery cuff are divided in the midline.
- The airway is then isolated, taking care not to disrupt the vascular supply to the trachea and bronchi, and the left main stem bronchus (the longer of the two bronchi) is dissected free.
- The left main stem bronchus is then divided by placing two TIA 30 staple lines, in succession, and transecting the bronchus between the staple lines. This should be done without compromising the carina but still preserving as much of the left mainstem bronchus as possible.
- The lungs are inspected for any missed pathology, surgical damage, and adequate cuff margins. The separated lungs are each placed in their own sterile plastic bags filled with Perfadex solution and no ice. After final examination of the lungs the sterile bag is sealed.
- The initial sterile bag or container is placed in a second sterile bag and this is filled with sterile ice slush to cover the lungs. The package is then placed in a third sterile bag and covered with sterile ice slush. This is then labeled and placed in an ice chest for transport. Any donor lymph tissue is placed in the ice chest as well. Pertinent documents, reports, or any radiographs are secured in or on the ice chest. The ice chest is closed securely for transport.
- The recipient lung team is notified that the procurement has been successful. Any further abnormalities are reported. An estimated time of donor arrival is communicated.

Alternative Practices

Ex vivo lung perfusion (EVLP)

- Donor lungs are placed in a sterile plastic device composed of a ventilator, pump, and filters. The pulmonary artery and left atria are cannulated, and the trachea is intubated. The circuit deoxygenates and filters the perfusate and the ventilator provides oxygen.

This allows for further assessment and monitoring of the lungs as well as protection and optimization.

Donation after cardiac death (DCD)

- Donation of organs from a donor after cessation of all cardiopulmonary function. This may be a patient who has suffered devastating and irreversible injury, who is near death and in whom further treatment is futile, but who does not meet formal brain death criteria.

- The procurement will occur at a time the family has decided to withdraw care. When life sustaining support is withdrawn, support is withdrawn, asystole is pronounced, death is declared, then the organs are immediately procured in the operating room.
    - Withdrawal of life-sustaining support is planned and performed at a time to facilitate procurement of organs.
    - After circulation has ceased for a period of several minutes (2-5 depending on local and institutional policies), death is declared.
    - The donor can be declared in the operating room or can be taken rapidly to the operating room, prepped and draped, and the procurement commences.

- The time from withdrawal of life-sustaining support to cardioplegia administration should be less than 30 minutes for donor lung grafts.

- DCD procurement can most easily be performed when the donor and recipient are in a common location, or alternatively using extracorporeal circulatory support devices.

Potential questions/alternative scenarios

Blood gases are poor upon arrival to procurement site

"On arrival to the donor site you review the latest arterial blood gas sent by the anesthesia team. They report PaO2 being 102 on FiO2 of 40% and PEEP 5."

- You are concerned about this discrepancy, and although the endotracheal tube appears to be correctly positioned above the carina on the last chest radiograph, you want to double check. You decide to perform a bronchoscopy at this time and in doing so note that the endotracheal tube has been inadvertently advanced into the right mainstem bronchus. You ask the anesthesia team to pull the endotracheal tube back. You also have them increase their FiO2 to 100% with PEEP 5 and you recheck arterial blood gases. This sample comes back with PaO2 of 318 and you are reassured that you are able to proceed with procurement.

"The cross-clamp is applied, and you start infusing the pulmoplegia solution. You inspect the lungs and note that the left lung is blanching much more than the right lung. You suspect that the right lung may not be receiving adequate perfusate. You confirm that the pulmoplegia is flowing well and so you suspect it may be due to the cannula position."

- Unequal distribution of pulmoplegia can compromise one lung. A pulmoplegia cannula placed too close to the bifurcation of the pulmonary artery, will usually favor the left main pulmonary artery, and the right lung will get less perfusate. The solution is to continually turn the cannula to the right and left side, thus manually perfusing both evenly. Or, to direct the tip of the cannula back towards the pulmonary valve (valve must be competent) and this will allow equal distribution of the pulmoplegia down the right and left pulmonary arteries.

- You should also add additional ice slush to each lung to further protect the organs.

Pneumonia suspected in donor lungs

"You arrive to the procurement facility and review the donor patient's history and physical documents. The chest radiograph from the previous day does not show any obvious consolidation. On bronchoscopy you find thick and purulent secretions in the right lower lobe that are re-pooling immediately after suctioning."

- In the case of procuring both donor lungs for a double lung implantation, signs of an infectious process can be discovered and subsequently managed after implantation, and

130

thus the donor organ can often still be accepted if the arterial blood gases and further inspection of the lung tissue is not concerning. In the single lung recipient or a tenuous recipient this should not be accepted. If after the pleura is opened and the lungs are inspected, there is poor compliance or obvious consolidation, then the organ should not be accepted.

Adhesions found upon lung inspection

"While performing inspection and palpation of the lungs you note that the left lung has many pleural adhesions to the chest wall."

- When there are minimal adhesions, and they can be easily released without traumatizing the lung during excision, then the donor organ can be accepted. These should be released by staying close to the chest wall, even extrapleural where the adhesions are dense, so that the lung parenchyma is not injured. If the adhesions are extensive then the procurement should be aborted. The procuring surgeon may contact the implanting team to discuss this decision-making process.

Anatomical variants

"When performing bronchoscopy, you are concerned that the anatomy of the right mainstem bronchus is not as expected. You are able to visualize the right upper lobe bronchus prior to the level of the carina."

- You should initially ensure the correct placement of the endotracheal tube. You must orient the bronchoscope to the membranous trachea and confirm the location of the carina. If you visualize the right upper lobe from the trachea, prior to reaching the carina, you must suspect a pig bronchus anatomical variant. You should stop and contact the implanting team at your home institution, since this makes implantation difficult. The bronchial anastomosis is one of the most vulnerable aspects of the implantation operation and can have many complications. A pig bronchus would require more complexity during implantation and may include patching or reimplantation techniques.
- When performing the inspection of the lungs and subsequent excision, any anomalous systemic or pulmonary venous drainage should be noted as this will also create difficulty during implantation.

Unexpected findings

"As you are inspecting the lungs there is an abdominal team proceeding with their procurement operation. An unsuspected tumor is found in the tail of the pancreas."

- This was biopsied and found to be a neuroendocrine tumor. Although these have an indolent course, and good prognosis when resected, the lungs are not accepted.
- Consider these expanded donor criteria:
  - Age >60 years
  - History of malignancy in certain specific cases can be accepted, such as thyroid tumor papillary carcinoma or low grade astrocytoma, if this has been treated and the patient has no evidence of recurrence on imaging.
  - Greater than 20 pack-year smoking history
  - Previous cardiothoracic surgery is no longer a contraindication for accepting donor lungs
  - Serology positive for treatable infections, such as Hepatitis C
  - Donation after death from drowning or hanging. This may cause significant pulmonary edema in the donor organ. If the arterial blood gases prior to procurement are adequate, these donor lungs may still be used, with no increase in complications for the recipient.

PART THREE – Summary
Procurement Checklist
Before Skin Incision

- ❑ Consent for Donation
- ❑ Blood type for donor and recipient, match, two accounts
- ❑ Brain death certification, two accounts
- ❑ Serologies
- ❑ Supplies

Lung
- ❑ Chest radiograph and CT imaging
- ❑ Bronchoscopy
- ❑ Arterial blood gases
- ❑ Ventilator settings of FiO2 100% and PEEP 5
- ❑ Limit IV fluids

Heart
- ❑ Electrocardiogram
- ❑ Echocardiogram
- ❑ Cardiac catheterization
- ❑ Inotropic and pressor requirements

Before Harvesting

Lungs
- ❑ Inspect and palpate for any nodules
- ❑ Selective arterial blood gases drawn from pulmonary veins
- ❑ Evaluation for atelectasis, recoil, and lung compliance
- ❑ Inspection for contusions, consolidations, edema

Heart
- ❑ Inspect for any pericardial effusion
- ❑ Evaluate contractility of the right ventricle and left ventricle
- ❑ Inspect and palpate for any coronary calcification
- ❑ Inspect and palpate for any aortic calcification

Pearls/pitfalls

- Be collaborative, cooperative, and respectful to all teams present during a procurement.
- Determine whether a more cosmetic Y-shaped incision is requested by family, funeral home, or donor organization prior to making incision.
- Determine the agreed upon locations for venting incisions and tissue cuffs among all procurement teams.
- Take care to identify any structural abnormalities of the heart.
- The azygous vein can be tied off, without being fully divided until the time of excision, to prevent any risk of hemorrhage or injury to the first branch of the right pulmonary artery.
- Do not forget to heparinize.
- Decide whether the left atrium will be vented through the interatrial groove or the left atrial appendage, or another site. There are risks and benefits to each method.
- Take care not to back-wall the aorta with the cardioplegia cannula.
- Do not apply the aortic cross-clamp before venting the left heart and ensuring decompression.
- Confirm adequate cardioplegia administration by rapid cessation of contraction and pressurization of the aortic root.
- Confirm adequate decompression of the left ventricle and address any signs of distention immediately by placing a sucker into the left ventricle.
- Ensure adequate cuff of the left atrium for both cardiac and pulmonary procurements.

132

- Ensure adequate cuff of IVC if there is an abdominal organ procurement and stay supradiaphragmatic when dividing this.
- Do not forget to perform a bronchoscopy upon initial assessment of the lungs.
- Identify any anatomic variants or structural abnormalities.
- Assess pulmonary venous saturations to evaluate the lungs.
- Examine the lungs within the chest, without entirely eviscerating them, so as to avoid injury or hemodynamic compromise.
- Do not over-inflate the lungs when attempting to resolve atelectasis.
- Do not divide the trachea and esophagus prior to excision, to avoid injury to either.
- The pulmonary artery cannulation site should be approximately 1.5cm from the pulmonary valve to maintain adequate length of pulmonary cuff and the pulmoplegia cannula tip should be directed towards the pulmonary valve to ensure even perfusion of both lungs.
- Confirm that both lungs blanch when pulmoplegia solution is given.
- When giving retrograde pulmoplegia, confirm that there is adequate return from the ipsilateral pulmonary artery.

Suggested readings

- Pasque MK. Standardizing thoracic organ procurement for transplantation. *J Thorac Cardiovasc Surg.* 2010;139(1):13-7.
- Powner DJ, Allison TA. Cardiac dysrhythmias during donor care. *Prog Transplant.* 2006;16(1):74-80.
- Dorent R, Gandjbakhch E, Goeminne C, et al. Assessment of potential heart donors: A statement from the French heart transplant community. *Arch Cardiovasc Dis.* 2018;111(2):126-139.
- Baran DA, Tallaj J, Hall S. Heart Failure and Transplantation Core Competency Curriculum. Version one, updated. *International Society for Heart and Lung Transplantation.* May 2017.
- Loor G, Shumway S, McCurry K, et al. Process Improvement in Thoracic Donor Organ Procurement: Implementation of a Donor Assessment Checklist. *Ann Thorac Surg.* 2016;102(6):1872-1877.
- Cohn LH, Adams DH. Heart Transplantation. Lung Transplantation and Heart-Lung Transplantation. Chapters 60 and 61. Cardiac Surgery in the Adult, Fifth Edition. 2018.
- Leard L, Dellegren G, Dilling D. Lung Transplantation Core Competency Curriculum. Second edition. *International Society for Heart and Lung Transplantation.* June 2017.
- Orens JB, Boehler A, de Perrot M, et al. A review of lung transplant donor acceptability criteria. *J Heart Lung Transplant.* 2003;22(11):1183-200.
- de Perrot M, Bonser RS, Dark J, et al. Report of the ISHLT Working Group on Primary Lung Graft Dysfunction part III: donor-related risk factors and markers. *J Heart Lung Transplant.* 2005;24(10):1460-7.
- Shigemura N, Bhama J, Nguyen D, et al. Pitfalls in donor lung procurements: how should the procedure be taught to transplant trainees? *J Thorac Cardiovasc Surg.* 2009;138(2):486-90.
- Tane S, Noda, K, Shigemura N. Ex Vivo Lung Perfusion: A Key Tool for Translational Science in the Lungs. *Chest.* 2017;151(6):1220-1228.

20. LUNG TRANSPLANTATION

Nathan Haywood, MD, J. Hunter Mehaffey, MD, MSc, and Alexander S. Krupnick, MD

Concept
- Patient selection and preoperative evaluation
- Single vs. double lung transplant
- Operative technique
- Use of mechanical circulatory support
- Postoperative care
- Potential questions/alternative scenarios
- Pearls/pitfalls

Chief complaint
"A 58-year-old woman with severe COPD is referred for lung transplant evaluation."

Patient selection
General selection criteria include pulmonary diseases that are life-limiting and lack possibility for improvement with medical therapy. Patients should have no medical contraindications, no active infection or malignancy, have adequate nutrition, be motivated to actively take part in the pre and postoperative process, and have an acceptable support system in place.

The most common indication for transplantation is obstructive lung disease (COPD/emphysema, alpha-1-antitrypsin deficiency) 37%, followed by interstitial lung disease (ILD) 30%, bronchiectasis (often related to cystic fibrosis) 19%, pulmonary artery hypertension (PAH) 4%, and other less common indications.

- *COPD/emphysema* – Referred when significantly hypoxic or hypercarbic, FEV-1 <25%, or have signs of secondary pulmonary hypertension

- *ILD* – Referred when significant hypoxia with minimal exertion, FVC <60%, DLCO <60%, or either drop by 10% over 6 months

- *Bronchiectasis* – Referred when hypercarbic, hypoxic with O2 dependence, FEV1 <30%, or frequent hospitalization

- *PAH* – Referred when RA pressure > 15 mmHg, failed pulmonary vasodilator therapy, declining exercise capacity

Contraindications to transplantation include uncompensated end organ failure (heart, kidney, liver, etc.) without opportunity for recovery, active malignancy, active substance addiction, and chronic active HBV/HCV/HIV.

Preoperative evaluation – Recipient
Any patient referred for lung transplantation needs to have comprehensive systems-based history and physical to identify past medical, surgical, and family history. A comprehensive exposure history, sensitization history, and substance abuse history (including smoking) should also be obtained.

In addition to surgical evaluation, patients require preoperative evaluation by transplant pulmonology as well as comprehensive psychosocial evaluation.

Patients referred for evaluation undergo additional extensive workup including comprehensive laboratory evaluation and testing to rule out additional comorbidity that would preclude transplantation.

Upon listing, patients are ordered according to the Lung Allocation Score (LAS), which is a complex scoring system that considers severity and usual time course of disease as well as probability of survival with and without transplant.

Preoperative evaluation – Donor

Brain dead (DBD) donors and cardiac death (DCD) donors have comparable outcomes. However, DBD donation is far more common. Potential donors undergo extensive evaluation. Acceptable findings include the following:

- ABO compatible and acceptable viral serology profile.
- CXR without significant infiltrate
- ABG with PaO2 >300 (with ventilator settings of FiO2 1.0 and PEEP 5)
- Lung size assessment with appropriate size match
- Bronchoscopy without sign of significant secretion burden or aspiration. Culture obtained with bronchoscopy

The use of ex vivo lung perfusion (EVLP) has emerged to increase utilization of marginal grafts especially from DCD donors. Basic tenants of EVLP include antegrade flushing with perfusate (i.e., Steen solution) at a max rate of 40% of cardiac output, gradual warming to 32° C, protective ventilation strategy, and intermittent recruitment maneuvers. It is initiated following routine procurement (see below) and a period of cold preservation. A benefit is that it allows for sequential perfusate gasses to evaluate for improvement in lung function. In addition to the EVLP method initially described in Toronto, the Transmedics Organ Care System™ is an FDA-approved and commonly utilized method. Normothermic lung perfusion is followed by cold preservation prior to implantation.

Unilateral vs. Bilateral

The majority of lung transplants are bilateral. The advantages of unilateral lung transplantation include shorter operative duration, and increased impact from donation (1 donor, 2 recipients). While no randomized controlled trials have been carried out, long-term survival appears to be superior with bilateral transplant. Ideal candidates for unilateral transplantation include older patients with interstitial lung disease, especially if there is a notable difference in function between lungs. Unilateral transplantation is contraindicated for patients with suppurative disease such as cystic fibrosis or bronchiectasis.

Index scenario (additional information)

"The patient has a remote 50 pack year history of smoking. Her FEV-1 is 25% of predicted and ABG revealed hypercarbia with PaCO2 of 55 mmHg. She does not have signs of additional uncompensated organ failure and has had recent negative lung cancer screening. She is listed for lung transplantation.
Two months following listing, an acceptable DBD donor became available. The patient accepted the offer for bilateral lung transplantation. "

Operative steps

Donor (please refer to Chapter 19 on Thoracic Organ Procurement for operative steps)

- Upon arrival at the implant center on back table, remove esophagus and aorta, separate lungs by dividing left atrium between PV orifices, PA at bifurcation, divide bilateral bronchi close to carina with fresh 15 blade. Prior to implantation, shorten donor bronchial length to one ring proximal to upper lobe takeoff to decrease risk of ischemic complication.

Recipient

- Communicate with anesthesia and OR staff to ensure double lumen ET tube, availability of TEE and bronchoscopy
- Perform bilateral anterolateral thoracotomy (if bilateral). Traditionally enter chest in 4th intercostal space but with ILD and small chest cavity 3rd intercostal space may be preferred. Ligate and divide bilateral internal mammary arteries. Perform clamshell

135

incision if heart operation at same time, significant cardiomegaly, or small chest cavity size limiting exposure

- Start with pneumonectomy of lung with worse function (contralateral lung on single lung ventilation)
- Perform pleural adhesiolysis with meticulous hemostasis
- Identify and protect critical structures including phrenic, vagus, and recurrent laryngeal nerve
- Divide PA using vascular stapler distal to truncus anterior branch on right and distal to branch to left upper lobe on left
- Divide pulmonary veins using vascular stapler at secondary branch points after it is mobilized from the pericardium
- Divide peribronchial tissue and sharply divide bronchus proximal to branch to upper lobe – it is important to resect any ischemic-appearing portion
- Remove lung
- Bring donor lung onto field and keep cool
- Perform end-to-end bronchial anastomosis with running 4-0 PDS using one suture for the membranous and one for the cartilaginous portion to ensure airtight anastomosis
- Either ensure adequate peribronchial tissue at site of anastomosis or wrap with well-vascularized tissue flap (pericardium or omentum)
- Place Satinsky clamp on proximal PA, trim staple line, and perform arterial anastomosis with running 5-0 proline
- Clamp left atrium and amputate recipient pulmonary vein stumps to create atriotomy cuff
- Perform pulmonary vein anastomosis with running 4-0 proline apposing intima to intima to exclude any atrial muscle
- Flush air prior to completing venous anastomosis by partially inflating lung and momentarily releasing the PA clamp
- Complete venous anastomosis
- Repeat above for contralateral lung
- Deflate lungs sequentially and assess for hemostasis
- Place bilateral large bore chest tubes, close sternum (if clamshell) with sternal wires, re-approximate ribs and close chest wall in layers
- Exchange double lumen for single lumen endotracheal tube and perform bronchoscopy to evaluate anastomoses
- Transfer to ICU

Adjunctive mechanical circulatory support

Some centers perform bilateral transplantation with intraoperative ECMO support. The use of ECMO instead of full cardiopulmonary bypass (CPB) allows for lower heparin use (50U/kg) and ACTs ranging from 180-200 secs. However, selective use of bypass or use of full CPB for lung transplantation is advocated at many centers with equivocal data.

Postoperative care

Patients are initially transferred to the cardiac and thoracic surgery ICU where multidisciplinary care is provided by the surgical, intensive care, and transplant pulmonology teams. Ventilator weaning strategy is initiated with care to limit significant barotrauma. Aggressive diuresis is performed over the first 48 hours to mitigate pulmonary edema. Initial strategies for immunosuppression often include induction with antilymphocyte/antithymocyte globulin or novel monoclonal antibody. Maintenance immunosuppression is accomplished with some combination of calcineurin inhibitor (tacrolimus, cyclosporine), cell cycle inhibitors (azathioprine, mycophenolate), and steroids.

Potential questions/alternative scenarios

136

"A 25-year-old DBD donor becomes available with best PaO2 of 290 mmHg, right-sided infiltrate on CXR, and moderate secretion burden. Are there strategies to improve and increase utilization of marginal lung donors?"

There is a relatively high rate of marginal lung function in available donors, which historically, has limited lung utilization to about 15-20% of available donors. One strategy to increase the use of marginal grafts is to initiate ECMO prior to implantation and have a low threshold to continue postoperatively to give the marginal lung time to recover. For marginal grafts from DCD donor, consider use of EVLP or Transmedics OCS™ (see above).

"A 22-year-old HCV positive donor becomes available. Is HCV positive to negative lung transplantation performed?"

The advent of antiviral agents directed against Hepatitis C has allowed the possibility of HCV positive to negative lung transplantation. Recipients are started on a four-week antiviral regimen hours after transplantation. Early studies have shown this strategy is effective at inducing sustained virologic response and reported cure rates are 100%. Thus the use of Hepatitis C donors is becoming routine in many centers.

"During procurement of a 22-year-old female DBD donor following drug overdose, you notice a right tracheal upper lobe (porcine) bronchus. What should you do?"

This represents the most common congenital bronchial anomaly. If it is a segmental bronchus, it can be oversewn. If the anomaly is a lobar bronchus, a donor lobectomy may be performed. Additionally, a modified anastomosis using secondary bronchus, right upper aberrant bronchus, and recipient bronchus can be attempted.

"On the backtable prior to bilateral lung transplantation for a 60-year-old male with COPD, you notice that the left pulmonary veins are completely separated without any associated atrial cuff. There is also a 0.5 cm defect in the right pulmonary artery 1 cm distal to where it was divided. What are some strategies to deal with poorly procured grafts?"

Pulmonary veins procured with inadequate cuff can cause significant anastomotic complications following implantation including bleeding. There are strategies for reconstruction using donor pericardium. If the pulmonary veins are connected but do not have enough atrial cuff to perform anastomosis, donor pericardial patch may be used to increase the size of the cuff. If the pulmonary veins are completely separate, vein intima can be circumferentially sutured to surrounding pericardium and the pericardium may be trimmed to create a new cuff. If there is a size discrepancy between veins (ie. injury at segmental level of superior vein), excess donor pulmonary artery may be used for reconstruction.

Pulmonary artery injuries are more common on the right side, which is usually inconsequential given the length of pulmonary artery on this side. In the above example it is likely that this portion of the artery will be trimmed prior to implantation. For more proximal hilar injuries, depending on the size of the defect, primary repair may be performed, or patch reconstruction may be performed with donor pericardium.

"Upon completing bronchial, arterial, and venous anastomoses during a unilateral lung transplantation for a 55-year-old female with ILD, you notice that the grafts are quite large compared to the recipient chest cavity. How do you downsize oversized grafts?"

This represents a case of poor size matching. If unrecognized, oversized grafts can cause significant complication following chest closure due to increased intrathoracic pressure, decreased venous return, and decreased cardiac output. Ideally, a size mismatch would be recognized prior to implantation and lobectomy could be performed on the back table. However, wedge resection of the lingula or right middle lobe with a stapling device may be performed if recognized following implantation.

"36 hours following bilateral lung transplantation for a 30-year-old male with CF, increased bilateral infiltrates are present on am CXR and ABG analysis reveals PaO2/FiO2 ratio of 250. What is the most likely diagnosis and how can it be treated?"

137

This patient is most likely experiencing primary graft dysfunction (PGD), which occurs in about 25% of lung transplants and is the main contributor to perioperative mortality. See the ISHLT grading system below:

- Grade 0 – PaO2/FiO2 ratio >300 without infiltrates on CXR
- Grade 1 – PaO2/FiO2 ratio >300 with infiltrates on CXR
- Grade 2 – PaO2/FiO2 ratio 200-300 with infiltrates on CXR
- Grade 3 – PaO2/FiO2 ratio <200 with infiltrates on CXR

The above patient has grade 2 PGD. The development of PGD is thought to most commonly be due to ischemia-reperfusion injury and the resulting inflammatory cascade. Treatment strategies include ICU level care with aggressive diuresis, lung protective ventilation, and inhaled vasodilators. Our institution currently has a trial underway to examine the use of A2A adenosine receptor agonist in lung transplant recipients to ameliorate ischemia-reperfusion injury.

"2 months following bilateral lung transplantation for COPD, a 53-year-old female presents to clinic with recent low-grade fever and shortness of breath. Laboratory analysis is significant for hypoxemia and leukocytosis. She is admitted and imaging shows bilateral infiltrates. She is pan-cultured, and no source of infection is identified. What is the most likely diagnosis? What do you need to confirm the diagnosis?"

The patient is most likely experiencing an episode of acute rejection, which can present similar to infection with fever, hypoxemia, and infiltrates on imaging. Bronchoscopy with transbronchial biopsy is recommended to confirm diagnosis and further rule out infection. Histologic findings suggestive of acute rejection include peribronchial macrophage and lymphocyte infiltration. Hallmarks of treatment include course of pulsed dose steroids with subsequent taper. Acute rejection rarely causes mortality. However, it is significantly associated with the future development of chronic rejection (bronchiolitis obliterans – irreversible scarring of terminal airways). In addition to cellular rejection the entity of acute antibody mediated rejection can occur due to preformed anti-donor antibodies. This diagnosis can be secured by biopsy and rising anti-donor antibodies detected by Luminex panel. The treatment involves B cell depletion through the use of Rituximab and plasmaphoresis to remove preformed antibodies.

Pearls/pitfalls

- Comprehensive preoperative workup including psychosocial assessment is necessary to evaluate patient candidacy
- Potential donors undergo extensive workup to evaluate for any precluding factors. EVLP can be performed to increase use of marginal grafts
- While bilateral transplantation is more common, ideal candidates for unilateral transplantation include older patients with interstitial lung disease, especially if there is a notable difference in function between the two lungs
- During procurement, ensure adequate atrial cuff around pulmonary veins. On back table, trim bronchus to one ring proximal to upper lobe take off to decrease risk of ischemic complication (relies on collateral circulation from PA).
- Poorly procured pulmonary vein/cuff and artery can be repaired with donor pericardium or excess donor pulmonary artery
- Start recipient pneumonectomy on the side with worse lung function. Routine use of ECMO during lung transplantation vs. selective cardiopulmonary bypass used for patients unable to tolerate single lung ventilation, refractory hypoxemia, significant pulmonary hypertension, and poor or difficult exposure
- Following bronchial anastomosis, ensure adequate peribronchial tissue coverage or cover with pericardium or omentum.
- PGD is the most common cause of perioperative mortality and should be treated aggressively with diuresis, lung protective ventilation, and inhaled vasodilators.

- Acute rejection is diagnosed with transbronchial biopsy. Steroids are mainstay of treatment. The risk of chronic rejection (bronchiolitis obliterans) is increased following an episode of acute rejection.

Suggested readings

- Brown LM, Puri V, Patterson GA. Lung Transplantation. Chapter 14. Sellke FW, del Nido PJ, Swanson SJ (Eds.). *Sabiston & Spencer: Surgery of the Chest.* 9th Edition 2016.
- Camp PC, Mentzer SJ. Overview of Lung Transplantation with Anatomy and Pathophysiology. Chapter 108. Sugarbaker DJ, et al. (Eds.) *Adult Chest Surgery.* 2nd Edition 2015.
- Bharat A, Patterson GA. Lung Transplant Technique. Chapter 109. Sugarbaker DJ, et al. (Eds.) *Adult Chest Surgery.* 2nd Edition 2015.
- Hayanga JWA, D'Cunha J. The surgical technique of bilateral sequential lung transplantation. *J Thorac Dis.* 6:1063-1069, 2014.
- Puri V, Patterson GA, Meyers BF. Single versus bilateral lung transplantation: do guidelines exist? *Thorac surg clin.* 25:47-54, 2015.
- Woolley AE, Singh SK, Goldberg HJ, Mallidi HR, Givertz MM, Mehra MR, et al. Heart and Lung Transplants from HCV-Infected Donors to Uninfected Recipients. *N Engl J Med.* 380(17):1606-1617, 2019.

21. ESOPHAGEAL CANCER

Anthony B. Mozer MD, MBA and David D. Odell MD, MSc

Adapted from 1st edition chapter written by Ryan A. Macke, MD, Roman V. Petrov, MD, and Manisha Shende, MD

Concept

- Understand the workup of esophageal cancer, including diagnosis and appropriate staging studies
- Understand the TNM staging system and treatment of early/late stage esophageal cancer
- Understand the indications for surgery, chemotherapy, radiation, and multimodal therapy
- Be aware of the multiple techniques used for esophagectomy, the key steps, and the pros/cons of each
- Understand the treatment of intraoperative and postoperative complications associated with esophagectomy
- Understand the role of the thoracic surgeon in palliation of esophageal cancer

Chief complaint

"You are referred a 63-year-old obese, white man with complaints of progressive dysphagia to solids and a 35-pound weight loss over the last 3 months."

Differential

The differential for dysphagia and weight loss is broad and should include a number of esophageal diseases including: esophageal cancer, esophageal motility disorder, GERD/peptic stricture, paraesophageal hernia, esophageal diverticulum, benign obstructing esophageal tumor (leiomyoma), and obstruction from external compression (aortic aneurysm, fibrosing mediastinitis).

History and physical

Most, but not all, patients presenting with symptoms of dysphagia and weight loss due to esophageal cancer will have locally advanced or systemic disease resulting in obstruction and inadequate oral intake. A complete physical exam should be performed focusing on lymph node basins that would be outside the routine field of resection (cervical, clavicular, and axillary), evidence of other distant disease (pleural or pericardial effusions, ascites, jaundice, headache or other focal neurologic symptoms), and signs of malnutrition. Important information obtained in a thorough history includes weight loss, smoking and alcohol use, long-standing GERD, Barrett's esophagus with or without dysplasia, hiatal hernia, regurgitation, hematemesis, dysphagia, odynophagia, and melena. The history and physical will give the surgeon an idea of histology (squamous versus adenocarcinoma), extent of disease, and functional status for surgical candidacy; however, much of the pertinent information needed for decision-making will be obtained in the diagnostic workup.

Tests

Work up of patients with suspected esophageal cancer includes a comprehensive constellation of imaging and invasive tests to establish the diagnosis, appropriately stage the disease, and assess for resectability.

- *Barium swallow.* Typically recommended as the initial study for evaluation of any patient with dysphagia. Most importantly, it will identify the location and extent of an obstructing lesion that may complicate upper endoscopy or endoscopic ultrasound (EUS) and provide help to make the diagnosis of other structural and functional disorders such as dysmotility, reflux, and hiatal hernia.

- *Upper endoscopy.* Provides direct assessment of the lesion and facilitates tissue biopsy to confirm the diagnosis. 6-8 biopsies of any suspicious or obstructing lesions should be performed to assess for malignancy. Anatomic landmarks should be assessed and documented including distances from incisors to cricopharyngeus/upper esophageal sphincter (~15cm), aortic arch (~25cm) and lower esophageal sphincter (~40cm). The location, length, extent of circumferential involvement, and degree of obstruction of Barrett's esophagus and tumor should also be documented for operative planning. A pediatric endoscope should be available for large, obstructing lesions. Fit patients with tumors at least 5 cm from the cricopharyngeus should be considered for resection, while cervical tumors < 5 cm from the cricopharyngeus are treated with definitive chemoradiation.

- *PET/CT.* Accuracy in excess of 90% for determining distant disease. CT alone may be used for this purpose but is less accurate and in the current era is rarely used alone for preoperative staging. May be limited in evaluation of regional nodal disease, as the lymph nodes may be "outshined" by the primary lesion. PET/CT is not sensitive for T staging and is limited in evaluation of brain metastases due to the high FDG-avidity of the brain.

- *EUS.* Serves as an adjunct to upper endoscopy and is the best available clinical tool for T and N staging. FNA of suspicious lymph nodes (short axis > 1 cm, round, hypoechoic) can be performed to confirm nodal disease by cytology. Large, obstructing tumors may not permit passage of the larger EUS scope. Rather than risk perforation, it is probably safest to omit the EUS when the scope cannot be passed easily beyond the lesion or attempt passage with a pediatric scope.

- *Bronchoscopy.* Should be performed at the time of resection in all patients with respiratory symptoms, all upper and mid-esophageal tumors, and squamous cell cancers (more likely to have transmural penetration and invasion into adjacent structures) to rule out airway invasion.

- *CT/MRI brain.* Only used if patient has focal neurologic symptoms to rule out brain metastases.

- *Physiologic testing.* Should include cardiac risk stratification (EKG, stress test), pulmonary function testing, and other tests based on patient comorbidities to assess candidacy for resection.

- *Laparoscopic staging and feeding access.* Although invasive, laparoscopy and/or thoracoscopy allows for visual assessment and tissue biopsy of lymph node basins to exclude occult distant malignancy, and should be considered for advanced tumors (T3, N+ disease). Laparoscopy is more accurate at confirming suspected celiac nodal disease than conventional imaging and facilitates preoperative enteral access by feeding jejunostomy placement, which is routinely practiced palliating dysphagia, overcome malnutrition, and offset the effects of induction therapy. Gastrostomy tube placement should be avoided due to compromise of the blood supply to the gastric conduit. Although there is minimal randomized trial data, ischemic preconditioning of the gastric conduit by arterial ligation or embolization is practiced by some groups but has not been shown to reduce anastomotic leak rates.

Index scenario (additional information)

"Barium swallow shows a partially obstructing distal esophageal mass. EGD shows a lesion located at the GEJ 40 cm from the incisors with proximal extension of BE to 38 cm. There is 1 cm of extension onto the cardia. Biopsy proves this to be a moderately differentiated adenocarcinoma. The lesion invades the muscularis propria only on EUS and there is no evidence of suspicious lymph nodes or distant disease on CT, PET/CT, or EUS. The patient is otherwise healthy. What is this patient's clinical stage and how would you manage this patient?"

Esophageal cancer is the 6th most frequent cause of cancer-related deaths worldwide, with a rising incidence in adenocarcinoma associated with the obesity epidemic. It is estimated that 30-40% of patients diagnosed with esophageal cancer will be resectable at the time of

141

presentation. Surgery provides the best local control and chance for cure. However, roughly 75% of patients recur distally following resection, suggesting the presence of occult distant disease at the time of diagnosis. As such, treatment of esophageal cancer typically requires a multimodal approach with chemotherapy and radiation therapy playing an important role, and all patients should be assessed for

surgical candidacy with a thorough review of comorbidities and physiologic workup.

Patients with high-grade dysplasia (HGD) or early, low grade esophageal adenocarcinoma limited to the lamina propria, muscularis mucosa and selected involvement in the superficial submucosa (cT1a/T1b, N0, M0) are preferentially treated with endoscopic mucosal resection (EMR), although an approximate 25% risk of occult nodal metastases has been reported for clinical T1bN0 disease. Ablative therapy is then used to eradicate any residual Barrett's metaplasia. Eligibility for primary endoscopic therapy in squamous cell carcinoma is limited to Tis and T1a tumors.

Patients with low-risk squamous or adenocarcinoma (cT1b-cT2, N0, < 2cm, well-differentiated) are recommended to undergo esophagectomy as primary therapy. Indications for neoadjuvant therapy, the modalities and dosages vary considerably between centers. While some centers favor chemotherapy alone to avoid radiation fibrosis, concurrent neoadjuvant chemoradiation has been shown by randomized controlled trial data to confer a survival benefit in patients with locally advanced squamous and adenocarcinoma (cT1b-cT2, N+ or cT3-T4a).

Adjuvant treatment with CRT or chemotherapy alone is indicated for patients who are found to have node-positive disease or are pathologically upstaged after resection. Postoperative radiation therapy risks damage to conduit blood supply and is discouraged at some, but not all, centers.

Commonly used first-line chemotherapy regimens include: Cisplatin (or Oxaliplatin) + 5-FU, Epirubicin + Cisplatin + 5-FU, and Paclitaxel + Carboplatin. Trastuzumab may be added in cases with overexpression of Her2-neu mutation. The dose of radiation varies from center to center, however 50 Gy is an accepted dose in the definitive, preoperative, postoperative, or palliative setting with patients receiving approximately 2 Gy/day, 5 days/week, for 5 weeks. It is not uncommon for patients receiving definitive CRT to be treated with higher doses (up to 60 Gy).

Once the patient has been cleared for surgery, three important decisions need to be made: choice of conduit, route of conduit, and surgical approach.

A gastric conduit supplied by the right gastroepiploic arcade is the conduit of choice in most centers, providing adequate length for an intrathoracic or cervical anastomosis and requiring only one anastomosis. Selective angiography of the celiac vessels should be performed in patients with prior gastric resection to assess the gastroepiploic arcade. Colon is the next best conduit in cases where the stomach is not usable due to distal tumor extension or disrupted gastroepiploic blood supply. The colon blood supply should be assessed with a CTA or mesenteric angiography and colonoscopy should be performed preoperatively to plan for colon interposition. The left colon, based off the ascending branch of the left colic artery, is most commonly used and provides a conduit with good length and matching diameter to the proximal esophagus. Disadvantages include need for multiple anastomoses (esophagocolic, gastrocolic, and colocolonic) and the tendency for conduit dilation in the long-term. While pedicled jejunum affords limited mobility for length, it is the conduit of choice in cases with extensive gastric but only distal esophageal involvement, where a total gastrectomy obviates the ability to perform gastric pullup and a roux-en-y esophagojejunostomy is performed. If the conduit is needed to reach the neck, the jejunum may be used as a free graft (supercharged jejunum), requiring microvascular techniques for the vascular anastomoses to cervical vessels. This technique is used in a few specialized centers and unless one is familiar with these techniques, it is probably unwise to mention during an examination.

142

Options for passage of the conduit include posterior mediastinal (native bed), substernal, transpleural, and subcutaneous routes. The posterior mediastinal route is the shortest and preferred path to reach the proximal esophagus for anastomosis and is used for immediate reconstruction. The substernal route is a longer route but is useful for delayed reconstruction when the native bed has been obliterated, such as occurs following esophageal exclusion. The transpleural and subcutaneous routes are rarely used.

Proximal and mid-esophageal tumors require transection of the esophagus high in the chest to obtain an adequate margin (ideally 5 cm from the primary tumor), necessitating a cervical anastomosis. It is also critical to note and resect beyond the proximal extent of any Barrett's esophagus, although a lengthy margin is not required. Although the extent and location does influence the surgical approach, outcomes are most impacted by one's own comfort based on operative experience. A *brief* description of some of the more commonly used esophagectomy approaches follows, along with pertinent pros and cons of each. Review of the anastomotic techniques commonly used is beyond the scope of this chapter, but it is recommended that the reader become familiar with at least one technique to articulate on examinations. Studies have failed to show an advantage in survival when comparing these different approaches. Intraoperative assessment of conduit blood supply has traditionally been based on surgical judgment, with one strategy being early tubularization or transection of the gastric conduit in pull-up cases to afford adequate observation time for tissue ischemia. Fluorescent perfusion-based imaging with indocyanine green (ICG) is a valuable adjunct available in some centers; however, high-level supporting evidence for improved outcomes is lacking.

Operative steps
Transhiatal esophagectomy (THE)
Pros: Do not need to reposition the patient, shorter operation time, decreased pulmonary complications by omitting a thoracotomy, ease of cervical leak management with less mediastinitis.

Cons: Limited and blind/blunt lymphadenectomy, higher blood loss, risk of injuring intrathoracic structures that cannot be clearly visualized, higher incidence of anastomotic leak.

- Supine position, head turned to the right, single lumen ETT

Abdominal phase
- Upper midline laparotomy, stage the abdomen to assure resectability, assess suitability of the stomach as a conduit.
- Divide left triangular ligament and retract left lobe of the liver.
- Divide the short gastric vessels and mobilize the omentum off the greater curvature, preserving the right gastroepiploic arcade.
- Divide the gastrohepatic ligament (watch for replaced left hepatic – preserve if replaced, dividing left gastric distal to the replaced take-off; divide if accessory). Divide the left gastric pedicle at its base, sweeping nodal tissue toward the specimen.
- Perform Kocher maneuver so that the pylorus reaches the hiatus.
- Open pharyngoesophageal membrane and dissect out the distal esophagus circumferentially (use narrow Deaver retractor through hiatus).
- Perform pyloromyotomy or pyloroplasty (optional).
- Place feeding jejunostomy (optional).
- Oversew inferior phrenic veins and after opening hiatus anteriorly (optional).
- Perform posterior esophageal mobilization by advancing hand palm up along esophagus to the level above carina. Stay close to the esophageal wall to avulse aortoesophageal vessels after they branch out before entering the wall to minimize

blood loss, which can be in excess of 1 liter during this phase (controlled with packing the mediastinum).

- Perform anterior mobilization by advancing hand palm down along esophagus (watch for membranous trachea (injury – blood in ETT, SQE, AL) and left atrium and pulmonary veins (injury – profuse BRB bleeding, hemodynamic instability). Mobilize lateral attachments of the esophagus in a similar fashion.
- Divide stomach along greater curvature (blue or purple GIA), fashioning the conduit. Stomach can be used as a narrow conduit (4-5 cm) or the whole stomach.

Neck phase

- Left neck incision along anterior border of the left SCM, divide the platysma, omohyoid, reflect straps, thyroid, and trachea medially and SCM, IJ, and carotid sheath laterally.
- Identify and expose the prevertebral fascia and mobilize the esophagus circumferentially with blunt dissection with two index fingers. After encircling the esophagus with a penrose for traction, dissect into superior mediastinum to the level of carina, meeting the dissection plane from below with blunt mobilization of the esophagus keeping close to NG tube to avoid injury to surrounding structures.
- Divide esophagus in the neck with a linear cutting stapler, incorporating one-inch penrose drain, secure penrose distally to the specimen and remove specimen retracting it inferiorly through the hiatus and abdomen passing it off the field. Send margins for frozen. Tamponade the mediastinum with sponges for hemostasis, if necessary (alternatively use 28F Argyle Saratoga sump tube with suction)
- Place the conduit into the plastic bag (camera sleeve works), secure to the penrose drain and retract into the neck, maintaining orientation (multiple methods used for passage of conduit, do what you know).
- Perform cervical anastomosis (hand-sewn single or double layer, EEA, side-to-side functional end-to-end, again do what you know).
- Place JP or penrose drain into the neck, bilateral chest tubes (optional if pleural space violation confirmed or anticipated), pull excess conduit back into the abdomen and secure to the hiatus, place NGT or pharyngostomy tube and close the abdomen.

Ivor Lewis esophagectomy (ILE)
Pros: increased LN yield, decreased neck morbidity (decreased risk of RLN injury), decreased leak incidence
Cons: lengthier procedure, harder to manage leaks causing more mediastinitis, increased pulmonary morbidity

Abdominal phase

- Supine position, double lumen tube (no lung isolation for abdominal phase).
- All steps of the abdominal phase are performed in the same fashion as the THE approach. However, once the conduit is made, the tip is sewn to the specimen and the specimen is passed through the hiatus for later retrieval in the chest.
- Close the abdomen. Place NGT. Turn the patient in full left lateral position and isolate the lung.

Thoracic phase

- Perform right posterolateral thoracotomy in 6th or 7th intercostal space.
- Mobilize the esophagus anteriorly (off the pericardium and carina, sweeping all lymphatic tissue with the specimen), divide the R vagus nerve close to the esophagus.
- Mobilize esophagus posteriorly off the aorta and spine (clip all aortoesophageal and lymphatic branches posteriorly). Make sure to avoid injury to the thoracic duct. If there is any concern of thoracic duct injury – perform prophylactic en mass ligation.

- Divide the azygos vein with vascular stapler (endo-GIA white or gold) and mobilize the esophagus up to the thoracic inlet, staying close to the esophagus to avoid injury to the airway or recurrent laryngeal nerve.
- Transect the esophagus above the azygos vein (performing a high intrathoracic anastomosis minimizes long-term problems of reflux). If there is concern about the proximal margin, an intraoperative endoscopy can be performed for confirmation.
- Pull the remaining specimen and attached conduit up into the chest and cut tacking suture. Pass the specimen off the table and confirm margins by frozen section.
- Pull the NGT back and perform the anastomosis (hand-sewn single or double layer, EEA, side-to-side, etc) If EEA performed, confirm two donuts and send them for frozen as final gastric margin.
- Advance the NGT into the mid-conduit position and connect to suction.
- Remove any redundancy in the conduit by pushing it back into the abdomen and secure to the hiatus with interrupted sutures.
- Place JP drain posterior to the conduit and bring it out inferiorly. Place one or two (posterior apical and basilar) 28 Fr chest tubes and close the chest.

Three-hole (McKeown) esophagectomy
Pros: Can be used to resect tumors in all locations, increased LN count.
Cons: Increased pulmonary complications due to thoracotomy, increased neck morbidity from cervical anastomosis, may need to perform staging laparoscopy first if question of resectability, requires repositioning, longer case.

Thoracic phase
- Double lumen intubation, right lung isolation.
- The chest part of the case is performed first, similar to the fashion described for the ILE, however the esophagus is not divided. The esophagus is mobilized from diaphragm to inlet and chest tubes are placed.

Abdominal and neck phases
- The patient is then repositioned supine, prepping in the neck as well.
- The abdominal and cervical portions of the case are carried out in similar fashion to the THE without the need for intrathoracic mobilization of the esophagus from the abdomen and mobilization of the proximal esophagus distally through the thoracic inlet.

Minimally invasive esophagectomy
There exist multiple combinations of laparoscopic and thoracoscopic and robotic-assisted techniques that have been described to mimic essentially any type of open esophagectomy. Frequently, these combinations include a mix of open and true minimally invasive steps, better described by the term "hybrid". Regardless of the technique used, the major goal is to minimize morbidity and mortality, blood loss, length of stay, and time to return to activities of daily living. There is now good evidence that has accumulated to support the use of these techniques; however, the procedures are complex and describing the details is beyond the scope of this chapter. The basic steps of the operation remain unchanged from the open predecessors of these MIE approaches.

"Following resection, the path report comes back as T2N1 with 2 of 18 lymph nodes positive. How would you counsel your patient at this point?"
Patients who are found to have lymph node involvement on final pathology have a poorer prognosis. The greater the number of lymph nodes involved, the poorer the prognosis (N1: 1-2 positive nodes, N2: 3-6, N3: > 6). Adjuvant CRT (for those who did not receive induction XRT) or chemotherapy alone should be offered to all patients with evidence of nodal disease, typically 4-6 weeks following resection.

"How would your management change if the preoperative EUS showed invasion beyond the muscularis propria, but without involvement of adjacent structures, and two suspicious periesophageal lymph nodes on EUS? What is this patient's stage? What if the patient had celiac nodal disease rather than periesophageal?"

Both patients have a clinical T stage of uT3 (u for EUS). Patients with T3 disease have an 80% chance of having lymph node involvement, although this may not be detectable on preoperative staging. An attempt should be made to confirm nodal involvement when suspicious nodes are seen on preoperative imaging. Periesophageal lymph nodes can be sampled with EUS-FNA and the aspirates sent for cytologic analysis. Nodes that are 1 cm or greater in the short-axis, round, and hypoechoic on EUS, > 1 cm in short axis on CT or PET, or with FDG-avidity on PET are considered suspicious and should be sampled when possible. Assuming the patient described has positive periesophageal lymph nodes, the clinical stage would be cT3N1 (clinical stage III). Celiac nodal disease is no longer considered M1 disease, as these nodes can frequently be resected with meticulous dissection. Laparoscopic staging allows for assessment of these nodes. Biopsies should be obtained to confirm metastatic disease within these nodes. Laparoscopy also allows for assessment of resectability. If the celiac nodes appear resectable and the base of the left gastric pedicle appears soft, then the patient may be a candidate for resection after induction therapy. If not, definitive CRT is the best option for the patient. Most centers offer induction therapy to patients with T3/resectable T4 and/or nodal disease. Some centers offer concurrent CRT while others favor chemotherapy alone, as radiation causes inflammation and fibrosis that may complicate resection.

"How would you assess the patient's response to induction therapy? What are the chances of this patient having a complete response to induction CRT? What if the PET/CT scan showed no evidence of disease, would you still resect? What if the histology was squamous cell instead of adenocarcinoma?"

It is recommended that patients be restaged with a PET/CT 4-6 weeks after completion of therapy to allow for completion of treatment effect and resolution of inflammation that may influence the PET scan. The use of EUS for restaging is controversial, as the accuracy is significantly diminished due to treatment effect. The patient should then proceed to resection if there is no evidence of nodal involvement outside the field of resection or distant metastases. Patients treated with definitive CRT who have evidence of persistent disease on post-treatment imaging may be considered for salvage esophagectomy in select cases.

Approximately 25-40% of patients will have a complete response to neoadjuvant therapy. Prognosis is significantly improved in this patient population. Even if restaging PET-CT scan shows no evidence of disease, patients with esophageal adenocarcinomas should still undergo resection. However, there is recent evidence supporting observation in patients with squamous cell carcinoma of the esophagus without evidence of residual disease (by post-treatment imaging and upper endoscopy with biopsy) owing to similar long-term survival in patients with or without surgical resection.

"How would your management change if during preoperative work up you discovered that the patient had an EF of 15%, had an MI 4 months ago, PFTs with a FEV1 of 35% and DLCO of 40%, and that he is wheelchair bound?"

This patient carries excessive risk for morbidity and mortality and is not an operative candidate. Patients who are found to be unresectable or are poor operative candidates should be offered definitive, concurrent chemoradiation therapy. Palliative radiation therapy can be offered for patients who cannot tolerate chemotherapy. Palliative chemotherapy alone does not prolong survival but can improve quality of life.

"What can you do for this patient's dysphagia? He is not able to eat and continues to lose weight."

A number of options exist to treat this patient's dysphagia and malnutrition. A feeding jejunostomy can be placed to provide enteral access for nutrition. If the patient responds to

CRT, swallowing will improve, and the tube can be removed. For patients who have dysphagia to saliva and liquids, something should be done to open the esophageal lumen and allow swallowing prior to beginning treatment. Upper endoscopy and gentle dilation (balloon dilation or Savary bougienage) may be enough to provide some palliation but runs the risk of perforation. Alternatively, the tumor can be debrided/debulked with Nd:YAG laser, photodynamic therapy, or intraluminal radiation (brachytherapy). These methods are also useful for controlling bleeding from friable tumors. Stenting has gained popularity as a palliative treatment for obstructing lesions. Balloon dilation is a good option for cases when the stenting apparatus cannot be passed beyond the lesion. A variety of covered metal (permanent) or plastic (temporary) stents are commercially available. Stents are typically placed with the assistance of fluoroscopy to confirm adequate positioning. Stent migration is a common problem, which is why some discourage the use of stents in patients who are to be treated with radiation therapy, as this local therapy can shrink the tumor and lead to migration. Perforation is less common but can be a catastrophic event in this ill population. Patients who have stents placed across the GEJ are more prone to reflux and should be treated with Carafate and BID PPI. Stents also provide a good option for palliation of malignant or postoperative tracheoesophageal fistulae (TEF). Stenting of both the esophagus and trachea is discouraged, as the radial force used to expand the stents can cause undue pressure and enlargement of the fistulous tract. Palliative esophagectomy with a substernal gastric pull-up is a reasonable option for patients in good health who have unresectable disease or for patients with TEFs that cannot be controlled with stents.

"You are referred another patient with a biopsy-proven, poorly-differentiated squamous cell carcinoma at 23 cm with invasion into the muscularis propria only and no lymph node involvement. How would you manage this patient?"
This level of invasion describes a clinical T2 tumor. Location of the tumor is a primary determinant of surgical approach. All types of esophagectomy can be performed for the treatment of distal esophageal cancers (Ivor-Lewis, McKeown, left thoracoabdominal, transhiatal, MIE). However, tumors extending more proximally than 25 cm require a proximal resection and cervical anastomosis. A transhiatal approach is less ideal for proximal tumors as tumor clearance and lymphadenectomy may not be adequately visualized. The McKeown, or 3-hole, esophagectomy is ideal for more proximal tumors such as the one presented in this scenario. Prior to proceeding with resection, bronchoscopy should be performed to rule out airway involvement, which would make the patient unresectable. Squamous cell carcinomas of the pharynx and very proximal esophagus (within 5 cm of the cricopharyngeus or about 20 cm from the incisors) are treated with definitive chemoradiation therapy, not resection.

"Bronchoscopy is negative for tumor invasion and EUS does not show invasion into adjacent structures. You are now doing a McKeown (3-hole) esophagectomy and as you are mobilizing the esophagus in the chest, you note that the tumor is adherent to the posterior membranous portion of the trachea. How would you proceed?"
Although the appropriate steps were taken prior to resection to rule out unresectable T4 disease, one should still be prepared for unexpected findings once in the operating room (especially on examinations!). Airway involvement makes this patient unresectable and the operation should be aborted. Addressing the patient's dysphagia and port placement for chemotherapy may be considered before leaving the operating room.

"Returning to the patient with T3N1 adenocarcinoma located in the distal esophagus, following CRT a restaging PET/CT scan shows resolution of FDG avidity in the periesophageal lymph nodes and residual, but decreased avidity in the primary lesion. EUS cannot be done because the tumor is too bulky to pass the scope. You proceed with an ILE and during the abdominal portion you find a suspicious lesion in the left lobe of the liver. How would you proceed? Say there is no liver lesion, but after completing the abdominal portion you are in the chest you find the tumor is adherent to the right inferior pulmonary vein. How would you proceed?"

147

Every esophagectomy should begin with a thorough search for distant disease or other evidence of unresectability. Laparoscopic staging prior to esophagectomy avoids a laparotomy in cases where distant disease is encountered. Peritoneal and serosal surfaces are carefully examined, with particular attention paid to the liver and omentum. The celiac axis is also assessed to make sure the base of the left gastric is not encased in tumor or there are true celiac axis nodes with tumor involvement that cannot be cleared, which would preclude resection. Suspicious lesions are biopsied and sent for frozen sectioning. If positive, the operation is aborted, and the patient is treated with palliative CRT.

The combination of CT and EUS will identify most cases where there is unresectable intrathoracic T4 involvement, but this may not always be the case. In cases where there is concern for tumor invasion into unresectable intrathoracic structures, it may be advisable to perform a staging thoracoscopy to evaluate the area of concern. Airway involvement can usually be ruled out with bronchoscopy. One should be prepared for a situation such as the one presented here regarding the pulmonary vein, particularly when beginning in the abdomen. You are committed at this point, having completed the abdominal portion of the case, so there is no turning back. One option is to leave the involved segment of esophagus adhered to pulmonary vein behind and perform a substernal gastric pull-up, although this might be an overly aggressive approach for some. The remainder of the esophagus is resected, the neck is prepared for a cervical anastomosis, the gastric conduit is brought up through a window created behind the sternum, and the cervical anastomosis completed. A partial upper sternotomy and resection of the left clavicular head is required to avoid compression on the proximal conduit. The patient is then treated with postoperative palliative chemotherapy and radiation (if not given for induction). Another option is to leave the segment of esophagus behind and exclude the patient. The remainder of the esophagus is resected, a cervical esophagostomy is brought out the left neck, the hiatus is closed, and a gastrostomy tube is placed in the tip of the conduit. The patient is then treated with palliative CRT. Finally, the tumor may be shaved off the vein and clips left to mark the area for targeted XRT. Regardless of how this problem is handled, the patient will not receive an R0 resection (it is an R2 resection) and prognosis is extremely poor.

Performing a right lower lobectomy in an effort to obtain an R0 resection may be performed at some high volume centers; however, this is likely too radical for examination purposes. T4 involvement that is considered resectable includes invasion of the pleura, pericardium, azygous vein, diaphragm, or adjacent peritoneum.

"You are referred another patient with short-segment BE and a small nodule within the BE at 37 cm that was biopsied and shown to be a moderately-differentiated adenocarcinoma. There was no mass seen on endoscopy. She would like to avoid surgery if possible. What would you offer this patient?"

Nodules or areas of ulceration within a segment of BE should raise the suspicion of HGD or invasive cancer. Endomucosal resection (EMR), which resects a piece of mucosa and submucosa, can be viewed as an extended biopsy. The specimen is then examined and can confirm histologic diagnosis, as well as depth of invasion. Beyond its diagnostic utility, EMR can also be definitive treatment for focal areas of BE with HGD (sometimes referred to as carcinoma in-situ) or intramucosal invasive adenocarcinomas (T1a). Extensive biopsies in the area of BE should be performed to assure that there are no other areas of HGD or invasive cancer. Multifocal disease (HGD or intramucosal cancer) is probably best treated with esophagectomy, although multiple EMRs may be performed. Following EMR, residual areas of BE are typically treated with radiofrequency ablation or other ablative therapies.

The primary early complication of EMR is bleeding, which is almost always treatable endoscopically. Strictures occur later, with a higher prevalence associated with multiple or repeat EMRs. Assuming the margins are negative, this patient will then need to undergo close surveillance with serial endoscopies, initially every 3 months for the first year, then annually.

"You do an EMR and the path returns as invasive adenocarcinoma with a positive deep margin. What is the T stage? What are the chances this patient has nodal involvement? What if the lateral margins are positive, but the tumor does not invade the submucosa?"

148

A positive deep margin implies that there is *at least* submucosal invasion of the tumor, making the patient *at least* T1b. Once the tumor invades beyond the lamina propria into the submucosa, the incidence of nodal involvement increased from < 3% for intramucosal tumors (T1a) to approximately 25% for tumors that invade into, but not beyond the submucosa (T1b). Patients with T2 lesions have nodal involvement in 25-50% of patients, while positive nodes are present in 75-80% of cases with T3 tumors. The patient should therefore undergo additional work up with CT, PET-CT, and EUS to complete staging. If additional staging reveals T3, resectable T4, or N+ disease, she should be treated with neoadjuvant therapy followed by resection. If she has only T1b or T2 disease, she should be offered resection. If the lateral margins are positive after EMR, but the deep margins are negative, the patient should undergo repeat EMR until lateral margins are negative.

"A patient is now POD 4 from a THE for a pT2N0 esophageal adenocarcinoma of the distal esophagus. He has a low-grade fever and a WBC of 13,000. The cervical wound is erythematous, and saliva is seen draining around the penrose drain. How would you manage this patient?"
Cervical anastomotic leaks are more common than intrathoracic leaks, theoretically due to more tension on the anastomosis. Fortunately, these leaks are easily managed with opening of the wound at the bedside, while avoiding more serious mediastinitis. The wound is irrigated, debrided, and dressed with wet-to-dry gauze. The patient is placed on broad spectrum antibiotics and antifungals. A clear liquid diet helps to clear debris intraluminally. Enteral nutrition is maintained with jejunostomy feedings or TPN if no enteral access is in place. Once the fever and leukocytosis have resolved and wound drainage is minimal, a barium swallow can be performed to confirm resolution of the leak. The diet is then advanced, and the patient monitored for signs of ongoing leakage. A barium swallow is not needed to confirm the leak if there is enough clinical evidence to suspect a leak. In most case, the wound should be opened without delay.

"The leak has resolved, and the patient is now at home, 10 weeks postoperatively, and is tolerating a regular diet. However, she complains of breads and meats 'sticking.' How would you proceed?"
Anastomotic strictures are common after esophagectomy, particularly after a leak. This patient should undergo upper endoscopy and dilation. The scope is advanced distally into the duodenum, a wire passed, the scope is removed, and serial dilations performed under fluoroscopic guidance with Savary or balloon dilators. Upper endoscopy is repeated to assess the stricture after every couple of increases in diameter of the dilators or when resistance is met. Blood on the dilator or mucosal tearing at the level of the stricture signifies adequate dilation. Serial dilations every few weeks may be required until maximal dilation has been reached and/or dysphagia resolves. Patients requiring serial dilations may be taught self-dilation with soft-tipped dilators (Maloney), with low risk of perforation with adequate education. Dysphagia that occurs later in the postoperative course should raise suspicion of local recurrence and any abnormalities noted on endoscopy should be biopsied.

"How would you monitor this patient for recurrence of her esophageal cancer?"
Surveillance protocols vary from institution to institution. Having a general idea of how you will follow these patients is necessary. Postoperatively, patients may be seen every 3-4 months for the first year, every 3-6 months for years 1-3, every 6 months for years 3-5, then annually after 5 years. Whole-body PET-CT scans are obtained at least annually for these visits. A CT of the chest, abdomen, and pelvis is obtained for all other visits. Any suspicious findings suggesting locoregional or distal recurrence on CT warrants a PET-CT scan and biopsy if the lesion is FDG-avid or has a suspicious appearance on CT. Suspicion of local recurrence is investigated with upper endoscopy and biopsy. An attempt should be made to confirm all suspected recurrences by biopsy.

Recurrent disease is treated with CRT or chemotherapy alone for palliation. Focal XRT may be considered for patients with painful metastases for palliation, even if treated with radiation previously. Very select cases of local recurrence may be considered for re-resection in good surgical candidates. Patients who were treated with definitive CRT that are found to have a resectable locoregional recurrent or persistent disease may be considered for salvage esophagectomy in select cases if they are deemed to be good surgical candidates.

"You have another patient who is POD 4 from an ILE for a pT3N1 esophageal adenocarcinoma located at 28-35 cm. He remains intubated and has failed weaning trials. He has had marginal blood pressure and poor urine output despite aggressive volume resuscitation. He is febrile to 102.1 this morning. Chest x-ray shows a RLL infiltrate and a right effusion. How would you proceed?"

This patient appears to be septic. There are a number of causes of postoperative infection following esophagectomy and all should be thoroughly investigated. Bronchoscopy should be performed, and BAL sent to rule out pneumonia. Urinalysis and urine culture should be sent for possible UTI. Blood cultures should be sent to rule out bacteremia and lines should be changed. The jejunostomy site should be checked for signs of infection. Peritoneal signs should raise suspicion of an enterotomy or leak from the feeding tube site or pyloric emptying procedure. However, first and foremost, one should be concerned about an anastomotic leak or conduit necrosis. A barium swallow cannot be obtained given the patient remains intubated. A CT scan would be helpful to evaluate for pneumonia, empyema, or a leak. However, sending a marginally unstable patient for a scan or barium swallow (if extubated) is unwise. The patient should be promptly brought to the operating room for an upper endoscopy or the endoscopy performed at the bedside to evaluate the anastomosis and conduit.

"The conduit is black."

Gastric conduit necrosis is a rare, but devastating occurrence with a high rate of mortality. However, prompt diagnosis and treatment may be lifesaving for this patient. Any periods of hypotension, evidence of hypoperfusion, fever, leukocytosis, or failure to progress should raise the suspicion of anastomotic leak or conduit necrosis. Imaging only wastes valuable time in these cases but can be carefully considered in patients who are stable. Prompt upper endoscopy is the gold-standard to rule out conduit necrosis. This patient should be taken to the operating room and the conduit taken down via thoracotomy. All necrotic conduit is resected. The remaining stomach is replaced in the abdomen and the proximal esophagus mobilized to the thoracic inlet. The chest is irrigated, and drains/chest tubes are placed. The patient is then quickly repositioned supine. The proximal esophagus is brought out the left neck and a cervical esophagostomy (spit fistula) is fashioned. A gastrostomy tube is placed in the tip of the remaining gastric conduit to decompress the stomach and a feeding jejunostomy is placed, if not already present. The hiatus is closed to prevent herniation of intraabdominal contents. If the patient is too unstable, the conduit is resected, the remaining stomach replaced in the abdomen, the hiatus is close from the right chest, and the proximal esophagus is mobilized. The patient is then brought back to the ICU to be resuscitated and the cervical esophagostomy and gastrostomy tube placed later, after stabilization. Gastrointestinal continuity can be reestablished with a substernal colonic interposition or gastric pull-up (if there is enough remaining stomach) months down the road once the patient is nutritionally replete.

Pearls/pitfalls

- A thorough preoperative workup is necessary to adequately stage patients with esophageal cancer and to assess resectability.
- Proximal and distal extent of the tumor plays an important role in determining the conduit that should be used and approach taken for resection.
- Chemotherapy and radiation play an important role in the multimodal management of esophageal cancer. Understanding the role of surgery, chemotherapy, and radiation is key to managing this patient population.
- Most patients who present with esophageal cancer will be unresectable. It is important to understand the surgeon's role in the palliative treatment of esophageal cancer.

150

- Morbidity and mortality rates following esophagectomy are significant. Understanding the more common and severe complications (i.e., anastomotic leaks, conduit necrosis, and anastomotic stricture) and having a plan of action is necessary.
- Know how to do at least one type of esophagectomy and be able to describe your preferred anastomotic technique.

Suggested readings

- Heger P, Blank S, Diener M, et al. Gastric Preconditioning in Advance of Esophageal Resection-Systematic Review and Meta-Analysis. *J Gastrointest Surg.* 2017 21:1523-32.
- Schuchert MJ, Luketich JD, Landreneau RJ. Management of esophageal cancer. *Curr Probl Surg.* 2010 Nov; 47(11): 845-946.
- Shapiro J, van Lanschot J, Maarten C, et al. Neoadjuvant chemoradiotherapy plus surgery versus surgery alone for oesophageal or junctional cancer (CROSS): long-term results of a randomized controlled trial. *Lancet.* 2015 16:1090-98.
- National Comprehensive Cancer Network. Esophageal and Esophagogastric Junction Cancers, Version 2.2019. Accessed 8/5/2019. https://www.nccn.org/professionals/physician_gls/pdf/esophageal.pdf

22. GERD AND BARRETT'S ESOPHAGUS

Michelle C. Ellis, MD, and Rishindra M. Reddy, MD

Concept

- Work up of gastroesophageal reflux disease (GERD)
- Medical management and surveillance of GERD and Barrett's esophagus (BE)
- Indications for operative intervention
- Options for operative approach
- Endoscopic management of BE

Chief complaint

"A 56-year-old man is self-referred to your office with complaints of long-standing heartburn, 'sour mouth,' and food sticking. His symptoms have persisted despite trying maximal doses of a number of 'acid-reducer' medications."

Differential

Gastroesophageal reflux disease (GERD), Barrett's esophagus (BE), hiatal hernia, paraesophageal hernia, esophageal motility disorder, esophageal stricture, eosinophilic esophagitis, esophageal cancer

History and physical

Typical symptoms of GERD include heartburn, regurgitation, and dysphagia. Atypical symptoms that have an established association with GERD include cough, laryngitis, and asthma. Additional extra-esophageal symptoms often linked to reflux include dental erosions, laryngitis, laryngeal polyps, and pulmonary fibrosis, though causation has not been clearly established. A history of recurrent pneumonias may be due to aspiration of refluxate, particularly at night. This history is important in elderly, frail patients or those with long-standing interstitial pulmonary disease, as an aspiration event may prove fatal and is a strong indication for surgical rather than medical management of GERD. A thorough review of the patient's medications is also prudent. Knowledge of whether H2 blocker or proton-pump inhibitors (PPIs) have been taken and if they provided any relief in symptoms has prognostic value when considering patients for anti-reflux surgery (ARS). It is also important to see how the medications are being taken (PPIs are not as effective if taken PRN, an appropriate course of medical management typically consists of 8 weeks of daily or BID PPI therapy). Any prior history of upper endoscopies and their findings is important as well. Knowledge of a history of BE and whether or not dysplasia was found on previous biopsies is another important piece of information.

Tests

- *Endoscopy:* may be normal in up to 70% of patients with GERD but needed to assess for presence and severity of any esophagitis, BE, stricture, or invasive disease, especially for those patients with alarm symptoms (dysphagia). Approximately 10-20% of patients with GERD seeking care will have a stricture or BE on endoscopy. Any abnormal appearing areas of mucosa should be biopsied.

- *Barium swallow:* provides delineation of anatomy including detection of hiatal hernia, strictures, or esophageal foreshortening. Suspect esophageal shortening in the setting of a large hiatal hernia (> 5 cm) or esophageal stricture. It is recommended that patients with symptoms of dysphagia undergo a barium swallow prior to endoscopy, which serves as a road map and may key the surgeon in on potential difficulties that may be encountered (i.e., tight stricture that may require a pediatric endoscope to pass, the possible need for dilation, retained food debris from a tight stricture or esophageal motility that may require the patient to be on clear liquids for a few days pre-endoscopy to clear the esophagus).

- *24-hour pH probe (Bravo) testing*: gold standard for diagnosis of GERD. A DeMeester score (abnormal > 14.7) is calculated based on 1) total percent time pH less than 4.0, 2) percent time pH less than 4.0 in the upright position, 3) percent time pH less than 4.0 in the recumbent position, 4) the total number of reflux episodes, 5) the total number of reflux episodes longer than 5 minutes, and 6) the duration of the longest reflux episode. Patients correlate symptoms with a diary of time spent in the upright/supine position as well as meal times. Neither the symptom of heartburn nor the presence of hiatal hernia is necessarily synonymous with GERD. Nocturnal reflux may be associated with a failure of medical therapy, GERD-related strictures, ulcers, or other complications.

- *Esophageal manometry*: provides information on esophageal peristaltic function and lower esophageal sphincter (LES) function during swallowing. Normal LES resting pressure is 15-30 mmHg. LES integrity depends on an adequate overall sphincter length (3-5 cm), as well as the presence of adequate (> 2.5 cm) intra-abdominal length. One must establish the presence of normal peristaltic function prior to surgical treatment, as abnormal peristalsis alone can contribute to symptoms and lead to inadequate symptom relief despite surgery. The amplitude of contractions (< 30 mmHg is considered low in most GI labs), percentage of peristaltic contractions (a normal esophagus will have 100% peristaltic contractions), and whether the esophagus is cleared with the contractions are all important pieces of information that will affect the decision to perform a partial versus a complete wrap during ARS.

- *Impedance monitoring*: useful in patients with non-acid reflux, assesses bolus transit through the esophagus thereby providing additional information on esophageal motility and function.

- *Gastric emptying test*: useful in diabetics or others in which delayed gastric emptying is suspected, also important for reoperations to document whether the vagus nerves are functioning or present (may have been inadvertently divided during a prior ARS).

- *Bernstein acid test*: largely historical, mild hydrochloric acid used to re-create reflux symptoms.

Index scenario (additional information)
"The patient's history and physical reveals long-standing heartburn and occasional dysphagia to meats and breads, especially after large or spicy meals. He has been self-treating with over the counter PPIs intermittently over the past five years with some relief. EGD demonstrates short segment BE without evidence of dysplasia on biopsy. 24-hour pH study demonstrates an average DeMeester score of 18 over a 2-day period. Manometry shows normal amplitudes throughout the esophagus, 100% peristaltic contractions, and complete bolus clearance. How would you proceed?"

Treatment/management
Symptomatic reflux that persists despite high dose, twice daily proton pump inhibitor therapy is the most common indication for ARS, followed by medication expense, and unwillingness to adhere to lifelong medical therapy. Other indications include endoscopically proven severe esophagitis or mucosal ulceration. These patients should first undergo medical management with BID PPIs for 6-8 weeks without interruption. The upper endoscopy is then repeated to gauge response to therapy. Ongoing or worsening esophagitis is an indication for ARS. Patients with complications of GERD, such as peptic strictures, BE, recurrent aspiration pneumonias, or interstitial lung disease without other known etiologies should be considered for ARS as well. ARS has not been shown to induce regression of BE with or without dysplasia. However, by removing the cause of the metaplasia, the risk of esophagitis and more BE should be decreased. Patients with known BE who undergo ARS should undergo surveillance upper endoscopies at the same time intervals as those who are not treated surgically (surveillance discussed below).

Whether a partial (Toupet or Dor) or complete (Nissen) fundoplication is performed, the principal goals of all ARSs remains the same: reduction/repair of any hiatal hernia if present, restoration of at least 2-3 cm of intra-abdominal esophageal length, closure of the widened hiatus, and re-establishment of the esophageal high pressure zone (fundoplication recreates the angle of His). If suspected, BE is identified on preoperative endoscopy (salmon-colored mucosa extending proximally from the squamocolumnar junction, aka Z-line), the patient should undergo biopsy to evaluate for dysplasia or invasive carcinoma. The presence of dysplasia is the greatest risk factor for future development of malignancy. The typical progression to invasive adenocarcinoma induced by GERD is esophagitis without metaplasia, metaplasia (BE) without dysplasia, low grade dysplasia (LGD), high grade dysplasia (HGD), and finally invasive adenocarcinoma. HGD is considered the immediate precursor to invasive cancer but is also a marker for esophageal cancer. Previous studies have shown that 30-40% of patients with HGD who undergo esophagectomy are found to have synchronous occult areas of invasive cancer elsewhere in the esophagus. The gold standard for endoscopic surveillance is the Seattle protocol, which entails 4-quadrant biopsies taken for every 1 cm of the areas of BE with additional biopsies of suspicious lesions as needed (i.e., areas of nodularity or ulceration). There is high intra-observer and inter-observer variation in the histopathologic diagnosis of HGD. Therefore, patients being referred for treatment of BE should have pathology reviewed to confirm the diagnosis. Surveillance should be performed every 3-5 years in those with BE and no dysplasia, every 6-12 months if LGD is present, and every 3 months if HGD is found and has been successfully treated with endoscopic mucosal resection (EMR) or consider surgical intervention. Mucosal directed therapies include radiofrequency ablation and EMR and have become first line therapy for HGD. EMR has the advantage of providing tissue for pathologic examination, aiding in identification of occult invasive cancer. Esophagectomy is now typically reserved for patients with invasive cancers, those requesting surgical intervention, those who fail endoscopic treatment, and those with HGD lesions not amenable to endoscopic mucosal directed therapies.

Operative steps

Open/laparoscopic fundoplication

Indications for minimally invasive approach are the same as open. Caution should be used in the setting of recurrent hernias or large hiatal hernias (> 5 cm), although some centers are approaching large hernias laparoscopically with good long-term results.

- *Port placement.* Varies by surgeon preference, but typically a 10 mm camera port 2/3 the distance from the xiphoid to the umbilicus, 5 mm right anterior axillary line port for a liver retractor, 5 mm right upper abdominal working port, 5 mm left upper abdominal working port, and a 10 mm left lateral subcostal working port. An upper midline laparotomy is made for the open approach.

- Gastrohepatic ligament is incised and a combination of blunt and sharp dissection is used to divide the phrenoesophageal membrane and mobilize the esophagus circumferentially from the crural attachments. Preservation of the peritoneal lining of the right and left crus is important, as this lining provides strength for closure of the hiatus (bites through the crus muscle alone, i.e., when the lining has been stripped, are more likely to pull through).

- The intrathoracic esophagus is mobilized up into the mediastinum from right to left pleura and pericardium to the pre-aortic plane. This maneuver can provide length to the esophagus to assure that there is at least 2-3 cm of tension-free, intra-abdominal esophagus, as GERD can lead to inflammation and scarring that may result in a shortened esophagus with time. If the esophagus is shortened and enough length cannot be obtained with intrathoracic esophageal mobilization, a Collis gastroplasty (wedge gastrectomy) may be performed to add esophageal length.

- Care should be taken to identify and preserve both vagus nerves during mobilization of the esophagus.

- A retro-esophageal window is then made for passage of the stomach in order to create the fundoplication.

- The short gastric vessels are then divided along the upper third of the greater curve of the stomach.

154

- The posterior hiatus is closed by re-approximating the crura with several interrupted sutures. Anterior sutures may be placed in cases of large hiatal defects due to large hiatal hernias.
- The upper third of the greater curve of the stomach is then passed through the retroesophageal window and "shoeshine" maneuver of anterior and posterior folds of fundus is performed to ensure there is no resistance and to obtain the desired bulkiness of the wrap.
- The fundoplication is then created over an esophageal bougie (51, 54, and 60 Fr most commonly used) with 3 interrupted sutures to create 2 cm fundoplication, or 4 sutures for a 3 cm fundoplication depending on surgeon preference. It is important to perform the wrap around the segment of intra-abdominal esophagus and not the gastric cardia, as wrapping around the stomach may lead to acid production proximal to the wrap, resulting in ongoing GERD symptoms despite the fundoplication.

Trans-thoracic fundoplication

Esophageal lengthening with a gastroplasty may be more easily performed from the chest, though the transthoracic approach may carry a slightly higher cardiopulmonary risk and postoperative pain issues than a laparoscopic approach. The transthoracic approach may also be useful for patients with prior transabdominal ARS, where a redo approach from the abdomen may be more difficult due to scarring. Some also prefer the transthoracic approach in the setting of a large hiatal hernia.

- The approach is typically via the left chest via thoracotomy through the 6th or 7th intercostal space.
- The inferior pulmonary ligament is divided, and the lung is retracted superiorly and anteriorly to expose the esophagus.
- A diaphragm retraction stitch may be helpful to expose the hiatus.
- The esophagus is dissected out from posterior mediastinum and encircled with a Penrose.
- The phrenoesophageal membrane is incised and any herniated stomach is returned to the abdomen after division of the short gastrics.
- A Collis gastroplasty is performed if necessary.
- Posterior crural sutures are placed but not tied; a 360° wrap is performed over an esophageal bougie, as described above, and returned to the abdomen. The crural sutures are then tied.

Potential questions/alternative scenarios

Mortality of both open and laparoscopic antireflux surgery is < 1%. Serious intraoperative complications include splenic injury, and gastric or esophageal perforation. Conversion to the open approach may be needed to aid in visualization or to safely address any of the above complications. Early postoperative complications include gas-bloat syndrome, dysphagia, or stricture due to an excessively tight wrap. Late complications include slippage of the wrap back into the chest, or failure of the fundoplication itself.

"You are doing a Nissen fundoplication and as you are dividing the short gastric vessels (or retracting the stomach), there is bleeding noted to be coming from the left upper quadrant. On further inspection, there is a capsular tear in the spleen. How would you manage this problem?"

Splenic capsular tears can often be managed with application of direct pressure for a period of a few minutes and can be additionally helped with applying one of a variety of topical hemostatic agents available to the area, for example Surgicel (Ethicon, Inc.). Persistent capsular or hilar bleeding may prove to be more difficult to control, necessitating conversion to open and direct control of surgical bleeding. If control cannot be gained with suture ligatures, formal splenectomy may need to be performed.

"You have a patient postoperative day three s/p Nissen fundoplication who is febrile and has peritoneal signs. During division of the short gastric vessels, the vessels were noted to be quite short. Energy was used for division of some of these vessels. How would you proceed? What if the patient had a Collis gastroplasty performed, but presented in the same manner?"

Any patient with peritoneal signs within the early postoperative period should warrant re-exploration to identify the source of either bleeding or perforation. Depending on severity of presentation, a preoperative imaging study such as an upper gastrointestinal contrast study (with water soluble contrast or thin barium) or CT scan can help to localize the areas of concern. Thermal injuries leading to perforation may not be limited to the stomach if care has not been taken during the initial operation to avoid resting the hot blade of the ligating device on nearby bowel. Thermal injuries tend to present a few days postoperatively. It is therefore important to fully evaluate the stomach and surrounding viscous structures for injury. Explorations may be carried out laparoscopically by an experienced minimally invasive surgeon, or by open laparotomy. Given the robust blood supply of the stomach, small perforations or thermal injuries can usually be repaired primarily or closed with an endoscopic linear stapler. Drains should be left near the area of injury after the abdomen has been thoroughly washed out. A patient presenting with these symptoms following an esophageal lengthening procedure (Collis) should raise concern for a leak from staple line of the Collis gastroplasty. Most leaks from the staple line can be managed with primary repair and drainage.

"You have a patient who is postoperative day one from a laparoscopic Nissen fundoplication. A Barium swallows is obtained, which shows delayed flow of contrast through a tight wrap. The patient complains of some dysphagia after starting a clear diet. How would you counsel this patient? What if her symptoms persisted beyond a week or two? What if they persisted after dilation?"

If at the initial operation the wrap was performed over an adequately sized esophageal bougie (the authors prefer a 54 Fr bougie), then early dysphagia and tight-appearing wrap on imaging can be attributed to local edema. If no or small sized dilator was used, an early re-exploration to create a looser wrap may be warranted. For those patients who had an adequately sized dilator used can often be managed with continued liquid diet and observation to allow the edema to resolve over time (up to 3 months). If dysphagia persists, endoscopic evaluation and dilation are warranted. The importance of an adequate preoperative work up is highlighted in a patient with prolonged postoperative dysphagia. If a motility disorder was excluded preoperatively in the patient with persistent postoperative dysphagia, then revision may be necessary to relieve an overly tight wrap that has not responded to dilation. Takedown of the wrap with a redo partial fundoplication (Toupet or Dor) should be performed in patients found to have esophageal dysmotility (i.e., low amplitude contractions).

"You have a patient who is two years s/p Nissen fundoplication. She now has recurrent heartburn and regurgitation. How would you work this patient up?"

Workup for recurrent symptoms in a patient that has previously undergone anti-reflux surgery is similar to the initial workup. A barium swallow study may provide useful information regarding whether the wrap remains intact and its location relative to the diaphragm (i.e., slipped Nissen). Manometry is useful as esophageal function may have changed over time. Fundoplications performed on foreshortened esophagi often recur due to the tension pulling the repair up into the chest, putting the crural stitches at risk. It is therefore important to carefully assess esophageal length prior to the initial operation with a barium swallow, as well as intraoperatively following mobilization of the esophagus. A Collis gastroplasty is needed if adequate tension-free length cannot be obtained.

Pearls/pitfalls

• 24-hour pH probe is the gold standard for diagnosis of GERD.

- Patients who fail medical treatment should also undergo a preoperative endoscopy, barium swallow, and manometry prior to any intervention.
- Patients with BE should undergo routine surveillance endoscopy. If HGD is identified, mucosal directed therapy is warranted.
- Gastroplasty in addition to fundoplication should be performed in the setting of foreshortened esophagus to prevent wrap slippage.

Suggested readings

- Sideris AC, Zheng YA, White A, Bueno R (2018). Surgical Techniques for the Treatment of Reflux Disease. Shields TW et al (eds), *General Thoracic Surgery*. 8th ed. Philadelphia, PA: Lippincott Williams & Wilkins. pp.1647-1659.
- Rice TW, Shay SS, Birgisson S (2016). Surgical Treatment of Benign Esophageal Diseases. Sellke FW (ed), *Sabiston and Spencer's Surgery of the Chest*. 9th ed. Philadelphia, PA: Elsevier. pp. 607-643.
- Rice TW, Goldblum JR. Management of Barrett's esophagus with high-grade dysplasia. *Thorac Surg Clin* 2012;22:101-107.

23. BENIGN ESOPHAGEAL DISEASE
Adnan M. Al Ayoubi, MD, PhD and Kalpaj R. Parekh, MBBS

Concept
- Rare (<1% of esophageal tumors), often asymptomatic and frequently identified incidentally
- Smooth muscle leiomyoma is the most common benign tumor
- Best classified based on tumor location within the wall of the esophagus
- Two thirds occur in the distal esophagus
- Treatment is reserved to symptomatic lesions and aimed to relieve obstruction or obtain diagnosis when increased suspicion of malignancy

Chief complaint
"A 52 years old female presents to clinic with complaints of dysphagia, which has been slowly progressing over the past several months. She also reports occasional feeling of food stuck in her chest."

Differential
Esophageal dysmotility disorders, esophageal mass (benign vs. malignant), diverticulum, hiatal hernia, GERD, esophageal stricture, vascular ring, neuromotor degenerative disorders. Benign esophageal lesions are classified based on their layer of origin. Most common lesions are summarized in the following table.

Origin	Lesion	Features	EUS Layer
Mucosa	Web	Mucosal membranous shelf, proximal esophagus. Project from anterior or lateral wall	1-2
	Shatzki's ring	Membranous shelf, distal esophagus. Encircles entire esophagus	
	Papilloma	Exophytic	
	Adenoma	Polypoid hyperplasia	
Submucosa	Granular cell tumor	Pale, firm	1-3
	Fibrovascular polyp	Rubbery, smooth, lobulated, elongated filling defects, proximal esophagus	
	Lymphangioma	Yellow, translucent	2-3
	Hemangioma	Reddish-blue, nodular	2-3
Muscularis	Leiomyoma	Fleshy, compressible, distal 2/3rd	4
Extraluminal	Inclusion cyst	Near tracheal bifurcation, filled with brownish fluid	4-5
	Duplication cyst	Typically, posterior, within the muscular wall, fluid filled and do not communicate with lumen. Submucosal mass on endoscopy, extraluminal compression on esophagram	

History and physical
Obtain a detailed history and physical exam, focusing on dysphagia including duration and progression of symptoms, intolerance of liquids vs. solids, associated weight loss, reflux, regurgitation of food, chest pain, retrosternal discomfort, cough, respiratory symptoms (aspiration).

158

Tests

- *Barium esophagram.* Best initial test for evaluation of the patient with symptomatic esophageal pathology. It helps determine location of lesion, size, contrast transit time, and luminal narrowing.
- *CT chest with oral and IV contrast.* Defines the borders of the lesion and its relationship to surrounding structures. Can be useful for smaller lesions and other extra-esophageal pathologies with similar symptoms such as vascular rings, lymphadenopathy, congenital and duplication cysts.
- *EGD.* Provides direct view to the intraluminal extension of the tumor and helps determine the degree of obstruction. Intramural lesions appear as submucosal bulges with normal overlying mucosa.
- *EUS.* Can be very helpful in establishing the diagnosis and is almost exclusively benign if the lesion appears homogenous, anechoic, or hyperechoic. Heterogeneous echoic lesions do not indicate malignancy but may be suggestive of malignancy particularly for larger lesions (>4 cm). EUS is very helpful to follow progression.
- *Biopsy.* Not universally recommended. Intraluminal and submucosal lesions may be biopsied; however, there is increased risk of brisk bleeding with hemangiomas. For intramural lesions like leiomyomas, FNA or forceps biopsy do not provide adequate material for appropriate pathologic evaluation, and a distinction between leiomyoma and leiomyosarcoma can be challenging even with complete resection; therefore, forceps biopsies are contraindicated if leiomyoma is suspected.

Index scenario (additional information)

"Contrast esophagram showed a smooth filling defect in the distal third of the esophagus. EGD/EUS was performed confirming the location of the lesion that was covered with normal appearing mucosa projecting into the lumen. EUS demonstrated a well circumscribed, hypoechoic lesion originating from the fourth layer, measuring 6 cm and uninvolved overlying mucosa. Patient was counseled for surgical resection. Describe your approach."

Both open thoracotomy and VATS from the left side are acceptable. The esophagus is exposed, mobilized, encircled, and the lesion identified by either palpation and/or EGD transillumination. A myotomy of the outer longitudinal muscle overlying the tumor is then made, and this can be smaller than the length of the lesion. Leiomyomas are typically gray-white, avascular, and smooth encapsulated lesions. Mobilization of the lesion can be performed using a combination of electrocautery as well as blunt and sharp dissections until the tumor is completely mobilized from the muscularis and submucosa. EGD may be used during dissection and provides excellent visualization of the mucosa preventing unnecessary damage and allowing for immediate detection of any mucosal injury by performing a leak/insufflation test. Next approximate the muscularis without tension using interrupted silk sutures. If the myotomy is long or the muscle layer is severely damaged during dissection, a flap of viable tissue may be required to buttress the repair and this includes a choice of any of the following: pleura, pericardium, omentum, diaphragm or pedicled intercostal muscle (one should harvest the pedicle and protect it during the thoracotomy if a difficult dissection is expected based on preoperative evaluation). This is thought to prevent mucosal bulging and formation of esophageal pseudodiverticulum, although it remains debatable. If the mucosa were injured during the dissection, I would repair it in two layers and use a buttressing flap as mentioned above. This may delay oral feeds and a consideration for NGT placement or feeding jejunostomy tube may be warranted depending on the extent of the mucosal tear.

"What if the lesion was in the mid esophagus?"
Follow a right-sided approach, either via thoracotomy or thoracoscopy. The azygous vein may need to be divided to improve esophageal exposure and mobilization.

What if the lesion was in the cervical esophagus?

Proceed with enucleation and closure of the myotomy through a left neck incision.

"What if the lesion was long, involved the gastroesophageal junction, and bore functional resemblance to achalasia?"
Still perform enucleation of the lesion and approximation of myotomy. I would more than likely need a buttressing flap and therefore do the resection via a thoracotomy and harvest a pedicled intercostal flap *a priori*. I would then reassess functional outcomes post-operatively. Esophagectomy is <u>NOT</u> indicated in the primary setting.

"What lesions would you resect endoscopically?"
This is limited to a small group of lesions arising from the mucosa, submucosa, or muscularis with intraluminal projection and/or polypoid pattern, typically less than 2 cm and may be pedunculated. Saline or ethanol injections of the mucosa are done to dissect the tumor free from the underlying submucosa, and the lumpectomy is performed using a snare wire and suction cylinder. Fibrovascular polyps, squamous cell papillomas and occasionally leiomyomas can be resected using this approach. Endoscopic mucosal resection (EMR) has been described for resection of symptomatic lipomas, granular cell tumors, as well as smaller hemangiomas. Sclerotherapy, fulguration, tumor enucleation, and esophagectomy have all been described for the treatment of hemangiomas depending on size and location. Biopsies are contraindicated due to risk of bleeding. Endoscopic needle decompression of inclusion and duplication cysts may be used to decrease lesion size and protect against life-threatening airway compression. This is typically followed by formal lesion surgical enucleation.

Pearls/pitfalls
- Benign esophageal tumors are mostly classified based on their location:
  - *Intraluminal*: adenoma, lipoma, fibrovascular, inflammatory polyps
  - *Submucosal*: hemangioma, granular cell tumor, neurofibroma
  - *Intramural*: leiomyoma, GIST, Schwannoma, rhabdomyoma
  - *Extramural*: cysts, duplications
- Leiomyoma is the most common benign tumor (75%) and arises most often from the muscularis propria in the distal 2/3rds of the esophagus
  - Smooth concave submucosal defect with no contrast delay on swallow
  - Normal overlying mucosa on EGD, homogenous on EUS, rarely undergoes malignant transformation
  - Difficult to differentiate leiomyoma and leiomyosarcomas
  - Avoid biopsy – extraluminal enucleation then more difficult
  - Difficult enucleation may be herald for sarcoma
  - Buttressing flaps encouraged but debated
- Leiomyosarcoma should be treated with esophagectomy

Suggested readings
- Overview: Anatomy and Pathophysiology of Benign Esophageal Disease. Sugarbaker DJ, Bueno R, Colson YL, Jaklitsch MT, Krasna MJ, Mentzer SJ (eds). *Adult Chest Surgery*. McGraw Hill. 2nd edition. 2015.
- Resection of Benign Tumors of the Esophagus. Sugarbaker DJ, Bueno R, Colson YL, Jaklitsch MT, Krasna MJ, Mentzer SJ (eds). *Adult Chest Surgery*. McGraw Hill. 2nd edition. 2015.
- Benign Esophageal Tumors. *Pearson's Thoracic and Esophageal Surgery*. Patterson GA, Pearson FG, Cooper JD, Deslauriers J, Rice TW, Luketich JD, Lerut AE (eds). 3rd edition. 2008.

24. ESOPHAGEAL MOTILITY DISORDERS
Marek Polomsky, MD, and Seth Force, MD

Concept

- Understanding symptoms and presentation of primary esophageal motility disorders
- Manometric characteristics
- Diagnostic work-up and indications for repair of achalasia
- Critical steps for repair of Heller myotomy with partial fundoplication
- Pitfalls and alternative solutions

Chief complaint

"A 48-year-old man presents with complaint of progressive dysphagia to both liquids and solids, accompanied by regurgitation."

Differential

The differential for his dysphagia includes motility disorders such as achalasia, nutcracker esophagus, diffuse esophageal spasm (DES), hypertensive lower esophageal sphincter (LES), ineffective esophageal motility (IEM), scleroderma, as well as hiatus hernia, esophageal diverticulum, peptic stricture, eosinophilic esophagitis, and esophageal cancer.

History and physical

A history investigating possible achalasia or other esophageal motility disorders should focus on eliciting classic symptoms of slowly progressive dysphagia for solids and liquids, regurgitation of bland undigested food, and chest pain. Other symptoms suggestive of achalasia include weight loss, aspiration with episodes of recurrent pneumonia or chronic cough, and heartburn. Comorbidities which may affect treatment algorithms include candidal esophagitis, malnutrition, and concomitant cancer, as well as previous thoracic or abdominal surgery. One must be careful to recognize patients that solely have gastroesophageal reflux disease (GERD), where an atypical presentation of reflux can mimic the symptomatology of achalasia. A physical exam focusing on the pulmonary and gastrointestinal systems should be made.

Tests

- *CXR.* A CXR can visualize the presence of a dilated fluid-filled esophagus (typically can see a right sided posterior mediastinal shadow), and the absence of a gastric bubble.
- *EGD.* When performing an EGD, one will often see a dilated esophagus with retention of saliva and undigested food, and a very tight LES making passage of the scope through it very difficult. It is performed to exclude obstruction from tumor or stricture (pseudoachalasia), or infections such as candidal esophagitis. Ringed contractions of the esophagus also suggest abnormal peristalsis that may be seen with other esophageal motility disorders.
- *Barium esophagram.* On a barium esophagram one can visualize a dilated esophagus with the presence of an air-fluid level, a characteristic "bird's beak" at the distal esophagus (from a non-relaxing LES), and aperistalsis. The esophagram can be normal in patients with early achalasia as opposed to patients with late stage achalasia, where a "sigmoid esophagus" may be present. Other motility disorders have characteristic appearances (i.e., corkscrew appearance seen with diffuse esophageal spasm [DES]).
- *Manometry.* Manometric characteristics of achalasia include absence of LES relaxation, elevated LES resting pressure (10-15 mmHg), aperistalsis of the esophageal body, and esophageal body pressurization. There have been variants of achalasia that have been described and it is not uncommon for patients with achalasia to have manometric results that do not meet all 4 criteria for the diagnosis. Type I (classic

161

achalasia) – impaired LES relaxation without significant pressurization within the esophageal body. Type II (compressive achalasia) – achalasia with esophageal compression (pressurization > 30 mmHg). Type III (spastic achalasia) – Achalasia with spastic contractions associated with rapidly propagated pressurization. The sine qua non for diagnosis of achalasia is failure of the LES to relax.

- *CT scan.* A CT scan can be useful to assess the integrity of the mediastinum, especially in end-stage achalasia or megaesophagus.

Index scenario (additional information)
"An EGD, barium esophagram, and manometry were performed with findings that were consistent with achalasia. The patient has no history of GERD and no previous surgeries. What is the optimal therapy for this patient?"

Treatment/management
The goal of therapy (both surgical and non-surgical) is to eliminate the outflow obstruction, thus relieving dysphagia, and maintain a barrier against gastroesophageal reflux. Medical therapy includes calcium channel blockers, oral nitrates, and sildenafil. Results of medical therapies are variable and have poor short-term results. Pneumatic balloon dilatation and endoscopic botulinum toxin injections are also alternatives but are rarely effective in the long-term. The most effective and common surgical therapy for achalasia is laparoscopic Heller myotomy with partial fundoplication, which has good long-term outcomes (> 90% relief of dysphagia more than 2 years). While there are no differences in outcomes, Dor fundoplication (anterior 180° wrap) is typically preferred to Toupet fundoplication (posterior 270° wrap) due to the preservation of posterior crural attachments and being technically easier to perform. Predictors of successful outcomes following Heller myotomy include increased magnitude of preoperative LES resting pressure, minimal degree of preoperative esophageal dilation or tortuosity, and the absence of earlier nonoperative interventions. Infections such as candidal esophagitis, caused by the chronic retained food and secretions in the esophagus, should be treated prior to surgery.

Operative steps
Laparoscopic Heller myotomy with Dor fundoplication
Goals – eliminate outflow obstruction, create a barrier against gastroesophageal reflux.

- Position patient supine in modified lithotomy position, general endotracheal anesthesia (GETA), Foley.
- Five working ports to access the upper abdomen, insufflate with CO_2, reverse Trendelenberg positioning.
- The gastrohepatic ligament is divided, making sure to look for a replaced or accessory left hepatic artery. If one is present, the gastrohepatic ligament is opened inferiorly and superiorly to the vessel and a clip is placed on the artery. 15-30 minutes is allowed to pass, and the left lobe of the liver is then assessed. If there is discoloration suggesting decreased inflow to the liver, the clip is removed, and the artery preserved throughout the dissection. If no ischemia, then the artery is an accessory branch and it can be divided (usually the case).
- Mobilize the esophagus of the right crus by opening the phrenoesophageal membrane. Do the same along the anterior arch of the hiatus, making sure to preserve the anterior vagus nerve. Carry dissection down along left crus to mobilize the esophagus. Division of the short gastrics facilitates dissection along the left crus. The posterior esophagus does not need to be mobilized if a Dor is to be performed, but circumferential mobilization of the esophagus is needed if a posterior Toupet is to be performed, in which case the posterior vagus nerve must also be sought out and preserved.
- Mobilize the intrathoracic esophagus by dissecting in the areolar plane within the mediastinum, dissecting the esophagus from the right and left pleura, as well as the anterior pericardium. Remember the vagus nerves will originate on the right (posterior vagus) and left (anterior vagus) as dissection is carried proximally in the mediastinum.

162

- Mobilize upper third of the gastric fundus by dividing the short gastric vessels.
- Mobilize the esophagus anteriorly at the hiatus by freeing up the gastric fat pad, going up into the mediastinum and clearing proximally at least 6 to 8 cm of GEJ (in preparation for a full Heller myotomy).
- With a bougie in place (45 or 50 Fr), perform a myotomy starting with blunt dissection using endoscopic Kittners to spread the longitudinal muscle. Then separate the circular muscle fibers from the mucosa, dividing with some type of energy device (hook electrocautery, bipolar, ultrasonic shears, etc.). The myotomy should extend proximally onto the esophagus for 4-5 cm through the GEJ (ensuring division of clasp fibers) and onto the anterior wall of the fundus of the stomach for 2-3 cm. Myotomy edges are carefully separated from the underlying mucosa for 40-50% of esophageal circumference.
- Perform intraoperative EGD to check for completeness of myotomy and to look for an unrecognized mucosal injury prior to proceeding to the fundoplication. Submerging the myotomy under water and insufflating assists with identifying mucosal perforations.
- To create the fundoplication, the mobilized anterior fundus is laid across the myotomy site and the left edge of the fundus is sewn to the left cut edge of the esophageal myotomy with three or four interrupted sutures, taking the highest stitch through the left crural pillar as an anchor. The right side of fundus is sutured similarly to the right edge of the cut esophageal muscle taking the highest suture through the right crural pillar to prevent torsion.

Potential questions/alternative scenarios

"A 59-year-old man with severe COPD, ESRD, and a previous laparotomy for gangrenous cholecystitis is diagnosed with achalasia. How would you manage this patient?"
This patient is not a good surgical candidate for surgical treatment of his achalasia, either through a laparoscopic or thoracotomy approach. Depending on the severity of his disease, medical therapy may be tried first. If this were to fail, endoscopic botulinum toxin injection is a reasonable alternative for this patient. Improvement in dysphagia following injection typically lasts 6 months or less and often times requires repeated injections for continued relief. The treatment is also expensive. Botulinum toxin injection should be avoided in patients who are surgical candidates because of the resulting submucosal fibrosis, however prior toxin injection does not rule a patient out for surgical treatment. This fibrosis may make attempts at surgical myotomy more difficult and increases the risk of intraoperative mucosal perforation. As achalasia is a progressive disease, this patient may eventually benefit from a percutaneous endoscopic gastrostomy (PEG) tube for enteral access.

"Your patient develops recurrent dysphagia following myotomy. How would you manage this patient?"
Perform an EGD and a barium esophagram to exclude an obstructing lesion, assess the integrity of the myotomy, and assess for esophageal dilation or tortuosity. Repeat manometry would be beneficial to assess for persistently high LES resting pressure (10-15 mmHg). If an incomplete (not extended proximally or distally enough or bridging muscle fibers are left behind) or a scarred myotomy is suspected, one can perform botulinum toxin injection, pneumatic dilation, redo myotomy, or in certain instances esophagectomy.

"Following completion of your myotomy you perform an intraoperative EGD and notice a small mucosal perforation near the GEJ. How would you proceed?"
Intraoperative mucosal perforation occurs on average 7% of the time and typically is located near the GEJ. If managed appropriately, this complication rarely has any significant clinical consequences. A small defect in the mucosa can be primarily repaired with absorbable suture. Subsequent buttressing with an anterior Dor fundoplication can provide further reinforcement. Endoscopy should always be done at the time of surgery to check for an adequate repair and to assess mucosal integrity. Postoperatively the patient should be kept NPO for 3-5 days, after which a swallow contrast study should be performed to assess for a

163

leak. If there is a leak, the patient should continue to be NPO with NGT decompression. Further management options include esophageal endoscopic stenting versus reoperation through the left chest or abdomen depending on the size of the leak and the patient's symptoms and clinical status.

"A 67-year-old patient presents with long-standing dysphagia and a dilated, tortuous esophagus. Manometry is consistent with achalasia. How would you manage this patient?"
A severely dilated and tortuous sigmoid-shaped esophagus (or megaesophagus) is suspect for end-stage achalasia. Even with esophageal dilation greater than 6 cm and a sigmoid-shaped esophagus, a myotomy can be first-line therapy. But often the esophagus can be so markedly dilated that standard Heller myotomy can be technically challenging and would not be sufficient to relieve outflow obstruction and permit for adequate esophageal emptying. In such circumstances, a transhiatal or a 3-hole esophagogastrectomy with gastric pull-up and cervical anastomosis can be performed. While patients who have a sigmoid esophagus and a prior failed myotomy are the best candidates for an esophagectomy. Esophagectomy as first-line therapy for achalasia - even in the setting of a sigmoid esophagus - is more controversial.

"A patient presents with severe spasmodic chest pain and dysphagia. You suspect the patient has an esophageal motility disorder. How would you work this patient up?"
After ruling out cardiac and other gastrointestinal sources of chest pain, non-achalasia primary esophageal motility disorders should be suspected. Manometric analysis should be performed. Disorders include nutcracker esophagus (100% peristaltic waves, distal esophageal amplitudes > 180 mmHg), diffuse esophageal spasm (simultaneous pressurizations in 20-90% of the swallows with the remaining swallows having prolonged contractions [> 6 seconds] and the presence of high-pressure amplitudes in the distal segment of the body), and hypertensive LES (resting LES pressure > 40 mmHg, 100% peristaltic contractions). First-line management of most non-achalasia motility disorders is medical therapy. A long myotomy followed by partial fundoplication is associated with good outcomes in these motility disorders when dysphagia and obstructive symptoms are the primary complaints and when the LES resting pressure is elevated with poor relaxation. The proximal extent of the long myotomy should be guided by manometric analysis and should extend past the abnormal and hypertensive contractions until normotensive esophagus is reached. If a myotomy needs to extend above the aortic arch, a right thoracotomy will be necessary.

"A 49-year-old woman with dysphagia also has history of Raynaud's phenomena and telangiectasias. What is the suspected diagnosis and how would you confirm this?"
A clinical diagnosis of scleroderma is suspected. Manometric characteristics include a hypomotile esophageal body in 100% of the swallows with a hypotensive LES. In contrast to achalasia, the LES does relax. Also, achalasia affects smooth muscle, therefore contractions in the more proximal esophagus (striated muscle) will be normal. Management is often times supportive therapy with aggressive anti-reflux medical therapy and dilation of strictures if they occur. If anti-reflux surgery is to be considered, one should perform a partial fundoplication given the impaired esophageal motility associated with scleroderma.

"A patient with long-standing GERD presents with dysphagia."
Diagnostic workup should include EGD, impedance-pH analysis, barium esophagram, and manometric evaluation. Mechanical obstruction may be secondary to peptic stricture, hiatal hernia, or adenocarcinoma. Patients with peptic stricture should be managed first with dilation, followed by anti-reflux surgery once the stricture is adequately dilated. Patients with GERD can also have ineffective esophageal motility
(IEM), presumably due to the progressive fibrosis caused by chronic inflammation. IEM is characterized by having at least 30% of the swallows with distal esophageal amplitudes < 30 mmHg, failed contractions that do not transverse the entire esophageal body, simultaneous waves with amplitudes < 30 mmHg, or absent peristalsis. Treatment consists of anti-reflux therapy or surgery, with reports of improved motility following cessation of the harmful reflux.

"A 72-year-old man with a history of GERD is referred to you with a barium esophagram that shows a 'classic' bird's beak appearance of the distal esophagus. He has had progressive dysphagia and a 20-pounds weight loss. He is being referred to you for surgical treatment of achalasia. How would you proceed?"

As stated above, make sure you confirm the diagnosis of achalasia with manometry and upper endoscopy. This patient's history is more suspicious for an obstructing distal esophageal cancer. Upper endoscopy must be performed preoperatively, and any suspicious lesions or strictures should be biopsied. Do not fall into the trap of doing a myotomy and fundoplication on a patient with an obstructing esophageal cancer.

"An 81-year-old woman with a history of achalasia and multiple prior pneumatic dilations is referred to you for dysphagia. Manometry appears consistent with achalasia. A barium esophagram shows only a mildly dilated esophagus and question of a filling defect in the mid-esophagus. What is the suspected diagnosis and how would you proceed?"

Remember that long-standing achalasia is associated with squamous cell carcinoma of the esophagus. This patient should undergo upper endoscopy and biopsy of the suspicious lesion. Should this prove to be a malignancy, the patient should undergo esophagectomy following appropriate staging and physiologic testing.

Pearls/pitfalls

- Four manometric characteristics of achalasia are 1.) absence of LES relaxation, 2.) elevated LES resting pressure, 3.) 100% simultaneous pressurizations with aperistalsis of the esophageal body, and 4.) esophageal body pressurization. While all 4 are not always present, the absence of LES relaxation must be present for the diagnosis of achalasia.
- Perform EGD to look for other associated pathology (pseudoachalasia, infection).
- Surgical therapy for achalasia consists of laparoscopic Heller myotomy with partial fundoplication.
- Length of myotomy should be at least 4 cm on to the esophagus and 2-3 cm on to the stomach.
- Check the completeness of myotomy and for mucosal injury with EGD at completion of myotomy.

Suggested readings

- Herbella et al. Surgical Treatment of Primary Esophageal Motility Disorders. *J GI Surg* 2008; 12: 604–608.
- Banki F and DeMeester TR. Surgery for Achalasia and Other Motility Disorders. Kaiser LR, Kron IL, and Spray TL. (eds) *Mastery of Cardiothoracic Surgery* (3rd edition). 2014; 199-212.
- Hong E and Liptay MJ. Achalasia. Franco KL and Thourani VH. (eds) *Cardiothoracic Surgery Review.* 2012; 1409-1411.

25. ESOPHAGEAL PERFORATION

Eric M. Krause MD, JD and Shamus R. Carr, MD

Adapted from 1st edition chapter written by Aaron J. Weiss, MD, and Andrew J. Kaufman, MD

Concept

- Causes of esophageal perforation
- Presentation, diagnosis, and workup
- Operative timing and options
- Pitfalls and alternative solutions

Chief complaint

"A 63-year-old previously healthy male with PMH significant for atrial fibrillation presents with substernal chest pain radiating towards the back after violent retching."

Differential

Esophageal perforation, acute coronary syndrome, thoracic aortic dissection, GERD, gastritis, pneumonia, tension pneumothorax and pericarditis. The most common causes of esophageal injury are: iatrogenic, Boerhaave's syndrome, tumor erosion, or external trauma. Iatrogenic injury to the esophagus occurs most commonly during flexible or rigid upper endoscopy and less commonly during surgical procedures. Boerhaave's syndrome arises from a rapid increase in intraluminal pressure from the patient vomiting with concurrent failure of relaxation of the upper esophageal sphincter. Cadaver studies have shown that as little as a 5 psi increase in intra luminal pressure is all that is needed to cause a perforation. If the perforation is due to a malignant lesion, then at best the patient has a T3 lesion with a minimum stage of IIB under the 8th AJCC guidelines. With the caveat that tumor cells have been spilled into the pleural space and mediastinum, possibly seeding one or both. External trauma is the least likely cause of esophageal perforation with most cases occurring as a result of high-speed motor vehicle crashes. Penetrating trauma rarely damages the thoracic esophagus due to its location; however, the cervical esophagus is more at risk.

History and physical

The history and physical exam should quickly alert the physician to the possibility of esophageal perforation. If stable and alert, the patient should be asked for timing, duration, location, and severity of chest/abdominal/back pain as well as any associated shortness of breath. As part of the history care must be taken when questioning about any recent esophageal procedures, emesis, ingestion of foreign material or trauma. If unable to directly question the patient, every effort must be made to obtain this information through the medical record or from that patient's contacts. A focused physical exam should be performed that includes vital signs, as well as lung, cardiac, and abdominal exams. At times, cervical crepitus can be felt along with a systolic crunching sound heard over left sternal border, known as Hammon's sign. Historically, according to Mackler a left thoracotomy was warranted if presented with an acutely decompensating patient who exhibits subcutaneous emphysema and thoracic pain that arose during or after vomiting. Physicians should be cautioned that this classic triad is not frequently present and that the presentation may differ based on several factors including the cause, the location, the size of the defect and the length of time elapsed since the onset of symptoms.

Tests

- *Labs.* A complete blood cell count, basic metabolic panel, liver function tests, troponin, INR/PT/PTT, type and screen, blood culture x2.
- *EKG.* To rule out an acute coronary syndrome or an arrhythmia.
- *PA and lateral X-ray, upright abdominal X-ray.* This is likely the first radiology that will be performed on a patient after presentation, but other studies are more sensitive

and/or more specific. Many signs suggest the possibility of an esophageal perforation and these include subcutaneous emphysema of the soft tissue surrounding the cervical spine, anterior displacement of the trachea due to air or fluid, widening of the superior mediastinum, the "V sign" which is emphysema in left lower mediastinum along the aorta and above the left diaphragm, mediastinal widening and the prescience of pleural effusions with or without an associated pneumothorax. For cervical esophageal perforations, a lateral neck X-ray may show air in the prevertebral fascia.

- *Esophagram.* An esophagram with water-soluble contrast is the test of choice when available and the patient is able to swallow because it is useful to both localize the perforation if present and to define any distal esophageal pathology prior to intervention. Unfortunately, it has approximately a 10% false-negative rate. If no leak is seen and clinical suspicion is high enough, the test can be repeated with thin (dilute) barium contrast, which is more sensitive for detecting small perforations.

- *Pleural fluid analysis.* Although rarely performed, a perforation can presumptively be diagnosed in the right clinical scenario with elevated pleural amylase levels or food particulate in the drainage.

- *CT scan of the chest with IV and PO water-soluble contrast.* A benefit of a CT with PO and IV contrast is that it can help localize the site of perforation better in 3 dimensions than an esophagram alone, but with a slightly higher false negative rate. However, another added benefit of the CT is that it can detect any concurrent extra-esophageal pathology, such as mediastinitis or metastasis. A CT scan with PO contrast can be performed on intubated patients by administering the contrast through an NGT placed approximately 20cm from the incisors.

Index scenario (additional information)

"The patient states that he began retching this evening without provocation and his chest pain coincided with his emesis. He says that his emesis was bilious with maybe some streaks of dark blood. He is normotensive with a slightly elevated temp at 38.0. Besides being tachycardic, the patient's cardiac exam is normal. The lungs are clear to auscultation bilaterally with tachypnea. No crepitus is palpated. His abdomen is soft, slightly tender in the epigastric region, nondistended, and without rebound or guarding. Troponins are sent and are negative. A CT scan with IV contrast is performed and demonstrates a left pleural effusion with pneumomediastinum. A follow up CT with PO contrast demonstrates contrast extravasation into the left pleural space. How would you proceed?"

Treatment/management

There are 4 primary principles for the treatment of esophageal perforation, regardless of its etiology. These are prevention of further mediastinal soilage, debridement and drainage of both the pleural and mediastinal spaces, initiation of broad-spectrum antibiotic coverage including anti-fungal coverage, and nutritional support.

- Immediate initiation of broad-spectrum antibiotics is paramount after the diagnosis is made and should not be delayed due to any interventions. Coverage should be guided by local antibiograms and must also include coverage for oral flora and yeast.

- The prevention of further soilage can be accomplished in multiple different ways with the most common being (in order): primary repair, stenting, and drainage. Rarely is an esophagectomy performed at the index operation.

- The debridement of the mediastinum is necessary to prevent overwhelming sepsis and death as antibiotics cannot easily penetrate mediastinal fluid collections. Decortication of the lung is necessary as the fully expanded lung can help with buttressing any repairs and to improve the patient's respiratory status.

- Nutritional support can be accomplished either through distal feeding access or TPN. The placement of distal surgical feeding access should be deferred until the patient is hemodynamically recovered and stable, and once further soilage is controlled.

- Ideally, surgical repair and debridement should be done within 24 hours as this is an inflection point for both morbidity and mortality.

Prior to proceeding to the OR the patient and or their family should be counseled as to the serious nature of their condition and that despite prompt interventions mortality is between 10–20%.

Operative steps
Primary Repair of a Distal Esophageal Perforation

- The patient will require general anesthesia with the ability to perform selective lung ventilation either through a double lumen tube or a bronchial blocker. The patient will also require an arterial line for hemodynamic monitoring and likely will need some form of central venous access as well.
- Generally, an EGD is performed first to localize the site of the perforation(s), determine if any distal obstructions are present and the integrity of the mucosa and its ability to undergo a primary repair.
- The patient should be positioned in right lateral decubitus (left side up) and the table should be flexed at the level of the anterior ischial spine. If the perforation localizes to the right of the esophagus and the right pleural space needs to be debrided, then it is appropriate to choose a right sided approach and left lateral decubitus positioning.
- A posterolateral thoracotomy is performed at the seventh intercostal space. If your entry is lower it is difficult to gain access to the entire mediastinum, and higher it is generally harder to perform your repair. If you intend to use an intercostal muscle flap to buttress your repair, it is best to harvest an intercostal muscle flap at thoracotomy as the muscle can be slightly damaged by the retractor if it is left in its natural position during the case.
- After thoracotomy, divide the inferior pulmonary ligament in order to retract the lung cephalad. The mediastinal pleura is opened along the entire length of the anterior and posterior esophagus.
- Localize the site and extent of perforation. A longitudinal myotomy both proximally and distally should be performed to fully expose the mucosal defect as it almost always extends beyond the muscular defect.
- After identifying and debriding the mucosal edges a primary repair using interrupted absorbable sutures is performed. A 45+ Fr Bougie or an EGD can be used to ensure that the esophageal lumen is not narrowed, although not entirely essential. As in all repairs, it is important to ensure that the repair is tension free. After the mucosal layer is repaired the muscular layer is closed using either interrupted or running non-absorbable suture.
- At this time any distal obstruction that exists should be dealt with if it was not already addressed. If a distal obstruction is not fixed the conditions that led to the perforation in the first place will continue to exist and the repair will be tenuous at best.
- At this point have the anesthesiologist pass an NG tube through the esophagus and into the stomach under tactile guidance from the operative field to ensure no disruption of the repair.
- The repair should then be buttressed, most commonly by using an intercostal muscle flap with the pleural side secured facing the repair. Other possible flaps include pericardial fat and omentum.
- The mediastinum and pleural space should be copiously irrigated, and hemostasis achieved. If desired the repair can be inspected at this time using an EGD. The repair can be further tested by filling the pleural space with fluid and insufflating while looking for bubbles in the operative field. If any are present, this would alert the surgical team to a residual defect that needs to be addressed prior to leaving the operating room.
- Multiple drainage tubes should be left in the pleural space including at least one tube juxtaposed to the site of the repair in case there is a postoperative leak.

- After the chest is closed it is up to the surgical team how to obtain access for nutritional support. Nutritional support options include a post-pyloric feeding tube, a surgical jejunostomy tube, or a central line for TPN. The decision on feeding access should consider the hemodynamic stability of the patient, since surgical feeding access is a semi-elective procedure and can be deferred until the patient is better resuscitated.

Minimally Invasive Debridement and Stenting a Distal Esophageal Perforation

- The patient will require general anesthesia with the ability to perform selective lung ventilation either through a double lumen tube or a bronchial blocker. The patient will also require an arterial line for hemodynamic monitoring and likely will need some form of central venous access as well.
- After the EGD is introduced and a full inspection of the esophagus and stomach has been performed, the perforation can be assessed for its suitability for stent coverage. To be suitable, the tissue must have enough integrity that it will not tear with the radial force of stent deployment and the perforation has to be less than 50% of the circumference of the intact esophagus.
- Stent deployment is performed using a guidewire and either fluoroscopic guidance or under direct visualization using a side by side technique.
- Ideally there should be at least a 2cm landing zone proximal and distal to the esophageal perforation in order to get an adequate seal and prevent stent migration.
- Stenting a very distal perforation has the potential unique complication of creating intolerable reflux by stenting open the GE junction. Similarly, with proximal perforations (those at or above 25cm from the incisors), many patients will have an intolerable sensation "in their throat" that only abates after stent removal.
- The decision to use either a fully covered or partially uncovered stent is left up to the surgeon and the clinical situation. The partially uncovered stents are less prone to migrate, but at the expense of providing less coverage area and possibly less of a complete seal.
- A completion EGD is required to ensure proper placement of the stent. It is also possible to make some positioning adjustments after deployment depending on the stent.
- The patient should then be placed in the appropriate lateral decubitus position based on preoperative imaging. If necessary, both sides can be done sequentially.
- The pleural space is then accessed for VATS debridement of the mediastinum with many surgeons beginning with a port in the 7th or 8th interspace in the mid-axillary line. Further ports can be inserted as needed.
- As in open repair multiple chest drainage tubes should be left in the pleural space including at least one tube juxtaposed to the site of the perforation in case there is a postoperative leak. Similarly, the decision about distal feeding access should be made at this time.

Potential questions/alternative scenarios

"What flaps can be used to buttress a primary repair of an esophageal perforation?"
Remember to plan for flap coverage and to alert the examiner to this, especially if you plan to use a muscle flap and are performing a thoracotomy. Multiple options exist for buttressing the repair and include in order of likelihood an intercostal muscle with pleura, pericardial fat pad, pedicled omentum, pedicled diaphragm, gastric fundus (abdominal esophagus only) and in extremely rare circumstances either rhomboid, latissimus dorsi muscles, or pleura alone.

"Instead of immediately sending the patient for the CT with IV contrast this is delayed, thereby delaying diagnosis by 48 hours. What would change about your operative strategy at this time?"
After 24 hours there is an increased risk of both morbidity and mortality, which is largely due to the decreased likelihood of a successful primary repair. Worse outcomes are also due to worsening mediastinitis with hemodynamic instability, prolonged inflammation degrading tissue integrity and increased need for extensive pulmonary decortications. Even with these

169

potentially slightly worsened outcomes, primary repair or stenting is preferred and should attempted over a drainage procedure if feasible.

If the patient cannot undergo a primary repair and they are not a candidate for stenting, a drainage procedure is the next best option. To perform this, the principles of primary repair still apply. The mediastinum and pleural space must be debrided, antibiotics must be rapidly started, nutritional support must be determined and a way to contain further mediastinal soilage still must occur. One option for this is a T-tube which can be placed into the defect creating a controlled esophagocutaneous fistula that allows for adequate drainage of the esophagus while giving the tissues around the site of perforation time to heal. This can be performed for both cervical and thoracic injuries. The patient should then have a complete decortication and chest tubes placed to ensure adequate drainage of the pleural space.

Only if the esophagus is clearly not viable should esophageal exclusion be considered at the index operation. If an esophagostomy is indicated, the esophagus is divided proximally and distally to the defect and the non-viable esophagus is resected. After extensive debridement and irrigation, drains are left in the former esophageal bed and the pleural space. The proximal esophageal remnant is then tunneled to above the clavicle, if possible, brought to the skin and sutured into place. If the patient is too unstable, an NGT can be left in the proximal stump with further management to be completed later. At the end of the drainage procedure, as before, feeding access can be deferred if the patient is too unstable. After the patient is stabilized a delayed reconstruction can take place with a completion esophagectomy followed by a substernal esophageal replacement, ideally gastric. If the stomach is not suitable to use, an iso-peristaltic colon interposition would be the next best option. The substernal route is the best option since it should be free of the extensive adhesions that would make a mediastinal pull up challenging.

"What should be done if there is an obstruction distal to the site of the perforation during a primary repair?"
Studies have shown that if primary repair is performed without treatment of a distal obstruction to the site of the perforation, failure of the repair will almost assuredly occur. Therefore, a surgeon is required to definitively deal with distal obstructions if the patient can tolerate it.

In the case of a paraesophageal hernia causing a distal obstruction, this must be reduced, and the diaphragmatic defect must be repaired. Similarly, a stricture/achalasia that is distal to the site of the perforation can be treated with open or thoracoscopic esophagomyotomy. If performed an incision is made opposite the site of perforation and should be carried distally past the obstruction and must continue onto the stomach. This should be carried through both muscle layers and care should be taken not to damage the mucosa/submucosa. If the patient has a long-standing history of stricture/achalasia with previous failed therapy, strong consideration should be given to performing a formal esophagogastrectomy with immediate gastric reconstruction.
If the patient is hemodynamically stable, it may be prudent to obtain a rapid full body CT scan while preparing the OR. This is because if the patient has obvious metastatic disease your operative management may change from completion esophagogastrectomy with immediate gastric pull up to exclusion and diversion.

"If the perforation occurred in the cervical esophagus, what surgical approach should be taken?"
For cervical perforations of the esophagus, as in distal perforations the same plan for anesthesia and EGD should apply. The incision should be made anterior to the left sternocleidomastoid (SCM) from the sternal notch to the level of the cricoid cartilage. After lateral retraction of the SCM and carotid sheath with concurrent medial retraction of the trachea and thyroid, use blunt finger dissection to encircle the esophagus and to expose the prevertebral space. Blunt finger dissection should be carried as caudal as possible in the paravertebral space and a Penrose drain should be left behind. Any anterior fluid

170

collections seen on preoperative imaging should also be addressed along with any pleural fluid collections. Often primary repair is not necessary and adequate irrigation and drainage will allow for the esophageal injury to heal on its own.

"What if the perforation were in the mid-esophagus?"

For injuries to the mid-esophagus, the approach is the same as for distal perforations, except that the approach is almost always through a right thoracotomy. It is very difficult to approach the mid-esophagus from the left chest due to the presence of the aortic arch.

Pearls/pitfalls

- Early diagnosis and treatment are of the utmost value to optimize outcome following an esophageal perforation.
- A variety of tests and imaging are useful in diagnosing an esophageal perforation with the gold standard being an esophagram with water-soluble contrast followed by thin barium if the initial study is negative and suspicion of perforation remains high.
- Operative intervention within 24 hours maximizes both the patient's chances of survival and chance of performing a successful primary repair. Buttressing of the repair should be performed and the surgeon can choose from many options.
- Stenting with thoracoscopic drainage is rapidly increasing in frequency with similar morbidity and mortality as open primary repairs with shorter lengths of stay; however, they have greatly increased risks of readmissions in the next 6 months.
- The etiology of perforation, clinical status of the patient, time from injury, extent of mediastinitis, and quality of tissue surrounding the injury should all be taken into account when determining whether primary repair is appropriate.
- Cervical perforations can typically be treated with drainage alone, assuming there is no leakage into the pleural space.
- Intrathoracic perforation should be approached on the side of extravasation of contrast or pleural effusion. If neither are present, distal perforations can be approached from the left or right, whereas mid-esophageal perforations are best approached from the right chest.

Suggested readings

- Raja Mahidhara and Richard K. Freeman. Esophageal Perforation. In: Joseph LoCiero III. Shields' General Thoracic Surgery. Philadelphia, PA: LWW.; 2018: 2961-2973
- Ory Wiesel and Jon O. Wee. Esophageal Stents. In: Joseph LoCiero III. Shields' General Thoracic Surgery. Philadelphia, PA: LWW.; 2018: 3445-3469
- Thornblade LW, Cheng AM, Wood DE, et al. A Nationwide Rise in the Use of Stents for Benign Esophageal Perforation. *Ann Thorac Surg.* 2017;104(1):227-233.

26. ESOPHAGEAL DIVERTICULA
Carlos J. Anciano, MD and Manisha Shende, MD

Concept
- Pulsion vs. traction diverticula (false vs. true)
- Anatomical level guides differential and intervention (Zenker's, mid-esophagus, epiphrenic)
- Minimally invasive and open approaches
- Concomitant underlying disorders
- Treatment aims to relieve distal obstruction, treat associated disorder, and avoid leakage at site of diverticulectomy and myotomy

Chief complaint
"A 72-year-old man arrives to your clinic with complaints of difficulty swallowing, sensation of food getting stuck in his throat, and occasional choking and regurgitation of food when eating."

Differential
Esophageal motility disorders (i.e., achalasia), neuromotor degenerative disorders, esophageal diverticulum, esophageal stricture/ring, GERD, hiatal hernia, cancer.

History and physical
Focus on evaluating dysphagia: patterns, progressiveness, saliva vs. liquid vs. solids. Look for regurgitation of digested or undigested meals, aspiration history, halitosis, and cervical bruits on swallowing. Changes in tone of voice and globus sensation suggest more proximal pathology. Respiratory issues such as new onset asthma, pneumonia, or pulmonary abscesses are commonly related. Up to 50% of proximal diverticula are associated with GERD. Progressive dysphagia or changes in symptom pattern may suggest progression of an underlying dysmotility disorder, hiatal hernia, or stricture. Chest pressure or spasm-like pain suggest more distal esophageal pathology and associated motor disorders. Loss of weight and old age should increase the suspicion of malignant disease.

Tests
- *Contrast esophagram.* Typically, the first step in the workup of dysphagia. Imaging should include views of the cervical esophagus to the stomach, as well as video cine recordings. Contrast pooling on post-swallow images will help to identify important characteristics of diverticula. Evaluate size, base/neck of diverticula, location and number of diverticula. Tertiary contractions, spasms, and esophageal quivering may suggest a motility disorder, but this is best confirmed with manometry. Evidence of reflux, rings, strictures, or filling defects should prompt further work up as well.
- *Manometry/pH studies.* Obtained selectively to determine etiology of diverticulum. A hypertensive upper esophageal sphincter and GERD are associated with Zenker's diverticula, while a number of motility abnormalities are commonly associated with epiphrenic diverticula.
- *CT scans.* Most useful for workup of mid-esophageal traction diverticula to evaluate for pulmonary or mediastinal inflammatory processes, such as granulomatous disease (i.e., TB, histoplasmosis). May also be helpful in planning operative approach (i.e., laterality).
- *EGD.* Perform carefully to avoid perforation. Can confirm presence and location of diverticulum, as well as evaluate for mucosal lesions. Therapeutically allows for dilation of strictures and allows for clearance of retained debris.
- *Labs.* Blood counts pointing to acute or chronic respiratory infections, blood losses, as well as nutritional status chemistries are useful.

"The patient's breath is foul as he speaks and states he sometimes regurgitates chewed up lunch when he goes to bed at night. Contrast esophagram shows a 4 cm posterior cervical outpouching with retained contrast on post-swallow scout. Where do you go from here?"

Treatment/management

This patient has a Zenker's diverticulum (a false, pulsion diverticulum). Given his symptoms, operative repair should be recommended. Patients with Zenker's are typically older (50% are > 70-year-old and 20% are > 80-year-old at presentation); therefore, it is important to assess cardiopulmonary reserve and nutritional status preoperatively. Once the patient has been deemed an adequate surgical candidate, one must then decide between endoscopic or open surgical treatment. Ankylosis of the jaw, cervical kyphosis, a prominent orbital arch, and a diverticulum < 3 cm (cannot fit stapler) or > 8-9 cm (creates a cloaca when stapled transorally) should prompt one to opt for an open approach. A narrow diverticulum neck with a larger pouch is an ideal candidate for endoscopic treatment with transoral stapling. Hiatal hernias and GERD are not uncommon in patients with Zenker's diverticula, with some proposing that there is compensatory tightening of the cricopharyngeus to protect from aspiration of refluxate, which then leads to the pulsion diverticulum. One must determine which pathology is more symptomatic (GERD/hiatal hernia vs. Zenker's), in which case the more symptomatic of the two is treated first. Treating both in the same setting significantly increases operative risk in a typically older patient population and should be avoided.

Operative steps

Diverticulectomy/diverticulopexy

Goals – relieve obstruction/high-pressure area/dysfunctional sphincter by cricopharyngeal myotomy, prevent collection of food debris within the diverticulum by pexy vs. resection.

- Supine patient with head slightly to right, ETT to prevent aspiration of retained debris. Left cervical oblique incision from hyoid to 1 cm above clavicle, retract sternocleidomastoid and carotid sheath laterally, larynx and thyroid medially.
- The omohyoid and middle thyroid vein may be divided for improved exposure.
- Avoid positioning retractors medially and dissect directly on the esophagus to minimize the risk of injury to the recurrent laryngeal nerve in the tracheoesophageal groove.
- Dissect out the diverticulum circumferentially to the base, which can be facilitated by placement of a 36-44 Fr bougie (probably safest to place over a guidewire to avoid perforation of the diverticulum).
- Cricopharyngeal myotomy is performed approximately 135° laterally, extending inferiorly at least 4 cm and proximally at least 2 cm on to striated muscle. The edges of the myotomy are separated approximately 90°.
- For diverticula < 2 cm, myotomy alone is sufficient treatment. Larger diverticula can be resected, most commonly done with a linear cutting stapler placed parallel to the long axis of the esophagus. The diverticulum may also be resected followed by hand-sewn reapproximation of the mucosa with 4-0 absorbable suture. Remnant omohyoid or strap muscle may be used to cover the repair. Salivary fistulae have been reported in up to 25% of patients undergoing diverticulectomy. Alternatively, pexy of larger diverticula to the more proximal prevertebral fascia prevents collection of debris within the lumen and has a significantly lower risk of fistulization.
- Retropharyngeal drain and layered, interrupted closure.

Transoral stapling

Goals – relieve obstruction with myotomy while creating a common channel between diverticulum and esophageal lumen to prevent collection of food debris.

- Supine patient, ETT to prevent aspiration of retained debris, shoulder roll, head slightly extended.

173

- Flexible esophagoscopy is performed first and a guide wire is placed in the true esophageal lumen for orientation.

- Rigid esophagoscopy is then performed with Weerda retractor. The top blade is positioned in the esophageal lumen while the lower blade is positioned in the diverticulum.

- The common wall between the true lumen and the diverticulum (which contains the cricopharyngeus) is centered in the view. A long stitch placed in the apex of the common wall aids with retraction during stapling.

- A linear cutting stapler with a dulled anvil tip is passed through the rigid esophagoscope. The stapler is positioned with the blunted end in the diverticulum and the cartridge in the true lumen. Serial firings may be needed for larger diverticuli.

Potential questions/alternative scenarios

"Now you are seeing a 54-year-old man complaining of crushing chest pain, dysphagia, heartburn, and regurgitation. After ruling out cardiac reasons for his chest pain, you obtain a Barium swallow, which shows a 7-8 cm outpouching in the distal esophagus. How would you manage this patient?"

This patient has an epiphrenic diverticulum (false, pulsion diverticulum). His symptoms of heartburn and spasm-like pain suggest a concurrent motility disorder, which are common in patients with epiphrenic diverticula. Epiphrenic diverticula, particularly small ones, will likely be asymptomatic or present with mild symptoms. Some surgeons argue that all epiphrenic diverticula should be treated surgically, while other believe that patients who are asymptomatic or with mild symptoms can be treated conservatively. Conservative, or medical management, consists simply of chewing food well and intake of adequate liquids with meals. Patients who are symptomatic should unquestionably be treated surgically. Common associated symptoms include dysphagia, chest pain, food retention, aspiration, and regurgitation. Since many patients with epiphrenic diverticula have an underlying functional or mechanical distal obstruction that contributes to the formation of the diverticulum, it may be unclear if the symptoms are due to the diverticulum itself or the accompanying esophageal pathology. For this reason, epiphrenic diverticula should always be addressed when other esophageal pathology is being treated surgically. Manometry will uncover underlying esophageal spasm, achalasia, or a nonspecific motility disorder that may affect the surgical plan. pH studies will identify GERD, which may have led to strictures or rings. EGD can visualize rings, strictures, areas of narrowing (external or internal compression), and allows for preoperative dilation. CT may assist with determining the best operative approach (chest or abdomen, left or right chest). A clear liquid diet may be required for a few days preoperatively to clear the esophageal lumen and diverticulum of debris. Treatment remains a myotomy extending proximal to the most cephalad diverticulum and distally past the area of incomplete relaxation (manometry guides). The myotomy is typically performed 90-180° away from the neck of the diverticulum. If further than 1 cm onto stomach (especially if non-relaxing lower esophageal sphincter), consider an anti-reflux procedure in the form of a partial fundoplication. When high amplitude contractions and spasm-like motility is present, it is best to perform a long proximal myotomy. Right-sided pouches need for long myotomy (proximal to the aortic arch), and higher epiphrenic diverticula should be approached from the right chest. Distal, smaller, or left-sided pouches may be approached from the left chest or abdomen. Favor an open, posterolateral thoracotomy approach unless extremely comfortable with VATS techniques. If the base is wide and the pouch small, myotomy alone suffices in most cases. For large diverticula, those with narrow necks, or diverticula in which the endoscope passes preferentially into the pouch, perform a diverticulectomy over a 50-54 Fr bougie with a linear stapling device. The esophageal muscle and/or pleura can be re-approximated to buttress the staple line. The myotomy should then be performed at least 90° away from the staple line. Be compulsive about elevating the muscle layer away from mucosa with right angle clamps or the energy device of choice before division to avoid injury to the underlying mucosa. If the mucosa is perforated, primarily repair with absorbable suture, buttress the repair, and rotate the site of myotomy. Local drainage (i.e., Jackson-Pratt) near the staple line in addition to chest tube drainage of the pleural space is recommended.

Contrast esophagram is routinely obtained in the early postoperative period before starting a diet. Save abdominal laparoscopic approaches for very small, distal diverticula, with distal manometry-guided targets (i.e., LES in achalasia). Approaching diverticula through the chest and performing abdominal fundoplication if symptoms of reflux in a second stage is also sometimes the preferred treatment plan. Aim to prevent recurrence, protect your suture line, and treat dysmotility. Injury to one vagus nerve is of little clinical significance, while bilateral injury may require a gastric emptying procedure.

"You walk in the office to meet a 43-year-old spelunker complaining of solid food dysphagia, stating that occasionally food 'won't go down' (while pointing to sternum). He reports occasional regurgitation of undigested food, as well as occasional blood-streaked emesis. How would you manage this patient?"

Contrast esophagram is the first test of choice for dysphagia, which in this case shows a 6 cm outpouching in the mid-esophagus. There seems to be contrast outside of esophagus, for which a non-contrast CT scan will help to clarify. The CT shows that the extra-luminal densities are actually calcifications in the mediastinum. This mid-esophageal (true, traction) diverticulum, demographics, hematemesis, and mediastinal findings should prompt the further imaging (CT scan). Granulomatous disease (i.e., histoplasmosis, TB) should be suspected. Treatment of symptomatic mid-esophageal diverticula remains myotomy and diverticulectomy with certain considerations. Hematemesis or hemoptysis raises concerns for erosions, airway-esophageal fistulae, vascular-esophageal fistulae, granulation tissue bleeding, ulceration and esophagitis. CT angiography is appropriate in surgical planning that may require vascular control as part of the plan. Chronic cough, changes in imaging such as bronchiectasis or airway to esophageal fistula should lead to anticipated pulmonary resection. All mid-esophageal diverticula should be approached from the chest via thoracotomy or a VATS approach if uncomplicated and the surgeons possesses the skill set needed. The level of the thoracotomy will depend on the exact location of the diverticulum; however, most can be approached through the right chest in the 5th or 6th intercostal space. Careful entry into the chest and consideration for intercostal muscle harvesting is needed. The myotomy should be carried at least 1 cm proximal and distal to neck of the diverticulum, 90-180° away from the neck. Pulmonary function testing preoperatively is also appropriate. Airway repair follows classic principles with interposition of live pedicle tissue (see other chapter on tracheoesophageal fistulae). Treatment of his primary pulmonary disease (histoplasmosis or TB) is also needed.

Pearls/pitfalls

- Pulsion diverticula (i.e., Zenker's, epiphrenic) are protrusions of the mucosa through a weak area in the muscle layers (false), potentiated by some anatomic or functional distal obstruction. Traction diverticula arise from inflammation of surrounding tissue that leads to pulling of all layers of the esophagus (true).
- For diverticula < 2 cm, myotomy suffices; resect large and narrow neck diverticula.
- Cancer in Zenker's diverticula is rare; most are squamous cell carcinomas resulting from neglect of the condition. When limited to the diverticulum, diverticulectomy suffices for long-term survival. Not having muscularis, further involvement requires a case-by-case, more aggressive approach.
- If a Zenker's patient is hoarse, document vocal cord exam before surgery and anticipate management in case of recurrent nerve injury.
- Diagnose motility disorders before treating the diverticula. If LES is normal on manometry, limit to < 1 cm gastric extent of myotomy. If compromised, extend > 2 cm and perform a partial fundoplication.
- If motility is normal, myotomy to 1 cm above level of most proximal diverticulum suffices.
- Ask Zenker's patient to open mouth and extend neck in clinic to see if they are candidates for transoral stapling.

175

- Suppurative lung disease with mid-esophageal diverticula require conscientious planning with PFTs, CTAs, esophagrams, cardiac clearance, etc.

Suggested readings

- Samson P and Puri V. Esophageal Diverticula. Locicero J, Feins RH, Colson YL, Rocco G (eds). *General Thoracic Surgery.* Lippincott Williams & Wilkins. 8th edition. 2018.
- Peracchia A, Bonavina L, Narne S, et al: Minimally invasive surgery for Zenker's diverticulum: Analysis of results in 95 consecutive patients. *Arch Surg* 1998; 133:695-700.

27. PARAESOPHAGEAL AND DIAPHRAGMATIC HERNIAS

Philip W. Carrott, MD, and Benjamin D. Kozower, MD, MPH, FACS

Concept

- Management of acute and chronic presentations of paraesophageal hiatal hernias
- Preoperative work-up
- Open and laparoscopic repairs
- Assessment of esophageal length
- Fundoplication options

Chief complaint

"You are asked to see a 70-year-old woman who was admitted overnight to the gastroenterology service for anemia and upper gastrointestinal bleeding. They performed an upper and lower endoscopy this morning and saw evidence of a large hiatal hernia with over half of her stomach above the diaphragm. Linear erosions were seen on the stomach mucosa at the hiatal narrowing, but there were no signs of ischemia."

Differential

Paraesophageal hiatal hernia (likely Type III by the classification of hiatal hernias), peptic ulcer disease, large epiphrenic diverticulum, esophagitis, tumor (GIST or gastric cancer)

History and physical

A thorough history usually uncovers multiple issues related to the hernia that have been evolving for some time. Hiatal hernias are long in evolution unless there is a congenital component to their origin (i.e., Bochdalek (posterior) or Morgagni (anterior) diaphragmatic hernias). The typical paraesophageal hernia patient will describe a spectrum of gastrointestinal and gustatory complaints including dysphagia, reflux, chest or abdominal pain, early satiety, decreasing meal size, regurgitation, and avoidance of late meals. In addition, patients with larger hernias will frequently complain of increasing shortness of breath that is often inaccurately attributed to aging rather than the dysfunction in respiration caused by mass effect of the hernia. Also, patients with paraesophageal hiatal hernias are often found to have occult anemia and GI bleeding from ulcerations/erosions caused by constriction of the stomach at the hiatus and movement in and out of the chest with respiration (Cameron lesions). As described in this patient, Cameron lesions are linear ulcers or erosions seen within the herniated portion of the stomach in patients with large paraesophageal hernias.

In the acute presentation, initial symptoms will more often be significant chest or abdominal pain due to ischemia. Patients may also present with nausea and inability to vomit due to complete or partial esophageal obstruction. Urgent nasogastric tube (NGT) decompression with or without endoscopy should be performed to relieve the intragastric pressure when possible. Signs of sepsis, unrelenting pain, or inability to pass a NGT suggests complete esophageal/gastric obstruction, typically from a volvulized intrathoracic stomach. This may lead to gastric ischemia or frank necrosis. Therefore, these signs should prompt emergent surgical intervention without any further delay for diagnostic studies. Patients who present acutely, but are stable and without signs of ischemia, are handled differently. Fluid resuscitation, electrolyte replacement, and appropriate diagnostic studies are carried out prior to proceeding to the operating room, typically during the same hospitalization. Chronic paraesophageal hernias that do not present with acute symptoms can be handled on an elective basis. Results of repair are significantly worse for patients who undergo repair in the setting of acute symptoms; therefore, elective repair of chronic paraesophageal hernias should not be delayed beyond a few weeks.

Tests

- *Imaging.* A contrast esophagram (a.k.a. barium swallow or UGI contrast study) is the cornerstone of diagnosis for paraesophageal hernias and should be obtained in most cases for diagnosis and definition of anatomy. Paraesophageal hernias are routinely imaged incidentally on CT scans and chest plain films, but these exams provide little additional information regarding the hernia not provided by the UGI. The one exception would be gastric wall perfusion seen on a contrast CT scan performed for abdominal pain, although this is not a necessary part of the work-up and is better assessed endoscopically. The UGI should be omitted in patients who present with signs of obstruction.

- *Labs.* Routine preoperative labs including CBC, BMP, and coagulations are typically all that are needed. Patients who present acutely frequently have electrolyte disturbances due to diminished oral intake and vomiting.

- *Endoscopy.* Routine endoscopy should be performed prior to any paraesophageal hernia repair to rule out other problems, such as esophagitis, Barrett's esophagus, malignancy, or ischemia. The timing of endoscopy either at diagnosis or prior to operative repair is not important. Upper endoscopy is particularly important for patients who present acutely, as signs of ischemia or necrosis will alter the operative plan.

- *Manometry/pH/impedance studies.* These esophageal function tests may be helpful in patients with a long history of reflux or regurgitation who may have esophageal dysmotility. The abnormal configuration of the esophagus likely produces some dysmotility and poor peristalsis, therefore some surgeons opt to forego these studies, assuming there is some degree of motor dysfunction. Large hernias may complicate the placement of probes needed to carry out these studies, in addition to making interpretation of the results more difficult.

Index scenario (additional information)
"The patient reports a 3-year history of anemia, the cause of which was not previously determined. She also reports that she feels full quickly and has occasional epigastric abdominal pain after meals. She was told that she had a hiatal hernia some years ago and was prescribed a proton pump inhibitor for reflux symptoms, although she no longer has regular reflux. The patient undergoes an UGI swallow study revealing a Type III giant paraesophageal hiatal hernia. How would you advise this patient?"

Treatment/management
Most patients who present with a paraesophageal hernia are symptomatic at the time of presentation. Indeed, in fit patients, if symptoms related to the hernia are affecting their daily life, such as early satiety, breathlessness, anemia, dysphagia, or significant reflux symptoms, the hernia should be repaired. The usual preoperative work-up for the patient's age and comorbidities should be undertaken as appropriate. Paraesophageal hernias may be classified as "giant" if over 50% of the stomach is herniated into the chest on preoperative imaging. The classification is well-known and relates to what is herniated, along with the location of the gastroesophageal junction (GEJ). Type I – sliding hernia of the GEJ, Type II – herniation of the fundus with the GEJ in the abdomen, Type III – both the GEJ and stomach are herniated into the chest, and Type IV – Type III with additional organs herniated into the chest. Type III is the most common "giant" paraesophageal hernia, and there is some debate as to the existence of Type II, since the GEJ is almost always herniated with the stomach. The most common method of primary repair for giant paraesophageal hernias is via laparoscopy, although key steps are the same for all approaches. Redo surgeries are possible via laparoscopy but may also be performed transthoracic with the Belsey Mark IV repair. The key steps include reduction of the hernia by dissection and removal of the hernia sac, establishment of adequate intra-abdominal esophageal length, hiatal closure, and a fundoplication of some sort to minimize reflux.

178

Laparoscopic repair

- Dissection begins at the hiatus, dividing the gastrohepatic ligament (pars flaccida). The sac is incised on the right crus, leaving the peritoneal covering on the crus, which provides strength for the hiatal closure.

- The sac is everted and blunt/sharp (with energy) dissection is carried out to divide the attachments of the sac to the mediastinum and mobilize the intrathoracic esophagus. The vagus nerves must be identified and preserved.

- Entry into the pleural space should be avoided when possible to avoid development of a tension pneumothorax due to insufflation. If the pleura is violated and a tension pneumothorax does develop, a pigtail pleural catheter or chest tube should be placed. A sustained positive pressure breath at the end of the procedure is usually sufficient to expel most of the insufflation and the chest tube is removed the following day.

- The short gastric vessels are divided along the upper third of the greater curve of the stomach in preparation for the fundoplication.

- The sac is completely removed from the mediastinum, typically from right to left, and excised. It is frequently easier to dissect the sac from the left crus after dividing the short gastric vessels.

- A bougie is then passed to assess the hiatus (54 or 56 Fr works for most patients). The right and left crus are then re-approximated with interrupted sutures beginning posteriorly (with the bougie pulled back in the upper esophagus). The authors use 0-Ethibond with or without pledgets, depending on the state of the crus. If the peritoneal lining of crus is stripped, the sutures are more likely to pull through the muscle and pledgets should then be considered.

- The bougie is replaced to assess the completeness of the closure. Occasionally anterior sutures are required for large hiatuses. Tight re-approximation of the crus should be avoided, as this will lead to postoperative dysphagia and possible obstruction.

- Esophageal length is then assessed. If there is less than 2 cm of intra-abdominal esophagus, Collis gastroplasty is undertaken with a thick tissue stapler to add the needed length.

- We typically perform a fundoplication with the neo-fundus by wrapping the esophagus anteriorly (180° - Dor). A 270° posterior wrap (Toupet) is also an option for patients with severe reflux. Some surgeons also perform a complete wrap (Nissen) but it is essential that it is truly a "floppy" wrap and that the patient has normal esophageal motility preoperatively. The stomach may also be secured to the diaphragm to help reduce the risk of recurrence.

Transthoracic hiatal hernia repair (TTHHR – Belsey Mark IV)

- Left anterior thoracotomy via the 6th or 7th intercostal space (should be based on preoperative imaging). If a re-do surgery, Chest CT scan should be obtained.

- Mobilize the sac anteriorly and posteriorly off the posterior pericardium and aorta/spine. It is frequently helpful to enter the sac if the anatomy is unclear.

- Excise the sac from the crus and stomach.

- Mobilize some fundus into the chest, usually dividing a few short gastric vessels.

- The right crus can be challenging to find as this is the deepest extent of the dissection. However, dissection of the hernia sac posteriorly will lead one to the right crus. The crus are grasped with a Babcock clamp and pledgeted 0-Ethibond sutures are placed in a horizontal mattress configuration to re-approximate the crus. These are left loose until the stomach is reduced to the abdomen.

- The fundoplication is performed by rolling the fundus up to the GEJ and securing it to the esophagus and itself. The needles are left on the second row of sutures so that they can be placed through the diaphragm anteriorly. The Belsey spoon may be used for retraction.

Open abdominal repair

- The basics of an open repair are the same for the above described laparoscopic approach.

- The Hill repair is used principally in the Pacific Northwest and is performed similarly to the laparoscopic method, but the fundoplication is performed with 5 silk sutures which are used to bring a small amount of fundus lateral to the vagus nerves around the esophagus, and then the sutures are passed through the crural repair posteriorly, anchoring the GEJ to the crural repair. A lengthening procedure is not typically needed as the repair can place some tension on the esophagus.

- Other fundoplications may be utilized in an open abdominal operation, as described above.

Potential questions/alternative scenarios

"Following mobilization of the esophagus, you determine that the esophagus should be lengthened. How is this determination made? Also, during laparoscopic repair you find that you and are having trouble closing the hiatus. How would you close a hiatus that won't come together?"

At least 2 cm of tension-free, intraabdominal esophagus is recommended to decrease the risk of recurrence. Extensive mobilization of the intrathoracic esophagus as proximal as the inferior pulmonary veins aids significantly in obtaining this length. However, the esophagus may be significantly shortened from a chronic paraesophageal hernia and/or from chronic reflux that leads to fibrosis and presbyesophagus. If full esophageal mobilization does not obtain enough length, a stapled wedge fundectomy (Collis gastroplasty) is most commonly used to lengthen the esophagus. The wedge should be performed with a bougie in place (typically a 54 or 56 Fr.) to avoid inadvertent narrowing of the esophagus. In order to determine if there is enough intra-abdominal esophagus, the GEJ must be clearly seen, which is most easily done by mobilizing the esophageal fat pad off the GEJ anteriorly.

The difficult hiatus is a problem without an easy solution. Polypropylene mesh has been used with some success, but there have been a number of reports of erosion into the esophagus. If there is too much tension on the crural repair, a biologic mesh such as acellular dermis or absorbable mesh should be used. In addition, it may help to start closing the hiatus anteriorly where there is a little less tension. During laparoscopic cases, a pneumothorax may be induced with insufflation to create a "floppy" diaphragm, which may permit adequate re-approximation of the hiatus. Adhesions to the liver and spleen should also be taken down to ensure the crus are not tethered laterally. Decreasing the insufflation pressure may also help to take tension of the hiatus.

"How would you treat Barrett's esophagus if found on preoperative endoscopy?"

Barrett's esophagus should be assessed with biopsy and histologic analysis. Biopsy-proven Barrett's should be followed with repeat endoscopies and biopsies. The recommended biopsies of 4 quadrants every centimeter of Barrett's should be performed yearly to look for dysplasia or cancer. Guidelines recommend surveillance every 1-3 years for uncomplicated Barrett's, with recommendations of either maximal PPI therapy or anti-reflux surgery for these patients. Patients with low-grade dysplasia should be followed every 6-12 months and high-grade dysplasia every 3 months if no eradication therapy (EMR, RFA, or esophagectomy) is carried out. Repair of a paraesophageal hernia and creation of a fundoplication does not alter the surveillance protocol.

"At laparoscopy, you see the stomach seems to enter the abdomen with the GEJ located intra-abdominally, but then herniate posteriorly through a separate diaphragmatic defect. How would you manage this?"

Other defects in the diaphragm are rarely seen but are possible in adults. Bochdalek (posterior paraspinal) and Morgagni (anterior parasternal) hernias can be closed primarily or repaired with Gore-tex mesh. The dissection can be disorienting since these defects have presumably been present since birth. Bochdalek hernias are more likely to involve the stomach. Much less is known about the natural history of these hernias, as they are most commonly found incidentally. Most surgeons recommend treatment for those that are symptomatic or those that appear to have incarcerated bowel or other abdominal viscera.

"The patient now has had 3 previous repairs and has recurrence of her paraesophageal hernia with the wrap from the previous surgery in the chest. How would you approach this hernia?"

Once a patient fails multiple redo antireflux surgeries/hernia repairs, the chance of a successful repair is less likely as the risk of recurrence increases with each redo operation. If this patient was unable to eat, unable to maintain their weight, or had other severe symptoms (significant abdominal pain or anemia from the hernia), many surgeons would offer the patient an esophagectomy. A roux-en-y "near" esophagojejunostomy may be another alternative if the patient has not lost a significant amount of weight already. If an esophagectomy is to be performed, there should he consideration for an intrathoracic anastomosis (Ivor Lewis or left thoracoabdominal approach) since the stomach may not be a suitable conduit due to the multiple reoperations. One should also be prepared to use an alternative conduit, such as colon, in these circumstances.

"A 45-year-old patient without previous surgery has a symptomatic hernia and a BMI of 39 with insulin-dependent diabetes and sleep apnea. How would you approach this patient?"

A patient that has significant reflux, a paraesophageal hernia, and morbid obesity qualifies for bariatric surgery and should be evaluated by a bariatric surgeon prior to consideration of paraesophageal hernia repair. The paraesophageal hernia would be repaired as usual, but a roux-en-y gastric bypass would benefit this patient more in the long-run. Most patients will gain weight following paraesophageal hernia repair since the repair restores normal function to their stomach. Some surgeons advocate a "near" esophagojejunostomy, which leaves only a small gastric pouch, thus removing all acid producing cells and preventing ongoing reflux.

"How would you follow these patients over time?"

Recurrence rates for paraesophageal hernia repairs range from 15-50%. Some surgeons do not offer routine postoperative follow-up of these patients, only seeing patients back in the office if symptoms recur. Due to the high recurrence rates, others chose to follow these patients annually or even more frequently with a barium swallow. Recurrence is more common after laparoscopic than transthoracic repair.

"A 76-year-old man presents with chest pain, nausea, and inability to vomit. The ED is unable to pass a NGT, which can be seen coiled in the chest. The patient has a history of a long-standing paraesophageal hernia. He has a low-grade fever, is tachycardic, and with marginal blood pressure. Upper endoscopy reveals patchy areas of ischemia in the stomach and an area suspicious for necrosis. How would you manage this patient?"

This is a life-threatening complication of paraesophageal hernias, and the patient must be operated on emergently. The most likely cause is gastric volvulus with resulting ischemia and progression to frank necrosis due to obstruction, distension, and decreased perfusion. If no frank necrosis is present, quickly reducing the hernia and performing a gastropexy (tacking the greater curve to the anterior diaphragm/anterior abdominal wall) may get the patient off the table quickly and to the ICU for resuscitation. The stomach can then be reassessed later endoscopically. Cases where there is gastric necrosis are more complicated. In these cases, the hernia may be reduced, and the area of necrosis is resected. Depending on the degree of resection, a gastrojejunostomy (BII or RNY) may be needed. This can be performed in a staged fashion if the patient is too unstable. In cases where the majority of the stomach is necrotic, a RNY is needed. If there is distal esophageal necrosis, the patient must undergo bipolar exclusion with resection of the necrotic stomach and esophagus. The esophageal

stump must be drained, either with a pharyngostomy tube or by placing a drain in the stump and bringing it out through the
abdominal wall. If time permits, a feeding jejunostomy is placed. Reconstruction with a substernal colon interposition can then be carried out in a delayed fashion once the patient has recovered.

Pearls/pitfalls

- Preoperative work-up should be thorough and include, at a minimum, UGI and upper endoscopy.
- Presentation with pain should have NGT placement or endoscopy to relieve possible obstruction.
- Urgent/emergent surgery for unrelenting pain or signs of ischemia.
- Must resect the hernia sac.
- Secure the stomach to diaphragm or anterior abdominal wall to prevent recurrence.
- Mesh is rarely indicated, but when truly necessary a biologic mesh is preferred.

Suggested readings

- Carrott PW, Hong J, Kuppusamy MK, et al. Clinical ramifications of giant paraesophageal hernias are under appreciated: making the case for routine surgical repair. *Ann of Thoracic Surgery* 2012; 94:421-8.
- Oelschlager BK, Pellegrini CA, Hunter JG, et al. Biologic prosthesis to prevent recurrence after laparoscopic paraesophageal hernia repair: long-term follow-up from a multicenter, prospective, randomized trial. *J Am Coll Surg* 2011; 213:461–468.
- Whitson BA, Hoang CD, Boettcher AK, et al. Wedge gastroplasty and reinforced crural repair: Important components of laparoscopic giant or recurrent hiatal hernia repair. *J Thorac Cardiovasc Surg* 2006; 132:1196-1202.

28. TRACHEAL STRICTURES AND FISTULAE

Michael P. Robich, MD, and Daniel Raymond, MD

Concept

- Diagnosis and workup of tracheal strictures and fistulae
- Management
- Conduct of the operations and pitfalls
- Managing complications

Chief complaint

"You are consulted by the MICU to see a 77-year-old woman with diabetes, respiratory failure due to pneumonia, and newly discovered bilious secretions from the tracheostomy. You are familiar with the patient as you placed the tracheostomy one month ago."

Differential

Gastroesophageal reflux disease, aspiration, tracheoesophageal fistula

History and physical

Patients at risk of developing a benign tracheoesphageal fistula (TEF) usually have risk factors including diabetes, corticosteroid use, immunodeficiency, infection, hypotension, prolonged intubation, neck trauma, caustic ingestion, foreign body ingestion, iatrogenic injury during tracheal or esophageal surgery, and granulomatous infections. High cuff pressures (30 cm of water (22 mmHg)) can impair mucosal blood flow and the concurrent presence of a nasogastric tube can contribute to development of a TEF. In ventilated patients, bilious secretions or tube feeds in the endotracheal tube or tracheostomy, gastric dilatation, and loss of tidal volumes are signs that may suggest a TEF. In non-ventilated patients, signs of TEF include persistent cough, fever, and dyspnea. Recurrent pneumonias are common in both groups of patients.

Tests

- CXR may demonstrate the endotracheal tube outside of the trachea and gastric dilatation.
- Contrast esophagography can identify the fistula. Water-soluble contrast should be avoided when TEF is suspected (iso-osmolar contrast is recommended if communication with the airway is suspected).
- CT scan may show a defect between the trachea and esophagus, as well as extra-luminal fluid collections.
- Direct visualization is the mainstay of diagnosis. Bronchoscopy will often reveal the defect. In ventilated patients the endotracheal tube must be withdrawn to examine the trachea at the point of contact with the balloon. Esophagoscopy can also be utilized to visualize the tracheal cuff protruding into the esophageal lumen.

Index scenario (additional information)

"The patient has bilious secretions and is noted to have volume loss on the ventilator. CXR shows a moderate-sized gastric bubble but is otherwise unrevealing. How will you manage this patient?"

Treatment/management

This is the classic picture for TEF. A bronchoscopy from above the tracheostomy (either transnasally or transorally) should be performed to examine the trachea with focus on the area where the balloon sits. Once the diagnosis is confirmed, a plan for management can be made. Esophagoscopy should be available as well for a thorough examination.

Spontaneous healing is rare in this situation and surgical intervention is usually needed. If non-operative treatment is to be attempted, the first step is to minimize further soiling of the airway. Keep the head of the bed elevated $> 30°$. The tracheostomy cuff should be repositioned distal to the TEF, but above the carina, with minimal cuff pressures. An adjustable flange tracheostomy tube or distal XLT tracheostomy (longer distal limb of tracheostomy) may be helpful in these situations. Endotracheal intubation with a single lumen tube may be required in cases where a tracheostomy cannot be adequately positioned. Efforts should be made to wean the patient from the ventilator, as the positive pressure provided by the ventilator keeps the tract open and minimizes the chance of closure. The patient's nutritional status needs to be aggressively optimized. Removal of the NG tube is important. Placement of a gastrostomy tube will allow continued enteral feeding and venting of the stomach.

If the patient cannot tolerate a period of non-operative management, covered tracheal or esophageal stents can be utilized as a temporizing measure to allow time for the patient to be optimized for surgical treatment, or in some rare cases may facilitate spontaneous closure. Stenting can cause extension of the TEF, particularly when both a tracheal and esophageal stent are used as the radial forces place unwanted pressure on the area of communication. Stenting should be used with caution and only by those with experience.

Once the patient has been optimized, an operative plan can be made. Preoperatively, a strategy to ventilate the patient needs to be made. If the fistula is small and will not require tracheal resection, the tube can be placed distally to allow repair. If tracheal resection is needed, proximal low tidal ventilation, distal high-frequency jet ventilation, double lung ventilation with distal airway isolation, or cardiopulmonary bypass can be utilized. In cases where primary repair or simple resection is not possible, esophageal exclusion (described in esophageal chapters) may be need to be performed as a last resort.

Operative steps

Takedown of TEF and primary tracheal repair

- *Incision*: a low collar incision with extension to the left. Subplatysmal flaps are raised.
- Dissect down to the tracheoesophageal groove, divide the left inferior thyroid artery to improve exposure. Dissection between the trachea and esophagus in the groove should be on the esophageal wall to avoid disrupting the anterolateral blood supply of the trachea and avoid injury to the recurrent laryngeal nerves.
- The fistula is identified circumferentially, sharply resected, and sent for pathologic analysis.
- The defects are debrided back to healthy tissue.
- The membranous tracheal defect is closed with interrupted 3-0 or 4-0 vicryl with the knots on the outside.
- The esophageal defect is closed in two layers (Mucosa- 4-0 vicryl interrupted, muscularis and adventitia- imbricating 3-0 vicryl interrupted).
- A sternocleidomastoid (SCM) flap is created by dividing the SCM distally and mobilizing an adequate length to cover the repair. The tracheal and esophageal repairs should be separated by the flap. The rotational flap is then sewn onto the esophagus with interrupted 4-0 vicryl.

Takedown of TEF and repair with tracheal resection

- *Incision*: collar incision for anterior approach to the trachea.
- The pretracheal plane is developed above and below the fistula and the trachea is dissected circumferentially at the level of the defect. Dissect bluntly on the trachea to avoid damage to the recurrent laryngeal nerves.

- A transverse tracheal incision is made below the fistula. The endotracheal tube is removed, a sterile tube is placed in the distal trachea, and cross-field ventilation initiated.
- The trachea is divided proximally, and the fistula is resected from the esophagus.
- The esophagus is repaired in two layers and a muscle flap placed.
- The trachea is then re-approximated end-to-end with interrupted 4-0 vicryl.
- A new endotracheal tube is placed distal to the repair.
- Postoperatively efforts should be made to extubate the patient as soon as possible.

Potential questions/alternative scenarios

"The TEF is large and won't be amenable to simple closure or resection. How will you manage?"

If the fistula is too large for the management strategies mentioned above, the defect can be dissected with a rim of esophageal wall. The rim of esophagus can then be approximated to re-create the membranous trachea with interrupted 4-0 vicryl. The esophagus is closed in two layers and a muscle flap placed. Reports have also described use of biologic prostheses, autologous pericardium, or aortic homograft to reconstruct the back wall of the trachea.

"A patient is found to have a left broncho-esophageal fistula. What is the appropriate surgical approach once the patient is deemed appropriate for surgery?"

The distal trachea, carina, and both mainstem bronchi can be approached via right thoracotomy or sternotomy. The defect should be resected and repaired as previously described. If extra length is needed to obtain a tension-free repair, the inferior pulmonary ligament can be taken down and a hilar release performed (opening the pericardium in a U-shape anterior to the hilum, curved under the inferior pulmonary vein, and posterior to the hilum). Neck flexion will also take tension of the anastomosis in the case of a tracheal resection. A sleeve resection with reconstruction can also be performed for bronchial fistulae. A muscle, pericardial, or pleural flap is placed to buttress the repair.

"A 67-year-old man presents one year after esophagectomy for esophageal adenocarcinoma with complaints of persistent cough, increased secretions, fevers, and chest pain. Bronchoscopy shows a TEF at the anastomosis and biopsy reveals cancer recurrence. How will you manage this patient?"

Malignant TEF is associated with esophageal, pulmonary, and tracheal cancers. Make sure to do an endoscopy and take biopsies to determine if there is recurrent cancer present. Malignant TEFs are often a sign of advanced disease with a poor prognosis and survival rates of less than 10% at 12 months. As such, management is geared toward palliation and avoiding significant morbidity. Covered tracheal and/or esophageal stents offer a reasonable management strategy. Esophageal exclusion with end cervical esophagostomy, gastrostomy tube for distal decompression, a feeding jejunostomy may be the only option in some cases to prevent ongoing soilage of the airway. Esophageal exclusion and bypass is often associated with significant morbidity and is generally not a good palliative option if other options exist. Chemotherapy and radiation may be of some benefit.

"The ER consults you to see a patient that was transferred from a rehab center with blood in the tracheostomy tube. The tracheostomy was placed 4 weeks prior to presentation. As you are examining the patient, massive bleeding from the tracheostomy begins. How will you manage this?"

The differential in this case scenario includes mucosal irritation from suctioning, tracheitis, bleeding tracheal granulation tissue, alveolar hemorrhage, and tracheoinnominate fistula (TIF). Given the history, and since it is a potentially fatal complication, one must presume that TIF is the diagnosis until proven otherwise. TIF is caused by erosion of an endotracheal tube balloon eroding into the innominate artery. It is usually caused by pressure necrosis by the tube. With the advent of lower pressure tracheostomy tube balloons, the incidence of TIF has decreased over time. However, when it does occur, the mortality is near 100%. Factors

185

that predispose to formation of TIF include: prolonged intubation, high cuff pressures to prevent air leak, poorly positioned tracheostomy, tracheostomy placed below the 4th tracheal ring, high-riding innominate artery, hypotension, sepsis, medical comorbidities (diabetes, infection, steroid use, malnutrition), and prior radiation. The peak time frame is 2-4 weeks after tracheostomy, with 75% occurring in the first month. Most patients, like the above example, will present with a small sentinel bleed, hours to days prior to massive bleeding.

In the case of TIF, over-inflation of the cuff balloon may *temporarily* tamponade the bleeding. This has been reported to be successful in 85% of cases. If this does not work, the tube can be slowly withdrawn while applying anterior pressure. If this maneuver fails, an oral endotracheal tube can be placed, and the tracheostomy tube removed. With the tracheostomy removed, digital pressure through the stoma can be applied to compress the innominate artery against the sternum as the patient is transported to the OR for immediate operative intervention.

Concurrent to the efforts to stop the bleeding, the operating room should be alerted, and volume/blood resuscitation initiated. The distal airway should be cleared, and diagnosis confirmed with bronchoscopy.

The choices for repair include simple ligation, resection of affected innominate artery, direct repair of the defect, and bypass of the fistula with a graft. Endovascular stenting has also been described. Because of the emergent and contaminated nature of the operation and the associated high mortality, ligation of the innominate artery is generally recommended. In cases where bleeding has ceased from the above-mentioned measures (i.e., this was a herald bleed), consideration can be given to CTA of the neck and chest to further delineate the anatomy prior to proceeding to the operating room; however, this should be done with caution.

Repair of tracheo-innominate fistula

- *Incision*: median sternotomy or partial upper sternotomy
- Innominate artery is exposed by dissecting the thymus and retracting the brachiocephalic vein
- Achieve proximal and distal control
- Ligate the artery

Index scenario (additional information)

"A patient presents following a complex postoperative course including tracheostomy after a major abdominal surgery. The patient was discharged ultimately to a rehabilitation unit and was de-cannulated in the unit over two months ago. The patient currently complains of progressively worsening dyspnea on exertion and stridor over last few weeks. How will you evaluate and treat?"

Differential

Post-intubation airway pathology includes benign strictures, granulomas, and tracheomalacia. Benign and malignant neoplasms, vocal cord dysfunction, prior airway trauma, and infection should also be considered.

Tests

- *CXR*: a high posteroanterior and lateral CXR can delineate some tracheal pathology, but CT scan shows more detailed information.
- *Dynamic airway CT*: can show highly detailed 3D reconstructions to demonstrate functional tracheal problems (i.e., tracheomalacia).
- *Laryngoscopy*: can be performed in the office setting on an awake patient for an initial assessment of the hypopharynx, vocal cords, and proximal trachea.
- *Bronchoscopy*: essential to make the diagnosis, plan treatment, and intervene as a definitive treatment or a bridge to definitive treatment.
- *Pulmonary function tests*: may see early flattening of the expiratory portion of the flow-volume loop (obstructive pattern).

"On bronchoscopic examination the patient has an anteriorly pointed, arrow-shaped stenosis that occurs at the level of the prior tracheotomy. How will you manage?"

Any patient with a history of endotracheal intubation developing symptoms of airway obstruction (wheezing, stridor, or exertional dyspnea) should be investigated for an obstructing tracheal lesion. Stomal stenosis is caused by enlargement of the tracheotomy and eventual healing with granulation tissue. As the granulation tissue contracts it narrows the tracheal lumen. The stoma can be enlarged due to leverage forces from equipment attached to the tracheostomy, a large tracheotomy at the time of insertion, or infection. Patients may present late, as they may not regain enough functional activity to manifest airway obstruction for some time. For a patient to be symptomatic at rest, the tracheal diameter is typically less than 30% of normal. Having the patient extend the neck or inspire rapidly may illicit stridor. Diagnosis can be made on laryngoscopy, which should be carried out prior to more invasive procedures requiring anesthesia.

Bronchoscopic evaluation of tracheal stenosis should be undertaken in the operating room with careful planning preoperatively by the surgical and anesthesia teams. The patient should initially be evaluated awake with local anesthesia and the anatomy should be confirmed. Intravenous anesthetic is provided without muscle relaxant until the airway is controlled, which may require suspension laryngoscopy and rigid bronchoscopy. The glottis and vocal cord function should be assessed in addition to the stenosis. If the tracheal lumen is less than 5 mm in diameter, dilation can be performed with graduated Jackson dilators. This will often provide only temporary relief, which can allow delay of the operation until the tracheal mucosa is healed and the patient is medically fit for surgery. If the stenosis is greater than 5 mm the bronchoscope should cross and will provide dilation. Gentle insertion of the tip of the bronchoscope into the stenosis with a rotatory motion and light pressure, typically allows it to advance past the stenosis. Other interventional pulmonary techniques such as balloon dilation, stenting, bouginage, or Nd:YAG laser debridement can be used (if you discuss this option remember to lower FiO2 to $\leq 30\%$ prior to using an energy source in the trachea). However, because the ischemic injury is full thickness, endoluminal therapies are not usually curative. Definitive treatment is resection of the affected area after careful assessment of the location and length of the stenosis. An anesthetic plan involving cross table ventilation, preservation of blood supply, and achieving a tension free repair are keys to success of the operation.

For patients who cannot tolerate tracheal resection or who have long strictures not amenable to resection, a redo tracheostomy may be needed. Care must be taken to make sure the distal end of the tracheostomy is distal to the stricture. The tracheostomy can eventually be exchanged for a tracheal T-tube. The soft, silicone T-tube is passed through the tracheostomy stoma and has three limbs: a shorter proximal limb that is directed toward the vocal cords; a longer distal limb that is directed toward the carina and should pass the stricture, and a short limb that passes externally through the tracheal stoma. When the external limb is uncapped, the patient can inhale/exhale through the T-tube. When the T-tube is capped, it acts as a stent, covering the stricture and allowing the patient to breathe and speak normally. It is important to measure the distance from the vocal cords to the stricture and from the carina to the stricture (done with flexible bronchoscopy). T-tubes with varying limb lengths are available or custom T-tubes can be ordered from the manufacturer. It is important to make sure the limbs are not too long, as uncontrollable coughing will be caused by irritation of the vocal cords or carina (depending on which limb is too long). T-tubes provide a good long-term option for inoperable patients, as they are better tolerated than tracheostomies, rarely cause stricturing, and allow the patient to speak and breathe normally. It is important to note that patients with T-tubes cannot be placed on mechanical ventilation, as a significant amount of the tidal volume will escape proximally out the nose and mouth (if necessary, the nose and mouth are sealed to prevent loss of volume, which is obviously not an option when the patient is awake). The T-tube is instead pulled out the stoma (easily done at the bedside) and

187

a cuffed tracheostomy is placed (making sure the distal tip passed distal to the stricture) through the stoma. Bronchoscopy and tracheal suctioning can be performed easily through T-tubes and there is little risk of migration.

Operative steps

- Low collar incision +/- upper hemisternotomy.
- Dissection is carried out immediately adjacent to the trachea to avoid damage to the recurrent laryngeal nerves. Circumferential dissection of the trachea is carried out only at the level of stenosis and not more than 1-1.5 cm of normal trachea. This will help preserve the lateral blood supply to the airway.
- Anterior and posterior mobilization of the trachea to the level of the carina is important to limit tension on the anastomosis.
- The stenotic segment can be identified by external abnormality or via transillumination during intraoperative bronchoscopy.
- The airway is divided sharply with care not to injure the esophagus posteriorly.
- The distal airway can be intubated with a sterile endotracheal tube and ventilator circuit.
- Ensure a tension-free anastomosis. The anastomosis is most commonly created with 4-0 vicryl or PDS in a running, interrupted, or combined fashion.
- The patient should be extubated in the OR.

Potential questions/alternative scenarios

"During a mid-tracheal resection, the anastomosis is under undue tension. How will you remedy this?"
Cervical flexion will provide enough tracheal length for most repairs. Some advise placing a stitch from the chin to the chest ("Grillo stitch") to maintain flexion postoperatively. Dissection on the anterior and posterior surfaces will preserve the blood supply and provide length. Suprahyoid laryngeal release will provide 1-1.5 cm of length, but postoperative dysphagia is a common sequela.

"Six weeks after tracheal resection a patient develops massive hemoptysis and dies. How could this have been prevented?"
A tracheoinnominate fistula can occur when the innominate artery is mobilized and subsequently erodes into the airway. An interposition muscle flap at the time of initial operation can be used to decrease the risk of this rapidly fatal complication.

"A 69-year-old patient with a tracheal stenosis presents in acute respiratory distress. Critical care is unable to intubate the patient. You are called for an emergency airway."
Patients with critical tracheal stenosis are at increased risk of obstruction from minimal amounts of secretions. Furthermore, a high-grade stenosis will prevent effective positive pressure ventilation. Thus, the patient must be kept spontaneously ventilating while be transported to the operating room. Use of paralytics prior to control of the airway will likely be lethal. During transport, preparations should be made for fiberoptic intubation, rigid bronchoscopy, jet ventilation, and emergent surgical airway placement. Start with mask ventilation first. Fiberoptic bronchoscopy can be performed, although in an emergency rigid bronchoscopy is often necessary to quickly dilate the stricture and establish an airway. Once the stenosis is dilated, place a tube exchanger (can ventilate through tube exchanger with jet as you pull out rigid), and a small ETT (pediatric). Once the patient is stabilized, further plans can be made for more definitive management. (redo tracheostomy, resection, T-tube placement, etc).

"You are asked to see a patient with multiple severe medical problems and a tracheostomy for 3-4 months. On bronchoscopy you note a circumferential distal stricture 3.5 cm proximal to carina, but distal to the tip of the tracheostomy. The patient is improving but

188

has required increasing vent support and has higher airway pressures. How will you manage?"

The most common post-intubation lesion is cuff stenosis, which occurs at the level of the sealing cuff (balloon). The radial pressure exerted from the cuff causes circumferential pressure necrosis, which can cause cicatricial scarring and stenosis. Large volume, low pressure balloons have helped decreased the incidence, however over-inflation can lead to damage of the trachea. This typically occurs within 3-4 cm of the cricoid cartilage and is a circumferential stenosis. Definitive management is resection with primary anastomosis. However, in patients that are poor surgical candidates or need mechanical ventilator support other options exist. A tracheostomy with a longer flange may be able to cross the narrowing as a temporary solution. Endotracheal stenting can also provide relief in the patient not fit for surgery. However, these stents tend to cause granulation tissue and the proximal and distal ends of the stent, essentially converting a single stricture into two. Focal circumferential stenoses of the trachea can be balloon dilated. The technique involves incremental inflation with frequent deflations to assess progress and check for injury to the airway. Topical application of mitomycin-C can retard restenosis. In stenosis involving only the cartilaginous rings of the trachea, balloon dilation should not be used as the risk of perforating the membranous airway is high. In the case where a stent in placed and the ends become obstructed by granulation tissue, options include serial debridement (YAG-Nd laser), serial dilations, or removal of the stent and placement of a T-tube to cover all the strictures segments.

Pearls/pitfalls

- A period of non-operative optimization of the patient's pulmonary and nutritional status should be instituted prior to repair of TEFs whenever possible.

- Try to extubate the patient as soon as possible after repair of TEFs or tracheal resections.

- Avoid injury to recurrent laryngeal nerve and have a low index of suspicion for nerve injury, which should be investigated with laryngoscopy.

- TIFs are life-threatening complications. Therefore, significant hemoptysis in a patient with a prior tracheostomy must be thoroughly investigated. Ligation of the innominate artery may be the fastest and safest way to save the patient's life.

- Patients presenting with tracheal strictures must be handled with caution, particularly when presenting acutely. Rigid bronchoscopy and the ability to jet ventilate is crucial. A plan is needed to do whatever is needed to obtain access beyond the stricture to ventilate. Once this is accomplished, planning for more definitive surgical treatment can take place.

- Options to treat tracheal strictures in the long-term include resection for focal strictures, while dilation, debridement, tracheostomy, and tracheal t-tube are options for more complex strictures (long, multiple) or inoperable patients.

Suggested readings

- Cooper JD, Grillo HC. The evolution of tracheal injury due to ventilatory assistance through cuffed tubes: a pathologic study. *Ann Surg*. 1969;169(3):334-348.

- Wright CD. Management of tracheoinnominate artery fistula. *Chest Surg Clin N Am* 1996;6:865–873.

- Wain JC Jr. Postintubation tracheal stenosis. *Semin Thorac Cardiovasc Surg*. 2009 Fall;21(3):284-9.

- Ott HC and Mathisen DJ. Tracheal Lesions. Sabiston and Spencer Surgery of the Chest. 9th edition. Sellke FW, del Nido PJ, Swanson SJ (eds). Ch 8: 132-149.

29. MALIGNANT LESIONS OF THE TRACHEA

Timothy J. Pirolli, MD, and William D. Ogden, MD

Concept

- Presentation and workup of tracheal tumors
- Differential diagnosis
- Principles of surgical resection
- Airway management during resection
- Postoperative care and adjuvant therapy

Chief complaint

"You are referred a patient with complaints of a cough and wheezing that's been getting worse for the last few months. The patient's pulmonologist told him he had a mass in his airway."

Differential

Primary malignant tumor of the trachea, metastatic tumor to trachea, benign tracheal mass, tracheal strictures, external compression of trachea by mediastinal mass, aspirated foreign body, adult-onset asthma

History and physical

A detailed H&P focusing on duration and progression of symptoms (hoarseness, cough, wheeze, stridor, dyspnea, hemoptysis, dysphagia) should be made. Other key components include examining the patient's functional status, a thorough review of systems, evaluation of comorbidities, medications and smoking/substance abuse history. A complete physical exam (focusing on the airway/lungs/lymph nodes/oropharynx) must be performed.

Tests

- *CXR.* Airway narrowing, mediastinal widening or evidence of metastatic disease.
- *CT scan of neck and chest.* May help delineate invasion of surrounding structures, metastatic disease. Critical for defining the length of the tumor.
- *Bronchoscopy (rigid or flexible) +/- biopsy.* Direct examination of tumor with tissue sampling if feasible. Length of the tumor is assessed, as well as distance from the vocal cords and carina.
- *Endobronchial ultrasonography (EBUS).* May assist in distinguishing primary tracheal tumor from external compression/infiltration of extrinsic tumor; may clarify extent of invasion.
- *Pulmonary function tests.* Evaluate for upper airway obstruction, flattening of expiratory and inspiratory phases, normal pre-operative assessment.
- *Basic labs:* CBC, BMP, INR/PTT.
- *PET scan/MRI brain/abdomen CT.* Examination for extra-tracheal sites of possible primary tumor or metastatic disease.
- *Upper endoscopy, esophageal ultrasound.* If concern for invasion into esophagus.
- *EKG/stress echo.* As part of preoperative cardiac workup if warranted.

Index scenario (additional information)

"A 61-year-old man with an 80 pack-year smoking history has been referred to you by his pulmonologist after increasing wheezing and coughing that was not responsive to bronchodilators prompted a workup that revealed a mid-tracheal mass. He has no other comorbidities except for hypertension. CT scan shows a tracheal mass measuring 2.0 cm long in the mid-trachea. PET scan reveals no metastatic disease. What further workup would you perform and what are his options?"

The patient has confirmed radiographic findings of a tracheal mass without evidence of distal metastases. The next step in the workup should be bronchoscopy (flexible +/- rigid) to examine the tumor, assess its length and resectability, and to biopsy the mass. Once a tissue diagnosis has been made, the decision on management must be addressed. Most tumors present as locally advanced disease at time of presentation. Most primary tracheal malignancies are either squamous cell carcinoma (SCC) or adenoid cystic carcinoma (ACC). Histology has prognostic importance for survival, with ACC and mucoepidermoid tumor having the best outcomes. SCC is more likely to present with hemoptysis, whereas ACC is more likely to present with obstructive airway disease. Survival in surgically resected patients is superior to non-resected patients in both major histologies. Lymph node involvement has been shown to result in decreased survival but does not preclude surgical resection. A standardized oncologic staging system has not yet been developed.

Surgical resection of the tracheal tumor should be considered for any patient who has a resectable tumor without metastatic disease and who would tolerate the surgery. Resectable tumors are typically less than 4.5 cm in length (MGH data), have minimal invasion into the mediastinum, are amenable to negative margins (although in ACC resections, positive margins may be accepted and respond to radiation therapy). No preoperative chemotherapy or radiation is warranted prior to resection of a tracheal tumor. Involvement of the larynx/subglottic tumors should portend a laryngotracheal resection and be performed at an experienced high-volume center or in conjunction with an otolaryngologist.

Tumors that are a direct extension or metastasis from other primary sites to the trachea are rarely resectable. Certain cancers such as some T4 NSCLCs and thyroid cancers that involve the airway may be amenable to resection only after a full metastatic workup is otherwise negative and the patient is an ideal surgical candidate. These surgeries are undertaken only if en-bloc resection of the tumor is curative.

Operative steps

Tracheal resection for a mid-tracheal tumor

Goals – resect the tracheal mass with negative margins with minimal disruption to tracheal blood supply and create a tension-free anastomosis.

- Adequate PIVs/central venous access is critical. Radial arterial line.

- Total intravenous anesthesia or slow induction of inhaled anesthetic agents is optimal to minimize risk of airway collapse. No muscle relaxants are given until the airway is secured. A rigid bronchoscope and jet ventilation equipment should be ready if collapse occurs prior to intubation. For intrathoracic tumors, cardiopulmonary bypass on stand-by may be warranted.

- Pre-incision bronchoscopy. Placing a 25-gauge needle percutaneously into the airway to define the upper/lower limits of the tumor under direct visualization may be helpful.

- Collar incision for upper/mid tracheal lesions (R thoracotomy or median sternotomy for lower tumors). Skin flaps are raised, strap muscles split, and the trachea is exposed with a pretracheal release from cricoid to sternal notch. The thyroid isthmus is divided and dissected off the trachea. The manubrium may need to be partially divided and retracted laterally.

- Define upper and lower borders of resection and dissect circumferentially around the trachea, staying close to trachea to minimize disrupting the main blood supply to the remaining trachea. Recurrent laryngeal nerves travel laterally in tracheoesophageal groove on each side. Avoid them. Pass a tape around the trachea. Remove any lymph nodes.

- Prior to excision of the trachea, a separate corrugated tubing setup should be passed off to anesthesia in preparation for cross-table ventilation. Tubing is connected to a flexible endotracheal tube (Tovell tube) and managed by the surgeon (assistant) on the field.

191

- Traction sutures are placed laterally on the trachea 1 cm below level of transection, incorporating 1-2 tracheal rings. Transect the trachea anteriorly between rings just distal to the tumor. Healthy cartilage should be present at the cut margin. Continuous suctioning of the airway is needed to prevent secretions and blood from passing into the distal airway.
- Communicate with the anesthesiologist as the ETT is withdrawn and Tovell tube is advanced into the distal airway through the tracheal incision by the surgeon. Jet ventilation may be used during this period.
- Circumferential dissection is carried out proximally and distally for a maximum of 1 cm dissection of the remaining trachea to maintain blood supply. Traction sutures are placed proximally. The trachea is then divided proximal to the tumor and the resected trachea/tumor is removed: maximum ~4.5 cm length (~8 tracheal rings). Send the specimen for frozen section of margins. Positive margins for ACC are accepted.
- The neck is flexed to assess tension on the airway and the traction sutures a retracted to bring the proximal and distal trachea together. Interrupted 4-0 coated Vicryl sutures (some use prolene) are placed starting at the midline posteriorly with the knots placed to lie outside of the trachea. Sequentially, sutures are placed on either side of the 1st suture 4 mm apart and 4 mm from the cut edge of trachea through cartilage. The sutures are clipped to the drape and continued around circumferentially without tying the knots until all sutures are placed. The anterior sutures are then placed in a similar fashion and the Tovell tube is removed as the endotracheal tube is advanced beyond the anastomosis. An alternative method is to advance the ETT beyond the area of resection into the distal trachea and place the sutures circumferentially without placing a Tovell tube.
- Neck is kept fully flexed and the anterior sutures are tied. If there is tension evident on the anastomosis, release maneuvers should be performed. The first maneuver should be the Montgomery suprahyoid release performed by dividing the hyoid muscles through a small horizontal incision and dividing the hyoid bone laterally, giving 1-2 cm more mobility. Other release maneuvers include a suprathyroid laryngeal, hilar (pericardial release for intrathoracic tumors), and inferior pulmonary ligament releases.
- Once the anterior sutures are tied and the tails cut, the posterior sutures are tied, working from lateral to the posterior midline on one side and then the other.
- A "guardian stitch" fashioned at the end of the case secures the underside of the chin to the chest at the level of the manubrium, keeps the patient's neck flexed and reminds them not to extend.
- Bronchoscopy after completion. Extubate immediately if possible, ICU care.
- Bronchoscopy of patient 1 week after surgery prior to discharge.
- Adjuvant therapy with 54-60 Gy of radiation 2 months postoperatively for most patients.

Potential questions/alternative scenarios
"What is the blood supply to the trachea?"
Lateral arcade of arteries arising from superior and inferior thyroid arteries (main supply of cervical trachea), internal thoracic arteries, and bronchial arteries (main supply of lower trachea).

"A patient presents with a life-threatening airway obstruction. She was previously diagnosed with a large, mid-tracheal lesion that you recently biopsied. The lesion is suspicious for malignancy and you are still awaiting the results. In the meantime, she presents in extremis. How would you manage this patient?"
If you do not have an airway, you cannot ventilate this patient. Therefore, emergency measures need to be carried out to obtain a patent airway. The patient should be transported to the OR immediately. IV sedation should be administered rather than general anesthesia. A rigid bronchoscope provides the best chance of establishing an airway in patients with an

acute obstruction due to intraluminal or extraluminal disease. If the tumor is not circumferential, the beveled tip of the rigid scope is advanced along the free area of tracheal wall, distal to the tumor. Jet ventilation may then be instituted to "catch up." Of note, it is useful to have a number of rigid scopes available, including pediatric rigid scopes, to facilitate passage (pediatric - 3.5, 4.0, 5.0, and 6.0 mm and adult - 7.0, 8.0, 9.0, 11.0, 14.0 mm sizes). Once the patient is stabilized, the rigid scope can be used to core out the tumor and to enlarge the lumen. Bleeding can be tamponaded with the rigid scope or with energy sources such as electrocautery, Nd:YAG laser, or argon plasma beam. These energy sources can also be used to perform additional tumor debridement (which may have been helpful at the time of biopsy in this patient), however, their use in the acute setting is unlikely to be tolerated as a low FiO2 is required to prevent combustion within the airway. A tube exchanger can then be passed through the rigid scope and an appropriately sized endotracheal tube passed over the tube exchanger after the rigid scope has been removed. If the tumor is circumferential and almost completely obstructive, the rigid scope is used to core out the lesion until a lumen is present and the scope can be advanced beyond the obstruction.

A note about acute airway obstruction from extrinsic compression/lesions. The rigid is still useful in this situation to obtain a patent airway, stenting the airway open and allowing ventilation distally. An airway stent may then be used in the acute setting to maintain airway patency (but should not be used in the acute setting for intraluminal lesions). Although measures such as tracheostomy and radiation can be useful tactics to provide airway patency, they should not be used in the acute setting. Elective resection may be carried out in the patient once airway patency is secured and workup is completed for surgical resection, should the tumor be resectable and the patient is an operative candidate.

"Which major histology has a better survival following resection? Which responds better to radiation therapy?"
Adenoid cystic carcinoid (as opposed to squamous cell) for both.

"You are referred a 79-year-old man with a 2 cm mid-tracheal tumor who presents with increasing dyspnea and hoarseness. He has ESRD, poorly controlled DM and ischemic cardiomyopathy with EF 30% and has PET-positive masses in RUL."
This patient is a poor operative candidate and surgical resection would not be curative (and would be very high risk). Tissue diagnosis is needed to confirm cell type of the tumor. Assuming this is a squamous cell carcinoma, he should only be offered radiation therapy (dosing of at least 60 Gy in daily fractions of 1.8-2.0 Gy). Measures may be needed to debride the tumor if his symptoms do not improve with radiation therapy. There have been no trials that define the role of chemotherapy as a treatment for unresectable disease.

"You are referred a patient with a biopsy proven SCC of the trachea measuring 2 cm and located in the distal trachea 2 cm proximal to the carina. What would your approach be to resection? What if it involves the carina?"
A median sternotomy provides good exposure to the distal trachea and gives access to the neck if release maneuvers are required. The sternum is opened, as is the anterior pericardium. The tracheobronchial bifurcation can then be accessed between the SVC and ascending aorta by opening the posterior pericardium. Distal tracheal tumors can also be approached via a right posterolateral thoracotomy, which is particularly useful if parenchymal resection is required in conjunction with a carinal resection. Carinal tumors have higher perioperative morbidity and mortality but can be undertaken by experienced surgeons.

"You are referred a patient with a long tracheal tumor measuring 6 cm in length? What are contraindications for resection?"
The trachea is approximately 11 cm long. Long tumors have been shown to be the most common reason why resection was not feasible. Some report resection of lesions up to 6 cm, but the risk of significant tension on the anastomosis is greater if greater than 4.5 cm is resected. Absolute contraindications for surgery include over 50% of tracheal length, multiple positive lymph nodes, mediastinal invasion of unresectable organs, a

mediastinum that has been irradiated with >60 Gy, and distant metastases for SCC. Distant metastases or mediastinal lymph node involvement requires tissue diagnosis, by mediastinoscopy, EBUS, percutaneous biopsy, etc.

"When is airway stenting appropriate?"
Airway stenting may be used to maintain airway patency in patients with aggressive, unresectable tumors that recur and obstruct the airway. Airway stenting is also a good option for the treatment of airway obstruction caused by external compression. However, stents constitute palliative therapy only and must be used in conjunction with tumor debulking (rigid bronch, mechanical coring, Nd:Yag laser, cryotherapy, argon beam, etc.). Montgomery T-tubes or metallic stents are used for symptom-relief and life expectancy is minimal.

"Following tracheal resection, your patient has significant laryngeal edema and is not able to be extubated. How would you manage this patient?"
Leave a small ETT and keep the patient intubated for 48 hours to allow for the edema to subside. Adjunctive measures include corticosteroids for 24-48 hours, fluid restriction, elevation of the head of the bed, and close monitoring in an ICU setting. The patient should be brought back to the OR 48 hours later and extubated with the help of anesthesia. If extubation is unsuccessful or the patient does not meet criteria for extubation, placing a tracheostomy tube two rings below anastomosis may be warranted. Consideration should be given to covering the anastomosis with a pedicled strap muscle flap for reinforcement.

"Another patient now 6 days after tracheal resection of a 3 cm lesion develops fever, crepitus over the neck and chest, and stridor. How would you manage this patient?"
Dehiscence of the tracheal anastomosis is of primary concern in this scenario. This suspicion should be immediately confirmed with flexible bronchoscopy. An endotracheal tube should be placed over the bronchoscope to avoid additional separation of the anastomosis and to assure adequate ventilation. A definitive airway is then established in the operating room with a tracheostomy distal to the anastomosis. The area surrounding the dehiscence is then debrided and drained. Finally, the defect is controlled with a muscle flap (i.e., strap muscles or sternocleidomastoid). Delayed re-operation may be attempted to revise the anastomosis once the patient has been stabilized and the infection is resolved. An alternative treatment in the short-term may be a covered stent for those patients who are not stable enough to undergo extensive reoperation early on. In this case, tracheostomy and drainage must be established prior to stenting. Esophageal injury should also be ruled out in this scenario (Contrast esophagram, EGD) should the bronchoscopy fail to show a dehisced anastomosis.

Pearls/pitfalls
- Tracheal tumors are uncommon, usually present as locally advanced disease, and appropriate patient selection for surgery is key to successful outcomes.
- Full evaluation of extent of disease including bronchoscopy and tissue diagnosis is essential for preoperative workup.
- IV induction of anesthesia, immediate intubation, and excellent communication with anesthesiologist is vital.
- Release maneuvers are critical to mobilizing trachea to avoid tension on the anastomosis (suprahyoid most common).
- Minimal circumferential dissection is critical in order to maintain the tracheal blood supply (located laterally); if needed, compromise oncologic principles of clear margins to favor a tension-free anastomosis.
- Avoid the recurrent laryngeal nerves! Never sacrifice both nerves if tumor is involved.
- Patients with unresectable tumors should receive radiation therapy or tumor debulking/stenting for palliation.
- Adjuvant radiation therapy is warranted for most tumors, especially with positive margins. ACC responds especially well.

194

Suggested readings

- Gaissert, HA et al. Treatment of tracheal tumors. *Seminars in Thoracic and Cardiovascular Surgery.* 2009; 21(3): 290-295.
- Gaissert HA and DJ Mathiesen. Primary Tumors of the Trachea. *Pearson's Thoracic & Esophageal Surgery.* 3rd Edition. Philadelphia: Churchill Livingstone, 2008. 312-320.
- Honings J et al. Clinical aspects and treatment of primary tracheal malignancies. *Acta Oto-Larynggoligca.* 2010; 130: 763-772.
- Macchiarini P. Primary tracheal tumors. *Lancet Onc.* 2006; 7: 83-91.
- Merritt RE and Mathieson DJ. Tracheal Resection. *Pearson's Thoracic & Esophageal Surgery.* 3rd Edition. Philadelphia: Churchill Livingstone, 2008:376-382.
- Wigle DA and S Keshavjee. Upper Airway Tumors: Secondary Tumors. *Pearson's Thoracic & Esophageal Surgery.* 3rd Edition. Philadelphia: Churchill Livingstone, 2008. 321-325.

30. MEDIASTINAL MASSES

Nakul Valsangkar, MD and Allan Pickens, MD

Adapted from 1st edition chapter written by Gabriel Loor, MD, and Daniel Raymond, MD

Concept

- Differential for a mediastinal mass by age, sex, and compartment involved
- Select appropriate diagnostic modalities
- Formulate a medical and surgical plan based on etiology
- Stage all malignant tumors
- Understand preoperative preparation, conduct of the operation, and manage postoperative complications

Chief Complaint

"A 61-year-old man is referred to your clinic after they were evaluated by their primary care physician for complaints of chest pain with exertion, non-productive cough, malaise and unintentional weight loss >10 lbs. The patient eventually undergoes a chest CT scan that identifies a 4.5 cm by 5 cm anterior mediastinal mass."

Mediastinal Compartments and Differential

The mediastinal space is divided into three compartments by the International Thymoma Interest Group (ITMIG) using multidetector CT scanning: prevascular, visceral, and paravertebral have recently been delineated in place of the older anterior, middle, and posterior compartments. The boundaries of these compartments are as outlined below.

Prevascular

1. Superiorly, thoracic inlet
2. Inferiorly, diaphragm
3. Anteriorly, posterior border/cortex of the sternum
4. Laterally, parietal mediastinal pleura
5. Posteriorly, anterior aspect of the pericardium as it wraps around the heart in a curvilinear fashion

Based on the boundaries as outlined above, the contents of this compartment include the thymus, fat, lymph nodes, and the left brachiocephalic vein, and therefore the most common masses found in this compartment are; thymic cysts, hyperplasia, thymoma, thymic carcinoma, and neuroendocrine neoplasms, germ cell neoplasms (teratoma, seminoma, non seminomatous neoplasms), lymphoma, metastatic lymph nodes, parathyroid adenoma, parathyroid carcinoma, and intrathoracic goiter.

Visceral

1. Superiorly, the thoracic inlet
2. Inferiorly, the diaphragm
3. Anteriorly, the posterior boundaries of the prevascular compartment
4. Posteriorly, a vertical line connecting a point on the thoracic vertebral bodies 1 cm posterior to the anterior margin of the spine

The middle mediastinal or visceral compartment can be divided into two major categories of contents.

1. Heart and associated vascular structures: superior vena cava, ascending thoracic aorta, aortic arch, descending thoracic aorta, intrapericardial pulmonary arteries, and thoracic duct;

2. Aerodigestive tract and associated structures: trachea, carina, esophagus, and lymph nodes. The extrapericardial pulmonary arteries and veins are not included this compartment.

Therefore, the common lesions in this visceral compartment include lymphadenopathy (lymphoma or metastatic disease), duplication cysts, tracheal lesions, bronchiogenic cysts, esophageal cysts, and pericardial cysts.

Paravertebral

The paravertebral compartment is defined as follows:
1. Superiorly, the thoracic inlet
2. Inferiorly, the diaphragm
3. Anteriorly, the posterior boundaries of the visceral compartment
4. Posterolaterally, a vertical line along the posterior margin of the chest wall at the lateral aspect of the transverse processes as noted above. This yields the following contents in the paravertebral compartment: the thoracic spine and paravertebral soft tissue associated neoplasms; neurogenic neoplasms that arise from the dorsal root ganglia/neurons adjacent to the intervertebral foramina such as schwannomas, neurofibromas, ganglioneuromas, paraganglianomas, and neurogenic sarcomas.

History and Physical

During the initial consultation, attention should be focused on symptoms and exam findings associated with Myasthenia Gravis (MG) with attention to pattern of ocular muscle weakness (diplopia, blurred vision), dysphonia, dysphagia, or progressive generalized weakness markedly noted more so at the end of the day. Whereas only 15%-20% of MG patients have a thymoma, 30% of patients with thymoma have MG. In addition, any history of fevers, night sweats, chills or malaise known as 'B' type symptoms should be elicited, as they are consistent with lymphoma or GCT. A complete physical exam must be performed, specifically looking for cervical and supraclavicular lymphadenopathy, inspiratory/expiratory stridor (indicative of dynamic airway compression) and decreased breath sounds or pericardial rub (indicative of pleural effusion or pericardial involvement). Obtain a detailed past medical history including prior malignancies, smoking history, prior chest surgery or radiation, history of cardiopulmonary disease, and details of significant comorbidities.

Other autoimmune disorders associated with thymoma include systemic lupus erythematosus, pure red cell aplasia, polymyositis, autoimmune myopathies, pernicious anemia, autoimmune thyroid diseases, rheumatoid arthritis, ulcerative colitis, dermatomyositis, scleroderma, Takayasu syndrome, autoimmune hemolytic anemia and cortical encephalitis. Mediastinal tumors are rare and a majority of these are asymptomatic. Age and gender along with specific imaging characteristics allow for a presumptive diagnosis in a majority of these patients. The most common mediastinal masses are thymic malignancy (35%), lymphoma (25%), teratoma (10%), and malignant germ cell neoplasm (10% - of which Seminoma; 40%, NSGCT; 60%).

Tests

- *Labs:* Beta human chorionic gonadotropin (B-HCG), alpha-fetoprotein (AFP) and lactate dehydrogenase (LDH) are elevated with non-seminomatous GCTs, but often normal with most seminomatous GCTs as well as thymomas or lymphomas. Notably, one-third of seminomas produce B-HCG but none make AFP.
- *Imaging:* When incidentally found, CT scan with IV contrast is the modality of choice and as outlined below has pathognomonic features for certain tumors. MRI without contrast is superior in distinguishing cystic from solid lesions and is used when IV contrast is contraindicated. 18-FDG-PET is not routinely used for diagnosis but rather for completion of staging and response to treatment particularly among lymphomas.
- *CT-guided core needle biopsy:* Although a CT-guided biopsy allows definitive tissue diagnosis in cases where medical management is the primary treatment (e.g., lymphoma and malignant germ cell tumors), this technique is plagued by a low

negative predictive value. In the event of an indeterminate diagnosis additional options for tissue diagnosis include: anterior mediastinotomy (Chamberlain procedure), video assisted thoracoscopic surgery (VATS), cervical mediastinoscopy. In the event of a clear presumptive clinical diagnosis, complete surgical excision is the ultimate diagnostic test.

Index Scenario (additional information)

"Further evaluation of the patient reports weakness that is most pronounced at the end of the day. This manifests as ocular weakness as well progressive dyspnea. He denies fevers, chills, night sweats, or any other 'B' type symptoms. He also denies other histories suggestive of CAD, HTN, or DM. The mass on CT appears lobulated without calcification, and it is centered on the left superior pole of the thymus. LDH, B-HCG and AFP are within normal range. What is the next step in the management of this patient?"

Treatment/Management

Age and sex are the most important clinical features which help narrow the diagnosis. Additional pathognomonic features on CT scan help confirm the diagnosis. For simplification of the approach we have divided the patients into three major groups by age and gender as listed below and the most common diagnoses in each group are discussed in detail with regards to medical and surgical management under the relevant heading.

 1. *Age > 40, Women, Men*

In men and women, the most common diagnosis is Thymoma (50%). Features suggestive of thymic paraneoplastic syndromes such as myasthenia gravis make the diagnosis certain. The next most common diagnosis is substernal goiter (10-30%) and this is obvious on CT scan. Rarely patients in this age group will have lymphoma (2-10%).

Thymoma

Thymoma is the most common anterior (previsceral) mediastinal mass in adults. Incidence is equal in males and females and usually in the third to fifth decade of life. Up to half of patients will be asymptomatic and the mass will be found incidentally. The other half may have pain, dyspnea, cough, hoarseness, or other associated syndromes (e.g., myasthenia gravis, red cell hypoplasia, hypogammaglobulinemia, SLE, rheumatoid arthritis, ulcerative colitis, thyroiditis). On CT, benign thymomas are usually <5 cm and appear well-circumscribed and round. Thymomas are malignant in 50% of patients and are usually >5 cm, irregular in shape, and may invade neighboring structures.

The treatment of thymoma is complete excision. This may require *en bloc* resection of structures to which the tumor may be adherent to (e.g., pleura, pericardium, innominate vein, SVC, lung). If both phrenic nerves appear to be involved, one nerve may be excised while the tumor is dissected from the other nerve; pathological frozen examination may help in differentiating the tumor from surrounding inflammatory reaction. Median sternotomy is the most common approach but cervical and VATS approaches are also described.

Masaoka staging system

•	*Stage I*	No evidence of microscopic extracapsular invasion.
•	*Stage II*	Microscopic or macroscopic invasion through the capsule into the surrounding fat or pleura.
•	*Stage III*	Invasion of adjacent structures (pericardium, great vessels, lungs).
•	*Stage IVa*	Pleural or pericardial metastasis.
•	*Stage IVb*	Lymphogenous or hematogenous metastasis.

Survival is based on stage. Stage I disease is completely encapsulated and has a 95% five-year survival. Stage II has microscopic invasion into mediastinal fat or mediastinal pleura (IIa) or through the capsule (IIb), and an 85% five-year survival. Stage III disease invades an adjacent organ and has a 70% five-year survival. Stage IV is metastatic to pleura or pericardium (IVa) or distant (IVb) and has a 50% five-year survival. Increased survival is reported with adjuvant and neoadjuvant therapy for stage III to stage IV disease with RT and cisplatin-based chemotherapy.

Myasthenia Gravis (MG)

MG is an autoantibody disorder with a prevalence of 5 to 12 per 100 000. The disease is twice as common in women and usually occurs in the second to third decade of life. For men, MG manifests in the sixth to seventh decade of life. The antibody targets the acetylcholine receptor (AChR), and binding causes decreased transmission of the action potential at the neuromuscular junction. Clinically, this manifests as decreased contraction of the muscle fibers, which results in weakness.

Symptoms are graded: (I) focal disease—ocular muscle weakness, (II) generalized mild to moderate disease, (III) severe generalized weakness, and (IV) life-threatening weakness—respiratory failure. After a physical examination identifying the level of weakness, an edrophonium (short acting anticholinesterase) test is confirmatory if the patient shows improvement. Assay for AChR antibody is also available.

The treatment of MG includes anticholinesterase therapy (pyridostigmine) and if needed, corticosteroids for immunosuppression. Plasmapheresis and IVIG are short-term therapies used for myasthenic crises, preoperatively, or intermittently in patients with poor control of MG despite immunosuppression. Thymectomy is indicated in patients with thymic hyperplasia or a thymoma. Thirty to 50% of patients with a thymoma have MG and 10% to 15% of patients with MG have a thymoma. Further, there is a role for thymectomy in any MG patient with early, generalized, moderate to severe disease, especially if refractory to medical management. Thymectomy should not be performed emergently for a myasthenic crisis/class IV disease.

Substernal Goiter

Intrathoracic goiter can appear as a mediastinal mass and is usually associated with cervical goiter. CXR frequently indicates tracheal deviation. Non-contrast CT shows enhancement of the thyroid gland because of its iodine content and confirms the diagnosis. Most intrathoracic goiters are removed from the neck, although an upper partial sternotomy in the form of a manubrial split may be required.

Operative steps

Thymectomy

Goals – explore, stage, total resection with surrounding fat, identify and preserve phrenic nerves

- Single lumen ETT, central venous catheter, arterial line, Foley catheter.
- Full median sternotomy, expose and explore the thymus, identify extent of disease.
  - o This operation can be performed also via a left or right VATS (thoracoscopic) approach depending on which side the dominant extent of the lesion lies.
- Open pleura bilaterally to assess for lung metastases and to identify the location of both phrenic nerves.
- Free up the right inferior horn of the thymus.
- Free up the right superior horn (resect the thymic-thyroid ligament).
- Ligate the lateral vessels coming from the mammary.
- Make a 1 cm incision above the right phrenic nerve on the mediastinal pleura, remove this superficial pleura and fat with the thymus.
- Repeat these steps on the left side.
- Divide the venous branches draining into the innominate vein.
- Carefully dissect both superior horns of the gland into the neck and divide small arterial branches from the inferior thyroid arteries.

"Postoperatively, the patient is extubated and doing well. 5 hours later you are called to evaluate the patient for generalized weakness and respiratory distress."
Identification of perioperative myasthenic crisis and its treatment is important. This patient may require reintubation for respiratory compromise. Postoperatively most thymectomy patients are extubated within 6 hours. This includes MG patients. Plasmapheresis may be required for MG patients exhibiting ocular weakness or respiratory weakness, although patients in acute distress warrant immediate re-intubation and plasmapheresis can then be initiated.

Potential questions/alternative scenarios
What if the patient is a 38-year-old woman and on further evaluation, this patient reports no weakness, malaise or fatigue? However, she does indicate some night sweats. Serum makers of LDH, B-HCG and AFP are within normal range. What is the next step in the management of this patient?
In this patient the diagnosis is less clear. A CT-guided needle biopsy should be performed.

"The initial CT-guided tissue biopsy is consistent with lymphoma." For ages 10-39 Women, what is the most common diagnosis:
The most common diagnosis in this group is Hodgkin's disease (HD), Non-hodgkin's lymphoma (NHL) (30-50%). For these tumors, the onset is slow and there are multiple matted lymph nodes, occasionally with the presence of 'B' type symptoms (fever, night sweats, weight loss, myalgia, arthralgia). In patients with heterogenous and calcified, bony appearing tissue in the mass, Teratoma is most likely (10-25%). Least likely is Thymoma (5-10%). Only 2-5% of this age/gender group get non-small cell germ cell tumors (NSGCT).

Primary mediastinal lymphoma
Primary mediastinal lymphoma is rare, causing only 5% to 10% of cases of anterior mediastinal masses. T-cell Non-Hodgkin's lymphoma is the most common; Hodgkin's (HD) and lymphoblastic lymphoma also occur in the mediastinum. The mediastinum is a common site for more disseminated lymphoma associated with mediastinal lymphadenopathy. A tissue diagnosis is necessary and may be accomplished with surgical biopsy via a cervical mediastinoscopy, anterior mediastinotomy, or thoracoscopic approach. Surgical biopsy yields a more reliable specimen for diagnosis than needle biopsy. HD is characterized by Reed-Sternberg cells under light microscopy. NHL is diagnosed also using light microscopy, cell surface markers, and flow cytometry. The primary modality for treatment is chemotherapy and radiation with CT or PET used to determine residual disease.

"You are referred a 36-year-old man with intermittent fevers and chest pain who is found to have a large mediastinal mass. Serum markers are pending. However, the initial CT-guided tissue biopsy is consistent with germ cell tumor. How will you proceed with the work up and management of this patient?" For ages 10 - 39 Men, what are the more common diagnoses:

Germ cell tumors
Germ cell tumors account for 10% to 15% of mediastinal masses. Males are affected more often. *Benign mediastinal teratoma* is the most common (60%) germ cell tumor in the mediastinum and affect men and women equally. They are usually asymptomatic but can occasionally become infected or rupture into the pleura or the airway (resulting in coughing of hair or sebum). Serum tumor markers are negative. Imaging indicates variable enhancement and well-circumscribed tumor with frequent calcification. Biopsy reveals well-differentiated tissue from more than one germ cell line. Surgical resection is the treatment traditionally using a median sternotomy but now more frequently via a robotic or VATS based approach.
Seminoma is the most common malignant germ cell tumor in the mediastinum and occurs far more frequently in males in the third to fourth decade of life. Serum tumor markers can reveal normal AFP and mildly elevated β-HCG levels. CT will reveal a characteristically

large, homogeneous mass with smooth borders. Seminomas tend to grow slowly and are sensitive to RT, which traditionally used to be the primary treatment. Currently however, cisplatin-based chemotherapy is used for primary disease and high response rates with an 80% cure rate have been reported. Any residual disease identified using PET imaging can either be resected or treated with additional chemotherapy.

Non-seminomatous germ cell tumors occur most often in young men 20 to 30 years old and are associated with elevated β-HCG (in 50%), AFP (also in 50%), and LDH. There are 3 main subtypes (in decreasing order of frequency): yolk sac carcinoma (most commonly associated with increased AFP), embryonal carcinoma, and choriocarcinoma (most commonly associated with β-HCG). These tumors tend to grow rapidly and compress neighboring tissues; thus, most patients are symptomatic at presentation. Tissue confirmation is the first step in management followed by three-drug chemotherapy as the first line of treatment (etoposide, ifosfamide, and cisplatin). Surgical resection is reserved for patients with normalizing tumor makers after chemotherapy. This paradigm is gradually shifting to a broader use of surgical resection after chemotherapy regardless of trend of the tumor markers.

"A 58-year-old woman presents with a history of recurrent cough. A CT scan shows a 4 by 6 cm cystic appearing mass adjacent to the right mainstem bronchi. What is your approach to this patient?"
The patient has a bronchogenic cyst, a middle mediastinal mass lesion

Middle Mediastinal Cysts
Most middle mediastinal masses are cysts. The management of these lesions is as follows:
Bronchogenic cysts are the most common cysts (60%) in the mediastinum and are associated with the airway, most often located posterior to the carina. The cysts have the histologic characteristic of the airway and lung. Most patients are symptomatic at time of presentation due to airway or esophageal compression. After tissue diagnosis is obtained, the treatment is complete transthoracic surgical resection.
Pericardial cysts are rare benign cysts that occur at the cardiophrenic angle, most often on the right. CT imaging is key to diagnosis as these cysts have a thin wall, are non-enhancing, and have a characteristic density like water. If symptoms arise, the treatment is surgical resection. Some argue all pericardial cysts should be resected because of the potential for rupture, erosion, or compression of the heart or great vessels.

"What if the lesion were asymptomatic?"
Surgical resection is indicated for children and young adults, specifically if there is impending alteration of anatomy. For adults with small, asymptomatic, well characterized cysts, serial radiologic examination with CT scan or MRI is acceptable. Resection can be offered to these patients if there is any change in the appearance, concern for infection, or onset of symptoms.

"A 55-year-old man presents to your clinic with bilateral lower back pain. After 3 months of physical therapy that did not change the symptoms, an MRI was ordered by his primary physician which showed a 4 by 5 cm mass at T8 near the left costovertebral junction. What is the approach to this lesion?"
The patient has a neurogenic tumor, a posterior mediastinal mass lesion.

Posterior Mediastinal Masses
Neurogenic tumors account for 15% to 20% of all mediastinal tumors and often present with pain or neurologic dysfunction. Arising from neural crest cells, the tumors can be divided into three main groups:
1. *Nerve sheath tumors.* Most common tumors overall, representing 40% to 70% of mediastinal neurogenic tumors. They usually present in the costovertebral sulcus. They tend to be benign with the two most common tumors being neurilemmomas (also called schwannomas) and neurofibromas. Neurofibrosarcomas are the

malignant counterpart and are differentiated from the benign ones by level of mitotic activity and lack of encapsulation.

2. *Ganglion cell tumors.* These tumors arise from the sympathetic chain and adrenal medulla. The benign tumor in this category is the ganglioneuroma, which can secrete vasoactive intestinal peptide (VIP). Ganglioneuroblastomas are malignant tumors that can present with metastases and are more common in children. These tumors are usually resectable.

3. *Neuroblastomas* are the most common solid extracranial malignancy in children and the most aggressive of the ganglion cell tumors. They can secrete VIP and catecholamines. Treatment of localized disease is surgical with adjuvant chemoradiation for residual tumor. Metastatic disease is treated with chemotherapy. Factors associated with poor prognosis in neuroblastoma are presence of metastatic disease, age (<18 months), degree of histologic differentiation, DNA ploidy, presence of residual disease, N-*myc* amplification, and high levels of neuronspecific enolase and LDH.

Paraganglionic tumors. These tumors arise from paraganglionic tissues in the costovertebral area and include pheocromocytomas (which produce catecholamines) and chemodectomas (hormonally inactive). Resection is the treatment of choice. Chemodectomas may also respond to RT. CT is the best imaging modality for these tumors. A percutaneous FNA biopsy may be obtained for tissue diagnosis (spindle cell neoplasm). Surgical excision, usually through a posterolateral thoracotomy, is the treatment of choice. The tumor capsule should be left intact if possible.

Pearls/pitfalls

- During thymectomy for thymic malignancies, any involved structures are resected *en bloc* with the mass.

- Phrenic nerve is always attempted to be spared. Bilateral phrenic nerve paralysis is a devastating complication

- For R1 resections during thymectomy, clips are placed in the field for consideration for adjuvant radiation therapy.

- *Myasthenia gravis*: Preoperative optimization with pyridostigmine, corticosteroids. immunosuppression. Plasmapheresis and IVIG are short-term therapies used for myasthenic crises, perioperatively

- *Germ cell tumors*: Know key differences between seminomatous and non seminomatous tumors.

- *Seminomas* reveal normal AFP and mildly elevated β-HCG levels. RT was the traditional treatment with Cisplatin-based chemotherapy now with surgical resection of residual disease.

- *Non-seminomatous germ cell tumors* have elevated β-HCG (in 50%), AFP (also in 50%), and LDH. Chemotherapy is the first line with surgical resection for patients with normalizing tumor makers after chemotherapy.

- *Lymphoma*: chemotherapy, surgery only for tissue diagnosis.

Suggested readings

- Sabiston and Spencer Surgery of the Chest, 9th Edition, Frank Sellke, MD, Pedro J. del Nido, MD and Scott J. Swanson, MD. 2016. Elsevier ISBN 9780323241267

- Pearson's Thoracic and Esophageal Surgery. Patterson MD, G. Alexander; Pearson MD, F. G.; Cooper MD, Joel D.; Deslauriers MD FRCPS(C) CM, Jean; Rice MDMD FACSMD, Thomas W.; Luketich MD, James D.; Lerut MD PhD, Antoon E. M. R. Churchill Livingstone 2008

- Carter BW, Benveniste MF, Madan R, et al. ITMIG Classification of Mediastinal Compartments and Multidisciplinary Approach to Mediastinal Masses. Radiographics. 2017;37(2):413–436. doi:10.1148/rg.2017160095

II. Adult Cardiac Surgery

31. CARDIOPULMONARY BYPASS PITFALLS

Juan G. Penaranda, MD, and Harold M. Burkhart, MD

Concept
- Establishing access for CPB
- Initiating CPB
- Maintaining CPB
- Separating from CPB
- Pitfalls that arise in each of the above steps

Chief complaint
"A 77-year-old diabetic man is undergoing a CABG AVR. Describe any preoperative workup relevant to CPB."

Differential
Non applicable

History and physical
Any patient requiring CPB needs to have a comprehensive systems-based history and physical to identify history of stroke, renal disease, coronary lesions, intestinal angina, respiratory problems, bleeding disorders, or peripheral vascular disease.

Tests
- Comprehensive labs (CBC, BMP, Coags, LFTs)
- Head CT if recent stroke
- Carotid duplex if stroke or bruits
- Mesenteric duplex if evidence of intestinal ischemia
- ABIs for evidence of peripheral vascular disease
- Coronary angio to identify critical lesions
- PFTs for history of respiratory problems
- Chest CT scan for any patient with calcification on CXR

These tests allow risk stratification, identification of lesions that require preoperative intervention and identification of lesions that modify the lowest acceptable MAP on CPB.

Index scenario (additional information)
"The patient has a creatinine of 1.7, and a carotid duplex showing a 60% asymptomatic left carotid lesion. Chest CT shows a normal appearing aorta without calcification."
This patient will require CPB in order to perform the combined CABG AVR. His MAP should be kept at the upper range of normal to ensure adequate renal and brain perfusion. A useful rule of thumb is MAPs = decade of age (i.e., 77 = 70-80 mmHg). Mild hypothermia (32-34° C) can be considered to decrease the tissue oxygen demand.

Operative steps
Cannulation
- Median sternotomy.
- Palpate the aorta for calcification.
- Ensure you are high enough to complete all your proximal procedures.
- Give Heparin (400 Units/kg).
- Place purstrings.
- Check your systemic pressure (ideally < 70 mmHg).

- Cannulate the aorta with a 21-24 F arterial cannula and secure the cannula.
- Check your line (assess the swing and line pressure with a test transfusion). Visualize the proximal aorta with the test transfusion.
- Cannulate the RA with a dual stage cannula that drains both the RA and IVC.
- Alternative venous cannulas include right angled IVC/SVC cannulas, 3 stage SVC cannula, or long femoral vein cannulation.
- ABC's - A: anticoagulate B: be sure you are high enough C: calcification.

Initiation
- Check your ACT and make sure you are > 480.
- Go on CPB - forward flow is initiated to ensure there is no obstruction.
- Empty out - drain the heart once forward flow is confirmed.
- Hold ventilation.
- Flush cardioplegia, specify your desired temperature, and complete any required dissection prior to cross clamp and arrest.
- Specify your temperature.
- ABC's - A: ACT B: breathing - hold ventilation C: circulation (forward flow and drainage, PAPs, CVP should be low).

Maintenance
- Check for asystole (clamp, antegrade/retrograde).
- Aortic vent on.
- Check for optimal MAPs (usually 50-80 mmHg) - higher age or greater atherosclerotic burden may require higher MAPs.
- Flow is usually 2.1-2.5 L/min.
- Assess perfusion via lactate, venous saturation, urine output.
- Cooling to mild hypothermia (32-34°C) may allow a decrease of flow and MAPs when needed.
- Check drainage - heart should be empty, CVP and PAP should be low.
- Check sats, ABG, oxygenation, visual inspection of arterial blood - should be bright red).
- ABC's - A: asystole B: breathing (oxygenation) C: circulation (forward flow, drainage).

Releasing the cross clamp
- Deair the left atrium and root.
- Administer hot shot cardioplegia (institution specific).
- Drop your flows, vent on, head down, release the clamp, resume your flows.

Weaning from CPB
In general, you need to be warm, have rhythm and be ventilating in order to come off.
A more detailed but useful mnemonic follows:
A - Anastomosis
B- Beat of the heart (fibrillation, pacing wires), Breathing - ventilation
C- Circulation (fill up the heart and eject), assess Contractiliy
D- Degrees (36° C)
E- Echo (function, valves, air), Electrolytes
F- Flows (gradually reduce while observing function and hemodynamics)
G- Gases (ABG)
H- Hypertension (vasodilate)
I - Inotropes

J- Juices (urine output throughout the case)

"5 minutes after the cross clamp is released the heart begins to over distend. You notice a lack of spontaneous contraction. What do you do?"

There are 2 considerations - one is that the valve has a leak of some degree and the second is that the heart is not ejecting to overcome any regurgitant volume. Usually the first maneuver will be to squeeze the heart to get it to decompress from the apex up towards the LVOT. Check your PAP which will give you a clue as to how effectively you are decompressing. Try to pace or tap the heart to encourage ejection but ultimately the solution may be to cross clamp.

"You attempt to pace but have no capture despite well placed leads. Anesthesia tells you there is 1+ central AI. Perfusion tells you that the potassium has been 7 meq/L and they have struggled to bring it down. The patient has not made urine during the case. You cross clamp the aorta, turn up the root vent and empty out the heart. After 10 minutes the potassium starts to decrease and the heart contracts."

Now you know the etiology. There is some leak, but it is hard to truly estimate it without contractility. Knowing the electrolytes is an important component of the weaning process as is the production of urine output. If the potassium does not decrease options include hemoconcentration, IV insulin and glucose, lasix, or bicarb. Usually the perfusionist can get the potassium down but it may take some time. Another option would be to vent the heart while you wait for the K to resolve. While you wait it would not be unreasonable to open the aortotomy and explore the aortic valve for any major defects especially if you were told that the AI was moderate-severe. But in the absence of something obvious and only 1+ AI, wait until you are ejecting to analyze the valve and decide on replacing or not. Once you are ready, release the cross clamp, pace prn, ventilate, fill up the heart, eject, wean your flows and check the echo carefully.

"A 60-year-old male patient has just undergone a mitral valve repair. You release the cross clamp. The heart begins to fibrillate. The echo does not demonstrate anything more than a trace to 1+ central aortic jet. You try to defibrillate but are unable to cardiovert. Describe your approach to defibrillating the patient."

Internal paddles are set at 10 - 20 Joules and gradually increased. If you cannot cardiovert give IV lidocaine and or amiodarone (150 mg IV) and try again. There are several issues that can make it hard to cardiovert: distention, air, low systemic pressures, electrolyte abnormality, poor oxygenation, and hypothermia. In addition, consider coronary ischemia or valvular incompetence. If the heart appears distended and or the PAPs are elevated, the initial step is to manually squeeze the heart while emptying out with CPB. If the heart continues to over distend then place a PA vent or LV vent. After placing the vent and decompressing the heart you should be able to cardiovert to sinus rhythm. Make sure the root vent is on to evacuate any air. Increase your perfusion pressures to > 75 mmHg both for improved coronary perfusion and to flush out any air that may have embolized. Give lidocaine and or amiodarone. Optimize your oxygenation, electrolytes and temperature. Check the echo to ensure that you do not have AI. Anything greater than 1+ warrants consideration for replacement (see previous scenario). On the differential, is damage to the non-coronary leaflet with placement of the mitral stitches. If this appears to be the problem by echo, arrest the heart and explore the aortic valve. If there is evidence of coronary ischemia as evidenced by ST changes or new regional wall motion abnormalities, then bypass with a vein graft. If you cannot defibrillate even after venting and reversing all the above then clamp, arrest and try again.

"Describe the components of the CPB machine."

Blood drains into the venous reservoir by gravity or vacuum assist. It is then pushed by centripetal or centrifugal pumps into the oxygenator/heat exchanger. It then continues to the arterial air filter and back to the patient.

206

"You are starting a mitral valve repair and ask the anesthesiologist to give the heparin. After the cannulas are in you ask your perfusionist if the ACT is adequate for bypass. He is having trouble and tells you a standard dose of heparin has been given and the ACT is only 200 seconds and is not going up. How do you deal with this issue?"

Antithrombin III deficiency is the most common reason for an inadequate ACT despite appropriate heparin dosing. An additional dose of heparin solves the problem in most cases. If the ACT does not respond appropriately to a second dose of heparin, one should consider administering either fresh frozen plasma or recombinant antithrombin III.

"You end up giving a dose of AT III and the ACT is now adequate for bypass. Soon after going on CPB, the perfusionist alerts you of a high aortic line pressure. What is your checklist for this situation?"

- Obstruction on the arterial circuit (kink in or clamp on line)
- Malposition of the aortic cannula
- Cannula too small for full CPB
- Evidence of aortic dissection: systemic pressure will be low, and the ascending aorta will be abnormal

"You checked the systemic pressure and it is normal. You inspect the ascending aorta and it looks normal without evidence of swelling or discoloration. You trace out the arterial line and there are no kinks in the circuit. Upon inspection of the cannulation site you notice there is an excessive angulation of the cannula suggesting that the tip is against the lateral aspect of the innominate artery. You reposition the cannula and the line pressure comes down. Your perfusionist now tells you there is poor venous return and a drop in venous reservoir volume after snaring the caval tapes. The right atrium is not distended, and the PAP is low. The CVP is elevated Your perfusionist lowers the CPB flow to protect the level of venous reservoir. What are some of the maneuvers to manage inadequate venous drainage?"

- Check for air locks
- Ensure good position of the venous cannula
- Elevate the level of the patient in relation to the reservoir if relying on gravity
- Use suction drainage
- Increase cannula size
- Reduce flows if still within ideal MAP range (may need to cool 32-34° C)
- Exclude other sources of blood flow into the heart especially in the setting of distention (aortic regurge - vent, azygous vein - adjust snares, left sided SVC - snare or cannulate)
- Consider other sites of volume loss (i.e., retroperitoneal or peritoneal hemorrhage) - check abdominal girth, H/H

"In this case the IVC right angle cannula has rotated before snaring the caval tapes and is now pointing towards the right atrium occluding the IVC drainage. You release the snare and reposition the cannula solving the problem. You also noticed that the SVC cannula was inserted into the azygos and reposition accordingly. After re-instituting CPB, your perfusionist cannot get the mean blood pressure above 40 mmHg. The anesthesiologist tells you the patient was on a high dose of ACE inhibitor preoperatively. What do you do next?"

Vasoplegia can be seen in patients on numerous antihypertensive medications, in particular ACE Inhibitors. In this situation, phenylephrine, norepinephrine, vasopressin or even methylene blue are options that can be used to increase the systemic pressure. This scenario may arise in the postoperative period as well.

"You placed a coronary sinus catheter for retrograde cardioplegia because the patient has moderate aortic regurgitation. As you start your retrograde infusion, the pressure within

the coronary sinus seems to be very low. You inspect the inferior aspect of the heart to make sure there has been no rupture of the coronary sinus or malposition of the catheter. You take out the catheter and the balloon is intact. You place the catheter in again and confirm its position by palpation. Despite this, the pressure remains low and the heart is not arresting. What are the causes of this problem?"

Inadequate retrograde cardioplegia delivery may be due to:

- Catheter displacement into the right atrium
- Rupture of coronary sinus
- Balloon rupture
- Persistent left sided superior vena cava (LSVC)

"You lift the heart to the right and discover a LSVC. You place a snare to occlude it since there is a large innominate vein and you are now able to arrest the heart."

If there is not a persistent innominate vein you can cannulate the LSVC separately.

"You finished your mitral valve repair and wean the patient off bypass. After a few seconds, the blood pressure drops, there is ST elevation on the EKG and the right ventricle distends. You suspect air has entered the right coronary artery. What are some of the maneuvers you use to overcome this problem?"

The right coronary ostium is anterior and susceptible to air embolism. It can be seen after valvular or other cardiac surgery and usually causes transient right ventricular dysfunction and distention. In this case, re-instituting CPB with a high perfusion pressure will help to support cardiac function and push the air through the coronary artery into the venous circulation. De-airing the heart through an aortic root vent will prevent further air migration into the coronary arteries. Consider evacuating air through the apex with a large bore needle if there is a large collection of air at the apex.

"The patient is now off bypass and you and the cardiologist are assessing the mitral valve repair with transesophageal echo (TEE). Your assistant points out to you that the aorta suddenly developed a bluish discoloration. Upon inspection, you notice there is an expanding hematoma in the ascending aorta. On TEE there is a dissection flap in the ascending aorta and the aortic valve is competent. What do you do now?"

The patient has developed an iatrogenic Type A dissection. Establish arterial access within the true lumen (axillary), cool, circ arrest, replace the ascending, resume flow (refer to chapter on iatrogenic aortic dissections).

"You are doing a mitral valve repair in a 42-year-old woman with asymptomatic severe mitral regurgitation. You performed aortic and bi-caval cannulation, instituted CPB and cooled to 32° C. After placing the aortic cross clamp and arresting the heart, the perfusionist alerts you of poor venous drainage. You notice a large amount of air in the aortic cannula. You are certain air has entered the aorta and suspect it has embolized to the brain. The level of the venous reservoir has gone down too low and air has been pumped into the arterial line. What do you do at this point?"

Even though massive air embolism after initiation of cardiopulmonary bypass is a rare complication (incidence less than 0.2% of cases), it has a high mortality and high incidence of neurologic injury. It most commonly happens if the blood level in the venous reservoir and oxygenator gets too low allowing air to be introduced into the arterial circuit. Rapid implementation of an algorithm may save the life of the patient or prevent significant neurologic damage.

A useful algorithm in this situation includes:

- *Perfusionist*:
    - Discontinue CPB
    - Clamp arterial and venous lines
    - De-air bypass circuit

208

- Add necessary volume to the reservoir
- *Anesthesiologist*:
    - Steep trendelenburg
    - 100% oxygen
    - Steroids/Barbiturates/Mannitol
    - Support circulation with vasopressors
- *Surgeon*:
    - Aspirate air from aortic root
    - Retrograde cerebral perfusion
- Reinstitute CBP and cool the patient down for cerebral protection
- Massage coronary arteries to displace air
- Complete surgical procedure and de-air heart in usual fashion
- Consider hyperbaric chamber postoperatively
- *ICU*:
    - Consider deep sedation for cerebral protection
    - Consider hyperbaric chamber

"You ask your perfusionist to stop the pump and clamp both the aortic and venous lines. You place the patient in trendelenburg and aspirate the air from the ascending aorta. Next you disconnect the arterial line from the cannula, de-air the line and connect it to the SVC cannula to start retrograde cerebral perfusion. 300 mL/min of flow directed up to the vena cava is started and after two minutes of perfusion you start seeing bubbles at the ascending aorta which are removed by an aortic root vent you have placed. You then reinstitute CPB and cool the patient down to 28° C for cerebral protection. You complete your aortic valve replacement quickly. The patient is weaned off bypass after 50 minutes and transferred to the ICU. The anesthesiologist gives steroids and barbiturates to the patient and keeps him in deep anesthesia for two days. A CT scan is performed and is negative for any intracerebral injury. The patient is discharged neurologically intact after 10 days in the hospital."

Pearls/pitfalls

- Patients undergoing CPB require a comprehensive workup to minimize the risk of end organ injury.
- *Phases of CPB are Induction > Maintenence > Seperation*: be familiar with critical elements of each of these phases.
- Target MAP is roughly equivalent to the patient's age (i.e., 63 year old = 60 mmHg, 83 year old = 80 mmHg).
- Air embolism, dissection, and venous perforations are major adverse events that can occur during CPB. Be prepared to anticipate, prevent and deal with these complications if they occur.
- Poor drainage can result from air locks, inappropriately positioned cannulas, persistent LSVC. An empty heart and poor drainage suggests loss of blood volume (i.e., retroperitoneal or peritoneal hematoma).

Suggested readings

- Bojar RM. Cardiopulmonary Bypass. Chapter 5. *Manual of Peri-operative care in adult cardiac surgery*, 4th Edition 2005.
- Millls NL, Ochsner JL. Massive air embolism during cardiopulmonary bypass: causes, prevention and management. *J Thorac Cardiovasc Surg* 80:708-717, 1980.
- Svensson LG and Crawford ES. *Cardiovascular and Vascular Diseases of the Aorta*. WB Saunders Company 1997.

32. MYOCARDIAL PROTECTION PITFALLS

Robert C. Neely, MD, Linda Mongero, CCP, James Beck, CCP, and Michael Argenziano, MD

Concept

- Cardioprotection strategies for the arrested heart during cardiopulmonary bypass
- Common errors and troubleshooting techniques
- Cardioplegia solutions

Chief complaint

"You are doing an aortic valve replacement on a 65-year-old man for severe aortic stenosis with moderate aortic insufficiency who has a history of previous triple vessel CABG (LIMA-LAD, SVG-PDA, SVG-OM). Discuss your options for cardioprotection."

In general, options for cardioprotection for an arrested heart include antegrade and retrograde delivery, continuous or intermittent. Types of cardioplegia include crystalloid or blood-based solutions that can be warm or cold. The most common practice is to use a solution that has a 1:4 blood to crystalloid ratio and is cooled to a temperature of 4° C and infused intermittently every 15-20 minutes.

This patient has important issues that influence the approach, namely a reoperation with prior LIMA conduit and the presence of moderate aortic insufficiency. Standard re-operative measures should be taken, including external pacing pads and prepped groins bilaterally in the event that emergent peripheral cannulation is needed for bypass (refer to redo CABG chapter).

In order to achieve adequate cardiac arrest with sufficient cardioprotection, one must ensure 4 things in this scenario - #1 excellent drainage through standard atrial, groin or bicaval cannulation (this can be augmented by an LV vent if needed) #2 ability to cross clamp the aorta - need enough room on the ascending for the placement of a cross clamp, axillary cannulation may be needed if the proximals are patent and high on the aorta #3 Identify the LIMA conduit - prior to arresting the heart, the LIMA should be clamped to prevent continuous perfusion during aortic cross clamping (NOTE: could avoid clamping LIMA in favor of cold bypass flow). #4 retrograde and antegrade cardioplegia access. Antegrade would perfuse the OM and PDA territories but not the LAD. Retrograde would perfuse the LAD territory. Adjunctive measures include moderate hypothermia (28-32° C) and direct cardioplegia down the vein grafts but again that would not supply the LAD territory.

In the setting of aortic insufficiency, a retrograde cardioplegia catheter should be inserted in order to ensure cardioplegia delivery. The downside of this approach is incomplete right heart protection when the tip of the retrograde cannula is distal to the middle cardiac vein. Direct retrograde insertion can circumvent this issue. The other downside is that if you get a perforation of the sinus during insertion you are in a difficult situation as the posterior part of the heart is likely to be stuck from the prior operation. On the other hand, any dissection that you do to facilitate retrograde insertion risks damage to the grafts. Do what you are most comfortable with but demonstrate thoughtfulness in either direction.

Index scenario (additional information)

"After cross clamping and delivering 500 mL of antegrade cardioplegia, you note poor distension of the aortic root, incomplete arrest, and left ventricular distension on transesophageal echocardiogram (TEE). How would you proceed?"

Switch to retrograde and turn on the aortic root vent. An aortotomy would also allow decompression. Another option is placing an LV vent in order to decompress the left heart as cardioplegia crosses the incompetent aortic valve and fills the LV. However, it may be difficult to get the vent in during a redo.

"You place an LV vent. The LV is decompressed but electrical activity persists. As planned, you give retrograde cardioplegia, but you note persistent activity and your perfusionist notes inadequate line pressure. You are unable to reliably palpate the retrograde catheter in the coronary sinus. Transesophageal echocardiography suggests the catheter is not in the coronary sinus. How would you proceed?"

Remember that this is a redo situation. Open the aorta (if you haven't already) and deliver additional antegrade cardioplegia directly down the vein grafts to get the best arrest that you can and cool to moderate hypothermia. Get around the cavas if you can and insert the retrograde catheter directly to get perfusion of the LAD distribution. The other alternative to getting excellent cardioplegia down the LAD territory is to cool to 20° and leave the L-LAD open.

"How do you ensure adequacy of retrograde cardioplegia delivery?"

Look for cessation of electrical and myocardial activity by checking the EKG and looking at the heart. Additionally, confirm with the perfusion team that you have adequate line pressure and flow. Most retrograde cannula tips have pressure monitor probes that report the pressure in the coronary sinus. A conservative upper limit of appropriate pressure is approximately 40 mmHg. This reflects a flow of 50-100 cc/min. Observe flow through the coronary veins and arteries during retrograde cardioplegia. Check the RCA and LCA ostia after the aorta is opened and retrograde is running to ensure adequate distribution of the retrograde to the right and left circulations. The myocardial temperature can also be a guide to the adequacy of cardioplegia delivery. You should note decreasing myocardial temperature assessed either manually or with a direct temperature probe.

Operative steps

Antegrade cannula placement

- Identify a favorable area on anterior curvature of ascending aorta with adequate room for aortic cross clamp cephalad and proximal anastomosis or aortotomy—if needed—caudad.
- Can check for plaque by palpation or evaluate with epiaortic ultrasound.
- Antegrade needle and cannula should be snared securely.
- After securing the line in place it must be flushed to deair. After cross clamping, run your induction dose and inspect the root for evidence of dissection and inspect the LV for distention. A fast arrest is a good sign.

Retrograde cannula placement

- A purse-string suture is placed in the inferolateral aspect of right atrium.
- Retrograde cannula is placed with a gentle L shaped curve and directed toward the orifice of the coronary sinus with guidance from the operator's opposite hand.
- The final placement is confirmed by palpation and/or transesophageal echocardiographic imaging, and further substantiated by distal pressure readings during infusion.
- Some cannulae have self-inflating balloons; others must be inflated manually. These balloons are rarely completely occlusive. This lack of complete occlusion is helpful in avoiding edema during CABG procedures when giving simultaneous cardioplegia down the retrograde catheter and a saphenous vein graft.
- If indirect retrograde placement is problematic, then direct retrograde placement can be used. This requires bicaval cannulation, caval snares for atrial isolation, small atriotomy, handheld retractor, identification of the coronary sinus ostium, purse string and direct placement of the coronary catheter. This is usually done with the clamp in place on the aorta.

211

- The standard catheters may be used for direct retrograde although an 8 mm flexible polystan catheter may be less traumatic. The purse string is secured which leads to occlusion of the coronary sinus. Thus, giving direct retrograde and cardioplegia down a vein graft simultaneously may theoretically lead to myocardial edema.
- Direct retrograde is a good way to ensure delivery down the right and left since the catheter is not advanced beyond the middle cardiac vein.

Potential questions/alternative scenarios

"How does the presence of a left sided Superior Vena Cava (LSVC) change your approach to cardioprotection?"

The presence of a left sided SVC poses an issue of volume returning to the right side of the heart (directly or via the coronary sinus) that is not drained by a venous cannula. This volume of blood then enters the pulmonary circulation and returns to the left atrium and ventricle and may cause distension. In addition, this blood is warmer than the cardioplegia solution and may negate cooling effects on the myocardium. The other issue is that in cases in which the LSVC drains into the coronary sinus, it is difficult to administer retrograde cardioplegia. In these cases, the LSVC can be occluded or cannulated directly and added to the venous drainage circuit. The latter technique is advisable if the LSVC is very large and is mandatory if there is an interrupted innominate vein.

"Upon infusing antegrade cardioplegia, the perfusionist notes high line pressure. What are your next steps in management?"

This raises concern for a dissection. Stop your antegrade flow. Check for kinks or clamps obstructing flow along the line, ensuring that the cardioplegia is flowing down the appropriate path to the aortic root. Also check to make sure that the pressure monitoring line is connected correctly. With regard to a potential dissection, visualize the aortic root and look for distension or discoloration/bruising around the cannula. Ask the anesthesiologists to visualize the ascending and descending aorta with transesophageal echocardiography. If dissection is confirmed start cooling with your original aortic cannula which is distal to the clamp (assuming the dissection is contained within the root. Prepare for a dissection repair (see chapter on Iatrogenic Aortic Dissection).

"After unclamping the aorta during a case with retrograde cardioplegia, you notice the myocardium is slow to regain electrical activity. Prior to placing pacing wires, what should you check?"

Check that the retrograde catheter is removed and/or that the balloon is down (if not automatically deflated after infusion) in order to allow for adequate coronary sinus flow.

"While sewing the distal anastomosis on a coronary artery bypass graft, you notice increase bleeding from the coronary arteriotomy, how do you proceed?"

The concern is that the arrested myocardium is getting perfused. First check that the aortic cross clamp is occlusive, and the aortic root vent is on. A possible explanation for mild bleeding at the arteriotomy site is the presence of collateral circulation. If unable to identify a correctable cause, monitor for signs of electrical activity and consider cold topical saline, cooling the patient (mild hypothermia - 32° C), reducing flows as tolerated or more frequent administration of cardioplegia solution.

"Discuss the principles of cardioplegic arrest, how this is achieved by components of the cardioplegia solution and name some common types of cardioplegia."

Minimizing myocardial oxygen demand is the primary principle of cardioplegic arrest. This is best achieved by rapid diastolic arrest after the aortic cross clamp is applied, thereby minimizing time of high ventricular work against a fixed afterload. Potassium is the most common electrolyte employed to produce diastolic arrest, and there are several common additional components, including sodium, citrate, and magnesium. Magnesium has been associated with decreased ventricular arrhythmias and improved cardiac performance in some studies. Histidine, Tryptophan, and Ketoglutarate (HTK) also comprises commonly used cardioplegia formulas. The cardioplegia solutions are cooled to 4° C which decreases myocardial oxygen consumption and diminishes contractile activity. Dextrose is used for glucose uptake and control of myocardial edema. Lastly, there are several iterations of blood and crystalloid ratios, but no evidence to support superiority, and preferences tend to be surgeon and/or institution specific.

"After placing the retrograde catheter, you encounter some dark blood emerging from behind the heart. You check and notice a perforation of the coronary sinus."
The rigid catheter can perforate the sinus especially in older and frail patients. If this happens, initiate cardiopulmonary bypass, cross clamp and arrest with antegrade. Repair the perforation directly with prolene suture or with a pericardial patch (see chapter on Venous Injuries).

Pearls/pitfalls
In general, there are a few things to consider when thinking about persistent activity which can be broadly grouped under "Access," "Collateral flow," and "Myocardial mass."

Access
- Are your retrograde and antegrade cannulas in place and properly connected?
- Is the retrograde too far and not protecting the RV despite antegrade?

Collateral flow
- Is the cross clamp completely occlusive?
- Is the right sided drainage adequate or do you need an additional cannula?
- Is there a persistent left sided SVC filling the right atrium?
- Is the left sided drainage adequate (is the root vent on or additional basket suckers in place; is there so much collateral flow that you need an LV vent)?
- Once drainage is optimized do you need systemic moderate hypothermia to 28-32° C to keep the residual collateral flow cool?

Myocardial mass
- Is the heart so hypertrophied that myocardial delivery of cardioplegia is inadequate - if so address all of the above and try topical hypothermia?

Suggested readings
- Chambers DJ and Fallouh HB. Cardioplegia and cardiac surgery: Pharmacological arrest and cardioprotection during global ischemia and reperfusion. *Pharmacology and Therapeutics*. 2010. Issue 127 (41-52).
- Levitsky S and McCully J. Myocardial protection. Sellke FW et al (ed). *Surgery of the Chest*. Saunders. 8th Edition.
- Mentzer RM, Salik Jahinia M, Lasley RD. Myocardial Protection. Cohn L (ed). *Cardiac Surgery in the Adult*. McGraw Hill. 2008.
- Sa et al. Is there any difference between blood and crystalloid cardioplegia for myocardial protection during cardiac surgery? A meta-analysis of 5576 patients from 36 randomized trials. *Perfusion*. 2012. July.

33. Vascular Injuries

Alykhan S. Nagji, MD, and John A. Kern, MD

Concept
- Recognition and control of venous injuries
- Strategies for repair of venous injuries

Chief complaint

"An 82-year-old man with previous mitral valve repair presents after extensive cardiology work-up which revealed severe mitral regurgitation (MR) with plans for mitral valve replacement. He has no significant medical comorbidities and his only surgical history is a previous mitral valve repair. He is symptomatic from his MR and a holosystolic murmur is heard radiating to the axilla. His TTE demonstrates an ejection fraction (EF) of 30%. What are his options and how would you proceed?"

Differential

Both the diagnosis and surgical need have been established. (refer to Mitral Valve chapter for details of work up, management and operative steps).

Tests
- Venous injuries related to mitral repair include AV groove disruption, injury to venous structures during sternal reentry, and coronary sinus tear with retrograde insertion. Some of these issues can be predicted ahead of time by reviewing the CT and cardiac catheterization.
- *CT scan*: determine the anatomy below the posterior table of the sternum (i.e., location and proximity of the innominate vein, vein grafts, atria, ventricle aorta, etc.).
- *Cardiac catheterization/plain films*: evaluate the mitral valve for MAC or crossing grafts.

Potential questions/alternative scenarios

"While performing your sternotomy, you encounter a significant amount of dark blood from the sternomanubrial junction."
- Remember this is a redo sternotomy and that by being higher up near the manubrium, this would be indicative of an innominate vein injury. Though you may be able to successfully control the innominate vein injury with direct pressure or sponge stick, the safest approach would be packing of the area along with having the sternum re-approximated so as to tamponade the bleeding.
- Cannulate peripherally (i.e., groin) and initiate cardiopulmonary bypass (CPB). This should decompress the heart and reduce the amount of bleeding from the injured innominate vein. Use of the pump suckers will help to capture any remaining blood. Once on CPB, reopen the chest and identify the injury. Carefully dissect out the innominate vein to achieve an adequate length without tension. This is key. Trying to repair it under tension will not work. Perform a repair with a Bovine or autologous pericardial patch using 5-0 or 6-0 Prolene suture (conservative approach). If the defect is small, a primary repair may be performed transversally without narrowing the vein. In a situation where the innominate vein is irreparable, it is safe to divide and oversew both ends of the vein. If the injury is far laterally this can be a big problem. Ligate the innominate vein down the middle to relieve tension. Try to repair the tear. If you cannot and the exposure is poor, consider a trapdoor incision (superior clavicular incision, anterior thoracotomy into the 3rd intercostal space across the sternum to meet with the median sternotomy, elevate the hemithorax to expose and repair the injury (ligate or primary).

"Let us say that you enter the chest without incidence. The previous repair used cannulation through the right atrial appendage. However, during this reoperation you decide to cannulate the superior vena cava (SVC) directly. While dissecting the SVC you create a large hole. You do not have any purse string sutures in yet."

- Initial management should be to tamponade the SVC injury. Proceed with inferior vena cava (IVC) and aortic cannulation and initiate CPB with vacuum assisted venous drainage so as not to get an air lock. This, along with the use of pump suckers through the SVC injury will help to clear the field. If the injury is visible, it may be possible to cannulate through the injury and fix the injury at the end of the case.

- If still unable to view the SVC injury, the injury may be more severe and would necessitate more proximal control on the SVC using a Rummel tourniquet. You should also consider placing a pump sucker in the azygos vein to help drain upstream of the injury. An alternative is to ligate the azygos vein.

- Once able to view and evaluate the extent of the SVC injury, repair either primarily (as described previously) or with a Bovine or autologous pericardial patch. Then replace your SVC cannula away from the injury or through the RA.

"You were able to successfully cannulate through your SVC injury and proceed with the remainder of your mitral valve repair. You decide to use standard retrograde cardioplegia, but have difficulty placing your coronary sinus catheter. When administering your first dose of cardioplegia, you notice bright red blood pooling in the pericardial well. You lift the heart and see the end of your coronary sinus cannula."

At this time, you should pull the coronary sinus catheter out and protect the heart using antegrade cardioplegia during the course of your mitral valve replacement. You may need to place a few horizontal sutures prior to proceeding with the case to control the bleeding. But once the procedure is completed, if the injured area is still bleeding or friable place a Bovine or autologus pericardial patch using 5-0 or 6-0 Prolene in a running fashion.

"Changing the scenario completely, you now have a 64-year-old female who is currently undergoing lead extraction. You are called emergently to the cath lab as the patient has just arrested and become hypotensive."

- Given that this was done under fluoroscopy, you should glean as much information from the cardiologist to help localize the injury in question. With these leads usually being heavily incorporated in the intima of the vessel wall there is a high likelihood of venous injury (in this case the SVC).

- Being that the chest is not open, you should cannulate via the groin and initiate CPB with vacuum assisted venous drainage. Once on CPB, open the chest and pericardium in the usual fashion. With the heart decompressed, identify the SVC and dissect enough length to obtain proximal and distal control from the site of injury. When identified, repair either primarily or patch as previously described.

- An alternative might be to open the chest right off the bat which decompresses the tamponade, apply manual compression of the injured vein, cannulate the aorta and RA and go on bypass.

"Taking another route, you have a 60-year-old man who underwent a CABG and AVR just 4 months ago and has presented to the emergency room with chest pain and was found to have a Type A dissection. The patient crashes and a decision is made to percutaneously cannulate using the femoral artery and vein. You decide to use a 25 Fr Multi-stage venous cannula. During your venous cannulation the wires and dilators pass easily. However, you have difficulty passing your venous cannula, but it passes, and you do have blood return. You complete your femoral cannulation and initiate CPB. When doing so, the patient continues to become hypotensive and you find there is decreased venous perfusion and low volume."

Goals are identifying the location of the injury, cannulating beyond it, and repair. Venogram if available for location otherwise rely on the history. At this time, you should be concerned about iliac vein injury. There are no clearly defined strategies to deal with such an injury. If the chest were open (not in this case) then you could centrally cannulate and repair the injury with aid of sucker bypass. Otherwise, gain access in the contralateral femoral vein and use this as your venous cannulation. Make sure to confirm placement and use a stiff wire. You should be beyond the injured iliac. Initiate CPB and decompress the heart. Repair the injured vein. If you have fluoroscopy you could try to get a wire across the injured vein and then a canula.

Bear in mind that the injury may be higher than the common iliac arteries (e.g., infrahepatic IVC). In this case you can try to cross the injury with a wire from the contralateral limb under fluoroscopy and stent the injury with your cannula. You would later need to explore the IVC through the abdomen for definitive repair. If you cannot cross the injury with a wire, then cannulate centrally to maintain distal perfusion while decompressing the venous system and plan for an abdominal exploration with local control and repair of the IVC injury. Sucker bypass can be used as an adjunctive maneuver. If you cannot or do not have time to cannulate centrally or peripherally then explore and repair the injury directly. This is obviously a very bad situation in the setting of an aortic dissection.

"You are called to the cardiac cath lab for an SVC rupture during balloon dilation for SVC syndrome."
Ensure an airway, IV access, and blood transfusion. Heparinize and perform an emergency median sternotomy. Aortic and bicaval cannulation with the SVC cannula placed through the RA and carefully traversing the injury. Initiate CPB and empty out the heart. Inspect the defect. Large defects require patch closure while smaller ones are amenable to primary repair as long as the SVC is not narrowed. In this patient with SVC syndrome a patch with autologus pericardium is ideal. Other strategies for dealing with a high or large SVC injury include clamping the SVC and establishing distal drainage for the head vessels (i.e., upper SVC or innominate vein). Autologous or porcine pericardium can be used to repair the injury. A large tube conduit with a dacron graft can also be considered. Also as noted above, you can certainly cannulate peripherally prior to opening the chest but it depends on the degree of hypotension. In this scenario the patient was essentially tamponading. Always inquire about any contraindications to femoral arterial cannulation prior to going down that route.

"An 81-year-old female patient is undergoing a mitral and tricuspid valve repair. Her tissues are noted to be very thin and frail. During bicaval cannulation the IVC purse string results in a large tear extending down below the diaphragm. How would you proceed?"
These injuries are not easy to control. The first step is to complete venous access and go on CPB as soon as you can. You can carefully pass the IVC cannula distal to the tear if you can see the distal extent. An occluding tape circumferential to the IVC and inferior to the injury may provide adequate exposure if there is room. Initiate CPB. Use fine prolene sutures or even a patch to repair the injury if you can see the distal extent from the mediastinum. Otherwise, go on with the SVC cannula and sucker bypass in the inferior pericardium. Have an assist manually control the bleeding in the IVC while you cannulate the femoral vein. You can try to traverse the injury with the femoral guide wire and then stent across with the cannula. If not at least establish drainage inferior to the tear. You can incise the diaphragm a bit from the mediastinum to expose the distal IVC but ultimately you may need to extend your midline incision into the abdomen and down along the right subcostal margin to expose and mobilize the liver infero-medially. This will allow exposure and repair of the retrohepatic IVC. Once the repair is done, readjust your drainage lines to ensure adequate exposure for your mitral and tricuspid repair.

"You are called to the cath lab because a patient who you were scheduled to perform a CABG on has had his RV punctured during an RV ablation. The pericardial drain placed in the cath lab is showing significant bloody drainage."

216

Transfer to the OR, emergent median sternotomy, place on CPB, arrest the heart and identify the puncture. Even if small, wide patch repair over the defect (autologous pericardium or other commercially available product). Bypass the original coronary lesions (usually with vein in emergency situations).

"You come off pump and are drying up after an ascending aneurysm replacement. You notice some continuous drainage from the left of the aorta. You retract the graft towards you and identify a 3 mm hole on the right pulmonary artery. What would you do?"

An injury to the PA can be lethal especially with a non-decompressed PA which has a paper-thin wall. Have a pump in the room. Identify where you will cannulate if needed. Since this injury is small you can attempt a small figure-of-8 or purse string suture (fine) to oversew.

"When taking the bite through the PA it tears and there is significant bleeding. You had previously cannulated with right femoral vein and right axillary."

Have an assistant hold gentle pressure over the tear. Give heparin and cannulate for CPB. In this case, sew an end - end graft to the prior axillary graft. Cannulate the atrium or femoral vein and go on CPB. The PA will decompress. Dissect the PA off the underside of the aorta and ensure it is well mobilized without tension. Close the hole primarily with adventitial reinforcement or sew a pericardial patch. You can tack the PA to the underside of the aorta for extra hemostasis.

"You are cannulated and ready to go on CPB for an AVR. After cross clamping and beginning antegrade cardioplegia you notice some bleeding under the arch of the aorta but are unable to localize a source. You check all your cannulation sites which are fine and there is still bleeding. You dissect further along the posterior backside of the arch and notice bleeding opposite to the aortic cannula."

To address what appears to be a perforation of the backside of the aorta from the cannula you will almost certainly need circulatory arrest. If the bleeding is under control and the forward flow is good, then cool with the existing cannula. Otherwise you might consider weaning off CPB and establishing axillary artery access. A small aortotomy and local repair should suffice to address the injury.

"After 20-minutes of cooling the temperature is 20° C. You stop the circulation, release the cross clamp and perform a transverse aortotomy near the injury which reveals a pinpoint tear opposite the aortic cannula. TEE showed no dissection and there is no grossly evident flap. You and are able to locally repair the tear with a horizontal mattress prolene stitch. You close the aortotomy, clamp distal to it and resume bypass. Circ arrest time was 6 minutes and you complete an uneventful AVR."

Pearls/pitfalls

- Perform the appropriate maneuvers to decompress the venous system in the presence of an injury.
- Consider peripheral cannulation when central cannulation would further exacerbate the problem or cannot be safely achieved.
- Have a low threshold to use Bovine or autologous pericardial patch to repair venous injures not amenable to primary repair.

34. STABLE ISCHEMIC HEART DISEASE

Charles M. Wojnarski, MD, MS, and Peter K. Smith, MD

Adapted from 1st edition chapter, "Stable Angina" written by Mark Kearns, MD, and Richard C. Cook, MD

Key Concepts

- Preoperative evaluation
- Indications for coronary artery bypass graft (CABG) surgery vs. percutaneous coronary intervention (PCI)
- Operative conduct
- General topics and evidence-base
- Conduit selection
- Patient scenarios and intra-operative complications

Patient Scenario: Chief Complaint

"A 78 y.o. male with new onset exertional chest pain presents to your clinic. His primary care physician ordered an exercise stress test which was grossly positive. He was then referred for left heart catheterization (LHC) which revealed 3-vessel coronary artery disease. The patient was told he needs bypass surgery and is here to for pre-operative evaluation."

General Considerations:

Patients with stable ischemic heart disease often present with exertional angina. At rest, coronary perfusion may be adequate; however, in the face of increased oxygen demand during periods of increased cardiac output, a supply-demand mismatch occurs as coronary vasodilatory mechanisms cannot overcome fixed, flow-limiting stenoses. Chest pain at rest, exertional angina not relieved by rest and new onset chest pain represent unstable angina, which should not be evaluated in the outpatient setting.

Guideline-directed medical therapy (GDMT) including lifestyle modification, statin therapy to achieve a low-density lipoprotein (LDL) level of 70-100 mg/dL, beta-blockade, aspirin and ACE inhibition in patients with left ventricular dysfunction, diabetes mellitus or chronic kidney disease should be initiated in all patients with stable ischemic heart disease. If non-invasive tests suggest high-risk coronary lesion(s), coronary interrogation with formal angiography or gated CT should be performed. A "Heart Team" approach to revascularization is recommended in patients with diabetes mellitus or complex multivessel coronary artery disease.

History and Physical

Patient comorbidities can have an important impact on choice of intervention and surgical planning. A history of diabetes mellitus, severe peripheral arterial disease, and symptomatic cerebrovascular disease should always be elicited. Previous chest, upper abdomen or extremity surgery or radiation may impact availability of arterial or venous conduit. Every effort should be made to obtain specific anatomic details of previous percutaneous interventions (PCI) and ascertainment of antiplatelet medication use is essential for the perioperative management of antiplatelet therapy.

The physical exam should be focused on findings that may impact operative plan or perioperative risk-stratification. A baseline neurologic exam should be documented. Cardiopulmonary examination should be performed to identify signs of heart failure, valvular abnormalities or COPD. Modified Allen's test with pulse oximetry should be performed for screening if radial artery conduit is to be used despite its high false-positive rate. Equivocal results should be further investigated with arterial duplex ultrasounography. Evidence of previous lower extremity vascular surgery or venous insufficiency should be further investigated with vein mapping study to determine saphenous vein suitability.

Laboratory investigations: Pre-surgical evaluation should include hematologic, biochemical and coagulation laboratory studies. Hemoglobin A1c (HbA1c) level should be obtained prior to surgery in patients with diabetes.

EKG: It is critical to establish a baseline electrocardiogram which can be referenced in the post-operative period. Rate, rhythm, axis-deviation or suggestion of LV hypertrophy should be noted.

CXR: Pre-operative radiographic chest examination should be assessed with attention to cardiac silhouette, presence of any pulmonary parenchymal disease and note should be made of any ascending aortic/aortic arch calcification. Occasionally a widened mediastinum may suggest an ascending aortic aneurysm. Note should be made of any pre-existing pleural effusions.

LHC: Coronary artery bypass grafting surgery cannot be done without proper angiographic assessment of the coronary anatomy, degree and location of stenoses, and general suitability for bypass grafting - all depicted by selective coronary angiography. Aortography, if performed, defines ascending aortic and root size, can be used to screen for aortic calcification, and may suggest the presence of aortic regurgitation. Careful observation of the aorta, root and valve plane during cinefluoroscopy may reveal calcification and affect decision making. Left ventriculography can inform one of LV function, LV chamber dilation and may be able to show aortic stenosis or mitral regurgitation. Anatomically, left main (LM) lesions $\geq$ 50% or non-LM coronary artery lesions $\geq$ 70% are hemodynamically significant.

Fractional flow reserve (FFR $\leq$ 0.80) is a physiologic determinant of hemodynamic significance of the cumulative effect of proximal coronary stenoses. FFR can be a useful adjunct to guide revascularization in angiographically intermediate coronary stenoses in patients with stable angina (Class 1) based on evidence from three large RCTs: DEFER, FAME, and FAME 2. It should be noted that the use of FFR to guide bypass grafting decision making is inferred from these PCI trials, and has never been studied directly. iFR (instantaneous wave-free ratio) is an emerging physiologic measurement which can also be used to determine hemodynamic significance of a lesion (iFR $\leq$ 0.89).

The SYNTAX score is the sum of the points assigned to each individual lesion identified in the coronary tree (divided into 16 segments) with >50% diameter narrowing in vessels >1.5mm diameter. A score $\geq$ 23 is considered is considered intermediate complexity and $\geq$ 33 represents high complexity disease. The Synergy between PCI with Taxus and Cardiac Surgery (SYNTAX) trial, assessed the optimal revascularization strategy for patients with previously untreated three-vessel or left main coronary artery disease. The trial showed the benefit of CABG over PCI regarding major adverse cardiac and cerebrovascular event at 5-years in patients with multivessel and left main coronary artery disease (26.9% vs. 37.3%, p<0.0001). At 10-year follow-up, the three-vessel disease subset had the patients whom underwent CABG had lower all-cause mortality (21.9% vs. 29.2%, p=0.007), especially among patients with a high SYNTAX score.

Gated cardiac computed tomography has emerged as a non-invasive option for imaging the coronary arteries. In certain patients, this can replace the need for LHC.

Echocardiogram: All patients undergoing CABG should have a pre-operative ECHO to determine LV and RV function and identify any valvular abnormalities that might be concomitantly addressed. Regional wall motion abnormalities may help determine the physiologic significance of borderline lesions.

Myocardial viability studies: Can be considered in patients with left ventricular ejection fraction (LVEF) $\leq$ 35% or those with ventricular dysfunction out of proportion to severity of coronary artery disease. However, a recent secondary analysis of the STITCH trial including 601 patients that had pre-operative viability studies showed that myocardial viability was not related to long-term benefit from CABG in patients with low LVEF. Viability was associated with improvement in EF post-operatively, but this did not translate into a survival benefit (test for interaction, p=.34). Therefore, the absence of myocardial viability does not obviate the survival benefit from CABG over medical therapy in patients with low LVEF.

Additional investigations: Generally, other studies are indicated by any major comorbidities of the patient and aid in risk-stratification. Any abnormality of the pre-operative CXR which may impact surgical plan should be followed up with a cross-sectional CT of the chest. This will help assess degree of aortic calcification as porcelain aorta will impact one's ability to place an aortic cross-clamp and may suggest an aortic no-touch, off-pump technique.

Carotid artery duplex scanning is reasonable in selected patients who are considered to have high-risk features (i.e., age >65 years, left main coronary stenosis, peripheral artery disease, history of cerebrovascular disease [transient ischemic attack, stroke, etc.], hypertension, smoking, and diabetes mellitus). Pulmonary function tests (PFTs) can be considered for patients with a history of pulmonary disease but are unlikely to impact operative management or candidacy. Most additional studies provide information for risk stratification and predicting major morbidity and mortality. The STS risk calculator should be used to counsel patients on individualized risks of operation. Predicted outcomes provided by the calculator include mortality, renal failure, permanent stroke, prolonged ventilation, sternal wound infection, reoperation, morbidity or mortality, short, long length of stay.

Patient Scenario - Additional Information

"On further questioning, the patient has diabetes mellitus type II (HbA1c 8.5%, on insulin), hypertension, hyperlipidemia, and is a former smoker. He has a 6-month history of exertional dyspnea and angina. You review his LHC which shows a chronic total occlusion (CTO) of his right coronary artery (RCA), a focal 80% proximal left anterior descending (LAD) artery stenosis and a 75% stenosis of a large first obtuse marginal artery (OM1). Echocardiogram reveals an LVEF of 45%, antero-lateral wall hypokinesis, but no valvular abnormalities. His SYNTAX score is 26 and STS predicted risk of mortality is 1.5%.

Indications for coronary artery bypass graft surgery:

The 2011 ACC/AHC Guideline on Coronary Artery Bypass Graft Surgery and 2012 ACCF/AHA/ACP/AATS/PCNA/SCAI/STS Guideline for the Diagnosis and Management of Patients with Stable Ischemic Heart Disease with 2014 Focused Update are the two main documents which outline the indications for CABG as they relate to PCI:

Indications for CABG that are associated with a survival benefit over medical therapy with or without PCI:

- Left main coronary artery disease (≥50% stenosis) and high complexity for PCI (SYNTAX score ≥33). (Class I)
- Three-vessel coronary artery disease (≥70% stenosis) and intermediate or high complexity for PCI (SYNTAX score ≥23). (Class I)
- Two-vessel coronary artery disease (≥70% stenosis) involving the LAD artery and intermediate or high complexity for PCI (SYNTAX score ≥23). (Class I)
- Patients with diabetes mellitus and multivessel CAD for which revascularization is likely to improve survival (3-vessel CAD or complex 2-vessel CAD involving the proximal LAD), particularly if a LIMA graft can be anastomosed to the LAD artery, provided the patient is a good candidate for surgery. (Class I)

Indications for CABG when PCI is noninferior to CABG and when PCI or CABG is preferred over medical therapy

- Left main coronary artery disease (≥50% stenosis) and low-to-intermediate complexity for PCI (SYNTAX score ≤32). (Class IIa)
- Three-vessel coronary artery disease (≥70% stenosis) and low complexity for PCI (SYNTAX score ≤22). (Class IIa)

- Two-vessel coronary artery disease (≥70% stenosis) involving the LAD artery and low complexity for PCI (SYNTAX score ≤22). (Class IIa)

Other indications for CABG:
- Clinically significant coronary artery disease (≥70% stenosis) in ≥1 vessel and refractory angina despite medical therapy and PCI. (Class I)
- Clinically significant coronary artery disease (≥70% stenosis) in ≥1 vessel in survivors of sudden cardiac arrest presumed to be related to ischemic ventricular arrhythmia. (Class I)
- Clinically significant coronary artery disease (≥50% stenosis) in ≥1 vessel in patients undergoing cardiac surgery for other indications. (e.g., valve replacement or aortic surgery) (Class I)

The 2016 Society of Thoracic Surgeons (STS) Clinical Practice Guidelines on Arterial Conduits for Coronary Artery Bypass Grafting provides additional procedural guidance:
- Internal mammary arteries (IMA) should be used to bypass the left anterior descending (LAD) artery when bypass of the LAD is indicated. (Class I)
- As an adjunct to left internal mammary artery (LIMA), a second arterial graft (RIMA or radial artery [RA]) should be considered in appropriate patients. (Class IIa)
- Use of bilateral IMAs (BIMA) should be considered in patients who do not have an excessive risk of sternal complications. (Class IIa)
- To reduce the risk of sternal infection with BIMA, skeletonized grafts should be considered. (Class IIa)
- As an adjunct to LIMA to LAD (or in patients with inadequate LIMA grafts), use of a RA graft is reasonable when grafting coronary targets with severe stenoses. (Class IIa)
- The right gastroepiploic artery may be considered in patients with poor conduit options or as an adjunct to more complete arterial revascularization. (Class IIb).
- Use of arterial grafts (specific targets, number, and type) should be a part of the discussion of the heart team in determining the optimal approach for each patient. (Class I)

It is worth mentioning that there is much controversy about the clinical trials that have led to the conclusions that PCI may be preferable or equivalent to CABG in patients with LM disease and low SYNTAX.

Patient Scenario – Treatment Plan

The patient in this scenario has a class I indication for coronary artery bypass graft surgery given his symptomatic, complex coronary artery disease. The presence of three-vessel coronary artery disease in this patient with diabetes and depressed LVEF further strengthens the case for CABG over multivessel PCI for survival benefit. A multidisciplinary heart team met to discuss the patient and determined that at age 78, choice of conduits would include a LIMA to the LAD and saphenous vein grafts to the remaining targets.

Operative Conduct: (Sample Operative Note)

Procedures:
1. Median sternotomy
2. Coronary artery bypass grafting x3: LIMA-LAD, SVG-OM1, SVG-PDA
3. Endoscopic saphenous vein harvest, right leg
4. Transesophageal echocardiography

Drains and Wires: 2 mediastinal 28fr chest tubes, 1 left pleural 28fr chest tube; atrial and ventricular epicardial pacing wires
Cross-clamp time: 62 min
CBP time: 84 min

Procedure in detail: The risks, benefits, complications, treatment options, and expected outcomes were discussed with the patient. Informed consent was obtained, and time out was performed. **Hemodynamic monitoring** lines and Foley catheter were placed. Following oral

221

endotracheal tube placement, general anesthesia was induced. The patient's skin was prepped with chlorhexidine-alcohol based solution from chin to toes. The chest, abdomen, groins and legs were draped in standard fashion. Transesophageal echocardiography demonstrated normal LV-RV function and no aortic valve insufficiency or other valvular abnormalities. **Median sternotomy** was performed. The left pleural space was opened. The left internal mammary artery was taken down as a pedicled graft using a combination of clips and cautery. Intravenous heparin was given at the appropriate dose to obtain anticoagulation sufficient for cardiopulmonary bypass (ACT ≥480). The LIMA was then transected distally, and flow was demonstrated to be excellent. The mammary bed was hemostatic. A left pleural chest tube was placed. The **pericardium** was then opened, and the pericardial cradle created. Concentric purse strings were placed, and the aorta was cannulated with an 18 Fr straight cannula. After adequate de-airing, this cannula was connected to the CPB circuit. A purse string was placed around the right atrial appendage and it was cannulated with a dual-stage venous cannula. **Cardiopulmonary bypass** was then initiated, and ventilation held. Perfusion temperature was allowed to drift to 32°C. A window was created in the left pericardium with care to preserve the phrenic nerve and the LIMA was fashioned to the appropriate length.

The **distal targets** on the posterior descending artery (PDA), first obtuse marginal artery (OM1) and left anterior descending artery (LAD) were then evaluated and marked. The IVC was encircled and a heart basket was then placed into the appropriate position. An antegrade vent/cardioplegia cannula was then placed in the ascending aorta. The aortic cross clamp was then applied, and the heart was arrested with 1200 cc of antegrade Del Nido cardioplegia. Topical iced-saline slush was employed as an adjunct for myocardial preservation. The **distal anastomosis to the PDA** was completed first. After exposing the PDA, the artery was opened and SVG was anastomosed to the coronary using 7-0 polypropylene suture in a standard running fashion. The anastomosis was checked for hemostasis which was excellent. The graft was sized and divided at appropriate length. The **distal anastomosis to the OM1** was completed next. After exposing the OM1, the artery was opened and SVG was anastomosed to the coronary using in the standard running fashion. The anastomosis was checked for hemostasis which was excellent. The graft was sized and divided at appropriate length. Next the anterior surface of the heart was exposed. **LIMA to LAD** anastomosis was completed in the standard running fashion. The anastomosis was checked for hemostasis which was excellent.

Antegrade cardioplegia vent was removed and two punches were made in aorta anteriorly. Proximal SVG anastomoses were performed with 6-0 polypropylene suture in running fashion. The aorta was de-aired and the cross clamp removed. **Examination** of all surgical sites revealed adequate hemostasis. Atrial and ventricular epicardial pacing wires were then placed. The patient was ventilated and successfully weaned off CPB. After a test dose of protamine, the patient was decannulated. Heparin was then reversed with protamine. Again, all surgical sites were evaluated for hemostasis which was excellent. **Post-bypass TEE** revealed preserved RV/LV function and no new wall motion abnormalities. Two mediastinal drains were placed. The sternum was closed using stainless steel wires and the incision closed in a standard fashion. A dry, sterile dressing was placed. At the end of the operation, all sponge, instruments, and needle **counts** were correct. The patient tolerated the procedure without complication and was transported to the intensive care unit in stable condition in normal sinus rhythm with epicardial pacer set to VVI backup rate of 50.

General Topics and Evidence-Base:
On-pump CABG (ONCAB) vs. Off-pump CABG (OPCAB)
In the United States, approximately 85-90% of coronary artery bypass graft surgeries are performed with the use of cardiopulmonary bypass. In the year 2016, the STS National Adult Cardiac Database showed 13% utilization of off-pump CABG. Off-pump and on-pump CABG have similar short-term outcomes. In the long term, OPCAB may have inferior outcomes compared to ONCAB, likely due to higher rates of incomplete revascularization. A

2018 systematic review of 30-years of literature comparing OPCAB and ONCAB by Gaudino, et al. summarizes the evidence best:

- "In the largest randomized comparisons (CORONARY [CABG Off or On Pump Revascularization] and ROOBY [Randomized On/Off Bypass] trials), there were no differences in the primary study end point at 30 days. In CORONARY, the primary composite outcome of death, nonfatal stroke, or nonfatal myocardial infarction (MI) was similar between OPCAB and ONCAB (9.8% versus 10.3%, $p=0.59$). In ROOBY, the primary composite outcome of 30-day death or major complications was similar between the 2 arms (7.0% versus 5.6%, $p=0.19$)."

- "At 5 years, there was no difference in the primary outcome in the CORONARY trial. In the ROOBY trial, however, 5-year survival was significantly worse in the off-pump group (15.2% versus 11.9%; $p=0.02$). Event-free survival was also significantly decreased in the off-pump group (31.0% versus 27.1%; $p=0.05$), along with MI and the need for repeat revascularization."

- "The available evidence suggests that OPCAB can be associated with better outcomes in high-risk patents. Elderly patients, patients with low EF, those with high neurological risk, women, and patients with end-organ failure may benefit from off-pump surgery, although the extent of this benefit remains unclear at present."

Bilateral Internal Mammary Artery (BIMA) vs. Single Internal Mammary Artery Revascularization:
The largest randomized-controlled trial comparing bilateral to single IMA revascularization is the ART trial (Arterial Revascularization Trial). 3,102 patients were randomly assigned to undergo either bilateral IMA or single IMA. In the intention-to-treat analysis at 10 years, was no difference between groups regarding all-cause mortality (hazard ratio [HR], 0.96; 95% confidence interval [CI], 0.82 to 1.12; $p=0.62$). Regarding the composite outcome of death, myocardial infarction, or stroke, there were 385 patients (24.9%) with an event in the bilateral-graft group and 425 patients (27.3%) with an event in the single-graft group (HR, 0.90; 95% CI, 0.79 to 1.03). A major criticism of the trial was high crossover: in the bilateral-graft group, 13.9% of the patients received only a single internal mammary artery graft, and in the single-graft group, 21.8% of the patients also received a radial artery graft.
The main disadvantage of BIMA grafting is a 2-3-fold increased risk of sternal wound complications. Known risks of sternal infection and malunion include nonelective procedure, age, uncontrolled DM (HbA1c >7%), obesity (BMI >40 kg/m^2), pre-operative hospital stays of >3 days, female sex, COPD, active smoking, immunosuppression regimen, and radiation mediastinal injury.

CABG in patients with diabetes mellitus:

The FREEDOM trial was a prospective, multicenter, randomized clinical trial that compared CABG to PCI with drug eluting stents in 1900 patients at 140 centers with diabetes and multivessel CAD. The primary outcome analyzed was a composite of death from any cause, nonfatal myocardial infarction, or nonfatal stroke. CABG had a lower 5-year rate of primary outcome (18.7%, n=147) as compared to PCI (26.6%, n=352; $p=.005$). The benefit of CABG over PCI persisted across all categories of SYNTAX score.

CABG in patients with low ejection fraction:
The Surgical Treatment for Ischemic Heart Failure (STICH) trial compared CABG with medical therapy in a group of patients with multivessel coronary artery disease and LVEF ≤ 35%. In the initial STITCH trial, CABG did not significantly reduce all-cause mortality (the primary outcome) as compared with medical therapy at 56 months (36% vs. 41%, $p=0.12$). However, recently published long-term follow-up of the STICH population (STITCHES) showed that after almost 10 years of follow-up, patients assigned to CABG, as compared with patients assigned to medical therapy, had lower rates of death from any cause (58.9% vs. 66.1%, $p=0.02$), of death from cardiovascular causes (40.5% vs. 49.3%, $p=0.006$), and of

death from any cause or hospitalization for cardiovascular causes (76.6% vs. 87.0%, $p<0.001$).

Intra-operative transit-time flow measurement (TTFM) of coronary bypass grafts:
A recent systematic review and meta-analysis of 35 relatively small prospective and retrospective studies showed that TTFM has a low sensitivity (0.25-0.46), but had excellent specificity for identifying abnormal graft flow (0.94-0.98).[17] Although not standardized, generally accepted cutoff values indicating abnormal graft flow are mean graft flow (MGF) <15ml/min for arterial and <20ml/min for venous grafts, pulsatility index (PI) ≥ 5 for both arterial and venous grafts, and diastolic filling percent <50% for both arterial and venous grafts. These parameters, in addition to surgeon judgement and clinical scenario may indicate need for intra-operative graft revision. Most commonly, addressing twisting or kinking of the graft and revision of distal anastomosis leads to resolution of abnormal flow patterns.

Myocardial temperature monitoring:
No large-scale retrospective or prospective randomized data exists on this topic and its use varies by institution and surgeon. If used, the probe is placed directly to the right of the LAD into the septum. Adequate cold cardioplegia supply to the myocardium is suggested by a septal temperature of 10-15°C. However, this tool should be used as an adjunct to other indicators of adequacy of delivery of cardioplegia including aortic root pressure, time to arrest and direct visualization of coronary content color change. In cases where proximal disease is severe and adequacy of antegrade delivery is in question, retrograde cardioplegia delivery through the coronary sinus can be considered. Myocardial protection as a topic is beyond the scope of this review but is a critical aspect of any coronary artery bypass procedure.

Perioperative anti-platelet therapy:
Aspirin (100 to 325 mg daily) should be administered to CABG patients preoperatively (Class I; Level of Evidence [LOE]: B). If aspirin was not initiated preoperatively, it should be initiated within 6 hours postoperatively and then continued indefinitely to reduce the occurrence of saphenous vein graft closure and adverse cardiovascular events (Class I; LOE: A).

For **elective** CABG, clopidogrel (Plavix) and ticagrelor (Brilinta) should be discontinued for at least 5 days before surgery (Class I; LOE B) and prasugrel (Effient) for at least 7 days (Class I; LOE: C) to limit blood transfusions. For **urgent** CABG, clopidogrel and ticagrelor should be discontinued for at least 24 hours to reduce major bleeding complications. Short-acting intravenous glycoprotein IIb/IIIa inhibitors (eptifibatide [Integrilin)] or tirofiban [Aggrastat]) should be discontinued for at least 2 to 4 hours before surgery and abciximab (Reopro) for at least 12 hours beforehand to limit blood loss and transfusions (Class I; LOE: B).

Guideline-directed post-operative medical therapy:
- **Beta blockers:** Beta blockers should be reinstituted as soon as possible after CABG in all patients without contraindications to reduce the incidence or clinical sequelae of AF (Class I; LOE: B). Beta blockers should be prescribed to all CABG patients without contraindications at the time of hospital discharge (Class I).
- **Statins:** All patients undergoing CABG should receive statin therapy, unless contraindicated (Class I; LOE: A). In patients undergoing CABG, an adequate dose of statin should be used to reduce low-density lipoprotein cholesterol to less than 100 mg/dL and to achieve at least a 30% lowering of low-density lipoprotein cholesterol (Class I; LOE: C).
- **ACE and ARB:** ACE inhibitors or angiotensin-receptor blockers should be initiated postoperatively and continued indefinitely in CABG patients who were not receiving them preoperatively, who are stable, and who have an LVEF less than or equal to 40%, hypertension, diabetes mellitus, or chronic kidney disease, unless contraindicated (Class I; LOE: A). Angiotensin-converting enzyme (ACE)

inhibitors and angiotensin receptor blockers (ARB) given before CABG should be reinstituted postoperatively once the patient is stable, unless contraindicated (Class I; LOE: B).

- **Insulin:** The use of continuous intravenous insulin to achieve and maintain an early postoperative blood glucose concentration less than or equal to 180 mg/dL while avoiding hypoglycemia is indicated to reduce the incidence of adverse events, including deep sternal wound infection, after CABG (Class I; LOE: B).

Conduit Selection:
Venous conduits
Reversed greater saphenous vein (GSV) is the most commonly used conduit in coronary artery bypass graft surgery with more 90% utilization in CABG surgery. It has a reported 10-year angiographic patency rate of 50-60%. GSV has a 1-year graft failure rate of 15-20%. The recently published REGROUP trial randomized 1150 patients to open vs. endoscopic vein harvest technique and found that in experienced hands, both techniques had similar rates of major cardiac adverse events (HR, 1.12; 95% CI, 0.83 to 1.51; $p=0.47$) through nearly 3 years of follow-up, with similar rates of wound complications.

Arterial conduits
The left internal mammary artery (LIMA) anastomosed to the LAD has a reported 10-year angiographic patency rate of >95% and 20-year patency of >90%. The 2011 ACC/AHC Guideline on Coronary Artery Bypass Graft Surgery recommends the following:

- If possible, the left internal mammary artery (LIMA) should be used to bypass the left anterior descending (LAD) artery when bypass of the LAD artery is indicated. (Class I; LOE: B)
- The right internal mammary artery is probably indicated to bypass the LAD artery when the LIMA is unavailable or unsuitable as a bypass conduit. (Class IIa; LOE: C)
- When anatomically and clinically suitable, use of a second internal mammary artery to graft the left circumflex or right coronary artery (when critically stenosed and perfusing LV myocardium) is reasonable to improve the likelihood of survival and to decrease reintervention. (Class IIa; LOE: B)

The right internal mammary artery (RIMA) has a reported angiographic patency of the RIMA at 10 years is 83-96% with patency directly related to the degree of proximal stenosis of the target vessel. Because the LIMA is preferentially anastomosed to the LAD, the RIMA is often anastomosed to a secondary target with less outflow than then LAD; furthermore, its trans-mediastinal course to left sided targets and higher rate of use as a free graft may also impact patency. A recent network meta-analysis of 4 randomized and 31 observational studies (n=149,902 patients) showed that use of saphenous vein (SV) was associated with higher long-term mortality compared with the RA (incidence rate ratio [IRR], 1.23; 95% CI, 1.12–1.34) and RITA (IRR, 1.26; 95% CI, 1.17–1.35). The risk of deep sternal wound infection (DSWI) for SV was similar to RA but lower than RITA (odds ratio [OR], 0.71; 95% CI, 0.55–0.91). There were no differences for any outcome between RITA and RA, although DSWI trended higher with RITA (OR, 1.39; 95% CI, 0.92–2.1). The risk of DSWI in bilateral internal mammary artery studies was higher when the skeletonization technique was not used.

The radial artery (RA) has a reported angiographic patency rate of 80-90% at 7 to 10 years of follow-up. The radial artery is muscular artery which is prone to spasm in the perioperative period in the setting of significant competitive flow from native coronaries. Therefore, the radial artery is only recommended to bypass left-sided coronary lesions with severe (> 70%) stenosis and right sided coronary lesions with critical (> 90%) stenoses. The recently published RADIAL patient-level pooled analysis of 6 randomized prospective trials (n=1305 patients) compared radial to SVG conduit as second conduit after LIMA-LAD and found a significantly lower rate of death, MI or repeat revascularization at 5 years (HR, 0.67; 95% CI, 0.49 to 0.90; $p=0.01$) and significantly lower risk of occlusion (HR, 0.44; 95% CI, 0.28 to

0.70; $p<0.001$) at mean angiographic follow-up of 50 months. In of the graft analyzed, 75% of targets were left circumflex, 25% were to RCA.

The right gastroepiploic artery (RGEA) has reported angiographic patency rate of 66% at 10 years – likely because it is most often used to graft right-sided lesions and requires a high level of experience to perform. Similar to the radial artery, it should only be used to bypass critical (> 90%) right-sided stenoses or severe (>70%) left-sided stenoses, as addressed by the 2011 ACC/AHC Guideline on Coronary Artery Bypass Graft Surgery contraindication to bypassing lesions not meeting these anatomic criteria (Class III, Harm). The GEA generally is used to graft the RCA but can be used for distal circumflex targets.

Patient Scenarios and Intra-operative Complications

"In which patient would you consider performing total arterial revascularization?"
Complete arterial revascularization may be reasonable in patients ≤ 60 years of age with few or no comorbidities. (Class IIb; LOE: C).[7] LIMA-LAD should be performed in every situation where LAD is to be bypassed. There are virtually no absolute or relative contraindications to utilizing the LIMA as one of the bypass conduits. Secondary target arterial conduits should be used only if the anatomic and physiologic criteria outlined above are fulfilled.

"When is coronary bypass indicated for patients undergoing non-coronary cardiac surgery?"
Coronary artery bypass grafting is recommended in patients undergoing noncoronary cardiac surgery with ≥50% stenosis of the left main coronary artery or ≥70% stenosis of other major coronary arteries (Class I; LOE: C).

"Your patient is found to have moderate aortic valve stenosis with a mean gradient of 28mmHg on preoperative echocardiography. He has no symptoms of aortic stenosis. Does this alter your operative plan?"
Patients undergoing CABG who have at least moderate aortic stenosis should have concomitant aortic valve replacement (Class I; LOE: C). Patients undergoing CABG who have mild aortic stenosis may be considered for concomitant aortic valve replacement when evidence (e.g., moderate–severe leaflet calcification) suggests that progression of the aortic stenosis may be rapid, and the risk of the combined procedure is acceptable (Class IIb; LOE: C). Please see Chapter 42 for management of ischemic mitral regurgitation at time of CABG.

"Your patient has a history of stroke and was found to have an 80% right carotid stenosis on preoperative screening carotid duplex. How does this change your management?"
In the CABG patient with a previous transient ischemic attack or stroke and a significant (50% to 99%) carotid artery stenosis, it is reasonable to consider carotid revascularization in conjunction with CABG. The sequence and timing (simultaneous or staged) of carotid intervention and CABG should be determined by the patient's relative magnitudes of cerebral and myocardial dysfunction (Class IIb; LOE: C). In the patient scheduled to undergo CABG who has no history of transient ischemic attack or stroke, carotid revascularization maybe considered in the presence of bilateral severe (70% to 99%) carotid stenoses or a unilateral severe carotid stenosis with a contralateral occlusion (Class IIb; LOE: C). A multidisciplinary team approach (consisting of a cardiologist, cardiac surgeon, vascular surgeon, and neurologist) is recommended for patients with clinically significant carotid artery disease for whom CABG is planned (Class I; LOE: C). Regarding specifics of concomitant carotid and coronary intervention please see Chapter 44.

"During the left internal mammary harvest, the anesthesiologist tells you that the patient is hypotensive to 60/40, unresponsive to fluid and vasopressors and has new ST changes. What are your next steps?"
Give full dose heparin. Take down the mammary retractor and replace with a sternal retractor. Open the pericardium and cannulate the distal ascending aorta, right atrium and go

226

on cardiopulmonary bypass. Once hemodynamic stability has been obtained, you may continue your internal mammary harvest and continue with the operation as planned.

Pearls/pitfalls

- Know the pathophysiology of stable angina and initial diagnostic and pre-operative workup of patients with coronary artery disease.
- Understand guideline-directed medical and surgical therapy for patients with coronary artery disease and know when CABG is indicated compared to PCI.
- Understand the key operative steps for coronary artery bypass graft surgery, the various conduits available for use, and know the strengths and weaknesses of each conduit in specific clinical/anatomic situations.
- Know the evidence-base for choosing specific conduits for bypass and their indications and contraindications.
- Be able to recognize intra-operative complications and know how to manage them.

Suggested readings

1. Fihn SD, Gardin JM, Abrams J, et al. 2012 ACCF/AHA/ACP/AATS/PCNA/SCAI/STS guideline for the diagnosis and management of patients with stable ischemic heart disease. *Circulation.* 2012;126:e354–e471.
2. Abu-Omar, Y., Mussa, S., Anastasiadis, K., Steel, S., Hands, L., and Taggart, D.P. Duplex ultrasonography predicts safety of radial artery harvest in the presence of an abnormal Allen test. *Ann Thorac Surg.* 2004; 77: 116–119
3. Cohn JD, Korver KF. Selection of saphenous vein conduit in varicose vein disease. *Ann Thorac Surg.* 2006;81:1269–74.
4. Götberg M, Cook CM, Sen S, et al. The Evolving Future of Instantaneous Wave-Free Ratio and Fractional Flow Reserve. *J Am Coll Cardiol.* Sep 2017, 70 (11) 1379-1402.
5. Mohr FW, Morice MC, Kappetein AP, et al. Coronary artery bypass graft surgery versus percutaneous coronary intervention in patients with three-vessel disease and left main coronary disease: 5-year follow-up of the randomised, clinical SYNTAX trial. *Lancet* 2013;381:629-38.
6. Panza JA, Ellis AM, Al-Khalidi HR, et al. Myocardial Viability and Long-Term Outcomes in Ischemic Cardiomyopathy. *N Engl J Med* 2019; 381:739-48.
7. Hillis LD, Smith PK, Anderson JL, et al. 2011 ACCF/AHA guideline for coronary artery bypass graft surgery: a report of the ACCF/AHA Task Force on Practice Guidelines. *J Am Coll Cardiol.* 2011; 58(24): e123-210.
8. Aldea GS, Bakaeen FG, Pal J, et al. The Society of Thoracic Surgeons Clinical Practice Guidelines on Arterial Conduits for Coronary Artery Bypass Grafting. *Ann Thorac Surg* 2016;101:801–9
9. D'Agostino RS, Jacobs JP, Badhwar, V, et al. The Society of Thoracic Surgeons Adult Cardiac Surgery Database: 2018 Update on Outcomes and Quality. *Ann Thorac Surg* 2018;105:15–23.
10. Gaudino M, Angelini GD, Antoniades C, et al. Off-Pump Coronary Artery Bypass Grafting: 30 Years of Debate. *J Am Heart Assoc.* 2018 Aug 21;7(16):e009934.
11. Lamy A, Devereaux PJ, Prabhakaran D, et al. CORONARY Investigators. Off-pump or on-pump coronary-artery bypass grafting at 30 days. *N Engl J Med.* 2012; 366:1489–1497.
12. Shroyer AL, Grover FL, Hattler B, et al. Veterans Affairs Randomized On/Off Bypass (ROOBY) Study Group. On-pump versus off-pump coronary-artery bypass surgery. *N Engl J Med.* 2009; 361:1827–1837.
13. Taggart DP, Benedetto U, Gerry S, et al. Arterial Revascularization Trial Investigators. Bilateral versus Single Internal-Thoracic-Artery Grafts at 10 Years. *N Engl J Med* 2019. 380:437-446.

14. Farkouh ME, Domanski M, Sleeper LA, et al., for the Freedom Trial Investigators. Strategies for Multivessel Revascularization in Patients with Diabetes. *N Engl J Med* 2012; 367:2375-2384

15. Velazquez EJ, Lee KL, Deja MA, et al. Coronary-artery bypass surgery in patient with left ventricular dysfunction. *N Engl J Med* 2011; 364:1607-16.

16. Velazquez EJ, Lee KL, Jones RH, et al. Coronary-artery bypass surgery in patients with ischemic cardiomyopathy. *N Engl J Med* 2016; 374: 1511-20.

17. Thuijs DJ, Bekker MW, Taggart DP, et al. Improving coronary artery bypass grafting: a systematic review and meta-analysis on the impact of adopting transit-time flow measurement. *Eur J Cardiothorac Surg.* 2019 Mar 25. pii: ezz075.

18. Dearani JA, Axford TC, Patel MA, et al. Role of myocardial temperature measurement in monitoring the adequacy of myocardial protection during cardiac surgery. *Ann Thorac Surg.* 2001;72:S2235–44.

19. R.D. Lopes, R.H. Mehta, G.E. Hafley, et al., for the PREVENT IV Investigators. Relationship between vein graft failure and subsequent clinical outcomes after coronary artery bypass surgery. *Circulation.* 125 (2012), pp. 749-756

20. Halabi AR, Alexander JH, Shaw LK, et al. Relation of early saphenous vein graft failure to outcomes following coronary artery bypass surgery. *Am J Cardiol.* 2005;96(9):1254-9.

21. Zenati MA, Bhatt DL, Bakaeen FG, et al., for the REGROUP Investigators. Randomized Trial of Endoscopic or Open Vein-Graft Harvesting for Coronary-Artery Bypass. *N Engl J Med.* 2019; 380:132-141.

22. Loop FD, Lytle BW, Cosgrove DM, et al. Influence of the internal-mammary-artery graft on 10-year survival and other cardiac events. *N Engl J Med.* 1986 Jan 2;314(1):1-6.

23. Sabik JF, Lytle BW, Blackstone EH, et al. Does Competitive Flow Reduce Internal ThoracicArtery Graft Patency? Ann Thorac Surg 2003;76:1490 –7.

24. Gaudino M, Lorusso R, Rahouma M, et al. Radial Artery Versus Right Internal Thoracic Artery Versus Saphenous Vein as the Second Conduit for Coronary Artery Bypass Surgery: A Network Meta-Analysis of Clinical Outcomes. J Am Heart Assoc. 2019 Jan 22;8(2):e010839.

25. Tatoulis J, Buxton BF, Fuller JA, et al. Long-term patency of 1108 radial arterial-coronary angiograms over 10 years. *Ann Thorac Surg.* 2009;88:23–9, discussion 29–30.

26. Deb S, Cohen EA, Singh SK, et al., for the RAPS Investigators. Radial artery and saphenous vein patency more than 5 years after coronary artery bypass surgery: results from RAPS (Radial Artery Patency Study). *J Am Coll Cardiol.* 2012;60:28–35.

27. Gaudino M, Benedetto U, Fremes S, et al. for the RADIAL Investigators. Radial-Artery or Saphenous-Vein Grafts in Coronary-Artery Bypass Surgery. *N Engl J Med.* 2018; 378:2069-2077.

28. Suma H, Tanabe H, Takahashi A, et al. Twenty years experience with the gastroepiploic artery graft for CABG. *Circulation.* 2007;116 Suppl 11:I188–91.

35. ACUTE MYOCARDIAL INFARCTION/UNSTABLE ANGINA

Basil S. Nasir, MBBCh, and James E. Davies, Jr., MD

Concept

- Initial management of patients with acute myocardial infarction (MI)/unstable angina (UA) with a focus on patients in cardiogenic shock
- Define roles for percutaneous coronary intervention (PCI) and coronary artery bypass grafting (CABG)
- Perioperative anticoagulation strategies
- Critical steps for CABG
- Potential pitfalls and alternate scenarios

Chief complaint

"A 63-year-old woman presents with acute onset crushing, substernal chest pain and dyspnea at rest lasting 1 hour. Her past medical history is significant for insulin-dependent diabetes mellitus, hypertension, and hyperlipidemia."

Differential

The initial distinction to make in these patients is stable angina versus acute coronary syndrome (ACS). The later includes unstable angina (UA) or non-ST elevation MI (NSTEMI) [often grouped together for management purposes] and ST elevation MI (STEMI). This further distinction is made on the basis of EKG tracing and cardiac markers. Symptoms occurring at rest rule out stable angina. Other potential diagnoses include acute aortic dissection and pulmonary embolism. In the event that all the above are ruled out, other pulmonary or gastrointestinal causes for the pain may be sought, including cholecystitis, pneumonia, peptic ulcer disease, etc. The initial management, including confirmation of the diagnosis as well as ruling out other pathology will be reviewed below.

History and physical

A full history should be undertaken with a focus on symptoms of chest pain, dyspnea or heart failure, and the chronicity of these symptoms. Assessment of past medical and social history to illicit risk factors for cardiac ischemia should also be performed. A full physical examination should be performed with attention to vital signs, neurological, cardiovascular and respiratory systems to help support the diagnosis and identify potential complications of MI or UA.

Differential

- *Laboratory studies.* Cardiac biomarkers are used to confirm the diagnosis of myocardial infarction. Complete blood count (CBC), coags, LFTs, blood gas, lactate and electrolyte panel including creatinine level should be obtained.
- *EKG.* EKG leads are placed in all 4 extremities with the ground typically in the right leg. Six precordial leads wrap around left thorax. Assessment for EKG abnormalities including ST changes, Q waves or T wave inversions may help delineate the myocardium at risk and the culprit vessel. EKG abnormalities in the inferior leads (II, III, aVf) and posterior findings (reciprocal changes in V1-2) suggest RV or RCA territory ischemia (or left dominant PDA disease). EKG abnormalities in the antero septal (V1-2), anteroapical (V3-4) or anterolateral (V5-6, I, aVL) suggest LV or LAD/LCx territory ischemia. Categorization of the myocardial infarction is based on ST changes and the initial clinical evaluation. Patients who present with angina-type symptoms for greater than 20 minutes with ST elevation > 1 mm in 2 contiguous leads or a new left bundle-branch block are diagnosed with an ST elevation myocardial infarction (STEMI). These patients are at greatest risk of transmural ischemia and are most often approached with PCI initially rather than CABG. Patients presenting with chest pain at rest lasting at least 10 minutes with elevated cardiac biomarkers or ST

elevation of 0.5 to 1 mm or ST depression greater than 0.5 mm or T wave inversion greater than 1 mm are categorized as having non-ST elevation myocardial infarction (NSTEMI). These patients are more likely to have subendocardial ischemia rather than transmural. NSTEMI and UA patients are often grouped together for management purposes. The goal of management in UA/NSTEMI is prevention of a transmural MI (ST elevations +/- Q waves). The EKG is also helpful in assessment of arrhythmias.

- *CXR.* Evaluate for pulmonary edema, congestive heart failure, or other pulmonary pathology. A widened mediastinum may be a clue to a diagnosis of aortic dissection/aneurysm. Look for calcification of the aorta which should then prompt a CT for further evaluation.

- *Transthoracic echo.* Evaluate global LV and RV function (EF%), regional wall motion abnormalities, valvular dysfunction, septum (VSD), and pericardium (effusions). Regional wall motion abnormalities may reveal the coronary territories involved in the infarct (i.e., posteroseptal/posterior/inferior/diaphragmatic free RV wall - RCA or left dominant PDA; anteroseptal/apical - LAD; lateral wall - LCx). Type of wall motion abnormality may suggest the stage of infarction (i.e., hypokinetic - early, akinetic - old, dyskinetic - could be either).

- *Myocardial viability studies.* These will rarely be obtained in a patient with STEMI but may be useful in patients with chronic stable angina or history of prior infarct. A reasonable indication for a viability study would be a history of ischemia with low ejection fraction (< 50%) and extensive akinesis on echo. This is especially true in a high-risk patient when it is unclear if revascularization will improve function or symptoms. Positron emission tomography (PET) scanning is the most common method used for this. If the PET shows decreased perfusion with preserved F-fluorodeoxyglucose (FDG) uptake, then this patient has viable myocardium that will benefit from revascularization. If there is extensive scar tissue as evidenced by decreased perfusion and decreased uptake, then the benefits of revascularization are questionable. MRI is another viability study that is being used.

- *Computed tomography (CT).* If the initial work-up for cardiac ischemia is negative, CT angio can be used to rule out pulmonary embolism, aortic dissection or other intra-abdominal pathology. CT is useful for ruling out ascending calcification if the CXR suggests excessive calcium.

- *Coronary angiogram*: gold standard for evaluating coronary lesions. Any lesion ≥ 70% is significant and thus a candidate for revascularization. Concomitant lesions > 50% may be reasonable to revascularize during open heart surgery for other issues. LM lesions ≥ 50% are significant. Physiologic studies may be used for questionable lesions. Fractional Flow Reserve (FFR) ≤ 0.8 is considered "significant."

Index scenario (additional information)
"History reveals similar episodes of chest pain in the past but lasting less than 10 minutes. Physical exam shows a diaphoretic woman with cool, clammy peripheries. Her heart rate is 120 beats per minute and blood pressure is 80/40 mmHg. The rest of the exam is unremarkable. Serum troponin levels are shown to be 10.2 µg/L (normal is < 0.1) and EKG shows ST elevation (> 1 mm) in leads V2 – V5. CXR is unremarkable."

Treatment/management
The diagnosis is cardiogenic shock secondary to an acute anterior STEMI. Initial medical therapy includes aspirin, nitroglycerin, morphine and supplemental oxygen. Heparin is often used as well especially in UA/NSTEMI patients awaiting surgery. Plavix is used if it is likely that a percutaneous intervention will be performed. If Plavix is given it is advisable to wait 5 days prior to CABG when possible (most applicable to UA/NSTEMI or stable angina). Ask about any other GPIIb/IIIa receptor blockers. Beta blockers, although indicated in patients with coronary ischemia, are contraindicated in this case due to hypotension. Appropriate venous access, with a central line if needed, is established. Invasive arterial monitoring and pulmonary artery catheters are helpful in guiding resuscitation.

230

Optimizing cardiac filling pressures should be undertaken by using fluid resuscitation or diuretics depending on the situation. Pulmonary capillary wedge pressures (PCWP) should be kept in the 16-22 mmHg range. Additional medical therapy includes use of inotropic agents such as milrinone, dobutamine or epinephrine to augment cardiac contractility once filling pressures are optimized. Vasopressors, such as phenylephrine or vasopressin, may be indicated, but they should be used with caution as they can cause an increase in afterload and other negative effects.

Intra-aortic counterpulsation

Use of an intra-aortic balloon pump (IABP) is helpful in cases of refractory shock despite initial medical management or in patients with major complications of myocardial infarction such as postinfarction ventricular septal defect (VSD) or acute papillary muscle rupture. It is also helpful for patients with UA/NSTEMI awaiting surgery.

The IABP is inserted via the femoral artery. The tip of the balloon should be positioned in the descending thoracic aorta just distal to the left subclavian artery. The position could be estimated at the time of insertion using the manubriosternal junction (angle of Louis) as an external landmark. Position could be confirmed by CXR, echocardiography or by fluoroscopy if placed at the time of catheterization. The IABP is set to inflate during diastole, just after the aortic valve closes, which is signified by the dicrotic notch on the arterial blood pressure tracing. The balloon deflates as late as possible during diastole, just before the aortic valve opens, which is marked by the onset of the R wave on the EKG tracing. By increasing coronary flow during diastole and decreasing afterload during systole the IABP improves myocardial oxygen supply and demand. Severe aortic insufficiency and peripheral vascular disease are contraindications for IABP.

Reperfusion strategies

Despite initial medical therapy and stabilization of the patient, establishing reperfusion of the ischemic myocardium is most important. Options include thrombolysis, PCI and CABG. In the setting of an STEMI, PCI is first line therapy. The goal should be door-to-balloon time of 90 minutes or less. In hospitals with limited access to interventional cardiology expertise, thrombolysis is a reasonable alternative. CABG has a limited role and has largely been replaced by PCI as first line therapy.

Once the culprit lesion is identified and treated with a balloon angioplasty, the decision must be made to proceed with PCI and intracoronary stenting or CABG for definitive revascularization. Emergency CABG is indicated in the following situation:

- Patients in whom primary PCI has failed or cannot be performed, AND…
- Coronary anatomy is suitable for CABG, AND…
- Persistent ischemia of a significant area of myocardium at rest and/or hemodynamic instability refractory to nonsurgical therapy is present.

OR…

- Patients with mechanical complication of MI including papillary muscle rupture, post-infarction VSD or left ventricular rupture. Note that these are late complications which typically occur 5 to 7 days following MI.

There are situations where emergency CABG may be preferred over PCI even in the setting of an acute STEMI and they generally revolve around scenarios where the lesions are not favorable for complete revascularization with PCI:

- Left main disease > 50% → PCI has become a reasonable alternative in the setting of an STEMI according to most experts although surgery is still the default option. If the patient's lesion is such that the anatomy is favorable for PCI, with a low syntax score, low chance of periprocedural complications and the patient is at high risk for CABG then PCI is the intervention of choice. Otherwise go to CABG.

- Left main equivalent (> 70% stenosis in the proximal left anterior descending (LAD) and circumflex arteries). Similar considerations to that discussed for LM (high risk patient, good anatomy, low syntax - consider PCI if its faster).
- Severe 3-vessel disease → CABG, especially if diabetic, reduced ejection fraction (EF) < 50%, high syntax score (> 32).

Operative steps
Coronary artery bypass grafting in the setting of acute MI and cardiogenic shock.

Note: Preoperatively, have a sense of the degree of end organ damage that has already occurred. Check lactate, LFTs, creatinine. If the patient has already suffered a significant amount of end organ injury, then stabilizing the patient with mechanical support (IABP versus ECMO versus VAD) may be reasonable until some reversal of end organ effects has occurred prior to surgery. If you decide to go to surgery, bear in mind that there is data suggesting waiting for at least 24 hours after the infarct has occurred prior to CABG unless you can revascularize within 6 hours of the infarct. There is some conflicting evidence regarding this issue and thus, the most prudent decision would be revascularize as soon as possible unless there is severe end organ dysfunction. The official ACC/AHA 2011 guidelines support emergent revascularization "irrespective" of the time from MI to CABG.

- Large bore peripheral intravenous access, radial arterial line, central venous line, pulmonary artery catheter, urinary catheter.
- General endotracheal anesthesia. Pre-induction IABP is recommended, especially in patients with reduced EF. Patients taken directly to surgery from the catheterization lab should have an IABP placed prior to transfer.
- Intraoperative transesophageal echocardiogram. Check for complications including ischemic mitral regurgitation (MR), left ventricular rupture, etc.
- Median sternotomy.
- Choice of conduit: Based on American Heart Association guidelines, use of the left internal mammary artery (LIMA) for LAD bypass is reasonable, even in the urgent setting. If the patient is unstable, and salvage surgery is undertaken, then vein grafts are acceptable because of the reduced time in harvesting the conduit.
- Open the pericardium, check the aorta for plaque and have lines available prior to LIMA harvest.
- Give heparin (400 units/kg).
- Arterial cannulation: Cannulation of the ascending aorta is preferred. Palpate the aorta and look for plaques. Epiaortic ultrasound is an adjunctive measure.
- *Venous cannulation*: two-stage cannula via the right atrial appendage.
- *Myocardial protection.* Place antegrade cardioplegia catheter/aortic root vent in the ascending aorta. Place a retrograde catheter in the coronary sinus. Remember to de-air cardioplegia lines prior to connecting them.
- Check activated clotting time (ACT). If ACT > 480 seconds, initiate CPB at normothermia or mild hypothermia.
- It may be helpful to identify targets for the distal anastomoses prior to cross clamping, as that may be difficult in the arrested heart, especially if targets are small.
- *Prepare for aortic cross clamp.* Reduce arterial flow. Apply cross clamp. Go back up to full flow (2.0-2.5 L/min/m^2). Arrest the heart with antegrade cardioplegia followed by retrograde cardioplegia.
- *Distal anastomoses.* Usually start with the right sided grafts. In the case of vein grafts, instillation of blood cardioplegia down the vein graft after finishing the distal anastomosis is encouraged. In general, 7-0 or 8-0 polypropylene suture is used in a

232

running fashion. For the LIMA graft, make sure the graft is occluded with a bulldog clamp while the heart is arrested to ensure adequate myocardial protection.

- *Proximal anastomoses.* Make sure that the vein grafts are not twisted and there is enough slack to allow for distension of the heart when it fills. Create aortotomy. In general, 5-0 polypropylene in running fashion is used.
- Remove aortic cross clamp. Consider terminal infusion of warm blood cardioplegia or "hot shot" in patients with left ventricular dysfunction prior to removing cross clamp.
- Check for hemostasis and wean from CPB.
- Give protamine.
- Place temporary atrial and ventricular pacing wires. Place chest tubes and close.

Potential questions/alternative scenarios

"Patient with acute NSTEMI, hemodynamically stable and meets indications for CABG."
Maximize the patient medically with heparin, ASA, oxygen, and IABP if refractory angina or low EF. Plan for urgent CABG. As mentioned above for revascularization in the setting of acute STEMI, some studies recommend waiting 1-3 days but ACC/AHA 2011 guidelines recommend revascularization irrespective of the timing between MI and CABG. Thus, in general proceed to the OR ASAP although you can afford a short delay of 24 hrs if the patient remains exceedingly stable. Outcomes may be better with the later approach.

"A 70 M patient is resuscitated from a witnessed cardiac arrest. Coronary angiography shows 3 V disease."
Urgent CABG is indicated for patients who have suffered a sudden cardiac arrest or life-threatening arrhythmia due to ischemic disease.

"Patient with inferior infarction and right ventricular involvement."
In general, similar considerations regarding timing of OR apply here as well. The assumption is that PCI has failed, or the patient has severe three vessel disease that is more amenable to CABG. Thus, CABG should be considered in an urgent fashion. The one caveat is that outcomes are poor in the setting of severe right heart failure, despite adequate revascularization and myocardial protection. In this setting, it may be preferred to delay CABG until the RV is optimized with inotropes, diuretics, or even mechanical support as needed depending on the degree of shock.

"Patient with recent MI and drug-eluting stent (DES), now presents for CABG."
The question of what do with a recently stented artery is controversial. If the stent is compromised, then it is reasonable to place a vein graft distal to the stent. If the stent is wide open without stenosis, any graft placed distal to it is likely to fail due to competitive flow. It is reasonable to leave that vessel alone, and just graft other compromised vessels.

"The above alternative patient is less than 1 year out from his DES placement. He is currently on clopidogrel and presents for urgent CABG 2 days after a NSTEMI."
Stopping the clopidogrel for 7 days carries a high risk for in-stent thrombosis since the DES is less than 1 year old (30 days in the setting of a bare metal stent). Performing surgery < 24 hrs after stoping plavix increases the risk of bleeding. The best scenario is to discontinue the plavix for 5 days in the elective setting or at least 24 hrs in the urgent setting. Short-acting antiplatelet agents, such as eptifibatide or tirofiban should be discontinued for at least 2 to 4 hours before surgery and abciximab for at least 12 hours before surgery. Clopidogrel is resumed shortly after surgery (usually the next day). If there is concern about in stent thrombosis due to an inability to resume plavix for any reason then it may be reasonable to place a vein graft distal to the stented vessel, regardless of patency. If you find yourself operating emergently on clopidogrel, there are no good options to reduce the risk of bleeding. Antifibrinolytic agents, such as aminocaproic acid, should be used. There is a higher risk of postoperative bleeding and increased transfusion requirements. Platelet transfusion is helpful

in this setting, even if the platelet count appears adequate, as native platelets are dysfunctional.

"Patient with history of MI. Echocardiogram shows akinetic myocardium."
In this setting dobutamine echocardiography, thallium imaging or positron emission tomography (PET) are useful. If hibernating myocardium is identified, then that region will benefit from revascularization. Infarcted myocardium will not.

"Seven days post-CABG, a patient complains of pleuritic chest pain and a fever. There is an associated lymphocytosis."
This likely represents postpericardiotomy syndrome, or if following an AMI, Dressler's syndrome. A pericardial rub may be present. The associated leukocytosis is predominated by lymphocytes or eosinophils. It is important to rule out other infectious complications, especially pneumonia. The diagnosis is one of exclusion. The treatment includes non-steroidal anti-inflammatory agents for 1 to 3 months. If this fails, then a course of steroids should be started. Colchicine has also been described in cases with persistent symptoms.

Pearls/pitfalls

- Distinguish between STEMI and NSTEMI/UA. The former is almost always treated with PCI while the later is more likely to be considered for CABG if anatomy is suitable (LM, 3V Dz).
- CABG is indicated in STEMI for failed PCI, mechanical complications of MI and cardiogenic shock if anatomy is unfavorable for PCI.
- If urgent CABG is indicated and the patient can be stabilized medically, it may be beneficial to delay surgery for 1-3 days.
- Pre-induction IABP placement is recommended for emergency CABG.
- If possible, stop plavix at least 24 hours prior to surgery and preferably 5 days before surgery.

Suggested readings

- Geroge I and Oz MC. Myocardial revascularization after acute myocardial infarction. Cohen LH (ed). *Cardiac Surgery in the Adult.* 2008;669-697.
- Hillis LD, et al. 2011 ACCF/AHA Guideline for Coronary Artery Bypass Graft Surgery: Executive Summary. *Circulation.* 2011;124:2610-2642.
- Antman EM, et al. ACC/AHA Guidelines for the Management of Patients With ST-Elevation Myocardial Infarction. *Circulation.* 2004;110:e82-e292.
- Jneid H, et al. 2012 ACCF/AHA Focused Update of the Guideline for the Management of Patients With Unstable Angina/Non–ST-Elevation Myocardial Infarction (Updating the 2007 Guideline and Replacing the 2011 Focused Update). *Circulation.* 2012;126:875-910.

36. MANAGEMENT OF THE PORCELAIN AORTA
Mark Joseph, MD, and Andy C. Kiser, MD

Concept

- Management of the Porcelain Aorta in relation to Coronary Artery Bypass Grafting (CABG) and Aortic Valve Replacement (AVR)
- Preoperative considerations
- Revascularization options
- Operative strategies and myocardial protection
- Pitfalls and alternative solutions

Chief complaint

"A 70-year-old man with previous h/o Hodgkin's lymphoma presents to his primary care physician with intermittent chest pain on exertion. CXR shows calcification of the aorta and is otherwise is unremarkable."

Differential

Angina, aortic stenosis w/aortic calcification, PE, dissection, mediastinal mass

History and physical

Clarify the duration and character of the chest pain to distinguish between possible etiologies. The calcium on the CXR raises concerns for a porcelain aorta although the CT scan is needed before establishing the diagnosis. Look for risk factors associated with this disease including atherosclerotic risk factors (diabetes, smoking, HTN, family history), radiation for Hodgkin's, renal failure/hemodialysis and aortic stenosis. Physical exam should focus on peripheral pulses, and cardiopulmonary exam.

Tests

- *EKG*: evidence of arrhythmias and previous or ongoing ischemia.
- *Echocardiography*: valve function and EF.
- Cardiac catheterization.
- *CXR*: look for other lung pathology.
- *CT scan*: CT scan is warranted in patients with strong risk factors for ascending aortic atherosclerosis or if there is evidence of aortic calcification on ECHO or CXR. Look for concomitant disease such as dissection or aneurysms.

Index scenario (additional information)

"Angiogram reveals significant 3 vessel disease: Left main (80%) and ostial LAD (80%), circumflex (75%) and mid RCA lesions (70%). Echo reveals AVA of 0.4 mm, peak gradient of 80 mmHg and mean gradient of 40 mmHg with a jet velocity of 4 m/s2. Diffuse circumferential ascending aortic calcification is noted on the CT scan. EF is 55%."

Treatment/management

There is a spectrum of ascending aortic calcification from multifocal patchy disease to diffuse involvement. The CT scan is helpful for preoperative planning although the final decision is made in the OR with careful palpation and the use of an epiaortic ultrasound. This patient meets criteria for CABG - AVR but is not likely to have a safe place to clamp and cannulate. In addition, he likely needs a LIMA-LAD, S-PDA and S-OM and thus needs room for proximals. If you can find a place to clamp and cannulate then that is a reasonable but unusual opportunity. Axillary artery cannulation affords you more real estate on the aorta for placement of the clamp. If you did find a safe place to clamp you may still have considerable difficulty finding a place for proximals. The safest and most reliable alternative is axillary artery cannulation, circulatory arrest, replacement of the ascending aorta, AVR, and CABG.

Operative steps

Goals – bypass coronary lesions, replace the aortic valve, protect the heart, and minimize manipulation of the aorta using a "no touch" technique.

- Central line +/- Swan, large peripheral IV's, arterial line, general endotracheal anesthesia (GETA), foley with temperature monitoring.
- Check the intraoperative TEE for evidence of AI or other unexpected pathology and to evaluate ventricular function.
- Median sternotomy, gentle palpation of aorta to determine extent of calcifications, and epiaortic ultrasound.
- Decide whether you can clamp or if you need circulatory arrest.
- Harvest the appropriate conduit depending on revascularization scheme (arterial and/or venous conduit).
- Heparinize (400 mg/kg), right axillary cannulation with a side graft, bicaval cannulation, retrograde coronary sinus catheter, once ACT is above 480, initiate cardiopulmonary bypass (CPB), (cool to 20°), place LV vent through right superior pulmonary vein (RSPV).
- While cooling you can perform the distal anastomoses with a stabilizer or simply wait.
- Once cool and EEG is silent, circ arrest, myocardial arrest, distal ascending graft anastomosis (may need limited endarterectomy to ensure a healthy aortic wall, consider felt reinforcement), deair the graft, clamp the graft, rewarm, hemostasis, inspect, resect and debride the aortic valve, complete any remaining distals, AVR, proximal ascending graft anastomosis and complete the proximal vein anastomoses from the new ascending graft.
- root vent, deair, unclamp, wean from CPB.

Potential questions/alternative scenarios

"You begin cooling and the patient fibrillates."

If you do have aortic insufficiency you will almost certainly fibrillate and over distend during cooling and you will have no place to clamp. Have an LV vent in place to protect you from over distending. You can attempt to defibrillate but it is often not helpful. IV lidocaine load can be tried as well. The key is to prevent overdistention until you are ready to circ arrest.

"Same patient but no need for AVR."

The most common approach in this setting is a beating heart CABG with or without axillary artery cannulation and CPB support. The decision to use support depends on how well the patient is expected to tolerate manipulating the heart and which vessels need to be grafted. An off-pump LIMA-LAD is a safe operation to describe. It involves harvesting the mammary, traction sutures on left side of the posterior pericardium, full heparinization, a commercially available immobilizer to stabilize the heart at the region of the LAD target, silastic vessel loops proximally and distally, and a shunt if needed. The patient must be adequately fluid resuscitated and potentially on pressors to tolerate the manipulation.

"The LIMA-LAD is completed off pump. How do you revascularize the Cx territory and the PDA with a porcelain aorta?"

An arterial graft (radial or free RIMA) fashioned as a Y off the LIMA or a RIMA in situ through the transverse sinus are options for a high OM. Options for the PDA include a RIMA in situ (may have issues with length here, usually reaches the RCA well), a SVG with proximal anastomosis to the innominate, carotid, subclavian, right axillary, or internal mammary arteries or the descending aorta; alternatively, if no SVG due to a prior CABG then consider an *in-situ* gastroepiploic artery (become familiar with this prior to suggesting it as an option).

"The circumflex and PDA disease is quite distal, the EF is 40% and you do not expect the heart to tolerate excessive manipulation for a completely off pump CABG. What are your options?"

Use right axillary and venous cannulation, go on pump to empty the heart while you use the stabilizers to graft your targets. You still have issues with needing long conduits to the lateral OM and PDA. Assuming no place on the aorta for a proximal, the best option may be a long RIMA in situ to the PDA and long radial from the LIMA to the lateral OM. Options for Y grafts include sizing and fashioning the end to side Y anastomosis first then completing the two distals or doing the distals first and then the end to side. Make sure the heart is full when sizing these arterial grafts. If you anticipate using the right axillary as inflow for a vein graft to the PDA in the not so uncommon event that the RIMA does not reach, then plan your axillary cannulation on the left. Other alternatives for the PDA or lateral OM include the in-situ gastroepiploic or a proximal vein off the descending aorta. The descending aorta can be accessed with an incision in the retropericardium. With the heart decompressed, elevate the heart out of the pericardial well and open the leftward pericardium behind the left phrenic nerve. Using a side biting clamp, the descending aorta can serve as an alternative for conduit inflow. Another alternative is to use the HeartString III (MAQUET, Wayne, NJ, USA) proximal anastomosis device if a small area of soft ascending aorta is available. Yet another option is a hybrid procedure with LIMA-LAD and stents to the PDA and/or circumflex. Always remember the significance of the lesion you wish to graft, the runoff and the distal target. A nonsignificant lesion on a nondominant right with excessive scar tissue, poor target and poor runoff is not worth the risk of "creative" coronary grafting strategies. Also remember that a sent is a reasonable option when appropriate.

Pearls/pitfalls

- Look for signs or risk factors for a calcified ascending aorta and get a CT scan if concerned.

- Need to replace the ascending with a graft if performing an AVR in the setting of a porcelain aorta.

- Beating heart CABG with or without CPB assist is an option for patients with a porcelain aorta in need of a CABG.

- For beating heart CABG where there is no space on the aorta for proximals anticipate alternative grafting strategies especially for the distal PDA and lateral circumflex. Hybrid procedures with LIMA-LAD and stents to the PDA and/or circumflex may be an option if the anatomy is favorable. Also consider the HeartString III device if you are comfortable and familiar.

- Axillary cannulation is preferred over femoral for same reason retrograde cardioplegia is preferred to avoid the "sandblasting" effect from the aorta towards the coronary ostia.

- If the ascending aorta cannot be safely replaced, consider a hybrid approach with LIMA to LAD and PCI +/-TAVR if both valvular and coronary disease are present.

Suggested readings

- Leyh R.G., et al. Management of porcelain aorta during coronary artery bypass grafting. *Ann Thorac Surg* 1999; 67(4):986-988.

- Mills N.L., Everson C.T.: Atherosclerosis of the ascending aorta and coronary artery bypass. Pathology, clinical correlates, and operative management. *J Thorac Cardiovasc Surg* 1991; 102(4):546-553.

- Sabik J.F., et al: Axillary artery: an alternative site of arterial cannulation for patients with extensive aortic and peripheral vascular disease. *J Thorac Cardiovasc Surg* 1995; 109(5):885-890.discussion 890-1.

- Sundt T.M., Barner H.B., Camillo C.J., et al: Total arterial revascularization with an internal thoracic artery and radial artery T graft. *Ann Thorac Surg* 1999; 68:399-405.

37. REOPERATIVE CORONARY ARTERY BYPASS SURGERY
Eric Griffiths, MD, and Gorav Ailawadi, MD

Concept
- Indications for redo coronary artery bypass grafting (CABG)
- Preoperative considerations
- Conduit choices
- Critical steps of redo CABG
- Pitfalls and alternative solutions

Chief complaint
"A 73-year-old man with history of CABG 12 years prior now has recurrent chest pain for 3 months and multivessel disease of both native arteries and vein grafts on repeat catheterization. He is referred to you for possible repeat surgical revascularization."

Differential
Recurrent CAD versus other non coronary etiologies. Reoperation is indicated in symptomatic patients with ischemia who have evidence of myocardial viability or who demonstrate large areas of myocardium at risk from progression of their disease.

History and physical
Confirm presence of symptoms, evaluate functional status. Identify comorbidities that may affect surgical risk: chronic obstructive pulmonary disease, end stage renal disease, peripheral vascular disease, stroke, or arrhythmias. On exam, evaluate carotid artery/bruits, quality of potential conduits such as vein and radial arteries, and signs of congestive heart failure. Obtain prior operative report.

Tests
- *EKG*: evaluate for arrhythmias, prior MI (Q waves), Bundle branch blocks indicating damage to conduction system.
- *Echo*: evaluate LV function, wall motion abnormalities, valvular function.
- *Cardiac catheterization*: review prior angiograms if possible.
    - Identifies location and degree of stenosis in native coronary, saphenous vein graft (SVG) and arterial conduits.
    - Injection of internal mammary arteries bilaterally should be performed to eval patency or for use as possible conduits.
- *Myocardial viability studies*: restored perfusion to ischemic or underperfused myocardium may lead to improved contractility. Revascularized scar tissue will not provide improvement.
    - Thallium scintigraphy.
    - Dobutamine stress echo.
    - *Positron emission tomography (PET)*: evaluates uptake of FDG as marker of cardiac metabolic activity.
    - Cardiac MRI.
- *CT chest*: evaluate relationship of sternum and underlying mediastinal structures including bypass graft locations, degree of aortic calcification.
- CT abd/pelv to evaluate femoral vessels for possible peripheral bypass.
- *Potential conduit studies*. Venous duplex and mapping for presence and adequacy of saphenous vein, Allen's test/arterial Doppler for radial conduit, cardiac catheterization to inject the mammary arteries and chest wall mammary duplex studies.

"The patient has hypertension, moderate COPD. ECHO shows EF of 45% with inferior and lateral wall motion abnormalities, and no valvular disease. Cardiac catheterization shows occlusion of SVG to PDA, 80% stenosis of SVG to OM, and patent LIMA to LAD, and 80% stenosis of proximal circumflex. Cardiac MRI shows viable myocardium in the inferior and lateral walls. How would you proceed?"

Treatment/management

The patient appears to be a candidate for surgical revascularization. Percutaneous coronary intervention (PCI) is an option for patients with discrete, focal disease with minimal myocardial areas at risk. This patient has an occluded SVG to an area with viable myocardium. This lesion is typically not accessible via PCI making it necessary for him to undergo redo CABG. Additionally, he has large areas of myocardium at risk and is a functional/active patient. Redo CABG has higher risk than primary revascularization with operative mortality rates ranging from 6.9-11% mostly due to increased risk of perioperative myocardial infarction (MI). Causes include incomplete revascularization, atheromatous emboli from diseased SVGs or aorta, damaged grafts, hypoperfusion through new grafts, or early graft occlusion.

Operative steps

- *Redo sternotomy*: increase risk due to adhesions to underlying structures including right ventricle, innominate vein, right atrium, aorta, lung and patent coronary bypass grafts.
- *Evaluate need for possible peripheral cardiopulmonary bypass*: closely adherent right ventricle, pulmonary artery or aorta (refer to Redo AVR chapter for alternative cannulation strategies).
  - If so, place femoral arterial and venous lines.
  - Axillary artery cannulation with end to side tube graft if warranted.
- Proceed with division of the anterior table of the sternum using oscillating saw, posterior table divided using Mayo scissors.
  - Avoid excessive traction on underlying structures.
  - Separate mediastinal structures from chest wall.
- Harvest the internal mammary artery (left, right, or both), if not previously used, may be performed after sternotomy, cannulation, or once on bypass depending on the stability of the patient.
- Intra-pericardial dissection.
  - Avoid excessive manipulation of venous bypass grafts "no touch technique." Avoids embolization of debri.
- Cannulation.
  - Once aorta dissected out, palpate or use epiaortic U/S for safe cannulation site as well as sites for proximal grafts.
  - Consider axillary or femoral bypass for excessive atherosclerotic disease.
  - Venous cannulation through right atrium using multistage cannula. If unable to clear safe site on atrium due to prior vein grafts or if adhesions to the right atrium are extensive, consider femoral venous cannulation or bicaval cannulation.
- Initiate CPB, dissect out the aorta to make sufficient room for antegrade and cross clamp.
- *Myocardial protection strategy*: combination of antegrade and retrograde cardioplegia. Antegrade cardioplegia alone may not protect areas supplied by patent pedicled internal mammary artery grafts and may dislodge debri in SVGs. Retrograde allows possible washout of coronary debri as well as access to myocardial areas of occluded arterial grafts. Protection of the right ventricle may not be complete with retrograde only cardioplegia. Clamping of patent arterial grafts ensures uniform cooling. If safe,

239

the LIMA can be clamped in tissue between left side of the aorta and medial surface of the left lung (check its trajectory on the CT scan). If this area is difficult to dissect, consider leaving LIMA patent. Do not risk injuring a patent LIMA. If intend to keep LIMA patent, use frequent antegrade and retrograde cardioplegia and consider cooling the patient to 28-30° C.

- *Revascularization strategy*: determine vessels/conduits to be bypassed and conduits to be used. Consider replacing older (> 5 yr) SVG when high degree of atherosclerosis is present. Must be individualized based on degree of stenosis, availability of conduit, and patient risk.
  - Avoid manipulation of SVGs to avoid embolization of atheroma.
  - Stenotic SVGs can be left in place or divided and replaced with new SVG.
  - When replacing stenotic SVG with arterial graft, should leave SVG in place in order to prevent hypoperfusion syndrome (worsening myocardial ischemia or infarction).
  - If possible, place left internal mammary artery (LIMA) graft to left anterior descending artery (LAD) or another large vessel perfusing a large ischemic region.
- *Distal sites of anastomosis*: may consider reusing prior distal site when replacing SVG with another depending on degree of disease present there. Otherwise consider "landing" on native coronary distal to prior anastomosis.
- Sites for proximal anastomosis may be limited due to prior involvement on the reoperative aorta.
  - Consider sequencing vein grafts to minimize number of proximal anastomoses.
  - Arterial free grafts can be anastomosed to the hood of new or old SVG due to lack of atherosclerotic involvement there or can be sewn to other arterial grafts for a "Y" type anastomosis.
- Arterial grafts.
  - LIMA to LAD if not previously performed.
  - Right internal mammary artery (RIMA) to right coronary artery/posterior descending artery or through transverse sinus to circumflex/proximal obtuse marginal. Transverse sinus is typically adherent and requires dissection. Also consider utilizing the RIMA as a free graft.
  - *Radial artery free graft*: affected by competitive flow, best if stenosis > 70% and used to a large vessel/large runoff territory.

Potential questions/alternative scenarios
"Patient fails to wean from bypass."
Check ABG, electrolytes (K+), assess degree of inotropic support, adequate volume and heart rate. Transesophageal echo (TEE) useful for assessing for old/new wall motion abnormalities, volume status of the heart, presence of unrecognized valvular dysfunction, and possible air in the aortic root. For visible air in the bypass graft, the vein can be clamped and deaired with a small 27g needle. A balloon pump may be necessary. These are longer operations on chronically ischemic hearts and patients are prone to myocardial dysfunction postoperatively. Myocardial protection must be as optimal as possible (refer to CPB pitfalls chapter).

Assess all grafts for adequate positioning (no kinks). Doppler assessment of new constructed graphs to check for patency. If poor flow with associated regional abnormality on TEE, grafts to that area should be reconstructed immediately. Revision can be performed by clamping and arresting the heart. Alternatively, if familiar with off-pump CABG techniques, can use cardiac stabilizer while on full cardiopulmonary bypass and revise the distal anastomosis (but be cautious, it went down for a reason, so you want to have optimal conditions the second time). If low cardiac output or regional abnormalities persist, then proceed to intra-aortic balloon pump placement (IABP). If IABP and inotropes fail, then consider placing mechanical ventricular support (ECMO, Abiomed, CentriMag, Impella, or other).

240

"No room on the aorta for proximal anastomosis."

Other locations for proximals include end- to- side anastomosis to patent arterial grafts, using the hood of patent old or new SVGs. Even occluded SVGs may have a patent hood that can be used. Consider using the RIMA in situ such that a proximal aortic site is not needed.

"You are doing the redo sternotomy and encounter bright red blood before sternum is open. You now see EKG changes."

Suspect coronary/graft injury. Heparinize and emergently place the patient on femoral bypass, open the sternum and expeditiously continue your dissection. If you can identify the injured coronary you can either repair, it or place a coronary perfusion catheter in the lumen to perfuse the area with warm blood. Continue operation. Replace injured vein graft.

"You heparinize, cannulate and dissect out the ascending aorta making enough room for cross clamping and antegrade access. The ACT is 480. Unfortunately, you injure the patent mammary while attempting to dissect it near the lung. Almost immediately you notice hemodynamic changes and regional wall motion abnormalities."

Initiate CPB, clamp and arrest the heart. Try to repair the injured mammary. If not, it will have to be replaced. Note that this illustrates the importance of being ready to clamp and arrest prior to dissecting out a patent mammary.

Pearls/pitfalls

- Review cath films, ensure myocardial viability in areas with diseased grafts.
- Thorough preoperative planning including op note, cannulation strategy and conduit assessment.
- Minimize manipulation of old SVGs.
- Make every effort to place LIMA on LAD if not done previously.
- SVGs that are bypassed by arterial conduit should be left in place.
- Be prepared to clamp and arrest when dissecting out a patent mammary.

Suggested readings

- Barreiro CJ and Bansal A. Reoperative coronary artery bypass surgery. Yuh D, Vricella LA, and Baumgartner WA (eds). *Johns Hopkins Manual of Cardiothoracic Surgery* 2007.
- Lytle BW. Re-do coronary artery bypass surgery. Little AG (editor). *Complications in Cardiothoracic Surgery: Avoidance and Treatment.* 1st ed. Blackwell Futura. 2004.

38. POST-INFARCTION VENTRICULAR SEPTAL DEFECT

Aaron J. Weiss, MD, and Joanna Chikwe, MD

Concept

- Presentation of post-infarction VSD and LV aneurysm
- Diagnosis and workup
- Operative timing and approaches
- Pitfalls and alternative solutions

Chief complaint

"A 65-year-old man was admitted to the hospital with chest pain and diagnosed with an acute anteroseptal myocardial infarction for which he underwent percutaneous coronary intervention. He was recovering on the floor four days later when he developed new chest pain and breathlessness."

Differential

Post-myocardial infarction ventricular septal defect, free wall rupture, tamponade, acute papillary muscle rupture, pulmonary embolism, aortic dissection/rupture, and ongoing ischemia/infarction.

History and physical

If patient is stable and alert, a short and focused history to elicit chest pain and dyspnea, calf or leg pain (possible deep vein thrombosis leading to a pulmonary embolism). Focused physical exam should include vital signs, a full neurological, cardiac with attention to new murmurs, lung, and extremities exam. In addition, one should focus on signs of right-sided heart failure (jugular venous distention (JVD), peripheral edema, etc.).

Tests

- *EKG.* Rule out ongoing or additional ischemic events, any arrhythmias.
- *Echo.* This is diagnostic. Color flow Doppler echocardiography shows the size and location of the VSD, ventricular function, mitral regurgitation, pulmonary artery and right-sided pressures, and rules out free wall rupture/tamponade.
- *Right heart catheterization.* Right heart catheterization shows a step-up in oxygenation between the right atrium and pulmonary artery (> 9% is diagnostic). Other information obtained includes an elevated pulmonary-to-systemic flow ratio (ranges from 1.4:1 to 8:1 and correlates with size of defect).
- *Left heart catheterization.* Most patients undergo this at the time of their initial presentation with acute myocardial infarction. In stable patients without a recent cardiac catheterization left heart catheterization will guide the decision to perform concomitant surgical revascularization. In unstable patients it is reasonable to omit this diagnostic modality.

Index scenario (additional information)

"On physical exam, patient is found to be hypotensive. There is a new harsh holosystolic murmur most prominent at the left lateral sternal border that radiates to the axilla and is associated with a thrill. Coarse breath sounds heard bilaterally. No JVD or peripheral edema noted. EKG shows no new changes from the EKGs performed since admission. Emergent echocardiogram performed at the bedside shows a large new anterior VSD."

Treatment/management

The natural history of untreated postinfarction VSD is poor (25% mortality rate within 24 hours, 50% mortality rate within one week, 80% within one month, 97% at 1 year). Postinfarction VSD is therefore an indication for urgent surgery.

Preoperatively, management should include reducing afterload to decrease the left-to-right shunt, maintain cardiac output and peripheral perfusion so as to avoid end-organ damage, and increase coronary perfusion pressure. These goals can be accomplished through the use of an intra-aortic balloon pump (IABP) as well as pharmacologic therapy with inotropic agents. As surgical mortality is directly proportional to duration of cardiogenic shock and multi-organ failure pre-operatively, current emphasis is on early surgical intervention. A small percentage of patients severely compromised by multi-organ failure may benefit from mechanical assistance such as biventricular support or ECMO for temporary salvage before more definitive surgery can be performed.

Operative steps
Repair of anterior septal rupture
- Arterial line, general endotracheal anesthesia, central line with large bore access (no pulmonary artery catheter), urinary catheter, transesophageal echocardiography (TEE).
- Median sternotomy, conduit harvest (saphenous vein, and left internal mammary artery in stable patients if coronary revascularization is planned), heparin 400 mg/kg, ascending aorta cannulation, bicaval cannulation, antegrade cardioplegia cannula, retrograde cardioplegia cannula, left ventricular vent through the right superior pulmonary vein, +/- systemic cooling to 25° C, once ACT is 480 initiate cardiopulmonary bypass (CPB), CO_2 insufflation.
- Deair antegrade line and run antegrade induction, followed by retrograde perfusion via the coronary sinus. Additional myocardial protection can be obtained by running cold blood cardioplegia during the VSD repair via retrograde coronary sinus catheter.
- Perform coronary bypasses: cardioplegia can be administered via the grafts prior to completion of the proximal anastomoses.
- Left ventricular transinfarct incision with infarctectomy is performed. Debride necrotic septal myocardium even enlarging the defect if needed. Place pledgeted interrupted horizontal mattress sutures around the defect. Pass the sutures through a felt strip then through the septum from right to left and then snap. Continue along the posterior rim. Along the anterior rim, pass the sutures from epicardium to endocardium. Then pass all the sutures symmetrically through a Dacron prosthetic patch. All sutures are pledgeted again and then tied down. Reapproximate the edges of the ventriculotomy with a double layer closure buttressed with Teflon felt or glutaraldehyde-preserved bovine pericardium.
- If used, biological glue is most effective if applied on dry myocardium in the decompressed, arrested heart i.e., prior to cross-clamp removal.
- Deair, wean from CPB, intraoperative TEE to assess for any residual VSD/shunt/left ventricular function/mitral regurgitation, if not already in place, an IABP may be necessary to help wean off bypass.

Potential questions/alternative scenarios
"On intraoperative TEE, the VSD appears to be apical. How would your operative technique differ?"
The same basic set-up as for an anterior septal rupture. Incision is made through the infarcted ventricular apex and the surgeon should debride any necrotic myocardium involving the left ventricle, right ventricle, and septum. Reapproximate the remaining apical portions to the apical septum using interrupted mattress sutures of 1-0 Tevdek passed sequentially through a buttressing strip of Teflon felt, the left ventricle, a second strip of felt, the septum, a third strip of felt, the right ventricle, and a fourth strip of felt. Tie these sutures down and then reinforce the closure with an over-and-over suture to ensure hemostasis.

"On intraoperative TEE, the VSD appears to be posteroinferior. How would your operative technique differ?"

Place the patient on CPB and arrest the heart. Retract the heart out of the pericardial well as you would for a bypass graft to the PDA. Trans-infarct incision is made through the left ventricle 1 cm lateral to the PDA. Debridement of necrotic left ventricular septal myocardium is performed. Inspect the mitral apparatus for any papillary muscle infarct. Less aggressive debridement of the right ventricle is performed as you only want to resect as much as necessary to achieve adequate visualization of the defect. If the posterior septum has separated from the free wall, it can be re-approximated primarily using a double-layered buttressed closure. Larger defects require patch closure as described earlier with the only difference being that the sutures are placed from the right side of the septum and from the epicardial side of the right ventricular free wall. Afterwards, a separate patch closure of the infarctectomy using Dacron graft maybe required versus a buttressed double layer primary repair depending on the size of the free wall defect. Primary closure of a large tissue defect has historically resulted in very poor outcomes. Check for hemostasis, deair, and wean from CPB.

"Is preoperative left heart catheterization necessary? And if CAD is found that necessitates bypass grafts, when should this be performed?"
It is controversial whether or not preoperative coronary catheterization is necessary. In patients with multivessel coronary disease, bypass grafts may increase both early and long-term survival. However, often the patient is too unstable to undergo a catheterization prior to surgery and thus necessitates an individual assessment of patient's hemodynamics and clinical situation. If bypass grafts are performed, they should be done before the repair of the VSD to optimize myocardial protection.

"Are there any other surgical techniques that might warrant consideration for repair of a VSD?"
Endocardial patch repair with infarct exclusion involves intracavitary placement of an endocardial patch to exclude infarcted myocardium while maintaining ventricular geometry. This technique excludes the VSD from the highly pressured left ventricle instead of closing it. Proponents of this approach argue that maintaining ventricular geometry enhances or at least preserves ventricular function.

"When would delayed repair of a VSD be acceptable?"
Patients with severe end-organ damage deemed too sick to undergo operative repair may be candidates for a delayed repair. Interval treatment may involve placement of a left ventricular assist device (LVAD) that theoretically will help improve end-organ dysfunction and allow for maturation of the infarcted tissue. A biventricular mechanical assist device may be necessary if the LVAD worsens the right-to-left shunt.

"What interventions may help a difficult wean from CPB following VSD repair?"
If an IABP was not inserted preoperatively, one should be inserted at this time to help reduce the afterload and improve coronary perfusion pressure. Pharmacologic adjuncts such as epinephrine and milrinone may help to augment contractility. Milrinone also improves diastolic function and reduces afterload. Other afterload reducing agents may be used as needed. If the patient is having decreased right heart function, the patient may benefit from inhaled prostaglandin or nitric oxide to help dilate the pulmonary vasculature and decrease the work of the right ventricle. A small percentage of patients may require a temporary ventricular assist device.

Pearls/pitfalls

- Discovery of a new onset post-infarction VSD requires urgent surgery.
- The greatest predictor of post-operative mortality is the length of time patients spend in cardiogenic shock pre-operatively.
- Echocardiography is the diagnostic test and is essential to adequately plan the surgical approach.

- The chances of successfully weaning from CPB are improved by expeditious institution of CPB with meticulous myocardial protection.
- The VSD should be approached via a transinfarct incision with meticulous debridement of necrotic myocardium to prevent delayed rupture.
- Inspect the mitral apparatus for any coexisting dysfunction or infarct of the papillary muscles.
- A tension-free closure is important, and therefore patch closure techniques are required for larger defects.

Suggested readings

- Mangi AA and Agnihotri AK. Postinfarction Ventricular Septal Defect. Spencer and Sabiston - *Surgery of the Chest.* 2010; 1449-1456.
- Gazoni LM. Mechanical complications of coronary artery disease. Mery CM and Turek JW. *TSRA Review of Cardiothoracic Surgery.* 2011. 282-289.
- Madsen JC and Daggett WM Jr. Repair of postinfarction ventricular septal defect. *Semin Thorac Cardiovasc Surg.* 1998. Apr;10(2):117-127.
- Arnaoutakis GJ, Zhao Y, George TJ et al. Surgical repair of ventricular septal defect after myocardial infarction: outcomes from the Society of Thoracic Surgeons National Database. *Ann Thorac Surg* 2012; 94: 436-44.

39. AORTIC STENOSIS

Alexander A. Brescia, MD, MSc, and G. Michael Deeb, MD

Adapted from 1st edition chapter written by Gabriel Loor, MD, and Douglas R. Johnston, MD

Concepts

- Indications for aortic valve replacement in the setting of aortic stenosis (AS)
- Diagnostic testing
- Treatment decisions (TAVR vs. SAVR)
- Preoperative considerations
- Options for annular enlargement
- Valve choices
- Surgical options and pitfalls

Chief complaint

"A 62-year-old man is referred to you by a primary care physician diagnosed with severe aortic stenosis by echo after presenting with a 3-month history of progressive dyspnea on exertion and chest tightness."

Differential

The diagnosis of severe AS has been established. Confirmation is important as well as ruling out concomittent pathologies that often coexist.

History and physical

A focused history to elicit symptoms of angina, syncope, or congestive heart failure (CHF) as well as fatigue or decreased exercise tolerance, which often precede more overt symptoms, is essential. Since asymptomatic severe AS is not an indication for intervention, establishing symptoms in a patient suspected of AS is crucial for decision making. A focused physical exam with emphasis on vital signs, heart, lungs, neuro exam, bruits, pulses, and peripheral edema is important. A classic crescendo-decrescendo (diamond shaped) systolic ejection murmur heard best at the 2nd right intercostal space should be appreciated.

Determining comorbidities [end-stage renal disease (ESRD), liver disease, pulmonary failure, bleeding disorders, stroke, peripheral vascular disease, etc.] is important to calculate a STS predicted risk of mortality/morbidity to help establish the most appropriate treatment algorithm.

Tests

- *EKG*: arrhythmias, LVH.
- *Echocardiogram.* Gradients are determined by continuous wave doppler peak gradient = 4(velocity)^2. The peak gradient is the maximum gradient present when simultaneous central aortic pressure is subtracted from LV systolic pressure, while mean gradient is the integral difference over the entire systolic ejection period (e.g. the area under the velocity curve). The aortic valve area (AVA) is determined by the continuity equation: Area = [(LVOT area) x (LVOT velocity)]/continuous wave velocity at the aortic valve. The indexed AVA is the AVA divided by body surface area (BSA). The dimensionless index (DI) is the ratio of the LVOT time-velocity integral to that of the aortic valve jet. Note that velocity is also influenced by cardiac output. Thus, patients may have low gradients because of low cardiac output (low flow).

  If low flow/low gradient AS is suspected and the patient has a normal LVEF ($\geq 50\%$), a stroke volume index ≤ 35 mL/min/m^2 will confirm the diagnosis. If the LVEF is < 50%, a dobutamine stress echo may be helpful. If the gradient is increased on stress echo and the AVA does not increase, this confirms the diagnosis of AS. However, if the gradient does not change and the AVA increases ≥ 0.3cm^2 or to ≥ 1.0cm^2, this confirms pseudo-AS. If the patient has a significant subvalvular gradient and asymmetric septal hypertrophy, a septal myectomy and the possibility of intervention on the mitral valve may be required (refer to HOCM chapter). In general, it is imperative to ensure that the echocardiogram is of excellent quality or have it repeated and interpreted by a cardiologist you trust.

- *Cardiac catheterization.* Virtually all patients evaluated for AVR should have evaluation of their coronary arteries for obstructive CAD. If the diagnosis of AS is uncertain by echo, the AV should be crossed for a hemodynamic AV study.

- *Coronary CTA.* For patients at low risk for CAD, coronary CTA may be performed to rule out obstructive CAD to avert a cardiac cath.

- *TAVR protocol CT scan.* All patients who are potential TAVR candidates should receive a TAVR CT scan, which will provide important anatomical information including valve morphology (TTE unreliable for morphology), aortic valve annular and LVOT sizing, coronary height and orientation, and sinus height and width sizing.

Diagnosis
The diagnosis of severe AS is defined as the presence of **any one of** the following:
1.) Mean AV gradient ≥ 40 mmHg
2.) Peak velocity across the AV ≥ 4 meters per second
3.) AVA ≤ 1.0 cm^2 or an indexed AVA ≤ 0.6 cm^2/m^2
4.) Dimensionless index ≤ 0.25
Confirmation of severe AS after referral is important as well as ruling out simultaneous pathologies such as obstructive CAD, aortic aneurysm, and mitral valve disease.

Index scenario (additional information)
"This patient is a diabetic, without syncope. Echo shows a valve area of 0.8 cm^2 and mean gradient of 45 mmHg and LVEF 60%. Cardiac catheterization shows no obstructive CAD. TAVR CT scan shows a tricuspid aortic valve with anatomy amenable to TAVR, no aneurysm, and no ascending calcification. What are his options and how would you proceed?"

Treatment/management
This patient meets AHA Class I indications for an aortic valve replacement (angina, CHF, severe AS). Deciding whether to perform SAVR or TAVR should be determined by 1.) anatomy (including valve morphology and annular size, aortic root dimensions, and vascular access), 2.) patient age and simultaneous medical conditions impacting long-term prognosis, and 3.) patient preference. In light of SAVR vs. TAVR trials, patient surgical risk profile no longer precludes patient eligibility from undergoing TAVR.

An STS risk score should still be calculated to inform shared decision making with patients and determine treatment options. For patients at prohibitive risk (STS score >15%), TAVR has shown survival benefit compared to medical therapy and SAVR should not be offered. For patients at high (STS score 8-15%), TAVR was found to be superior at 3 years in the CoreValve trials and non-inferior at 5 years in both the CoreValve and PARTNER trials. For intermediate (STS score 4-8%) and low (STS score <4%) risk, TAVR has been shown to be non-inferior to SAVR at 2 years in the Evolut and PARTNER trials. Risk of permanent pacemaker implantation is higher after TAVR, while risk of bleeding, atrial fibrillation, and re-hospitalization is higher after SAVR. The current patient is likely low surgical risk. In choosing between TAVR vs. SAVR in a 62-year-old low-risk patient, the surgeon should discuss the likelihood of additional procedures over the patient's remaining life span, especially if bioprosthetic SAVR or TAVR is performed. As part of this discussion, valve type and durability should be highlighted.

247

Surgical valve choices include bioprosthetic and mechanical. Patients < 60 years old may benefit from mechanical valves given the lower reintervention rate (up to 98% freedom from reoperation at 25 years) compared with tissue valves. Also, mechanical valves have been associated with superior survival at 15 years follow-up compared to bioprosthetic valves in patients 50 to 70 years old. However, they are associated with a 1-2%/year thromboembolic rate and 1-2%/year bleeding rate from systemic anticoagulation. For older patients (> 70 years old), a bioprosthetic valve offers excellent long-term durability with minimal thromboembolic and bleeding risks (90% freedom from structural valve deterioration [SVD] at 15-25 years). Bioprosthetic valves should be considered in younger patients with a desire to avoid long-term anticoagulation, provided reoperation can be expected with a low mortality rate. If this 62-year-old patient chooses a bioprosthetic SAVR, he should be counseled to expect either a redo surgical operation or a transcatheter valve-in-valve (VIV) operation in 8-15 years. Short-term outcomes of transcatheter VIV procedures have been reported with excellent outcomes if the patient does not have patient-prosthesis mismatch from the primary SAVR. Surgical aortic valve bioprosthesis design and structure will influence the degree of technical difficulty for future VIV procedures. Stentless valves and stented wraparound valves pose additional technical challenges to the operator at the time of VIV implantation. This should be taken into consideration at the time of primary SAVR if a future VIV procedure is anticipated.

Transcatheter valves have shown similar mid-term outcomes and are anticipated to have similar 10-year durability to bioprosthetic surgical valves, though outcomes beyond 10 years are not yet available. The impact of suitability of future TAV-in-TAV based on patient anatomy and the ability to access the coronary arteries for future treatment is unknown and controversial. This consideration is a particularly important component in determining treatment for this 62-year-old low risk patient, for whom multiple future procedures will be necessary if a bioprosthetic valve is implanted at the index procedure. In addition, mid- and long-term durability of TAV-in-SAV and TAV-in-TAV are currently unknown.

Alternative scenarios/treatment decisions

"Cardiac catheterization in the same patient showed 3-vessel, obstructive CAD including a severe proximal LAD lesion."
Patients with concomitant CAD should be evaluated as CABG vs. PCI candidates. In this case, the severe proximal LAD lesion and obstructive 3-vessel disease are an indication for CABG. In assessing CAD, a SYNTAX score > 22 in the setting of 3-vessel disease strongly favors surgery over PCI. If the patient has not yet undergone CT, they should have an aortic protocol gated CT scan performed to assess the aorta prior to surgery. This patient should be counseled on receiving a mechanical vs. bioprosthetic SAVR. Patients opting for mechanical valves should not have contraindication to lifelong anticoagulation and must be socioeconomically capable of anticoagulation therapy.

"In the same patient, TAVR CT shows a Sievers Type 1 functional bicuspid aortic valve with right to left fusion."
In dealing with patients with bicuspid valves, STS risk score is important. For patients with a functional bicuspid valve at low surgical risk, TAVR has not been approved for use. In patients at intermediate surgical risk, it is important to assess for associated ascending aneurysm, which would be a strong indication for surgery if > 4.5 cm. For patients < 65 years of age, patients should be advised there is an approximate 57% of a 2nd procedure, 18% chance for a 3rd procedure, and 2% for a 4th procedure in their lifetime. Therefore, strong consideration should be given for surgery with a mechanical prosthesis or surgical bioprosthetic valve since the outcomes with future TAV-in-SAV are more predictable than TAV-in-TAV. Additionally, future reoperative open surgery will be less complex after a primary SAVR versus TAVR. For patients at high risk without associated aneurysm or CAD and with anatomy suitable for TAVR, shared decision making incorporating patient preference should be prioritized in deciding between TAVR and SAVR. Prohibitive risk patients should undergo TAVR.

248

"An 82-year-old patient with 2-vessel severe, obstructive CAD (RCA & circumflex), severe symptomatic AS, extremely poor functional status, and a 12% STS risk of mortality."

With a 12% risk of mortality, this patient is at high-risk for SAVR and the randomized TAVR trials show the patient would benefit from staged PCI and TAVR procedures. A SYNTAX score < 33 in the setting of 2-vessel disease favors PCI over CABG and should be performed in conjunction with TAVR. However, TAVR CT scan and full work-up should be undertaken to assess anatomic suitability for TAVR, followed by shared decision-making with the patient. If the patient requests surgery, a SAVR + 2-vessel CABG could be performed with a bioprosthetic valve.

"Patient is 78-year-old, ESRD, inactive, EF=30%, and the EOAI is 0.8 with a highly calcified root."

This patient's age, low EF and ESRD will more than likely calculate an STS-PROM in the high-risk category and TAVR would be more appropriate if the anatomy is suitable. If the STS-PROM falls within the intermediate range of risk, then SAVR with a mechanical valve should be considered due to the poor durability of a bioprosthetic valve in ESRD secondary to early calcification.

The resultant EOAI (cm^2/m^2) for SAVR is an important component for this patient and can be determined by sizing the valve, checking the EOA for the valve using the manufacturer published (IFU – Information for Use) chart and dividing the resultant EOA by the patients BSA. An EOAI < 0.85 suggests a small aortic root with the risk of moderate patient prosthesis mismatch (PPM) for EOAI 0.65–0.85, and severe PPM for EOAI < 0.65.

In this patient who is elderly with a poor EF and calcified root, a moderate amount of PPM through SAVR would be preferred over the longer cross-clamp time and technically more challenging aortic root procedure. However, if anatomically acceptable, a TAVR should be favored, since the randomized trials show PPM occurs significantly less for TAVR than SAVR and would minimize the concerns for PPM and the morbidity of SAVR. Patient education and shared decision making is critical for this patient.

"A 70-year-old female undergoing workup for 3V CABG is found to have moderate AS on echo – would you replace the aortic valve at the time of the CABG?"

This scenario represents a Class IIa indication (i.e., weight of evidence is in favor of usefulness). The decision to replace the valve hinges on the risks involved with the added procedure and the benefits of a longer interval free from reintervention. In general, it is prudent to replace moderate AS at the time of CABG for reasonable candidates with minimal comorbidities especially in the setting of a highly calcified valve, fast progression, or patients younger than 70 years of age.

"Patient is 75-year-old asymptomatic with severe aortic stenosis on echo. How would you determine the timing of surgery?"

The prognosis for patients without symptoms is excellent but it falls significantly once symptoms develop. Watchful waiting with medical management including risk factor modification and statin therapy is appropriate for most patients. However, some require surgery based on specific indications and others require additional testing to elicit symptoms. Patient with severe AS unintentionally limit their activity to minimize or eliminate symptoms and it is important to perform a monitored stress test to determine the status of the patients claim of asymptomatic. Patients with atypical or vague symptoms may undergo a stress echo. Inappropriate hemodynamic response, dizziness, or chest discomfort signifies a positive test and provides grounds for AVR.

Immediate indications for surgery in this patient would include: a low gradient (< 40 mmHg) severe AS with LV dysfunction (< 50%) and contractile reserve; critical AS, a velocity of ≥ 5 m/sec or a MVG > 50 mm/Hg; evidence of severe LVH (LV thickness > 1.6 mm); and patients undergoing another open heart procedure (i.e., CABG, mitral valve surgery).

Goals: relieve obstruction, replace the valve, protect the heart and coronaries, and prevent embolization.

- Large bore IV, arterial line, general endotracheal anesthesia (GETA), pulmonary artery catheter (optional), Foley catheter – watch for v-fib on induction.

- Intraoperative TEE to confirm/re-evaluate valve or other unexpected pathology.

- Minimally invasive approach via partial sternotomy or mini thoracotomy as well as full median sternotomy are acceptable approaches. Pericardial stay sutures palpate the aorta or use epiaortic ultrasound to evaluate for calcifications to determine aortic cannulation site.

- Heparin (400 u/kg), aortic cannulation, 2-stage venous cannula, retrograde cardioplegia cannula (not mandatory), once ACT is 400 initiate CPB, dissect aorta from PA, insert antegrade cardioplegia cannula.

- De-air antegrade line, clamp, and run antegrade induction, follow with retrograde. Intermittent doses of retrograde with occasional doses directly down the right coronary (depending on duration and whether good retrograde flow is noted coming from the RCA).

- Venting strategies:
    o LV vent through right superior pulmonary vein
    o LA vent
    o Floppy-tipped pump sucker dropped through the valve into the LV
    o PA vent

- Aortotomy – define the RCA, small transverse aortotomy anterior midline 1 cm above the RCA. Extend laterally towards and superior to the LCA ostium, then medially in an oblique fashion towards the middle of the noncoronary sinus. Place stay sutures as needed.

- Inspect and resect the valve along the annulus.

- Completely debride the calcium from the annulus, patch or primary closure of any defects with autologous pericardium, irrigate copiously and size the valve. When sizing the valve, check the EOA for the specific chosen valve type using the manufacturer published IFU chart and dividing the resultant EOA by the patients BSA to evaluate for PPM.

- Place horizontal mattress sutures along the annulus (2-0 braided pledgeted (infra-annular), unpledgeted mattress, or figure-of-eight stitches).

- Pass them through the valve ring, seat the valve.

- Check the pledgets, LCA ostium, RCA ostium.

- Tie the valve down under the left coronary ostium, then the right ostium, and make sure both coronary ostia are patent prior to completion of tying.

- Irrigate, check LCA and RCA ostium again, and close the aortotomy with a running prolene suture.

- De-air by valsalva and compressing the heart prior to closing the aortotomy, assess rhythm, pacing wires, wean from CPB, assess the valve by TEE.

"The patient has v-fib on induction."
Secure the airway and ventilation, initiate CPR immediately, assistant preps while you scrub. Drape, give heparin, and perform an emergent median sternotomy. Aortic and venous cannulation. Initiate cardiopulmonary bypass (CPB), assess flows and drainage, and proceed with AVR. Alternatively, you can initiate immediate percutaneous femoral CPB to immediately perfuse all organs, assess flows and drainage, and proceed with AVR.

"You are unable to arrest the heart."

250

A slow arrest is not uncommon in a hypertrophied heart. Go systematically down your algorithm for persistent activity – check the cross clamp to ensure you are completely across, check your drainage (distention, elevated pulmonary artery pressures) and improve it if necessary (a pre-clamp LV vent through the right superior pulmonary vein is advantageous in avoiding this issue). AI may be underestimated by echo. When in doubt or if AI is suspected open the aorta and give direct ostial cardioplegia. Add topical ice, consider systemic cooling to mild-mod hypothermia (30° C).

"The intraoperative TEE shows a moderate perivalvular leak."
Define the anatomy on TEE carefully, clamp, arrest, open the aorta and reassess the valve, if you identify an obvious gap you can place a horizontal pledgeted suture or be prepared to remove and replace the valve. Be certain that complete decalcification of the annulus is achieved prior to inserting the valve since retained calcium can lead to not properly seating the valve causing para-valvular leak. Consider the patient's condition. A trivial leak in an 85-*year-old* patient should probably be left alone.

"When you release the cross clamp, the heart distends."
Most often this occurs in the setting of paravalvular leak. With a mechanical valve the washing jet AI may be enough to distend the heart if it fibrillates. Turn flow down, compress the heart, defibrillate, or place a vent and defibrillate. If the heart remains asystolic and distended after defibrillation, place epicardial pacing wires and begin pacing. This issue can usually be avoided by placing an LV vent prior to the initial cross-clamp. If unable to obtain a rhythm the possibilities include electrolyte abnormality such as hyperkalemia or poor protection. If unable to restore rhythm with the heart empty, clamp and re-arrest the heart (see chapter on CPB pitfalls).

"You determine that only a 19 mm St Jude Biocor will fit into this patient. The EOAI assuming a BSA of 2.2 m^2 is 0.59. What are your options?"
Options include upsizing with a stentless root (if familiar with this technique), root enlargement, total root replacement, or acceptance of PPM with a valve that yields the greatest EOA. In this patient with relatively good quality tissue and few comorbidities the longer clamp time is likely worth the added EOA.

- *Root enlargement procedure - Nick's procedure*: Extend the aortotomy into the nadir of the noncoronary sinus and base of the anterior mitral leaflet with the goal of obtaining a size that is 1 or 2 increments larger than the original. Use autologous pericardium (or other commercially available products i.e. CorMatrix, Perigaurd) to patch and enlarge the opening. Place sutures along the left and right coronary sinuses as usual. Seat the valve. Pass non-pledgeted sutures outside in through the patch and into the sewing ring for the non-coronary portion and tie. Complete the aortic closure with the patch.

- *Root enlargement procedure - Manouguian procedure*: Another enlargement alternative whereby the aortotomy is extended posteriorly through the commissure between the left and non-coronary cusps into the interleaflet triangle and carried into the anterior leaflet of the mitral valve. The left atrium is opened in this process and must be closed as well.

- *Total root replacement*: Root replacement with a homograft or a stentless bioprosthesis with upsizing and coronary reimplantation. You can usually place a larger homograft/stentless root than a standard bioprosthetic/mechanical valve and the hemodynamics are better. However, a mechanical valve total root may be favorable in a younger patient. If anticoagulation is contraindicated or not preferred, then perform a stentless or a homemade stented bioprosthetic root replacement, which may be more amenable to future VIV procedures.

"You take your Nick's annular enlargement too far into the anterior leaflet of the mitral valve and the patient has moderate MR on TEE after coming off pump"

Examine the mitral carefully on TEE, clamp, re-arrest the heart, expose the mitral valve through either the left atrium or right atrium and transseptal approach, and make every effort to repair the mitral valve. While the Nick's annular enlargement allows an increase by more than one valve size, its main risk is extending too far on the anterior mitral leaflet. For surgeons not comfortable with the Nick's or Manouguian annulus enlargement procedures or for very small EOAIs, a total root replacement may be a safer option.

Pearls/pitfalls

- Replace symptomatic severe AS (velocity $\geq$ 4 m/s, mean $\geq$ 40 mmHg, AVA $\leq$ 1.0 cm^2, indexed AVA $\leq$ 0.6 cm^2/m^2, dimensionless index < 0.25).
- Replace asymptomatic severe AS only IF low gradient with < 50% EF, critical AS (velocity $\geq$ 5 m/sec or MPG $\geq$ 50 mm/Hg), severe LVH, concomitant cardiac operation, fast progression, severely calcified.
- Determination of SAVR vs. TAVR by anatomy, concomitant pathology, patient age, and patient preference
- Patients > 70-*year-old* – generally bioprosthetic SAVR or TAVR rather than mechanical SAVR
- Assess the aorta intraoperatively for calcifications that may change clamp/CPB strategy.
- Irrigate debris and check the LCA and RCA ostia after seating the valve.
- Patient-prosthesis mismatch (PPM) – EOAI < 0.85 $\rightarrow$ consider root enlargement procedure or total aortic root replacement.

Suggested readings

- Brzezinski A, Koprivanac M, Gillinov A, Mihaljevic T. Pathophysiology of Aortic Valve Disease. In: Cohn LH, Adams DH, editors. Cardiac Surgery in the Adult, 5e New York, NY: McGraw-Hill; 2018. Chapter 26.
- Al-Atassi T, El Khoury G, Boodhwani M. Surgical Treatment of Aortic Valve Disease. In: Selke FW, del Nido PJ, and Swanson SJ, editors. Sabiston and Spencer Surgery of the Chest, 9e Philadelphia, PA: Elsevier; 2016. p. 1334-1349.
- Diaz R, Hernandez-Vaquero D, Alvarez-Cabo R, Avanzas P, et al. Long-term outcomes of mechanical versus biological aortic valve prosthesis: Systematic review and meta-analysis. J Thorac Cardiovasc Surg 2019 Sep;158(3):706-714.
- Duncan A, Moat N, Simonato M, de Weger A, et al. Outcomes Following Transcatheter Aortic Valve Replacement for Degenerative Stentless Versus Stented Bioprostheses. JACC Cardiovasc Interv 2019 Jul 8;12(13):1256-1263.
- Ranganath NK, Koeckert MS, Smith DE, Hisamoto K, et al. Aggressive tissue aortic valve replacement in younger patients and the risk of re-replacement: Implications from microsimulation analysis. J Thorac Cardiovasc Surg 2019 Jul;158(1):39-45.
- Rahhab Z, El Faquir N, Tchetche D, Delgado V, et al. Expanding the indications for transcatheter aortic valve implantation. Nat Rev Cardiol 2019 Sep 16. [Epub ahead of print]

40. AORTIC VALVE REGURGITATION

Bogdan A. Kindzelski, MD, MS and Douglas R. Johnston, MD

Adapted from 1st edition chapter written by Juan G. Penaranda, MD, and Harold M. Burkhart, MD

Concept

- Diagnosis of severe aortic regurgitation
- Indications for aortic valve replacement and repair
- Preoperative Considerations
- Operative Strategy
- Transcatheter options
- Pearls/pitfalls

Chief complaint

"A 64-year-old man with known aortic valve regurgitation has been followed by his local cardiologist for the last 5 years. On echocardiogram this year there is severe aortic valve regurgitation with an ejection fraction of 45%, a left ventricular end-systolic dimension (LVESD) of 50 mm and a left ventricular end diastolic dimension (LVEDD) of 65 mm."

Differential

The diagnosis has been revealed to you. Rule out other concomitant valvular pathology or coronary artery disease, which may change your approach.

History and physical

Focused history to establish presence of symptoms and functional class is the first step. Ask about symptoms such as exertional dyspnea, syncope, orthopnea, paroxysmal nocturnal dyspnea, angina, and palpitations. Ask about prior history of endocarditis, rheumatic fever, aortic dissection, trauma, congenital valve anomalies such as bicuspid aortic valve to help determine the etiology of the AR. Focused cardiopulmonary physical exam to document the presence of diastolic and systolic murmurs, displaced apical impulse, signs of CHF or pulmonary edema, widened pulse pressure and its classic peripheral signs (water-hammer, Quincke Pulse, Duroziez sign).

Tests

- *EKG*: may reveal left ventricular (LV) hypertrophy and/or arrhythmias.
- *CXR*: an enlarged cardiac silhouette may suggest LV dilation or aortic root enlargement.
  - *Echocardiography*. Confirms the diagnosis, assess the etiology of AR and assess valve morphology, provide semiquantitative and quantitative estimates of AR severity, assess LV dimensions, mass, and systolic function and assess aortic root size. Most commonly the AI is graded as 1-mild, 2-moderate, 3-moderately severe 4-severe. In addition, echo is critical to assess valve morphology. In particular bicuspid morphology is generally more amenable to repair, especially with more normal sized roots. The jet direction in these patients is critical
- *Coronary angiography*: to be done in patients with significant risk factors for coronary artery disease or those older than 40 years of age in whom aortic valve replacement (AVR) is considered. Rule out or identify any coronary anomalies that may alter your cardioplegia strategy and/or require root replacement techniques.
- Cardiac catheterization with root angiography and measurement of LV pressures is indicated when echocardiograms are inconclusive or discordant with physical findings.
- *CT scan*: optional test, however if echo demonstrates any signs of aortopathy or in younger patients with concern for connective tissue disorder or bicuspid valve, then this test is critical to assess the presence of concomitant aortic root pathology or

dissection. In older patients with calcium noted on echo, CT can determine the extent of calcium burden (porcelain aorta) and whether there is a safe area to crossclamp. CT should also be considered in patients who may be considered for minimally invasive aortic valve surgery. CT should be considered mandatory prior to revision sternotomy.

- *Cardiac MR*: optional test, allows for evaluation and quantification of aortic regurgitation and its impact on LV function as well as aortic root and ascending aorta pathology. Especially useful in the presence of suboptimal echocardiograms.
- *Exercise testing*: valuable in assessing functional capacity in patients with minimal or equivocal symptoms.

Index scenario (additional information)

"This patient denies any exertional dyspnea, orthopnea, paroxysmal nocturnal dyspnea, chest pain; he revealed a previous syncopal episode 40 years ago. Past medical history is remarkable for hypertension and COPD. On physical exam there is a displaced apical impulse and a grade IV/VI diastolic murmur in the mid left sternal edge and a wide pulse pressure. EKG demonstrates NSR with non-specific intraventricular conduction delay. CXR reveals cardiomegaly. Echocardiogram demonstrates ejection fraction of 45%, severe aortic valve regurgitation with regurgitant volume of 77cc, LVEDD is 65 mm LVESD is 50 mm, mild tricuspid and mitral regurgitation, with max aortic root and ascending aorta dimensions of 40 and 38 mm, respectively. There is no evidence of abscess, vegetation, or dissection. A CT scan was not performed because his creatinine was 1.8 and the echocardiographic findings did not suggest aortic root pathology. What are the treatment options at this time and how do you counsel the patient regarding valve option?"

Treatment/management

Surgical management of AR most commonly involves aortic valve replacement (AVR). In highly selected patients, an aortic valve repair by an experienced surgeon at a high-volume center may be an option. Note: See the general recommendations regarding valve choices in the aortic stenosis chapter. Aortic root pathology is discussed in other chapters (Aneurysmal disease and Dissections). Severe AR is defined as by the following echocardiographic/angiographic parameters:

- Jet width ≥ 65% of LVOT;
- Vena contracta > 0.6 cm;
- Holodiastolic flow reversal in the proximal abdominal aorta
- Regurgitant volume ≥ 60 mL/beat;
- Regurgitant fraction ≥ 50%;
- Effective regurgitant orifice ≥ 0.3 cm2;
- Angiography grade 3+ to 4+;
- In addition, diagnosis of chronic severe AR requires evidence of LV dilation

Considerations should include: size of root, possible reimplantation, bicuspid valve and potential for repair.

According to AHA/ACC 2014 Guidelines, indications for AV replacement/repair for chronic AR include:

- *Class I*
    - Symptomatic patients with evidence of severe AR
    - Asymptomatic severe AR with LV dysfunction (LVEF < 50%)
    - Asymptomatic severe AR while undergoing other cardiac surgery.
- *Class IIa*
    - Asymptomatic severe AR with normal LVEF (≥50%) and with evidence of dilated left ventricle LVESD > 50mm

- Progressive AR (Vena contracta $\leq$ 0.6cm, RVol < 60ml/beat, RF < 50%, ERO <0.3cm^2) undergoing other cardiac surgery
- *Class IIb*
  - Asymptomatic severe AR with normal LVEF ($\geq$50%) and with evidence of dilated left ventricle LVEDD > 65mm in a low risk surgical candidate

Importantly, there is ongoing discussion to decrease the LVESD cutoff in patients with asymptomatic severe AR due to better post-operative outcome and LV remodeling in those who undergo earlier surgery. Other echocardiographic parameters, such as left ventricular global longitudinal strain, have shown prognostic value and benefit in targeting patients with earlier surgery, improving outcomes.

Operative steps
Aortic valve replacement
The surgical steps for aortic valve replacement for aortic regurgitation are similar to those for aortic stenosis (see chapter Aortic Stenosis), although a few considerations should be mentioned.

- *CPB and myocardial protection.* Any degree of AI carries the risk of distention once if the heart fibrillates. This is especially true for severe AI. Therefore, cooling should never be begun until the aorta is freed for crossclamp and retrograde cardioplegia access is obtained You will rarely get arrest with antegrade. Thus, an LV vent for decompression during CPB may be considered, room to clamp the aorta, room for the aortotomy and retrograde cardioplegia access should all be ensured in the event that the heart distends during CPB. The same applies for circulatory arrest cases or any case where a patient has even moderate AI. Direct ostial coronary delivery is an option once the aorta has been crossclamped and the aortotomy performed.

- *Exposure.* An LV vent catheter can be considered and helps to keep the operative field dry and prevent distention. Other options include placement of a pulmonary artery vent or simply use a pump sucker across the aortic valve into the left ventricle.

- *Aortotomy.* Usually an oblique aortotomy towards the middle of the non-coronary sinus will provide adequate exposure. It will also allow aortic root enlargement if needed. In the cases where the ascending aorta needs to be replaced, the aorta should be transected just above the sinotubular junction. Transverse aortotomy, preserving the sinotubular junction, should be used when the plan is valve repair.

Potential questions/alternative scenarios
"The heart continues to eject and begins to distend shortly after initiating CPB."
Prior to initiating bypass make sure you are ready for the possibility of ventricular distention. If this occurs, you will need to arrest the heart immediately. Prior to initiating CPB, establish retrograde cardioplegia access. If there is a question about the location of the retrograde catheter then be prepared for direct retrograde insertion which requires bicaval (IVC and SVC) cannulation from the onset. After establishing retrograde make room for the aortic cross clamp and identify a reasonable site for your aortotomy. Now initiate CPB. Next, cross clamp the aorta and give induction cardioplegia through the retrograde catheter. In order to vent during this phase of induction, turn on the aortic root vent (assuming you had time to place it) or make the aortotomy. Once the retrograde is complete, finish the aortotomy, identify the coronary ostia carefully and give induction cardioplegia directly down the coronaries. For the remainder of the case give retrograde every 15-20 minutes or alternate between retrograde and direct ostial perfusion as you wish.

"The retrograde cannot be established or the position is questionable."
Cannulate the IVC and SVC separately. Make room for the aortic cross clamp and identify your aortotomy site. Once CPB is initiated, place the LV vent, clamp, make the aortotomy and give direct cardioplegia down the ostia. With the heart arrested, snare the SVC and IVC,

make a right atriotomy and place the retrograde catheter directly in just past the opening of the coronary sinus. Continue induction cardioplegia through the retrograde. Direct retrograde can also be established prior to cross clamping and this is desirable if heart function is poor or there is any question about placement of the retrograde.

"During placement of the retrograde catheter you get dark blood behind the heart. You confirm a small coronary sinus perforation. How is your cardioprotection scheme altered?"
Retrograde will be unreliable in this setting. The safest option is to initiate CPB, clamp and give ostial cardioplegia throughout the case. If the operation is lengthy you might consider small coronary catheters for intermittent perfusion without having to pause for the handheld perfusion catheters every 15 minutes. Coronary sinus perforation should be repaired using a patch.

"Intraoperative transesophageal echocardiogram shows a tricuspid aortic valve with prolapse of the right cusp. After making the aortotomy and inspecting the valve you confirmed the TEE findings. What are your surgical options at this time?"
Aortic valve replacement with a mechanical valve or bioprosthesis is the safest answer in this scenario. Aortic valve repair can be performed for a variety of aortic valvular pathologies. Techniques entail commissural figure-of-8 suspension sutures, cusp repair with commissuroplasty, free-margin plication or resection, annulus repair with resuspension, cusp tailoring or replacement of the cusp with autologous pericardium, and root reimplantation or remodeling for annuloaortic ectasia. Isolated cusp perforations can be repaired with an autologous pericardial patch. A CLASS (Commissure, Leaflet [cusps], Annulus, Sinus, Sinutubular junction) scheme should be used when assessing the aortic valve apparatus intraoperatively, subsequently performing the indicated repair. Importantly, calcified or stenosed aortic valves are difficult to repair and have a higher chance of residual AR. Repair techniques should only be utilized by surgeons with extensive experience at high volume-valve centers. Studies have shown similar early mortality and morbidity compared to conventional valve replacement with approximately 10% of patients requiring reoperation at 10 years. Furthermore, not requiring anticoagulation for mechanical prostheses, is an added benefit for younger patients in whom a bioprostheses may provide limited durability.

"Patient fibrillates and arrests while cannulating the right atrium. You attempt to defibrillate but the heart dilates, and you are unable to cardiovert back into sinus rhythm."
Quickly institute cardiopulmonary bypass, empty out and defibrillate. If unable to empty out due to severe AI, cross clamp and open the aorta. Decompress the heart with a sucker through the aortic valve and localize the coronary ostia to give antegrade cardioplegia with an ostial cannula. Once heart is arrested, perform the aortic valve replacement.

"After AVR, you are unable to close the aortotomy secondary to the large prosthesis putting tension on the aortotomy suture line."
The aortotomy should be closed utilizing a bovine or autologous pericardial patch to insure no tension on the suture line.

"You remove the aortic cross clamp and immediately notice that the left ventricle dilates. There is significant ventricular ejection while trying to come off bypass and once you are off bypass the pulse pressure is significantly wide. What would you do at this point? The TEE shows severe periprosthetic regurgitation with reversal of flow in the descending aorta, the regurgitant jet is coming from the noncoronary sinus. How do you manage this situation?"
Peri-prosthetic leaks should be dealt with in the operating room. It is important to differentiate prosthetic versus peri-prosthetic regurgitation. It is vital to quantify and localize the leak as this will dictate your approach. Leaks from the non-coronary sinus may be amenable to direct suture repair while other locations may require removing the prosthesis in order to fix the problem.

"You go back on pump, arrest the heart and reopen the aorta. There is a small gap in the non-coronary sinus after probing and inspecting the valve. You are able to place an everting mattress suture from outside of the aorta into the sewing cuff solving the problem. As you finish your case your chief resident calls you from the other operating room. He had done a mitral valve repair with a triangular resection and a complete annuloplasty ring. As he came off bypass, he noticed severe aortic valve regurgitation on TEE. The jet appears to be originating from the left coronary cusp on short axis view. He is puzzled and wants your advice."

Aortic regurgitation is an uncommon but known complication from mitral valve procedures. The aortic valve cusps can be entrapped with the sutures used for the mitral repair/replacement. TEE can help diagnose this problem in the operating room.

"You go back on CPB and arrest the heart; you open the aorta with an oblique incision and notice the left cusp has been retracted with an annuloplasty stitch. You then reopen the left atrium, cut the offending suture, and place one more annuloplasty stitch avoiding the aortic valve. Before closing the left atrium, your final inspection of the aortic valve revealed an intact valve. You close the aorta and come off bypass. TEE shows trivial aortic and mitral regurgitation.

A 77-year-old male with symptomatic, native AR presents to your clinic for possible surgical intervention. His PMH is significant for HTN, HPL, COPD on 2L of O2, ESRD on hemodialysis, and significant calcifications in the ascending and descending aorta noted on CT scan. He was deemed a nonsurgical candidate at an outside institution. Is there an alternative option for this patient?

SAVR remains the gold standard in patients with native AR, however TAVR has been shown to be a potential option for nonsurgical candidates with symptomatic AR. Nonetheless, for patients with AR, the lack of extensive valvular or annular calcification presents challenges to transcatheter approaches. In these patients, a self-expanding prosthesis is used due to larger annular sizes and lack of calcification. TAVR for native AR has been shown to be effective in the short term at reducing AR and improving quality of life in nonsurgical candidates, albeit with the tradeoff of a significantly higher 30-day mortality rate (10-13%) compared with TAVR utilized for AS patients.

Pearls/pitfalls

- Replace or repair the aortic valve in the setting of severe AR if symptoms are present or there is evidence of LV dysfunction or LV dilatation (LVEDD 6.5 cm or LVESD 5 cm). Delaying surgery compromises outcomes
- Anticipate how AI can alter your cardioprotection strategy. Ensure retrograde access. Cardioplegia directly down the coronary ostia is an alternative.
- Prior to initiating bypass be prepared for LV distention. Make room to clamp the aorta, identify your aortotomy site, establish retrograde cardioplegia and anticipate the need for an LV vent. Have ostial plegia catheters available.
- Concomitant root pathology (> 4.5-5 cm) should be addressed in good surgical candidates at the time of the operation.
- Aortic valve repair techniques include commissural figure-of-8 suspension sutures, cusp repair with commissuroplasty, free-margin plication or resection, annulus repair with resuspension, and root reimplantation and can provide similar results as conventional AVR without the need for anticoagulation when done at high volume valve centers.
- Symptomatic acute aortic regurgitation should be taken care of expeditiously since the ventricle has not had time to develop any adaptation to overcome the increased volume load. This may lead to rapid clinical decompensation.
- TAVR with a self-expanding bioprosthesis may be considered as an option in selected patients with AR who have no surgical options

257

Suggested readings

- Nishimura RA, Otto CM, Bonow RO, et al. 2014 AHA/ACC Guideline for the Management of Patients with Valvular Heart Disease: A Report of the American College of Cardiology/American Heart Association Task Force on Practice Guidelines. *J Am Coll Cardiol* 2014;63:e57
- Anwaruddin S, Desai ND, Szeto WY, et al. Self-Expanding Valve System for Treatment of Native Aortic Regurgitation by Transcatheter Aortic Valve Implantation (from the STS/ACC TVT Registry). Am J Cardiol. 2019.
- Dujardin KS, Enriquez Sarano M, Schaff HV et al. Mortality and morbidity of aortic regurgitation in clinical practice: a long term follow up study. *Circulation* 1999;99:1851-1857.Ducharme A, Courval JF, Dore A, Leclerc Y, Tardiff JC. Severe Aortic Regurgitation immediately after Mitral Valve Annuloplasty. *Ann Thorac Surg* 1999;67:1487-89.
- Yang L.-T., Michelena H.I., Scott C.G., et al: Outcomes in chronic hemodynamically significant aortic regurgitation and limitations of current guidelines. J Am Coll Cardiol 2019; 73: pp. 1741-1752
- Zeeshan A, Idrees JJ, Johnston DR, et al. Durability of Aortic Valve Cusp Repair With and Without Annular Support. Ann Thorac Surg. 2018;105:739-74
- Anwaruddin S, Desai ND, Szeto WY, et al. Self-Expanding Valve System for Treatment of Native Aortic Regurgitation by Transcatheter Aortic Valve Implantation (from the STS/ACC TVT Registry). Am J Cardiol. 2019.

41. REOPERATIVE AORTIC VALVE REPLACEMENT

J Hunter Mehaffey, MD, and Kenan W Yount, MD

Adapted from 1st edition chapter written by *Leora Yarboro, MD, and John A. Kern, MD*

Concept

- Discuss the common indications and preoperative workup for Redo AVR
- Operative Planning including Surgical vs. Transcatheter Approach
- Potential pitfalls and management

Chief complaint

"A 65-year-old man with history of prior aortic valve replacement now presents with dyspnea on exertion."

Differential

The differential in this patient includes structural valve disease, endocarditis, valve thrombus or pannus formation, coronary artery disease, and primary pulmonary disorders such as progressive COPD. Certain conditions such as bicuspid aortic valve, rheumatic disease, young age at the time of replacement with a bioprosthetic valve, and endocarditis can lead to early native valve failure. Stented pericardial valves tend to fail by aortic stenosis of the biologic prosthesis and tend to last longer than porcine valve. Smaller valves resulting in patient-prosthesis mismatch (size < 23 mm or EOAI < 0.85) show trends of earlier re-stenosis and limit future options for valve-in-valve transcatheter approaches. Stentless valves (*e.g.*, Toronto valve) have largely fallen out of favor because of early deterioration; in these cases, the mechanism is usually insufficiency rather than stenosis. Although structural valve deterioration is rare for mechanical valves, mechanical valves in the aortic position may still fail due to endocarditis, pannus formation, stroke, or intolerance of anticoagulation. Although mechanical valves have generally been favored for patients < 55 years-old, they do limit a patient's lifestyle and future TAVR options.

History and physical

A focused cardiopulmonary history and exam is important. Focus on surgical scars and prior vein harvest sites. Listen for new murmurs, JVD and assess femoral and pedal pulses as this may be important in determining alternative cannulation strategies. Determining a patient's risk and life goals are important given that the mean 30-day mortality after redo AVR approaches 7.1%. Compared to TAVR, redo AVR is associated with a lower incidence of vascular complications and perivalvular leak at the expense of a higher short-term stroke rate, atrial fibrillation burden, AKI, and major bleeding. As transcatheter technologies develop, the risk-benefit analysis associated with this decision is likely to change.

Tests

- TTE (May consider TEE if concern for endocarditis)
- Coronary imaging
    - Look for coronary artery disease that may require CABG; also look for any ostial left or right coronary disease)
    - Fluoroscopy study if concern for mechanical valve thrombus/pannus
- CTA chest/abdomen/pelvis
    - Looking for transcatheter options, root size, STJ width, coronary heights, and access options. These measurements may also help carefully plan a redo open AVR if necessary.
    - For patients going on for redo open AVR, important to access femoral access in case cardiopulmonary bypass is required prior to redo sternotomy or emergently. Also assess for any concomitant aneurysmal disease.

- o Standard review of anatomic proximity to bone for redo (innominate vein, aorta, RA, RV).
- o For patients with endocarditis, can help clarify the extent of a root abscess (determining whether bovine patch or homograft may be required) or aorto-mitral curtain involvement.
- Carotid duplex
- Pulmonary function testing (PFTs)
- Vein mapping (if previous CABG)
- U/A & blood cultures
- Lab: CBC, BMP, LDH (hemolysis), renal insufficiency, T&C
- Obtain previous operative note
    - When was the last operation?
    - What was the manufacturer and size of the last valve?
    - What exactly was the procedure? Was there a root enlargement or other root procedure performed?
    - History of previous CABG? What were the conduits? Do the conduits cross the sternal midline?

Index scenario (additional information)

"Patient has isolated aortic regurgitation on TTE with no significant coronary artery disease."

The next step is to decide whether the patient would best be suited for valve-in-valve TAVR or redo AVR. Early complication rates from valve-in-valve (ViV) TAVR are acceptable and lower than what would be predicted for redo AVR. The durability of ViV TAVR remains to be determined. The above testing and a heart team evaluation will help make the decision. Endocarditis is an absolute contraindication to TAVR. Mechanical valves preclude ViV TAVR.

If the patient had a prior bioprosthetic valve, it is important to know what the initial gradient was leaving the OR and what the gradients were during the first 1-2 years after the first AVR. If the gradients were always high, then it indicates the patient may have had too small of a valve placed during the index AVR and that they would not be an optimal candidate for ViV TAVR; instead, they may need a redo AVR with a root enlargement. Other flags for caution for ViV TAVR may increase the risk of possible coronary obstruction include inadequate or effaced sinuses, low coronary heights (*e.g.*, < 10 mm), or a prior surgical valve in which the leaflets are on the outside of the frame rather than the inside of the frame (*e.g.*, St. Jude Trifecta). While there is technology to reduce the risk of coronary obstruction in these scenarios, patients at high risk for coronary obstruction need to have a compelling reason not to proceed with redo AVR.

Prior bioprosthetic valves < 23 mm are challenging in that they may require the smallest size TAVR valve to be placed inside of them or they require fracturing of the surgical valve (via high pressure balloon dilation). Again, while such maneuvers have been performed successfully, if you are considering putting in the smallest available TAVR valve or fracturing a prior SAVR valve, then the patient must have a compelling reason not to proceed with redo AVR. Similar technical challenges for ViV TAVR include a narrow STJ or a small root.

One important footnote is that the labelled size of surgical bioprosthetic valve refer to the external diameter of the sewing ring—thus the landing zone of the native valve annulus measured by the surgeon at the time of initial AVR. However, for ViV TAVR, the internal diameter of the sewing ring, the struts, and the leaflets is the more relevant dimension because the TAVR valve is being landed inside (rather than outside) the old surgical valve. The internal diameters of prior SAVR valves can be found from various industry sources and mobile apps, but prior SAVR internal diameter must always be confirmed by CTA or TEE; operative notes notoriously have errors. Fortunately, many patients carry a card in their wallet with the surgical valve information.

Finally, if the prior bioprosthetic valve has failed due to AI rather than AS, then there needs to be a compelling reason not to proceed with redo AVR as currently approved TAVR systems are designed for AS rather than primary AI, although some systems that target AI are under investigation. Finally, other considerations for deciding on ViV TAVR vs redo AVR include the patient's access options, concomitant pathology (e.g., co-existing aneurysm > 5.5 cm, multivessel CAD better treated with CABG), age and life-expectancy. All patients being evaluating for ViV TAVR vs redo AVR deserve careful consideration by a multidisciplinary heart team.

By the same token, there are several risk factors that should lead on to strongly consider ViV TAVR over redo AVR if the former is feasible. These include older age (e.g., > 75-80 years-old) prior CABG with patent LIMA (especially if near the sternum), heart failure with reduced ejection fraction (HFrEF), poor conditioning, calcified ascending aorta, and renal failure. Such risk factors can severely affect the early and long-term survival and recovery from redo AVR.

It is debated whether self-expanding valves or balloon expandable valves are best for ViV TAVR, although there is some bias in real world practice for self-expanding valves in ViV scenarios. First, self-expanding valves have slightly more favorable post-TAVR gradients, which is important given that the valve area is being reduced by putting a valve inside a valve. Second, the higher pacemaker risk of self-expanding TAVR valves is less of a concern for ViV procedures since the conduction system is somewhat protected by the old bioprosthetic valve. Third, the aorta may be calcified in redo settings and thus the self-expanding valve may be less likely to traumatize a root that is calcified; this is also important if there is any concomitant aneurysm or if a root enlargement procedure was performed during the index TAVR. Fourth, self-expanding valves do not require rapid pacing for deployment, which may be relevant if the patient has a sicker ventricle due to recurrent AS. One caveat to these biases is that the taller nitinol stent in the current iterations of self-expanding valves (e.g., Evolut R & Evolut Pro) may complicate future coronary access if the patient has CAD.

In conclusion, at present, redo AVR remains the treatment of choice for younger patients at low surgical risk with severe structural valve deterioration.

Operative steps
- Perioperative monitoring
  - TEE, PA catheter, cerebral oximetry, Foley with temp probe, arterial line, R2 pads.
  - Review CT scan for areas of concern – proximity of aorta/right ventricle/innominate vein/atrium/grafts. Check for excessive ascending aortic calcification.
  - Prep legs in case of coronary injury and need for vein.
  - As with any AS case, the scrub nurse should be ready to go and the fellow/attending should be in the room and ready to quickly start given hemodynamic instability.
- Cannulation
  - Develop a plan for potential alternate cannulation sites – axillary vs. femoral
    - Be sure to at least prep in the right axillary access site during draping.
    - While it is not always necessary, it is probably safest practice to either have the femoral vessels exposed, or percutaneous wire access in case of

emergency <u>prior to opening the sternum</u>. At the very minimum, small (4F) sheaths should be placed in the femoral vessels.

- Be able to discuss which patients you would go on bypass for prior to opening the sternum (*i.e.*, CT scan demonstrates live grafts in close proximity to sternum or previous aortic injury on entry). A reasonable approach would be the following:
  - *Structures a safe distance away*: expose the femoral vessels or access percutaneously prior to sternotomy (if you injure something you can heparinize and cannulate).
  - *Structures in proximity*: Depending on cannulation strategy (axillary vs. femoral), have vessels ready to go (wires in, graft sewn, etc). This can be done using small doses of heparin.
  - *Critical grafts under the sternum, aorta close to the sternum, high PA pressures with RV close to sternum*: go on bypass vein prior to sternotomy (if you injure something you can empty out and even drop flows as needed) - the main drawback to fully heparinizing and cannulating prior to the dissection is bleeding. One area of discussion/debate is whether to cool here. Cooling can result in fibrillation (~28-32C) which can be difficult to deal with in a redo with an undissected heart.
  - *Calcified aorta*: refer to porcelain aorta chapter.
  - o Other reasons to cannulate peripherally electively prior to or after sternotomy deal with "real estate" - usually the ascending aorta can be safely cannulated distal or lateral to the prior cannulation site, but if you do not have enough room because of live grafts or it proves too hazardous to expose then cannulate the axillary artery/fem artery. If the atrium is stuck, then proceed to femoral venous or (if additional drainage needed) bicaval cannulation.
- Myocardialprotection
  - o Prefernces vary but some combination of anterograde, retrograde and ostial cardioplegia. If you abandon a retrograde catheter, you will be limited to repeated handheld doses unless you use longer duration (*e.g.*, del Nido) cardioplegia. If due to adhesions you cannot dissect enough of the heart out to confirm retrograde catheter placement, there is always the option to directly place it (which requires bicaval cannulation).
    - *Aortic insufficiency* further necessitates both retrograde cardioplegia to obtain arrest and an LV vent to prevent distension. If there is no or minimal AI, an LV vent is not needed, but other options to facilitate a bloodless field include a PA vent or simply using a Ross tip pump sucker across the aortic valve into the LV.
  - o Cool to 32-34°C.
- Dissection
  - Dissect out the right atrium and ascending aorta for cannulation
  - Heparinize, cannulate, clamp, arrest.
  - Previous aortotomy site may be calcified. Open just proximal or distal to it. The prior operative note may indicate whether the prior aortotomy was lower or higher than desired for optimal exposure. Excise valve sharply using a Kocher to help stabilize the valve. Remove all sutures with blade. Use a freer-elevator to gently remove valve. Vigilantly identify and remove all pledgets. Examine the root after removal for any inadvertent injury.

262

- Valve
  - Size annulus after debriding pannus. Determine whether root enlargement or repair is necessary with a bovine suture. If a bovine patch is needed, it may be more prudent to take bites outside to inside the aorta such that any pledgets around the patch end up outside the aorta rather than inside the aorta. Place annular sutures and tie down valve.
- Close aortotomy
- Place pacing wires (consider a-wires if complete heart block)
- Post-op
  - Redo AVRs have significantly longer operative, bypass and cross clamp times. Consequently, they may have variable degrees of vasoplegia and cardiogenic shock requiring resuscitation. They also have higher rates of heart block so make sure you have well placed and reliable wires.

Potential questions/alternative scenarios
"Patient fibrillates during initial dissection."
- Two things that cause this include bovie electrocautery and CPB with an incompetent valve. Thus, preoperative planning for this scenario is critical, particularly if you know the patient has at least moderate AI.
  - Have external defibrillator pads on the patient prior to prepping. If you do fibrillate prior to having the heart dissected, shock with external pads at 100-200 Joules.
  - Try to avoid going on CPB until the heart is dissected out. Try to avoid electrocautery near the LV during the initial dissection until you are ready to go on pump and arrest. Keep cautery low (<45).
  - If the patient becomes hemodynamically unstable, cannulate (centrally or peripherally) and go on pump immediately. If the heart then distends, decompress manually or with an LV vent until you are able to clamp and arrest.
  - Ideally, an LV vent could be placed through the RSPV. However, in an emergent scenario (when the heart distends and defibrillates before you have the heart dissected out) options include (1) stabbing LV apex (if enough exposed) or (2) clamping the aorta and performing an aortotomy combined with direct handheld cardioplegia to achieve arrest.

"Patient with previous CABG."
Preoperative cardiac catheterization is crucial in these patients.
- If a prior LIMA is patent, have the choice to keep it patent and use frequent antegrade and retrograde cardioplegia and consider cooling the patient to 28-30°C. If you choose to clamp the LIMA, do not risk injuring it during your dissection. If you absolutely had to reduce LIMA flow for myocardial protection, from the left pleural space you can place a tonsil across all tissue where the LIMA is expected to be and that may be enough to slow down the flow, obviating the need to specifically isolate and clamp it. You must be ready to clamp and arrest prior to attempting patent LIMA dissection because any injury will require immediate CPB support and myocardial protection.
- You will likely need to mobilize previous grafts to allow for aortotomy. If unable to mobilize graft and it is still patent may need to transect and perform bypass. The proximal can be to the aorta or hood of the vein graft and the distal can be to the vein graft or a new distal. Ligate the old graft.

"Unable to access the root and get exposure of the valve through your aortotomy"
Consider aortic transection to enable exposure and allow better access to the old valve.

"Tear in aorta/outflow tract when removing old valve."

263

Valve may be incorporated, or previous dissection may have been extensive. Be prepared with bovine pericardium or even homograft for reconstruction if necessary.

"Right Coronary ostia injured during excision of valve."
Be prepared by prepping in the legs on all redo operations. Perform bypass. Reference cath to be sure that bypass is distal to any native disease.

"You notice significant RV dysfunction coming off bypass."
Always assume any regional functional problem coming off bypass is a coronary problem. Coronary problems are obviously life-threatening and cannot be ignored. If you've proven to yourself that the problem is not air in the coronary, the safest plan is to assume you've obstructed to the right coronary with your newer, larger valve and thus proceed with an expeditious vein graft to the right coronary artery. Do not instead try to reopen the aorta and re-replace the valve. This situation also highlights the importance of ensuring you can see the os of both coronary after the valve is lowered into place. This can also be double-checked by giving retrograde cardioplegia and looking for blood return from the os.

"After redo-AVR, you find it difficult to close the aortotomy due to tension on the aorta."
In redo settings, the aorta can be less compliant and thus a large prosthesis can place undue tension on the suture line. If this is the case, augment your closure with a bovine pericardial patch to minimize tension on the suture line.

"You instead have a 77-year-old patient with a mechanical valve that has failed and 2+ MR with no obvious mitral abnormalities."
The patient probably has functional mitral regurgitation that is accentuated by severe AS. The safest option is performing an expeditious redo AVR and seeing if the mitral regurgitation will decrease thereafter. If were to persist several weeks afterwards, there are other options down the road one could consider for functional mitral regurgitation (*e.g.*, MitraClip).

Pearls/pitfalls
- Valve type, valve size, implantation technique, and root enlargement during the first AVR can affect the technical success of either a redo AVR operation or ViV TAVR procedure.
- The differential diagnosis of the failed prior surgical valve must be considered, and it is critical to rule out (1) high gradients as a result of patient prosthesis mismatch (PPM) and (2) endocarditis if the patient is being considered for ViV TAVR.
- Redo AVR is still the treatment of choice for younger patients with favorable risk factors.
- Review echo and cardiac catheterization to ensure no other procedures or evaluation is necessary.
- CTA Chest/Abdomen/Pelvis is critical for planning. If it cannot be obtained due to renal disease (in which case they are likely better suited by ViV TAVR), then non-contrast CT ± TEE at the very minimum.
- Obtain and study previous operative note.
- Discuss mechanical vs. tissue valve preoperatively.
- After reviewing the CTA and patient's BSA, have an idea of what size valve the patient currently has and what their anatomy can accommodate, as well as what size the patient needs or can tolerate.
- Careful preoperative planning for cannulation and myocardial protection is critical, particularly if re-entry will be difficult or if AI is present.
- Have the femoral vessels exposed or accessed before sternotomy and have cross-matched blood in the room (typically 4 units).
- Injury to coronary arteries → bypass with vein grafts.
- Increased risk of heart block postoperatively → place v-wires and maybe even a-wires.

264

- Be prepared for complications, *e.g.*, need for aortic root enlargement/replacement.
- Any complication that can occur during primary AVR is more likely to occur in a redo.

Suggested readings

- Hirose H, Gill IS, Lytle BW. Redo-aortic valve replacement after previous bilateral internal thoracic artery bypass grafting. Ann Thorac Surg 2004;78(3):782-785.
- Potter DD, Sundt TM, 3rd, Zehr KJ et al. Operative risk of reoperative aortic valve replacement. J Thorac Cardiovasc Surg 2005;129(1):94-103.
- LaPar DJ, Yang Z, Stukenborg GJ et al. Outcomes of reoperative aortic valve replacement after previous sternotomy. J Thorac Cardiovasc Surg 2010;139(2):263-272.
- Kaneko T, Vassileva CM, Englum B et al. Contemporary outcomes of repeat aortic valve replacement: A benchmark for transcatheter valve-in-valve procedures. Ann Thorac Surg 2015;100(4):1298-1304; discussion 1304.
- Ejiofor JI, Yammine M, Harloff MT et al. Reoperative surgical aortic valve replacement versus transcatheter valve-in-valve replacement for degenerated bioprosthetic aortic valves. Ann Thorac Surg 2016;102(5):1452-1458.
- Lau C, Gaudino M, Mazza A, Munjal M, Girardi LN. Reoperative aortic valve replacement in a previous biologic composite valve graft. Ann Thorac Surg 2016;102(5):e477-e480.
- James Edelman J, Khan JM, Rogers T et al. Valve-in-valve tavr: State-of-the-art review. Innovations (Phila) 2019:1556984519858020.
- Sedeek AF, Greason KL, Sandhu GS, Dearani JA, Holmes DR, Jr., Schaff HV. Transcatheter valve-in-valve vs surgical replacement of failing stented aortic biological valves. Ann Thorac Surg 2019;108(2):424-430.
- Webb JG, Murdoch DJ, Alu MC et al. 3-year outcomes after valve-in-valve transcatheter aortic valve replacement for degenerated bioprostheses: The partner 2 registry. J Am Coll Cardiol 2019;73(21):2647-2655.

42. Functional Mitral Regurgitation

J Hunter Mehaffey, MD and Kenan W Yount, MD

Adapted from 1st edition chapter "Ischemic Mitral Regurgitation" written by *Kenan W. Yount, MD, MBA, and Gorav Ailawadi, MD*

Concept

- Primary mitral regurgitation (MR) is caused by a primary leaflet abnormality. Usually this is the result of degenerative disease.
- By contrast, secondary MR (the focus of this chapter) occurs when structurally normal valve leaflets are unable to coapt completely, owing to a distortion of either (1) the annulus or (2) the subvalvular apparatus.
    - ○ Annular dilation as a result of dilated cardiomyopathy results in Type II MR, which is frequently referred to as "functional" mitral regurgitation.
    - ○ Subvalvular distortion (usually tethering of the posterior leaflet) can occur as a consequence of left ventricular (LV) remodeling as the result of ischemic heart disease (*e.g.*, prior inferior myocardial infarction).
- Either mechanism is essentially a disease of the LV rather than the mitral valve itself.
- Patients who have LV dysfunction and secondary MR have a much worse prognosis than patients with either abnormality in isolation.
- It is controversial whether myocardial revascularization alone will be enough for some of these patients.
- It is controversial whether addressing the MR will be of value for some of these patients.

Chief complaint

"A 60-year-old female with a past medical history significant for hypertension, dyslipidemia, coronary artery disease, and non ST-segment elevation myocardial infarction treated medically 3 years ago presents with increasing shortness of breath. She describes a history of fatigue and shortness of breath worsened by exertion. She denies recent anginal episodes."

Differential

Acute coronary syndrome, HFrEF, structural valve disease, COPD

- *Other diagnoses to consider:* acute postinfarction ischemic MR (with or without papillary muscle rupture; see "Alternative Scenarios"); ischemic CAD with concomitant MR as a result of other etiologies (*e.g.*, degenerative mitral valve disease, rheumatic disease, endocarditis).

Carpentier's classification system - describes the mechanism of MR.

- **Type I** involves normal leaflet motion—MR results from LV enlargement and subsequent annular dilatation (*e.g.*, functional MR).
- **Type II** involves leaflet prolapse (*e.g.*, degenerative MR; acute papillary rupture after MI)
- **Type III** involves leaflet restriction and is further subdivided into **IIIa** (restriction during systole and diastole) and **IIIb** (restriction during systole alone). Rheumatic disease classically results in Type IIIa whereas chronic ischemic disease is Type IIIb.

Differential secondary MR

- *Functional MR:* Type I mechanism. Dilated cardiomyopathy producing global LV dilation resulting in annular enlargement. These patients may have severely depressed LV *function* (usually LVEF < 35%), hence the term "functional."

- *Ischemic MR:* Type IIIb mechanism. Prior myocardial infarction or ischemic remodeling resulting in <u>asymmetric</u> ventricular remodeling, most often affecting the inferior and lateral LV wall. Although it can be seen with global LV remodeling, the distinguishing feature usually involves substantial disruption of the subvalvular apparatus, especially **downward and lateral (*i.e.*, apical) displacement of the posteromedial papillary muscle** leading to leaflet tethering. Note that the term "ischemic" MR classically refers to a chronic condition rather than acute papillary rupture after an MI.

- These two entities lie along a clinical spectrum given the heterogeneity of ischemic heart disease. Although they cannot be completely separated, clarifying the mechanism will help determine surgical management because the degree of LV dysfunction, chamber remodeling, and valvular complex disruption differ with each.

History and physical

A focused history and physical should clarify any recent history of acute coronary syndrome (ACS) or angina. Most patients have symptoms of congestive heart failure (CHF) due to worsening LV function and moderate-to-severe MR in the setting of known or unknown prior MI. Consequently, it is necessary to obtain a history of prior cardiac interventions, prior imaging, and progression of current symptomatology. Comorbidities, such as diabetes, pulmonary disease, kidney disease, cerebrovascular disease, and peripheral arterial disease impact surgical outcomes. These patients tend to be high-risk with operative mortality approaching 5-10%.

Tests

- CXR may show pulmonary edema and an enlarged cardiac silhouette. Also assess for calcification of the aorta and arch which would warrant a CT.

- EKG may show changes of a prior inferior MI.

- Transthoracic echo (TTE) may show evidence of prior MI and LV dysfunction. Given the primary mechanism is leaflet tethering in ischemic MR, the regurgitant jet will be directed *toward* the restricted leaflet; annular dilatation, however, will cause the jet to appear central. Grade – 1 = mild, 2 = moderate, 3 = moderately severe, 4 = severe.

- Transesophageal echo (TEE) is the study of choice to clarify the mechanism of regurgitation. The grade of MR may be lower on TEE intraoperatively due to anesthesia and ventricular unloading. Rely on the estimated degree of regurgitation preoperatively by TTE but ensure that you have a TEE prior to any intervention to give the best anatomical detail and clarity.

- Coronary angiography may show significant multivessel CAD; look for an occluded vessel with inferior wall motion abnormality on the left ventriculogram. Clarify right versus left dominance (left dominance is more problematic if the circumflex were injured during mitral valve surgery).

- Viability testing may identify patients most likely to benefit from valve intervention. MR in the setting of inferior scar tissue or a tethered posterior leaflet is unlikely to improve with CABG alone while MR in the setting viable myocardium may improve with CABG alone.

Index scenario (additional information)

"Left heart catheterization revealed multivessel disease: there is left main disease (~ 70% stenosis) and proximal LAD stenosis; the RCA is occluded but the LAD target and OM targets appear acceptable. MRI shows good viability anteriorly but there is concern for non-viable scarred myocardium inferiorly. A more recent TTE shows LVEF to be estimated at 30-35% with pulmonary hypertension, severe mitral regurgitation, and inferior wall motion abnormality. TEE shows a restricted and tethered posterior mitral leaflet and confirms severe mitral regurgitation."

Treatment/management

The benefit of surgical revascularization (CABG) is clear, provided the patient has suitable coronary targets affected by high-grade proximal lesions resulting in ischemic but viable myocardium.

This patient has severe MR and thus expert consensus still favors simultaneous correction of the severe MR at the time of CABG. The question of which surgical strategy has been the subject of substantial research.

Historically, mitral valve repair (MVr) with a reduction annuloplasty (slightly undersized, complete ring, e.g., 28-30 mm) was favored over mitral valve replacement (MVR) for secondary MR based on its relatively lower perioperative morbidity and mortality; the presumed benefits of preserving the subvalvular apparatus to help preserve LV function; and less need for re-intervention given the risk of bioprosthetic structural valve deterioration. Annular reduction for a Type I mechanism was thought to decrease wall stress and improve LV function. For patients with a Type IIIb mechanism, this approach proved insufficient due to the more localized pattern of geometric deformation, possibly explaining their higher rates of recurrent MR postoperatively. Subvalvular interventions to reposition the posterior papillary muscle toward the septal annulus have been employed and reported on retrospectively but have largely fallen out of favor. Most practitioners do not perform ancillary subvalvular interventions in the setting of IMR.

A large randomized trial conducted by the Cardiothoracic Surgical Trials Network (CTSN) dramatically changed clinical practice by comparing MVr vs. chordal sparing MVR at the time of CABG for severe MR. This trial showed no significant differences in LV remodeling, survival, or outcome at 1 or 2 years. Additionally, there was a significantly higher rate of recurrent MR in the MVr cohort, which thus predisposed MVr patients to recurrent heart failure, atrial fibrillation, repeat interventions, and repeat hospitalizations. Of note, is that at 2 years, mortality approached 20-25% in both groups, confirming the overall poor prognosis of this patient group regardless of surgical strategy. Thus, replacement for this patient population gives you the best chance of leaving the operating room with a single pump run and no MR.

Given these data, most surgeons now favor a chordal-sparing mitral valve replacement (MVR) at the time of CABG for severe MR. A bioprosthetic valve is logical given that most patients in whom replacement is favored in these settings will not experience valve degeneration in their lifetime.

One caveat is that in some situations (e.g., at the time of an apical incision such as an LVAD or Dor) some surgeons may instead employ a simple Alfieri suture for predominantly Type I mechanism secondary MR.

Operative steps

- Swan-Ganz catheter placement should be considered in these patients given their LV dysfunction and pulmonary hypertension.
- Intraoperative TEE is imperative to clarify the mechanism of MR and determine the quality of the repair, but it is *not* reliable in judging the severity of MR. Go by the preoperative grade.
- Median sternotomy is the classic approach for combined mitral valve-CABG.
- Bi-caval cannulation is routine. Some practitioners favor femoral cannulation for the IVC.
- Myocardial Protection: After the aorta is cross-clamped, antegrade cardioplegic arrest followed by intermittent retrograde cardioplegic infusion is wise for a diseased left ventricle. Practitioners are divided on whether to incorporate del Nido during coronary operations and thus try to avoid broaching that discussion on a board exam. Regardless of the order of the grafts, all distal anastomoses should be performed prior to mitral

268

valve replacement to avoid excess manipulation of the heart after MVR, as that predisposes to AV groove dissociation. When RCA disease is present, consideration should be given to prioritizing that graft first to enable periodic antegrade delivery to the RV since it may be inadequately protected by retrograde alone.

- After completion of the distal CABG anastomoses, expose the mitral valve via left atriotomy. The left atrium is usually dilated enough in these patients to approach the valve from Waterston's (or Sondergaard's) groove rather than necessitating a transseptal approach. That said, some surgeons may prefer a right sided approach.

- Everting pledgeted sutures through the annulus in a horizontal fashion. The anterior portion is usually approached last as it is the most difficult to expose. Closely spaced sutures (some practitioners overlap sutures) may prevent dehiscence. Size according to both inter-trigonal and anterior leaflet size using the manufacturers sizer. Sutures are then placed through the sewing ring and secured to the annulus with either hand-tie or Cor-knot.

- After valve replacement, close the left atriotomy. Some surgeons leave a temporary LA or LV vent in place prior to tying down the left atriotomy closure.

- Proceed with proximal anastomoses.

Potential questions/alternative scenarios

"The same patient presents but has more diffuse coronary disease with less obvious targets and a global dilated cardiomyopathy with an LVEF of 15%."
Such a patient primarily has LV disease and should instead be considered for LVAD. If the decision is made to proceed instead with an LVAD, it is more controversial whether to address the mitral valve at the time of LVAD. Replacement of the valve would require arresting the heart and thus many practitioners instead favor an Alfieri suture via the LV apex after apical coring (if they choose to address the MR at all during the LVAD operation).

"A 70-year-old male presents with 2^+ MR, and 3 vessel CAD each with > 70% stenosis. Would you perform a CABG or CABG MVR? He has a history of poorly controlled diabetes, COPD and ESRD."
This patient has moderate IMR with multivessel CAD. Options include surgical revascularization alone versus concomitant mitral valve repair. Few surgeons would replace the mitral valve in the setting of only moderate MR. The CTSN trial looking specifically at moderate MR at the time of CABG found that concomitant MVr resulted in longer operative times, longer hospitalizations, higher rates of atrial fibrillation, and higher rates of stroke; however, it resulted in less MR at 1-2 years with but without any favorable effect on LV reverse remodeling. Surgical correction thus introduces a higher perioperative risk in the setting of an already higher predicted operative mortality operation for only moderate. In a patient who has these many comorbidities one would certainly be justified in doing the most expeditious operation with least risk, which in this case is a CABG alone. Perhaps MitraClip would be an option down the road for that patient if the MR progresses.

For a healthier individual who can tolerate a ring annuloplasty or Alfieri suture, doing so may decrease the incidence of worsening MR in the future. In that scenario, a viability study may help guide the decision: irreversible disease from infarction would seemingly benefit more from a concomitant MV intervention. Judgement also comes into play with 2^+ MR. As a rule of thumb, $3-4^+$ should get a replacement unless you have good reason to limit cardiopulmonary bypass time and the patient just barely makes 3^+ MR.

"The patient experiences recurrent severe MR one year after the operation."
The patient's coronary anatomy should be re-evaluated, and any ischemic disease addressed. Repeat TEE is warranted to clarify the mechanism of the progressive MR.

If the mechanism is secondary: Strong consideration must be given to maximizing guideline-directed medical for heart failure (*e.g.*, increasing beta-blockade, ACE/ARB). Consideration should also be given for Cardiac Resynchronization Therapy (CRT) if indicated (*e.g.*, wide

QRS in setting of low EF). The MIRACLE trial revealed that CRT not only induced reverse remodeling but also reduced the degree of IMR at 12 months, likely by correcting dyssynchrony between the posterior papillary muscle and the lateral LV wall. The degree of MR should then be reassessed once maximal heart failure therapy has been achieved.

If severe MR persists despite these interventions, the patient should be considered for a percutaneous mitral valve repair (such a patient is almost certain to be high or prohibitive risk for re-operation). Any decision to intervene warrants a detailed assessment of frailty and comorbidities that will potentially limit the patient's lifespan and quality of life independent of their MR. In this scenario, a TEE could determine whether the patient has anatomy suitable for a MitraClip procedure.

The COAPT trial showed significantly lower rates of hospitalization for heart failure at 2 years and lower all-cause mortality at 2 years in patients undergoing MitraClip for secondary MR The results are in contrast to the MITRA-FR trial conducted in Europe, but the criticism of MITRA-FR has been that it included substantial numbers of patients with less severe degrees of MR and patients in whom medical therapy may not have been maximized. Consequently, for patients who have heart failure symptoms truly refractory to maximal medical therapy with a high degree of mitral regurgitation and severe LV dysfunction not amenable to LVAD, MitraClip can certainly be considered.

If the mechanism is instead primary: Assuming the patient is symptomatic and a good operative candidate, he may be a candidate for re-operation. This sometimes is approached from a right thoracotomy if prior CABG has been performed and the bypass grafts are patent. However, such a patient's comorbidities may render them high or prohibitive risk for re-operation, in which case, MitraClip can certainly be considered.

"A 68-year-old male presents with worsening chest pain that began acutely 2 days ago. He had some improvement initially and did not come into the hospital. He now presents with worsening chest pain and increasing shortness of breath. A coronary angio shows a 70% mid circumflex lesion and an 80% RCA lesion. He is left dominant with the circumflex giving off the PDA. His echo shows a ruptured posterior papillary muscle. He is on moderate doses of epinephrine and levophed with PAP of 50/20 and cardiac index of 2.0. His EF is estimated at 50%. His blood pressure is 80/40 mmHg. Physical exam reveals bilateral crackles and a new holosystolic murmur. His CXR shows acute pulmonary edema. How would you proceed."

At least 25% of patients develop either a new mitral murmur or have TTE evidence of MR after an acute MI. Usually, these are transient alterations that ultimately resolve, but MR can be persistent in approximately 1-5% of patients as a result of papillary muscle ischemia. Papillary muscle rupture is increasingly rare with today's focus on rapid revascularization after acute STEMI. Nevertheless, it still carries a mortality approaching 50-75% without surgical intervention and 20-25% with surgical intervention. Major contributors to mortality are advanced age, the duration of preoperative shock, the presence of other cardiovascular comorbidities, and operative delay. Postoperative morbidity can result from peripheral organ failure and stroke. Acute IMR occurs 2-7 days (mean 4 days) after MI. Patients present with acute dyspnea due to pulmonary edema and cardiogenic shock. A new holosystolic murmur with the above history could be seen in either an acute VSD or acute IMR. Unlike an acute VSD, MR is best heard at the apex rather than the left sternal border and does not have an associated thrill.

The posteromedial papillary muscle is more vulnerable because of its single blood supply (RCA for right dominant or circumflex for left dominant) compared to the dual blood supply of the anterolateral papillary muscle (LAD and circumflex). Papillary muscle rupture results in flail leaflet. Unlike acute VSD, acute IMR is more commonly associated with acute inferior STEMI.

- *Tests*: EKG may show signs of inferior MI whereas an acute VSD may show conduction abnormalities. A bedside TTE may demonstrate flail mitral leaflets and a mass attached to the chordae, representing the ruptured papillary muscle.
- *Preoperative Stabilization*: Acute MR can rapidly result in pulmonary edema and multisystem organ failure from reduced forward flow. Inotropes (*e.g.*, milrinone), and vasodilators (*e. g.*, nitroprusside, nitric oxide) can stabilize the patient's hemodynamic status; by contrast, volume overload or increased afterload would worsen the patient's MR. Intubation and mechanical ventilation may be required for respiratory failure. Diuretics may reduce pulmonary edema, but caution should be taken not to create prerenal azotemia. Mechanical support with an intra-aortic balloon pump (IABP) should be strongly considered. Some patients may need to be stabilized with ECMO if they have already progressed to severe end organ dysfunction and there is question over whether that is salvageable with an operation.
- *Role of PCI/CABG*: Pre-operative cardiac catheterization is often performed at the time of diagnosing the MI. This may occur a few days prior to the papillary rupture in which case a stent or angioplasty was likely performed or the cath may be done at the time of diagnosing the MR if the patient presented in a delayed fashion. If the patient's coronary lesions have not already been addressed, then a CABG and MVR should be done. Otherwise proceed to an MVR alone unless there is suspicion for stent thrombosis (EKG with evolving infarct) in which case the cath should be redone.
- *Operation:* Papillary rupture is an emergent situation, and intervention should not be delayed unless the patient is prohibitive risk. Mitral valve repair for papillary muscle rupture is rarely possible. Re-implanting a ruptured papillary muscle into recently infarcted LV tissue can result in repair failure, prolonging bypass time in a patient who has already been in shock. Consequently, mitral valve replacement with chordal preservation if possible is preferred.

Pearls/pitfalls
- **Carpentier Classification:** Critical to understanding mitral regurgitation mechanism.
- **Severe MR with symptomatic CAD:** Combined CABG-mitral valve replacement.
- **Moderate MR with symptomatic CAD:** Combined CABG-mitral valve repair will decrease MR severity more than CABG alone, but it may have no effect on survival. Consequently, preoperative risk factors, viability, and symptoms should help guide the decision to add mitral valve repair to a CABG.
- **Severe MR with Dilated Cardiomyopathy:** Maximize medical therapy/consider percutaneous repair vs LVAD/transplant.
- **Acute MR from papillary muscle rupture:** Surgical emergency; few would find fault with valve replacement.

Suggested readings
- Carpentier Classification: Stone et al. Section on "Primary versus secondary MR" within "Clinical Trial Design Principles and Endpoint Definitions for Transcatheter Mitral Valve Repair and Replacement: Part 1: Clinical Trial Design Principles." *J Am Coll Cardiol.* 2015 Jul 21;66(3): pages 282-284 only.
- Severe MR with symptomatic CAD: Goldstein *et al* for CTSN. Two-Year Outcomes of Surgical Treatment of Severe Ischemic Mitral Regurgitation. *N Engl J Med* 2016; 374:344-353.
- Moderate MR with symptomatic CAD: Michler *et al* for CTSN. Two-Year Outcomes of Surgical Treatment of Moderate Ischemic Mitral Regurgitation. *N Engl J Med* 2014; 371:2178-2188
- Severe MR with Dilated Cardiomyopathy: Stone et al for COAPT. Transcatheter Mitral-Valve Repair in Patients with Heart Failure. N Engl J Med 2018; 379:2307-2318.

- Acute MR from papillary muscle rupture: Carrott, Gardner, Kron. Section on "Acute Ischemic Mitral Regurgitation" within "Chapter 56: Surgery for Complications of Myocardial Infarction." *Mastery of Cardiothoracic Surgery* 2014, 3rd edition. pages 548-551.

43. NON-ISCHEMIC MITRAL VALVE REGURGITATION

Jordan P. Bloom, MD, MPH and Serguei Melnitchouk, MD, MPH
Adapted from 1st edition chapter written by *Jennifer M. Worth, MD, and Chittoor B. Sai-Sudhakar, MD*

Concept

- Etiology and pathophysiology
- Indications for mitral valve intervention in the setting of primary mitral regurgitation
- Preoperative evaluation
- Mitral valve repair techniques
- Management of complications
- Pearls / Pitfalls

Chief complaint

"A 68-year-old woman is referred to you with a 4-month history of shortness of breath after being diagnosed with severe mitral regurgitation by echocardiography."

Differential

Differentiate primary vs. secondary valvular disease. Primary or organic mitral regurgitation is a result of an intrinsic valve abnormality. These include the entire spectrum of the degenerative mitral valve disease (ranging from fibroelastic deficiency to Barlow's valve), congenital malformations, inflammatory diseases, bacterial endocarditis, calcification, trauma, and tumors. Secondary or functional mitral regurgitation is due to problems with the heart resulting in secondary annular dilation. The most common etiology is ischemia with subsequent ischemic cardiomyopathy; other causes include dilated cardiomyopathy, hypertrophic obstructive cardiomyopathy, myocardial sarcoidosis, endomyocardial fibrosis, and myocardial tumors.

History and physical

It's important to elicit any symptoms of angina or heart failure in addition to comorbid conditions which all affect survival. Focused physical exam including vitals, neurologic exam, heart/lung sounds, peripheral exam including pulses and edema. The holosystolic murmur of MR best heard in the left lateral decubitus position at the apex and radiates to the axilla. If the murmur radiates toward the aortic area the pathology is likely a flail PL; whereas if the murmur radiates toward the spine or axilla, it is likely a flail AL. The murmur of functional MR is variable and has poor correlation between intensity and severity (due to LV dilation, variable volume status, etc.).

Tests

- *EKG*: look for evidence of previous infarcts, cardiomegaly; may see left atrial (LA) enlargement or atrial fibrillation.
- *CXR*: may see cardiomegaly, LA enlargement, and/or pulmonary edema.
- *Echo*: severe MR documented by a vena contracta width of ≥ 0.7 cm, effective regurgitant orifice (ERO) ≥ 0.4 cm^2, regurgitant volume (RV) ≥ 60 mL, regurgitant fraction (RF) $\geq 50\%$, and an effective regurgitant orifice/jet area (ERO) $> 40\%$ of LA area. 3D echo is a useful modification to enable better visualization of functional and anatomic relationships to help plan operations. Transesophageal echocardiogram (TEE) gives much clearer images and is typically used to classify the mechanism of valvular dysfunction (Table 39-1) and document the severity (Table 39-2). It also provides a much better assessment of mitral valve, aortomitral curtain, and/or aortic root involvement in endocarditis cases.

Table 39-1. Carpentier's Functional Classification of Mitral Valve Dysfunction.

Dysfunction	Leaflet Motion	Common Etiologies
Type I	Normal leaflet motion	Annular dilation due to ICM/DCM, perforation in endocarditis, congenital cleft

273

Type II	Increased leaflet motion (leaflet prolapse)	Valve prolapse due to FED, myxomatous degeneration, Barlow's valve, Marfan syndrome, endocarditis, trauma
Type IIIa	Restricted leaflet motion in diastole (restricted opening)	Leaflet thickening due to rheumatic disease, radiation, carcinoid, lupus
Type IIIb	Restricted leaflet motion in systole (restricted closure)	Leaflet tethering due to ICM, DCM

Table 39-2. Mitral regurgitation severity.

	RV	RF	ERO
Mild	< 30 mL	< 30%	< 0.2 cm^2
Moderate	30-59 mL	30-49%	0.2-0.39 cm^2
Severe	> 60 mL	> 50%	> 0.4 cm^2

- MR is commonly graded on a scale of 0-4: 0 = none/trivial; 1 = mild, 2 = moderate, 3 = moderate-to-severe, and 4 = severe

- *Cardiac catheterization*: look for evidence of coronary artery disease and dominance. It is important to know whether the patient has a right or left dominant coronary circulation for the rare case of trouble coming off cardiopulmonary bypass and/or lateral/inferior wall hypokinesis. MAC can also typically be seen on LHC.

- *ECG gated CTA:* alternative modality (supplanting coronary cath) to screen for coronary artery disease in low-risk patients. Also helpful in cases of MAC to assess proximity of calcium to the left circumflex artery.

Index scenario (additional information)
"The patient is not diabetic and has shortness of breath with moderate activity. Echo shows vena contracta of 0.6 cm, EF 55-60%, and mild dilation of the LA in the setting of P2 leaflet prolapse. The MR is graded as 3-4+. What are treatment options and how would you proceed?"

Treatment/management
This patient has moderate-to-severe symptomatic primary MR and thus meets criteria for mitral valve intervention (Class I recommendation). Modern options for mitral valve regurgitation include surgical repair or replacement and catheter-based approaches (reserved mostly for high-risk patients) such as the MitraClip or transcatheter mitral valve replacement (TMVR) via transfemoral or transapical approach. Most commonly, mitral valve surgery is performed through either a full sternotomy or a right mini-thoracotomy. Some programs use either total endoscopic or robotic platforms for even smaller incisions.
Mitral valve repair has become the standard of care for such patient and results in the most favorable survival profile. Criteria favoring mitral valve repair include chordal rupture in a limited portion of the posterior leaflet with normal anterior leaflet or a simple prolapse of the posterior leaflet. In addition, ruptured chordae to the anterior leaflet, myxomatous degeneration, or leaflet perforation/chordal rupture from endocarditis. Valve repair should follow Carpentier's principles including preservation or restoration of full leaflet motion, creation of a large coaptation surface, and stabilization of the annulus.

Operative steps for mitral valve exposure via median sternotomy
- Place a large bore IV, arterial line, GETA, PA catheter, Foley catheter.
- Check intraoperative TEE for mitral anatomy. Confirm the direction and complexity of the jet, the presence of a flail segment or leaflet prolapse. Anteriorly directed jet is due to posterior leaflet prolapse and posteriorly directed jet is due to anterior leaflet prolapse. The TEE gives you a sense of the feasibility for repair. Also consider patient

factors and your tolerance for a second pump run if the repair fails. For this you need to consider comorbidities, age, etc.

- Median sternotomy, pericardial stay sutures, palpate the aorta for calcifications ± epiaortic ultrasound.
- Heparin (400 mg/kg), aortobicaval cannulation, antegrade and retrograde cardioplegia catheters placed. Initiate CPB once ACT is 480. Administer antegrade cardioplegia to achieve diastolic arrest (while periodically ruling out LV distention). Cooling to 34 C is sufficient for the majority of cases. Consider cooling to moderate hypothermia (28-32° C) for a better myocardial protection in more complex/prolonged cases. In cases of transseptal approach, dissect and encircle the IVC and SVC while snaring them with tourniquets. The exposure is a matter of choice. The following describes the most common left atriotomy (paraseptal) approach via Sondergaard's (Waterston's) groove:
  - Use scissors or cautery to expose the roof of the left atrium along Sondergaard's groove. Be careful not to get into the RA. This step can be done prior to arresting the heart but is easier done while on bypass with the RA decompressed. After heart is arrested, an incision is made in the middle of the dissected area – away from pulmonary veins while leaving a sufficient rim of LA tissue at the groove for a later closure. LA incision is extended in a curvilinear fashion superiorly and inferiorly to allow placement of retractor blades. Stay away from the pulmonary veins and the right atrium. A flexible pump sucker is placed into the left inferior pulmonary vein to keep the operative field dry. Self-retaining or handheld retractors are used to aid the exposure.
- Perform valve analysis and determine pathology:
  - Annulus (dilated, calcified - atrial versus ventricular calcification)
  - Leaflet tissue (prolapse - which segment?, flail, redundant myxomatous tissue or limited fibroelastic degenerative tissue)
  - Chordal attachments (primary - margin, secondary - underside, tertiary - annulus)
  - Height of the posterior leaflet (ideal is 2/3 anterior and 1/3 posterior or less than 1.5 cm posterior leaflet).
- Goals – Repair valve if technically feasible, otherwise replace with mechanical valve if less than 60 year-old (needs to be explained to the patient preoperatively). Use a bioprosthetic valve in patients > 60 yo, women of childbearing age, or if contraindication to warfarin exists.

Valve repair

- Carpentier's principles of valve repair include preservation or restoration of full leaflet motion, creation of a large coaptation surface, and stabilization of the annulus.

- A ring or a band annuloplasty are considered necessary adjuncts to reinforce most repair techniques. Some surgeons place the annuloplasty sutures first to aid the exposure. Start with posteromedial trigone and work counterclockwise using non-pledgeted braided horizontal mattress sutures. Make sure you get the fibrous trigones (appear as "dimples" and are one stitch above the corresponding commissures). In case an annuloplasty band is used instead of a complete ring (a band and a complete ring are equally effective for repair of primary mitral regurgitation), one would not place sutures between the trigones along the base of the anterior leaflet, while placing decent anchoring stitches in the trigones themselves and travelling from one trigone to another.

- Neighboring structures: avoid deep (and outside the annulus) stitches in the area of posteromedial commissure/right trigone (conduction tissue); avoid deep stitches along the base of the anterior leaflet while travelling from the right trigone to the left (aortic valve); avoid deep bites near the base of P1 scallop and instead angle the needle toward the ventricle (away from the atrium) to avoid injuring circumflex artery. One can also

275

injure the coronary sinus with a deep retraction stitch outside the annulus of the P3 scallop, while trying to obtain a better visualization of the latter.

- Mitral valve prolapse is a spectrum of disease. Therefore, in fibroelastic deficiency, where there is paucity of tissue, one should either use neochords or do a very limited triangular resection. In Barlow's valve, where there is excess tissue in almost all scallops, one needs to perform quadrangular resection with a sliding plasty to remove excess tissue from the posterior leaflet. When there is excess tissue in height and width in one of the scallops (e.g. myxomatous degeneration of P2), one either performs a limited quadrangular resection with a sliding plasty or a triangular resection with reduction of leaflet height ("butterfly technique"). When performing resectional techniques, it often helps to place a silk suture around the healthy chordae that flank a diseased segment and resect only the diseased segment. Cut edges of leaflets are then reapproximated using interrupted or running non-absorbable suture.

- When performing neochordal repair technique (either for anterior or posterior leaflet prolapse), one places a CV-4 (or CV-5) PTFE suture either as a figure of eight or as a pledgeted horizontal mattress stitch through the head of a papillary muscle. Both suture ends are then brought twice through the free edge of the prolapsing segment (each time from the ventricular side to atrial side). It is much easier to place the neochords before the annuloplasty ring is tied. Once the ring is tied, the left ventricle gets insufflated with saline and the length of the neochords is adjusted so that there is a tight seal between the coapting leaflets without any residual leaflet prolapse. Then, the sutures are carefully tied (without excessive tension) in order to avoid inadvertent overcorrection with subsequent result of leaflet tethering. Most frequently one needs to place two (or even three, four) sets of PTFE sutures (using both papillary muscles) in order to reliably repair a wide P2 or A2 prolapse or a bileaflet prolapse. Only in an isolated focal prolapse one set of neochords might be sufficient.

- Chordal transfer can be used to repair anterior leaflet prolapse as well. In this case, a portion of posterior leaflet is excised and transferred ("flipped over") along with its primary chords to the prolapsing segment of the anterior leaflet. Obviously, one then needs to reconstruct the posterior leaflet in a standard fashion and that is the major drawback of this repair technique. Secondary chord transfer can be used as an adjunct technique to strengthen the anterior leaflet edge in addition to the neochords. In this technique, a strong secondary chord is cut from the undersurface of AL and transferred to the leaflet edge, where it is affixed with non-absorbable suture. In addition to strengthening the neochordal repair it also helps to correctly estimate the desired neochordal length.

- Commissuroplasty is frequently employed to repair commissural prolapse. In this technique both commissural edges are sutured together with either a running suture or with a series of imbricating horizontal mattress sutures (preferred), thus placing the prolapsing tissue below the coaptation plane. One is judicious about the extent of closure to avoid creating mitral stenosis and is therefore cognizant to choose the largest acceptable annuloplasty ring in such cases.

- In cases of leaflet thickening or retraction (such as in IIIa), one sometimes needs to extend the height of either anterior or posterior leaflet. For this a glutaraldehyde-treated autologous pericardium is tailored in a semilunar (posterior leaflet) or an ovoid (anterior leaflet) shape. The leaflet is detached at approximately a 3-5 mm distance from the annulus and incision has to be extended from one commissure to another in order to achieve effective height extension and non-restricted leaflet motion.

- Size the annuloplasty ring (or band) to match the height of the anterior mitral leaflet (not the intertrigonal distance) and upsize if possible while performing insufflation of the left ventricle with saline solution (saline test). Band and ring sizes typically range from 26 to 40mm. A larger ring/band helps prevent systolic anterior motion (SAM) and has lower transmitral gradients due to a larger mitral valve area (MVA). Sew the band and tie the sutures. Some perform a final saline test at this point and do an "ink test" along the coaptation line in order to assess whether the ink line is not too high on the anterior leaflet (ideally should be at the transition between the clear and rough zones of the anterior leaflet to avoid SAM) and confirm presence of sufficient coaptation depth along the posterior leaflet.

- After deairing and closing the left atrium, remove cross clamp and wean from the CPB. Assess the valve with TEE and have a low threshold to convert a repair to a replacement if left with 2-3+ MR. Be aggressive with re-repair even in the setting of a mild MR in younger patients. Use judgement, but mild MR in a frail elderly patient is acceptable. Incidentally, the older the patient and the more the comorbidities, the more you might consider mitral valve replacement with a tissue valve, especially in the setting of a complex valve pathology.
- The usual checklist after a mitral valve repair involves checking:
    - 6-lead ECG (rhythm, conduction abnormalities, evidence of ischemia)
    - Residual MR (trivial or mild (in some cases) are acceptable)
    - Transmitral gradient (should be less than 5 mmHg)
    - Rule out presence of SAM
    - Rule out lateral/inferior wall hypokinesis
    - Rule out new eccentric AR
    - Assess presence of air and deair accordingly via aortic root

Valve replacement

- Detach the anterior leaflet approximately 3 mm from its base from commissure to commissure. Prepare two leaflet edge segments for chordal sparing valve replacement by dividing the anterior leaflet in the middle and resecting excess leaflet tissue while leaving strong primary chords along with the corresponding leaflet edge segments. Those two segments will be anchored by valve sutures to the corresponding commissures on either side. Attempt to preserve the entire posterior leaflet with its chords to mitigate risk of AV groove disruption and resect only excess or prolapsing tissue as needed. One is to avoid leaving too much chordal tissue behind, especially in the setting of small left ventricles. Some small series suggest that excess chordal tissue might contribute to higher incidence of tissue valve thrombosis due to increased flow turbulence. On the other side, judicious chordal sparing technique is associated with a better postoperative long-term left ventricular function and remodeling.
- If calcium is encountered in the subannular space, debride only if necessary, for the valve to lie flat and well opposed to the annulus or to facilitate suture placement ("respectfully resect"). Atrial decalcification can be done safely but the more you debride the ventricular calcification the greater the risk of AV groove disruption or circumflex injury. If you debride the calcification extensively including the ventricular calcium, you need to sew a pericardial patch (autologous or bovine) that saddles the annulus and covers the entire area of decalcification. In terms of annular suture placement, both everting (pledgets on the atrial side) and non-everting (pledgets on the ventricular side) horizontal mattress suture placement techniques are generally acceptable for regular mitral valve replacement cases. However, in the setting of decalcification or mitral annular calcium (MAC), a non-everting technique (pledgets are on the ventricular side) is strongly advised in order to further mitigate AV groove disruption.
- Bioprosthetic valves should be oriented with the post well out of the outflow tract. To accomplish that, two posts face the trigones and the third post divides posterior annulus in the middle. Mechanical valves are usually implanted in an anti-anatomic position in which the hinge lines are orthogonal to the native mitral commissures. Alternatively, a mechanical valve can be implanted in anatomic position in which the hinge lines are parallel to the native mitral commissures. Some studies using vector flow mapping to assess hydraulics of the left atrium found the formation of blood flow in the form of vortex, where both leaflets of a prosthetic valve positioned in an anti-anatomic orientation would receive equal initial opening force due to symmetric orientation of the leaflets relative to the atrial vortex. In contrast, in anatomic position the posterior

leaflet often demonstrates subtle delayed opening and early closure, a phenomenon also known as "lazy" leaflet. Also, of importance is to assess the leaflet clearance and strive for absolutely no interference from the subvalvular apparatus. Occasionally, if despite all measures one of the leaflets is immobile on TEE after coming off the CPB, one needs to rearrest the heart and turn the valve 45 degrees to either side.

- Close atriotomy with a running prolene suture, irrigate, deair, and wean from CPB.

Potential questions/alternative scenarios

"A 60year-old woman presents for follow up of her known mitral regurgitation. She has minimal symptoms which in no way disrupt her activities of daily living. She is very active. When would you offer an asymptomatic patient an MVR."

According to the guidelines, patients with chronic severe MR (3-4+) should be offered surgery if the patient experiences mild-moderate LV dysfunction with an EF less than 60%, moderate PHTN (PAP > 50 mmHg at rest), new onset atrial fibrillation, or an end systolic ventricular dimension (ESD) greater than or equal to 40 mm. Asymptomatic patients with preserved LVEF and > 95% likelihood of successful repair may be offered surgery for chronic severe MR.

"A 56-year-old female patient with a heart murmur presented to the ED with worsening dyspnea and hemoptysis. Four days prior she endorsed an intense workout during which she experienced severe precordial chest pain. On presentation she was tachycardic, with elevated JVP and bilateral RALS. There was a grade IV pansystolic murmur best heard at the apex. A CXR revealed bilateral pleural effusions. What is the most likely diagnosis and how would you manage?"

This is a classic scenario for exercise-induced acute chordal rupture resulting in severe MR and subsequent heart failure. Patients with MVP are at an increased risk. Other diseases such as rheumatic heart disease and infectious diseases such as endocarditis can also cause chordal rupture. Blunt chest trauma is another rare cause of this problem. Patients should be taken to the operating room for urgent mitral valve repair to avoid long term consequences of acute MR in a non-accommodated LA. Acute chordal rupture has degenerative etiology and needs to be differentiated from the papillary muscle rupture due to ischemia as the management differs.

"A 59-year-old male was admitted with an acute onset of shortness of breath. Physical exam reveals bilateral rales and a systolic murmur. Chest X-ray shows right lung opacification in the setting of leukocytosis. Echocardiography shows severe mitral regurgitation (MR) in the setting of a flail PL."

As in the previous scenario, this is a case of an acute mitral regurgitation due to an acute chordal rupture and it requires an urgent corrective mitral valve surgery. Patients who present this way are commonly misdiagnosed as having "atypical pneumonia" and are treated frequently with antibiotics. They invariably decompensate quickly if the MR is not addressed immediately and have high risk of mortality. Almost all cases of mitral disease-associated unilateral pulmonary edema is right sided and thought to be due to flow reversal into the pulmonary veins during systole.

"What are the different approaches to expose the mitral valve and when would each be considered?"

Table 39-4. Mitral valve exposure

Standard Approach	
Left Atriotomy (paraseptal)	• Most common approach to MV • Via Sondergaard's (Waterston's) groove • Incision of choice for mini-thoracotomy and robotic platforms
Transseptal Approaches	
Vertical transseptal	• **Incision via fossa ovalis** • Feasible with a large LA in the setting of a chronic MV pathology • Reduces risk of PPM, easier closure
Extended superior transseptal (Guiraudon)	• Vertical transseptal incision is extended superiorly onto the dome of the left atrium • Risk of damaging the SA nodal artery (higher risk of PPM) • Generally, a better exposure for a deep chest anatomy / wide AP diameter • Approach of choice in the setting of previous AVR or aortic root replacement • Can be easily extended and connected with an aortotomy incision for a "Commando" operation (e.g. endocarditis, radiation case)
Horizontal transseptal (Dubost)	• Very uncommon • Can be considered in the setting of a hostile anatomy between the aortic root and LA dome (e.g. presence of calcified aortic homograft, etc.) • Difficult closure, risk of narrowing right superior pulmonary vein, risk of transseptal incision progressing and tearing AV node area, high risk of PPM
Alternative Approaches	
Transaortic	• Aortotomy is extended onto the dome of the left atrium • Useful in endocarditis cases when both aortic and mitral valves need to be replaced (transaortic Commando) • Exposure can be challenging; in which case the incision can be connected to the extended transseptal incision
Left atrial appendage	• Very uncommon • Requires left thoracotomy • Alternative approach after multiple previous re-operations
Transventricular	• Can be utilized if entering the LV for another reason (e.g ventricular aneurysmectomy or LVAD placement)

"Your patient being evaluated for a mitral repair had a previous AVR complicated by a wound infection and mediastinitis requiring flap closure."

Right anterolateral thoracotomy approach - 4th intercostal space centered in the anterior axillary line. Femoral venous and arterial cannulation. Be familiar with alternative strategies to arrest the heart since you may not be able to clamp and deliver antegrade so easily in this case. Options include fibrillatory arrest under moderate hypothermia or endoballoon (both require competent aortic valve).

"Anesthesia gives the patient nipride to make room for more volume when coming off the pump. The patient becomes hypotensive and 3+ MR is noted with encroachment of the anterior leaflet onto the LVOT. What is the treatment?"

279

This patient has systolic anterior motion (SAM) of the mitral valve which was accentuated by the increased ventricular systolic contraction in the setting of an underfilled ventricle. The treatment of choice here is to wait while the volume rolls in. May also consider adding a beta blocker to reduce the vigor of the systolic contractions once the volume is optimized. Inotropic support and/or reduced afterload will make things worse.

"Describe SAM and options for correcting it after an attempted mitral repair."
The line of coaptation after a reduction annuloplasty and leaflet resection/repair typically gets displaced just a bit more anterior (towards the LVOT) than it did before. The anterior leaflet can obstruct the LVOT during systole creating a gradient. As the anterior leaflet gets sucked into the LVOT during systole (Venturi effect), the posterior leaflet prolapses towards the atrium causing an anteriorly directed jet. Thus, the two main worrisome components of SAM are regurgitation and high LVOT gradient. If the posterior leaflet is left > 1.5 cm in height after repair the risk for SAM is greater. If the patient has a small hyperdynamic ventricle the risk for SAM is greater. If the ring is undersized too much, then the risk of SAM is also greater because the line of coaptation bulges anteriorly. First ensure that you are not simply underfilled as described in the prior scenario. Otherwise, treatment strategies aim to reduce the posterior leaflet height if it is clear that that is the culprit. Folding valvuloplasty of the edge of the posterior leaflet with interrupted horizontal pledgeted sutures, changing a triangular resection into a quadrangular with sliding annuloplasty, and placement of a larger ring are all options for reducing the posterior leaflet height. A more aggressive maneuver is to replace the valve. Another simple fix in a frail high-risk patient that may not tolerate a second pump run is an Alfieri stitch.

"What are the pre- and intra-operative SAM risk factors?"
- Tall posterior leaflet (>15mm)
- AL:PL ratio ≤ 1.3
- Aorto-Mitral Plane Angle < 120 deg
- Coapt – Septum Distance < 25mm
- Interventricular septum (IVS) thickness > 15mm
- Small and hyperkinetic LV
- Anterior displacement of papillary muscles
- Small prosthetic ring

"After a mitral valve replacement, a significant amount of bright red blood is seen welling up behind the heart once the cross clamp is released!"
Atrioventricular dissociation after mitral valve replacement. Often occurs after completion of CPB or a few hours after procedure. Patients have massive intrapericardial hemorrhage which can be a lethal event. Rupture occurs in the LV near the AV groove posteriorly. Tends to occur more in women with small LVs. Generally considered to be a technical error from a) too much traction on the annulus during excision of the valve or insertion of prosthesis; b) tearing of the annulus after the new valve is in place when the heart is lifted manually; c) penetration of stitches in the posterior left AV groove; d) perforation from papillary muscle excision; e) perforation of AV groove during calcium debridement (especially with ventricular calcium). Go back on CPB and re-arrest. Re-open the LA, remove the prosthesis and inspect the ventricle. An appropriately sized pericardial patch is secured over the area of perforation with a running prolene suture and interrupted pledgeted sutures as needed. The valve is reimplanted and the operation is completed as previously described. If the initial operation was a mitral valve repair, the valve must be replaced if there is an AV groove disruption. This is necessary because the PL tissue is now used to buttress the patch repair and reduce tension on the suture line of the patch repair by providing additional chordal support beyond the repair.

"ST changes are noted along the lateral leads and the patient becomes hypotensive requiring high dose epinephrine and norepinephrine. What has happened?"

280

The differential may include postcardiotomy syndrome with cardiogenic shock from reperfusion or poor protection. However, the most likely culprit in the setting of a valve replacement is damage to the coronary especially with the isolated lead changes. Go back on, harvest a segment of vein, arrest and bypass to a distal OM.

Note that a valve causing excessive traction on the circumflex can lead to delayed myocardial ischemia and even LV rupture secondary to erosion of the strut through an infarcted LV free wall. This is seen most often in women with a small LV or when the LV is weakened after an infarct. Special care needs to be taken to ensure the safety of the circumflex artery and if any question is raised, a marginal branch should be bypassed using a SVG prior to coming off cardiopulmonary bypass.

"After opening the left atrium, there is much more blood than is expected despite a floppy sucker in the RSPV. You cannot see anything, what are the possible explanations?"

First, check that the aortic cross clamp is completely around the aorta and tight enough to occlude flow. Next, explore the septum for an ASD. This is typically able to be accomplished via the left atrium although sometimes to repair may require a right atrial incision.

Pearls/pitfalls

- Know the indications for mitral valve surgery.
- Know the different exposures for the mitral valve and when you would choose one over the other.
- Know the major complications of the procedure - circumflex injury, AV disruption, aortic regurgitation.
- Recognize SAM and its treatment (medical - volume, betablocker; surgical - posterior leaflet height reduction, upsizing the band/ring size).
- Know how to deal with a calcified mitral annulus.

Suggested readings

- Kouchoukos NT and Kirklin JW. Kirklin/Barratt-Boyes *Cardiac Surgery: Morphology, Diagnostic Criteria, Natural History, Techniques, Results, and Indications.* Philadelphia, Pa: Churchill Livingstone, 2003.
- Yuh, DD, Vricella LA and Baumgartner WA.*The Johns Hopkins Manual of Cardiothoracic Surgery.* New York: McGraw-Hill Medical Pub, 2007.
- Carpentier, A., Adams, D. and Filsoufi, F., 2010. *Carpentier's Reconstructive Valve Surgery.* Maryland Heights, Mo.: Saunders/Elsevier.

44. REOPERATIVE MITRAL VALVE REPLACEMENT

Cynthia E. Wagner, MD, and Gorav Ailawadi, MD

Concept

- Indications and outcomes for reoperative mitral valve surgery
- Considerations for re-repair vs. primary replacement
- Considerations for bioprosthetic vs. mechanical valve replacement
- Operative details specific to redo mitral valve surgery
- Complications of mitral valve surgery

Chief complaint

"A 70-year-old woman with a 3-month history of dyspnea on exertion is referred by her cardiologist after a TTE showed severe MR due to leaflet prolapse, mitral annular calcification, mild pulmonary hypertension, and LVEF 55%. The patient underwent mitral valve repair for leaflet prolapse ten years ago."

Differential

The diagnosis has been established and should be confirmed with a detailed H&P and appropriate tests. In the absence of an echo report, the differential diagnosis for these symptoms in a patient s/p valve repair would include recurrent MR, MS, AS, AI, cardiomyopathy, CHF, pulmonary hypertension, stable/unstable angina, or primary pulmonary disease.

History and physical

A thorough history to establish functional status, assess for comorbidities (HTN, HLD, DM, AF, CAD, carotid disease, PVD, CKD), and determine all prior surgeries or procedures. Detailed operative reports from all prior cardiac surgeries should be obtained. Some patients will not recognize stent placement (cardiac or aortoiliac) or pacemaker placement as surgery and should be asked directly about these procedures, as they will guide further work-up and may impact plans for cannulation. A history of trauma to the right chest should be inquired about if a right lateral thoracotomy is planned. Medications should be reviewed and indications for anticoagulation should be questioned, as this may impact choice of valve prosthesis if mitral valve replacement (MVR) is planned. Social factors, including family planning in younger female patients, occupation, and hobbies, should be identified that may increase bleeding risk from anticoagulation for a mechanical valve. All patients should be asked about prior stroke and residual deficits prior to cardiac surgery. A focused physical examination should follow, assessing for heart rate and rhythm, murmurs, bruits, bibasilar rales, and lower extremity edema, and noting all prior surgical incisions. In select patients, assess fall risk and frailty with grip strength and 15 ft walk test.

Tests

- EKG to assess for AF.
- CXR to assess number of sternal wires, may show cardiomegaly and cephalization of pulmonary blood flow.
- Non-contrast chest CT to assess distance between posterior sternum and anterior RV as well as extent of aortic calcification and mitral annular calcification, and CTA chest to identify course of patent grafts if patient has undergone prior CABG.
- CTA abdomen/pelvis to assess vessel caliber and tortuosity if femoral cannulation is planned.
- Preoperative TEE to better visualize mitral valve pathology is essential in determining mechanism of MR, especially if re-repair is planned, and may identify thrombus in the LA appendage if patient has AF.

- Cardiac catheterization should be routine, as undiagnosed CAD may result in perioperative morbidity or the need for further reoperation and is essential in determining patency of grafts in patients who have undergone prior CABG.
- Consider right heart catheterization in patients with severe LV or RV dysfunction or symptomatic patients in class III-IV CHF.
- Carotid duplex in high-risk patients.
- PFTs in select patients.
- Obtain prior operative report to include year of surgery, details of operation, valve exposure, possible location of grafts, manufacturer of valve.

Index scenario (additional information)
"The patient has had progressively worsening MR and LV function on annual TTE and has been asymptomatic on a diuretic and an ACE inhibitor until recently. She does not have AF and does not require anticoagulation for any pre-existing disease. She has HTN, hyperlipidemia (HLD), and DM, and a preoperative cardiac catheterization shows severe multi-vessel CAD. This prompts a carotid duplex prior to cardiac surgery. A chest CT shows a mildly dilated RV immediately posterior to the sternum and an ascending aorta with minimal atherosclerotic disease. A CTA abdomen/pelvis is done in anticipation of femoral cannulation prior to redo sternotomy."

Treatment/management

This patient meets criteria for a reoperative mitral valve surgery according to current ACC/AHA guidelines.

Table 40-1. Indications for intervention in mitral valve disease.

Symptomatic patients with moderately severe to severe MR (3-4+) or moderate to severe MS
Asymptomatic patients with severe MR with any of the following conditions: • LVEF < 60% • LV end-systolic diameter > 40-45 mm • PHTN with PASP > 50-60 mmHg New-onset AF

Mitral valve repair eliminates the risks associated with MVR, including bleeding, thromboembolic events, and prosthetic valve endocarditis. Re-repair is associated with lower mortality compared to replacement at reoperation and may be attempted on previously repaired mitral valves unless severe calcification of the leaflets, annulus, and subvalvular apparatus or extensive leaflet destruction from endocarditis is present. However, this requires a high comfort level with redo repair strategies - it is never wrong to replace especially during a redo. Etiology of valve disease dictates durability of repair. After primary mitral valve repair, freedom from reoperation at 10 years is 95% in patients with degenerative valve disease vs. 53% in patients with rheumatic valve disease. Early failure after repair (< 2 years) is often the result of technical failure, while late failure after repair (> 2 years) is often due to progression of native valve disease. Repair without ring annuloplasty is a predictor of recurrent MR and need for reoperation. Most first-time reoperations after mitral valve repair result in replacement, for which preservation of the subvalvular apparatus should be attempted as this has been shown to reduce operative mortality and preserve LVEF. Major factors to consider in discussions regarding bioprosthetic vs. mechanical MVR include patient age, life expectancy, comorbidities, and bleeding risk from anticoagulation. Bioprosthetic valves will deteriorate, and the rate of structural valve deterioration and need for reoperation are inversely related to patient age at implantation. Mechanical mitral valves require lifelong anticoagulation (INR goal of 2.5-3.5), and the risk of hemorrhagic stroke is 2-4% per patient per year. The rate of thromboembolic complications (1-3% per patient per year) and the risk of prosthetic valve endocarditis are similar between bioprosthetic and mechanical valves. Although mechanical valves do not structurally deteriorate, they are prone to paravalvular leaks and undergo nonstructural dysfunction (pannus formation). The average time to reoperation after primary MVR is similar between bioprosthetic and mechanical valves (mean 11.5 years), though the durability of a mechanical valve can extend years beyond that of a bioprosthetic valve. The majority of bioprosthetic valves are replaced for structural deterioration and most mechanical valves are replaced for paravalvular leak. The operative mortality of redo MVR is approximately 4.7%. There is no significant difference in operative mortality after redo MVR in patients receiving bioprosthetic vs. mechanical valves (5% vs. 4.4%). Mortality rates have decreased in recent years due to earlier intervention prior to significant LV dysfunction and advances in operative techniques and perioperative care.

Operative steps

- Consider femoral or axillary arterial cannulation and femoral venous cannulation prior to redo sternotomy if RV is adherent to chest wall. (refer to Redo AVR chapter for cannulation algorithm).

- Redo sternotomy is the most common approach for reoperative mitral valve surgery and demands preoperative identification of patent grafts from prior CABG, proximity of heart to posterior sternum, and RV dilatation. A median sternotomy is necessary in the setting of concomitant CABG or AVR. However, a right lateral thoracotomy is an alternative approach in select patients undergoing exclusive mitral valve surgery (tricuspid valve may also be visualized with this approach).

- Myocardial protection is commonly achieved with cardioplegic arrest with antegrade and/or retrograde cold blood cardioplegia. Strategies for myocardial protection will need to be altered in patients with a patent LIMA-LAD from prior CABG. DHCA or ventricular fibrillatory arrest may be feasible in select patients undergoing exclusive mitral valve surgery without significant AI.

- Standard left atriotomy is begun in Waterston's interatrial groove and extended inferiorly to provide optimal exposure of the mitral valve. A transeptal approach through a right atriotomy is a common alternative in patients with significant adhesions undergoing reoperative mitral valve surgery.

- In patients undergoing MVR after repair, all attempts should be made to preserve native leaflet tissue and associated chordae tendineae during MVR, as disruption of the continuity between the mitral annulus and LV apex has been shown to result in decreased LV function postoperatively. This can be accomplished by imbrication of the leaflet tissue to the annulus.

- Care must be taken when resecting valve sewing rings to avoid removal of excess annular tissue and subsequent disruption of the atrioventricular junction. There are several options for mitral annular reconstruction, including bovine vs. autologous pericardial patch reconstruction or suture placement across the atrioventricular junction to restore a fibrous mitral annulus.

- In patients presenting with a paravalvular leak after MVR, consider percutaneous closure devices or open repair with pledgeted reinforcing sutures or a bovine pericardial patch prior to excision of a competent valve (though most often these patients require redo MVR). Read the prior operative report carefully. These types of minimally invasive options may be ideal for patients who had a very difficult initial operation with annular reconstruction.

- Determining valve competency with saline test and intraoperative TEE following repair is crucial in identifying need for immediate revision, as residual MR (> 1+) at the completion of surgery is a risk factor for recurrence of moderate/severe MR and need for reoperative mitral valve surgery, and cumulative risk of mortality increases with each reoperation.

Potential questions/alternative scenarios

"The patient requires high-dose pressors as they are weaned from CPB. This pressor requirement persists into postoperative day 1 and a TTE shows a lateral wall motion abnormality. Discuss the complication."

The distance between the posterolateral mitral annulus and the circumflex artery is 2-4 mm. Patients are at risk for postoperative MI if sutures are placed too wide or deep around the posterolateral annulus during MVR or ring annuloplasty.

"The patient is unable to be weaned from CPB without external V-pacing. The monitor shows complete heart block. Discuss the complication."

The AV node is deep to the posteromedial commissure. Care must be taken to avoid placing sutures too deep around the annulus during MVR or ring annuloplasty.

"Discuss the risks, management, and prevention of prosthetic valve endocarditis (PVE)."

Risk of infection is greatest during the first three postoperative months and decreases thereafter to < 1% per patient per year after the first postoperative year. Early PVE (within the first 2 mos) is often caused by virulent *Staphylococcus* infections and has a higher mortality than late PVE, often the result of *Streptococcus* infections. Infection is localized to the sewing ring of mechanical valves, resulting in abscess formation and dehiscence, while infection of bioprosthetic valves occurs on the leaflets and leads to vegetations and leaflet perforation. Indications for and timing of surgery should be individualized and based on response to antibiotics and hemodynamic stability (refer to Endocarditis chapter). Despite improved outcomes after surgery, PVE continues to carry a high mortality rate, and in patients with prosthetic heart valves, the AHA currently recommends prophylaxis with amoxicillin or cephalexin prior to dental procedures, invasive procedures of the respiratory tract involving biopsy, or excision of infected soft tissues.

"The patient agrees to undergo bioprosthetic MVR. She asks if a third operation will be likely."

In patients receiving bioprosthetic valve replacements, the freedom from reoperation at 15 years is 80%. Bioprosthetic valves in the mitral position are exposed to increased hemodynamic stress during systole compared to bioprosthetic valves in the aortic position and undergo deterioration at a higher rate. Currently, younger patients are receiving bioprosthetic valves due to improvements in valve design and durability and options for transcatheter   valve-in-valve   implantation.

Pearls/pitfalls

- Considerations in reoperative surgery include alternative strategies for cannulation, surgical approach to the mitral valve, and myocardial protection.
- Mitral valve repair at primary surgery and at reoperation is associated with lower mortality compared to MVR and should be attempted if possible (this requires a high comfort level with redo repair strategies - it is never wrong to replace especially during a redo).
- Choice of bioprosthetic vs. mechanical MVR should be based on individualized risk of reoperation vs. anticoagulation.
- MVR with leaflet/chordal sparing is associated with improved outcomes but do not compromise your outflow.
- The mitral annulus is near the circumflex artery and AV node.

Suggested readings

- Acquired disease of the mitral valve. Sabiston and Spencer - *Surgery of the Chest*, 8th edition. 1207-1240.
- Reoperative valve surgery. Cohn L (ed). *Cardiac Surgery in the Adult*. 3rd edition. 1159-1174.
- Nardi et al. Survival and durability of mitral valve repair surgery for degenerative mitral valve disease. *J Card Surg.* 2011 Jul;26(4):360-6.

- Suri RM et al. Recurrent mitral regurgitation after repair: should the mitral valve be re-repaired? *J Thorac Cardiovasc Surg.* 2006 Dec;132(6):1390-7.
- Potter et al. Risk of repeat mitral valve replacement for failed mitral valve prostheses. *Ann Thorac Surg.* 2004 Jul;78(1):67-72.

45. MITRAL STENOSIS

Marek Polomsky, MD, and Robert A. Guyton, MD

Concept

- Indications for mitral valve replacement (MVR) in setting of mitral stenosis (MS)
- Preoperative conditions
- Valve choices
- Critical steps of MVR
- Pitfalls and alternative solutions

Chief complaint

"A 53-year-old immigrant man presents with a diagnosis of mitral stenosis. His primary care physician heard a diastolic apical heart murmur, and subsequent echocardiogram revealed severe mitral stenosis."

Differential

The diagnosis of mitral stenosis is established. Differential causes of mitral stenosis include rheumatic heart disease (majority), congenital malformation, infective endocarditis (IE), mitral annular calcification, rheumatologic disorders, endomyocardial fibrosis, conditions that obstruct the mitral valve (left atrial myxoma, cor triatriatum), and prosthetic valve complications (thrombosis, calcification).

History and physical

A focused history is performed to elicit symptoms of dyspnea and hemoptysis, as well as chest pain and hoarseness, which occur less frequently. Symptoms are brought on by any situation that increase the transmitral pressure gradient (exertion, stress, exercise, tachycardia, fever, infection, atrial fibrillation (AF), pregnancy). Many patients deny symptoms because progression of disease is very slow, thus there is a gradual decrease in activity and exercise tolerance. MS can present with complications such as AF, pulmonary edema, embolic events, IE, and right heart failure. One should ascertain whether there is a prior history of rheumatic heart disease (if treated and which kind of antibiotics) and if the patient is an immigrant from another country. A complete physical should be performed focusing on the cardiovascular exam with presence of murmur (low-pitched diastolic rumble most prominent at the apex), opening snap of the mitral valve heard at the apex, and signs of right heart failure indicative of advanced disease. Pinkish blue patches on cheeks ("mitral facies") may be present from vasoconstriction due to low cardiac output.

Tests

- *EKG.* An EKG is performed to assess for any arrhythmias (particularly AF). In addition, a broad p-wave that is notched with increased amplitude ("p-mitrale") from left atrial (LA) hypertrophy or enlargement may be present.
- *Echo (M-mode, two-dimensional and color Doppler flow mapping).* Echocardiography is used to assess morphology of the valve apparatus and subvalvular structures (chordae and papillary muscles), measurement of valve orifice, Doppler transvalvular gradient and valve area (calculated from diastolic velocity curve), coexisting mitral regurgitation, pulmonary pressures, systolic function, exclusion of LA thrombus, and size of LA, left ventricle, and right ventricle. Transesophageal echo (TEE) is generally preferred over transthoracic echo (TTE).
- *Cardiac catheterization.* Cardiac catheterization is performed in order to assess the coronaries, mitral valve gradient, and pulmonary artery pressures.
- *CXR.* LA enlargement, a calcified mitral annulus, and pulmonary vasculature congestion or cephalization may be visible on a CXR. If aorta appears calcified check CT.

287

- *Stress echo (exercise or dobutamine stress echo).* A stress echocardiogram is used to objectively evaluate exercise activity, which is important for provocation of symptoms in inactive patients, and to assess pulmonary artery pressures with exertion.

Index scenario (additional information)

"The patient had history of rheumatic heart disease as child, and after diagnostic work-up was found to have very calcified severe MS (valve area 0.8 cm^2) with severe pulmonary hypertension (70 mmHg). He is mildly symptomatic."

Treatment/management

This patient meets criteria for mitral valve replacement. Surgery (MVR) is indicated (2006 ACC/AHA guidelines) in patients who are found to have moderate-severe MS (MV area < 1.5 cm^2), NYHA class III or IV symptoms, and the valve is not amenable to either percutaneous mitral balloon valvuloplasty (PMBV). In addition, mildly symptomatic patients (NYHA II) with severe MS and pulmonary hypertension (PAP > 50 mmHg at rest, > 60 with exercise) who are not candidates for valvulotomy are considered for surgery. Severe PHTN, however, raises a red flag. It is hard to tell whether this will be readily reversible or not. It is worth a chance, but care must be taken in the postoperative setting. PMBV is not appropriate if there is presence of LA thrombus that persists despite anticoagulation, mitral valve is nonpliable or severely calcified, or if there is moderate-severe mitral regurgitation (MR). Wilkins score > 8 predicts failure with valvuloplasty (leaflet mobility, thickening, calcifications, subvalvular apparatus). Mechanical prosthesis is recommended in this patient, and in patients that present young (< 65 yo) especially with long standing AF. A bioprosthetic valve would be indicated in patients who are elderly, who cannot have warfarin, or who are not compliant.

Operative steps

Mitral valve replacement

Goals – relieve obstruction, replace the valve, protect the heart/coronaries, prevent further clot formation and embolization.

- Place central line with Swan-Ganz catheter, arterial line, general endotracheal anesthesia (GETA), foley.
- Assess mitral valve via TEE.
- Perform median sternotomy. Palpate for aortic calcifications +/- epiaortic US.
- Systemic heparin, aortic cannulation, 3-stage venous or bicaval cannulation, retrograde cardioplegia cannula.
- Initiate cardiopulmonary bypass (CPB) once ACT level appropriate (400-600), +/- cooling (28-32° C).
- Cross-clamp, run cold blood antegrade cardioplegia, followed by retrograde.
- Vertical left atriotomy incision in Sondergaard's groove anterior to the right pulmonary veins (or use exposure of choice).
- Place sump vent into LA in dependent position near left superior pulmonary vein.
- Inspect the mitral valve.
- *Note*: perform any necessary afib procedures such as left atrial appendage excision/ligation/ MAZE at this time to avoid manipulating the heart too much after the prosthesis is in place.
- Excise calcified leaflets leaving 1-2 mm of leaflet tissue along the annular circumference, dividing chordae along tips of papillary muscles (preserve subvalvular apparatus and papillary muscle-chordal-leaflet attachments whenever possible, but not at the expense of outflow tract obstruction in a small ventricle). Usually the posterior leaflet can be salvaged to maintain continuity while the anterior is resected.

288

- Size the valve, place horizontal mattress sutures 8-10 mm apart (usually with pledgets) around the annulus, everting (atrium –ventricle) for mechanical valve, and non-everting for bioprosthetic valve (ventricle-atrium) or calcified annulus.
- Pass sutures through sewing ring and seat the valve. Mechanical valve should be in anti-anatomic position, bioprosthetic valve with largest leaflet facing the left ventricular outflow tract (LVOT) avoiding outflow obstruction. Use a dental mirror to double check.
- Tie down sutures and start rewarming if cool.
- Close left atriotomy with 3-0 or 4-0 prolene, leaving LV vent.
- Give hot shot cardioplegia before releasing the cross-clamp, deair, wean from bypass, and assess valve by TEE, leave pacing wires.

Potential questions/alternative scenarios

"Patient is a pregnant female."

In previously asymptomatic female, elevations in heart rate and cardiac output during pregnancy can increase the transmitral gradient which can lead to symptoms. Medical management should be the first line of therapy, and if fails then anatomically suitable valves can undergo PMBV. Mitral valve surgery during pregnancy is associated with an increased maternal and fetal risk. Females with MS planning to become pregnant should have their MS treated prior to conception.

"Patient has a non-calcified and pliable mitral valve."

The patient is candidate for PMBV or open commissurotomy and valve repair. Patients who have pliable and non calcified valves, with little or no subvalvular fusion and no calcification in commissures, absence of 3+ or 4+ MR (moderate - severe MR), and no LA thrombus are candidates for PMBV or open commissurotomy and valve repair. If there are not any contraindications, PMBV should be performed first. Extent of valve pathology dictates PMBV vs. open commissurotomy and repair ("soft" rheumatic changes without extensive subvalvular pathology are amenable to PMBV). In addition, patients who are at high surgical risk from comorbidities to undergo MVR should be considered for PMBV.

"In what order would you proceed with concomitant AVR, TVR, or CABG."

Distal coronary anastomoses are performed first, which avoids lifting of the heart after mitral prosthesis is placed and allows using the bypass grafts for cardioplegia. Aortic valve leaflets are excised, and then perform MVR. Then perform AVR. TVR is performed after MVR, and it can be performed after removing the cross-clamp.

"A 64-year-old female with ESRD has severe mitral annular calcification (MAC)."

Patients with ESRD are at increased risk for MAC. The degree of MAC influences the surgical approach. Mild amounts can be handled by placing the sutures in an inverted manner (ventricle → atria) around or even through the calcium (if soft enough). Moderate amounts can be debrided until you have a smooth symmetrical surface for the prosthesis to attach. You can then take the inverted sutures along the posterior half of the annulus and pass them through a pericardial patch or felt strip before going through the sewing ring for additional reinforcement. Greater degrees of MAC may require radical debridement of the calcified annulus down to epicardial fat followed by reconstruction with a pericardial patch (autologous pericardium or glutaraldehyde-fixed bovine pericardium) that saddles/sandwiches the annulus. The patch is attached to LV endocardium on the LV side and atrial tissue on the LA side. Valve sutures would then pass through the patch going from the LV to LA and then the sewing ring. Other alternatives include seating the mitral prosthesis at the intra-atrial level with the aid of a Dacron collar. Be sure you are familiar with these approaches before describing or performing them.

"You discover AV groove rupture."

Atrioventricular groove rupture can occur if the sutures are placed too deep, if there is excessive retraction, if the heart is massaged too vigorously at time of deairing, or if there is overly aggressive debridement or decalcification of the posterior leaflet and annulus. If an AV groove rupture is discovered rearrest the heart if not already cross-clamped and close the full extent of the tear with a pericardial patch. The patch should be secured by sutures into healthy myocardium for a tension-free repair, with careful placement of sutures near coronary vessels.

"After coming off bypass EKG changes are noted in the lateral leads with lateral wall motion abnormalities and depressed ventricular function."
A circumflex artery injury is suspected which can happen if sutures are placed too deep along the posterior annulus. In order to fix this problem, a RSVG to the circumflex artery distribution will be needed.

"After removing cross-clamp you see increased LV distention."
An aortic valve injury may happen when sutures are placed too deep across the anterior annulus, thus injuring the non-coronary or left aortic valve cusps. It is recognized once one removes the cross-clamp and sees the LV distend due to aortic insufficiency, which can be visualized on TEE as well. Re-arrest the heart, open the aorta and left atrium, and after inspection remove the offending suture or possibly the whole mitral prosthesis. The aortic cusp will need to be repaired or replaced.

"Conduction block post-op."
A conduction block can happen if one takes sutures too deep near the posterior commissure and right trigone where the AV node and Bundle of His can be injured. Often with radical debridement there is no other room to place sutures. If the conduction disturbance does not improve after several days post-op, a permanent pacemaker will be needed.

"When coming off bypass you note increased gradients across the left ventricular outflow tract (LVOT)."
LVOT obstruction can occur from the prosthesis if it is a high-profile mechanical valve, large stented biologic valve posts, or even from low-profile valves that are not properly seated. Typically, one will need to replace the valve with a lower profile valve. In addition, if one leaves the mitral anterior leaflet unresected with chordal sparing techniques, systolic anterior motion (SAM) can occur due to retained anterior leaflet and chordae, especially if there is septal hypertrophy. In general SAM usually improves if one stops inotropes, volume loads, adds beta-blockers, and adds vasopressors (increasing afterload). Occasionally one may need to perform an aortotomy with transaortic excision of the offending subaortic mitral tissue, and myectomy.

"Perivalvular leak on the postoperative echo."
Most small leaks will stop after protamine administration. If there is a significant leak, then you will have to go back on bypass and fix or re-implant the valve.

"How would you manage patients postoperatively after MVR."
Close attention should be paid to patient's respiratory status and pulmonary pressures. If a patient develops or has elevated pulmonary artery pressures signifying severe pulmonary hypertension, more aggressive diuresis than usual will be needed. Right ventricular function may be compromised necessitating ionotropic and pulmonary vasodilatory therapy. Be very careful with volume overload on these patients. Run them high (inotropes) and dry (diuretics). Anticoagulation (AC) therapy will need to be initiated for mechanical valves (goal INR 2.5-3.5).

Pearls/pitfalls

- Mitral valve replacement is indicated for moderate-severe MS (MV area $< 1.5 \text{ cm}^2$), NYHA class III or IV symptoms, and the valve is not amenable to either percutaneous mitral balloon valvuloplasty (PMBV) or open commissurotomy.

- Mildly symptomatic patients (NYHA II) with severe MS and pulmonary hypertension (PAP > 50 mmHg at rest, > 60 with exercise) who are not candidates for valvulotomy are considered for surgery. Patients with severe MS and new onset afib are also considered for PMBV or replacement.

- Tissue valve in patients > 65 yo, sinus rhythm, and who cannot take or are non-compliant with warfarin.

- *Order of concomitant procedures*: distal coronary anastomosis $\rightarrow$ debride aortic valve $\rightarrow$ MVR $\rightarrow$ AVR $\rightarrow$ TVR (can be done w ccx removed).

- Overly aggressive debridement or retraction/lifting of the heart can lead to AV groove rupture.

- Deep valve sutures can cause injury to the circumflex artery, aortic cusps, and conduction system.

Suggested readings

- Yun KL and Miller DC. Acquired valvular heart disease: mitral valve replacement. *Mastery of Cardiothoracic Surgery* 2007. 378-390.

- Gallegos RP, Gudbjartsson T, and Aranki S. Mitral valve replacement. *Cardiac Surgery in the Adult* 2012.

- Bonow RO et al. ACC/AHA 2006 Guidelines for the management of patients with valvular heart disease. A report of the American College of Cardiology/American Heart Association Task Force on Practice Guidelines (Writing committee to revise the 1998 guidelines for the management of patients with valvular heart disease). *JACC* 2006. 48:e1.

46. Arrhythmia Surgery

Clauden Louis, MD, Daniel Ryan Ziazadeh, MD, Peter Knight, MD

Clauden Louis, MD, Daniel Ryan Ziazadeh, MD, Peter Knight, MD

Concept
- Subtypes
  - Paroxysmal Atrial Fibrillation (PAF)
    - AF intermittently with each episode less than 1 week
  - Non-Paroxysmal Atrial Fibrillation (NPAF)
    - Persistent AF - lasting longer than 1 week
    - Longstanding Persistent AF - continuous AF of greater than 1 year
    - Permanent AF - AF that cannot be electrically cardioverted
- Surgical pitfalls and indications for ablation

Key terms: Non-Paroxysmal Atrial Fibrillation (NPAF), Paroxysmal Atrial Fibrillation (PAF), MAZE, Cryoablation, Radiofrequency Ablation

Chief complaint

A 61-year-old female with long-standing atrial fibrillation following failed EP ablations presents for further evaluation and consultation regarding definitive management of her arrhythmia.

Differential

Non-Paroxysmal Atrial Fibrillation (NPAF), Paroxysmal Atrial Fibrillation (PAF), Premature atrial contractions, Premature ventricular contractions, Atrial Flutter

History and physical

Any patient being considered for arrhythmia surgery needs to have a comprehensive system-based history and physical to identify history of stroke, renal disease, coronary lesions, respiratory problems, bleeding disorders, or peripheral vascular disease. This can usually be performed prior to intervention as arrhythmia surgery is typically an elective procedure. Concomitant cardiac comorbidities must be ruled out.

Tests
- Biochemical Profile (CMP, LFTs)
- CBC
- Cardiac Enzymes (Troponin, CK, LDH)
- BNP
- EKG
- ECHO (TTE +/- TEE)
- Cardiac catheterization

Index scenario (additional information)

Upon further evaluation of her transthoracic echocardiography, imaging reveals that in addition to long-standing atrial fibrillation she also has severe mitral regurgitation. What is the definitive management available for this patient?

Treatment/Management
- The objective of intervention for AF, either stand-alone or concomitant, depends on whether the patient has PAF or Non-PAF.
  - Paroxysmal AF - "Isolate the Triggers."
  - N-PAF - "Interrupt the Drivers."
- In the treatment of this lesion a Bi-Atrial Maze with LAA ligation should be considered. Bi-atrial MAZE surgical procedures are more effective than left-sided

procedures in eliminating AF as the addition of right atrial lesions increase likelihood of normal sinus rhythm. (Barrett et al)., Sole Left-Sided Maze Procedure are incomplete as RA drivers are not intervened upon. Additionally, right-sided ablations are important for the prevention of atrial flutter.

Indications
1) Atrial fibrillation resistant to drug Tx
2) Intolerance to drug Tx
3) Six months of atrial fibrillation w/ enlarged atrium
4) High risk for thromboembolism (eg hypercoagulable state)
5) Contraindication to anticoagulation
6) Patients who have suffered a stroke on Coumadin

Key maneuver is pulmonary vein isolation (majority of atrial fibrillation foci located in pulmonary veins) MAZE can be done off cardiopulmonary bypass (cryolesions, RF ablation) Success rate – 70%

Contraindications
Relative
- None

Operative steps – Cox Maze IV
Conduct of operation varies significantly depending on what else needs to be done
- Aortobicaval cannulation
- Pulmonary Vein Isolation and Ablation (can be done outside the heart using Atricure RF device or inside the heart using cryo).
  - o Ablation of the right pulmonary veins (RPVs)
  - o Ablation of the left pulmonary veins (LPVs).
  - o Must obliterate Ligament of Marshall
    - Fetal left SVC that stretches across the base of the LA appendage near the LSPV
- Snare SVC/IVC
- Arrest heart (not mandatory)
- Open left atrial appendage (LAA)
- LAA to left superior vein lesion
- Exclude LAA: clip or surgical ligation
- Left atriotomy
- Construction of the floor lesion of the box
- Construction of the roof lesion of the box
- Coronary sinus lesion
- Mitral valve lesion
- Vertical right atriotomy
- Tricuspid valve lesion
- Superior vena cava lesion
- Inferior vena cave lesion

What is the cryoablation energy source?
- Nitrous Oxide – Atricure (CryoICE)
  - o Reaches probe temperatures of -60^0C
- Argon Gas – Medtronic (CryoFlex 10S)
  - o Reaches probe temperatures of -150^0C
- Both devices feature a 10 cm malleable probe with insulation sleeve

What is the purpose of the box lesion?

- Adding the roof and floor lines to create a Box Lesion does two things.
    1. It isolates 80% of the triggers that induce PAF
    2. It interrupts at least some of the macro-reentrant circuits that sustain N-PAF
- If a given patient has N-PAF that happens to be sustained by some of the reentrant circuits that are interrupted by the Box Lesion, this alone might cure that patient's N-PAF.
- This occurs infrequently but may account for the reported 20-45% 5-year success rate of catheter ablation for N-PAF.

Potential Questions / Alternative Scenario

While dissecting the transverse sinus, you inadvertently see a dark collection of blood begin to pool. What have you likely injured?

There is a concern for injury of the right pulmonary artery (RPA).

Potential questions/alternative scenarios

A 61-year-old female with a 7-year history of mitral regurgitation and long-standing atrial fibrillation underwent a concomitant mitral valve repair with ring annuloplasty and a Cox Maze IV procedure with left atrial appendage ligation. She returns 2 weeks later to the clinic with symptoms of palpitation and found to be in atrial flutter with a heart rate of 160 beats/min. What is the likely cause of her symptoms?

"Peri-Mitral Flutter"

Failure to interrupt conduction across the Left Atrial Isthmus allows the development of so-called "Peri-Mitral Flutter", the most common mode of failure of surgery for AF. This is due to an incomplete lesion line involving the mitral valve annulus. A catheter-based intervention by EP colleagues may assist in completing this ablation line.

- Lesions sets not connected such as transmural ablation of the epicardium and endocardium of the coronary sinus to the level of the mitral annulus can lead to flutter
- A large macro-reentrant circuit develops just above the mitral valve annulus thus it's important to perform both the mitral line to prevent conduction across the atrial myocardium and the coronary sinus lesion to prevent conduction across the coronary sinus.
- Coronary sinus conduction occurs in a small subsegment of patients. Thus, all patients undergoing arrhythmia surgery require ablation to both the mitral isthmus and the coronary sinus lesion. One must collapse the CS during cryoablation, a circumferential lesion can be assured.
- As the CS is collapse an "iceball" is created by the cryoprobe on the epicardium that can also be seen as an "iceball" on the endocardium of the left atrium, as the LA is opened. Preventing postoperative Peri-Mitral flutter is done by placing both the mitral line and the CS lesions in the same plane.

Potential Complications / Alternative Scenarios

While preforming the Cox Maze IV with cryoablation, you notice a cryolesion across the pericardial surface of the right atrium of the heart. What complication can you expect post operatively and how can this mistake be avoided in the future?

- It is wise to protect the right phrenic nerve while performing cryosurgery in either the right or left atrium. The handle of the cryoprobe can sometimes be inadvertently resting on the right phrenic nerve and cause temporary right hemidiaphragm paralysis. Special care should be taken at all times of the procedure to avoid this complication.

Potential Questions / Alternative Scenarios

After completing the Cox-Maze IV, you notice that there is a discontinuous lesion due to a fold in tissue. The cryoprobe is no longer sterile. You determine that the line appears good enough. After rewarming, you notice that the patient is still in A-Fib.

Why did the procedure fail?

- The Maze is unforgiving, with even a minor slip in technique. Even a single break in the line can preserve a macro reentry circuit and the entire procedure will fail.
- Incoming waves of atrial activation will find even the slightest break in the line. The lesions must be uniformly transmural (full thickness), and contiguous. Unfortunately, even cryoablation and bipolar RF clamps are not full proof. Gaps in the ablation line create islands of scar that can result in iatrogenic flutter.
- Tissue folding is a sign of poor technique and will always create a line with multiple breaks. The clamp will only ablate through the folded section, creating an air tissue interface in the unfolded sections with no contact or ablation.

Potential questions/alternative scenarios

Instead of using the cryoprobe for pulmonary vein isolation in a patient with PAF, you have selected the Atricure Synergy Bipolar RF clamp. You believe that you have effectively created contiguous, transmural lines of ablation. However, after rewarming, you again notice the patient is in A-Fib. Your scrub tech notices some char on the clamp but does not mention it to you. Why did the procedure fail?

- Effective operation of the RF clamp depends on perfect contact between the tissue and the electrodes. Char is an isolator that disrupts this contact and prevents the underlying tissue from appropriately heating. A break in the line, will render the procedure ineffective.
- Surgeons may sometimes confuse char as a sign of high heat reaching the tissue surface, but this is incorrect. The surgeon and scrub tech must be vigilant in removing char from the clamp. It is recommended to clean the clamp after every three ablations. Repeated ablation over an area of char will just produce more char.

Potential questions/alternative scenarios

After cannulation, normothermic cardiopulmonary bypass is instituted prior to left pulmonary vein isolation. The heart is retracted to the patient's right to expose the left atrial appendage and left pulmonary veins. When this retraction is performed, the Ligament of Marshall is stretched taught and is easily identified near the left superior pulmonary vein. The ligament is divided with a cautery. Immediately afterwards, a device is seen protruding through the left atrial appendage.

- Although very rare, the exposure required for Ligament of Marshall may compromise the position of the LV Vent. It is necessary to expose and divide the Ligament of Marshall to obtain passage behind the left pulmonary antrum for left sided pulmonary vein isolation.

Potential questions/alternative scenarios

After completing the Cox Maze IV with placement of the AtriClip, you come off cardiopulmonary bypass. The anesthesiologist notices a small pouch with clot in the appendage. What is the likely cause of this problem?

- The Atriclip was likely not placed at the base of the appendage. The Atricure AtriClip is a left atrial appendage exclusion system that is indicated for occluding the left atrial appendage and creating a left atrial appendage line that circles around the conical structure of the base of the appendage. It should be placed under direct visualization and in conjunction with other cardiac surgical procedures. Direct visualization requires the surgeon to be able to see the heart directly with or without camera assistance.
- Improper placement will leave behind a small pouch that is often a source of thrombus. Alternative techniques include left atrial appendage amputation that was

295

traditionally one of the remaining cut and sew lesions in the Cox Maze IV. In rare circumstances, amputation can lead to bleeding through the suture line or from tributaries at the AV grove near the coronary sinus from improper dissection.

- Amputation will remove many of the potential macro reentry circuits but not the ones at the base. If amputation is preferred, the base needs to be anchored to the left pulmonary vein isolation.
- One advantage of placing the clip on the LAA at this juncture is that you can visualize your isolation from the inside of the left atrium during concomitant mitral valve surgery.

Potential Questions / Alternative Scenarios

In the above scenario, following securing of the AtriClip or amputation of the LAA, the patient is noted to have EKG changes with T-wave inversions in the lateral leads. What are your concerns?

- There is likely inadvertent injury to the left circumflex coronary artery causing myocardial infarction at the time of LAA isolation.
- Normally, the LAA orifice is at the level of the frenulum between the left pulmonary vein orifices and it is located several centimeters from the mitral valve annulus. In addition, the circumflex coronary artery is normally located far away from the LAA orifice in the AV groove near and slightly below the coronary sinus.
- In some patients, the LAA orifice is located nearer the MV annulus and is in the plane of the LIPV orifice. In addition, the proximal circumflex coronary artery, or just one segment of it, can lie unusually close to the base of the LAA.
- For the high lying LCX, this close juxtaposition of the proximal LCX with the LAA can pose a danger when closing the LAA from the endocardium. The position of the circumflex cannot be seen from the endocardial view. In the situation described here, it is likely that the LAA orifice is unusually low and the circumflex is unusually high, setting up a potential for injury.

Potential questions/alternative scenarios

After completion of the classic right atrial appendage line, you come off cardiopulmonary bypass and notice that the patient is in complete heart block. What caused this?

- The only remaining place in the right atrium where a macro-reentrant circuit can form is around the base of the RA appendage.
- While damage to the AV node during the Maze procedure is nearly impossible, this is the one line in which it can occur. If the cryoprobe is positioned too posteriorly, it can inadvertently damage the pacemaker complex and result in permanent pacemaker dependency.
- The SA node can also be injured. To prevent this from occurring, the final RA lesion is placed from the distal end of the vertical atriotomy to the tip of the RA appendage. It is extremely important to place this lesion as far anteriorly as possible to avoid injury of the pacemaker complex.
- The modified RAA line has been advocated as a simpler, safer, and faster approach to accomplish the same results. It consists of the vertical atriotomy and IVC line segment and anchor to form a line from the IVC to the tip of the RAA.

Potential questions/alternative scenarios

"A 57-year-old woman with a history of obesity and atrial fibrillation (AF) was treated initially with antiarrhythmic medications and was not compliant due to the side effects. She underwent 2 catheter ablations for persistent afib with a short period of relief but now returns with recurrent palpitations, generalized weakness and dizziness for more than a week. It has been 4 months after catheter ablation and the cardiology refers her to you for a surgical alternative?"

Differential

296

The diagnosis was established initially by the cardiologist. Recognizing other associated diseases will be important for planning surgical interventions. Also, review the EKG carefully to ensure that the rhythm is labelled correctly.

History and physical Attempt to determine the pattern of afib (paroxysmal - spontaneous conversion, recurrent - requires ECV/antiarrhythmics or persistent), medications (anticoagulation, antiarrhythmics), and complications of afib (stroke, peripheral emboli). Identify signs and symptoms of diseases that predispose to a high recurrence rate after catheter ablation: hypertension, hypercholesterolemia, persistent AF, or obstructive sleep apnea. Predisposing factors include age, male sex (because of the tall stature), hypertension, hyperthyroidism, chronic kidney disease, alcohol, PE, obesity (BMI > 30 kg/m2) and family history. Ask about any known ischemic or valvular issues.

Tests

- Labs: CBC, BMP, Coags.
- 12 lead EKG to establish the rate and rhythm.
- 24 Holter monitoring especially if the patient is currently in sinus rhythm.

CT scan or MRI: pulmonary vein protocol in patients with a failed catheter ablation (to rule out pulmonary stenosis).

Echo: complete valvular assessment, septal anatomy, right and left function, and left atrial size. Severely dilated left atrium decreases the likelihood of achieving sustained sinus rhythm.

Left heart catheterization: for IHD and for establishing coronary anatomy (left dominant patients are at slightly increased risk of injury to their coronary arteries while ablating close to the coronary sinus).

Electrophysiological mapping: which utilizes the combination of pace/anatomic/activation mapping to identify potential sites for ablation.

Index Scenario (additional information)
"The patient has normal electrolytes, no valve abnormalities and evidence of persistent afib on 24-hour holter monitoring with a rate between 70 and 90. Her cardiac catheterization is normal."

Index scenario (additional information) "The patient has normal electrolytes, no valve abnormalities and evidence of persistent afib on 24-hour holter monitoring with a rate between 70 and 90. Her cardiac catheterization is normal. "Treatment/management Indications for catheter or surgical ablation include paroxysmal (PAF), persistent or recurrent AF in patients who do not tolerate or have failed antiarrhythmics. Catheter ablation is usually attempted first once or even twice prior to referral for surgery unless the patient is undergoing surgery for a concomitant lesion. This patient has failed medical and catheter-based interventions and is thus a candidate for standalone surgical ablation. Options include pulmonary vein isolation (works well for PAF), or Cox MAZE IV (cut and sew or the modified ablation protocol). For this patient Cox MAZE IV will give her the greatest chance of sinus rhythm control.

Potential questions/alternative scenarios
"A 65-year-old female with a history of PAF is undergoing an AVR and is noted to have PAF."

This is an excellent indication for pulmonary vein isolation (PVI). PVI can be used as a standalone procedure for PAF especially in patients with comorbidities who need a limited operation. However, it is not as complete as the Cox Maze IV and is not as successful for persistent or recurrent AF. PVI is very often used for PAF in patients undergoing valve surgery with good results.

Pulmonary venous isolation (PVI)Median sternotomy, aortic and single stage venous cannulation. Initiate CPB and perform the right sided lesions first. Right sided lesions: carefully get around the right superior pulmonary vein (RSPV) and right inferior pulmonary vein (RIPV) with blunt and sharp dissection. Stay away from the phrenic nerve. The bipolar RF jaws are inserted around the right sided pulmonary veins and then clamped on the atrial tissue to avoid pulmonary vein stenosis.

297

Left sided lesions: now arrest the heart and get around the left sided pulmonary veins in a similar fashion. Identify and divide the ligament of Marshall. Here you must make sure that you are away from the circumflex artery on the AV groove when clamping on the left atrial tissue. Excise/ligate LAA: excise and suture or occlude the LAAL with a variety of commercially available devices. Perform the AVR. "A 58-year-old male is undergoing a mitral valve repair and has a history of PAF." For this patient the PVI is best performed when the left atrium is opened with a single cryoablation catheter. Bipolar devices can be used for the inferior and superior connecting lesions to prevent injury to the esophagus. But remember to excise or exclude the LAA prior to repairing or replacing the mitral valve. You do not want to lift on the heart after the mitral is completed due to the potential for AV groove disruption. "The same patient has a history of persistent afib." There are a few different ways to do this. It is reasonable to plan for left and right sided lesions (Cox Maze IV) as well as LAAL as described above. Make the left atriotomy through Sondergaard's groove, address the left sided lesions, LAAL, repair/replace the valve and make a separate right atriotomy for the right sided lesions. Alternatively, perform the mitral through a transseptal incision. The one risk with the transseptal is that if the mitral exposure is not great and you need an extended transseptal then you risk injury to the artery supplying the SA node.

Potential questions/alternative scenarios
"A 59-year-old diabetic, hypertensive male patient with chronic kidney disease is suffering from persistent atrial fibrillation. She had an intracranial bleed while on warfarin and other class 1 and 3 anti arrhythmics. How would you proceed?"
This patient is at increased risk of intracranial hemorrhage with CPB. Thus, catheter ablation with best medical management may be her best option. "On electrophysiologic mapping a patient is a suitable candidate for minimally invasive PVI, but a thrombus is discovered intraoperatively on
TEE, how will you proceed?"
The minimally invasive PVI will be converted to an open procedure.

Potential questions/alternative scenarios
"A 57-year-old obese, female who is a known case of atrial fibrillation (AF) was treated initially with antiarrhythmic drugs and she was non-compliant due to the side effects, this was followed by a catheter ablation procedure but she is still having occasional palpitations 2 months after catheter ablation?"
If she is highly symptomatic and antiarrhythmics are not effective or tolerated a second attempt at catheter ablation after careful electrophysiologic mapping can be attempted. If this fails wait for 3 months and proceed with surgical management.

Pearls/pitfalls
- Dissecting transverse sinus RPA
- Lesions sets not connected (CS epi and endo) to mitral annulus can lead to flutter
- Phrenic nerve to cryoablation
- Discontinuous lesions due to fold in tissue
- Discontinuous lesion due to char on bipolar clamp (measuring tissue impedance and there is no conduction)
- LV vent prior to LPV isolation
- LAA not on base
- Oversew LAA hitting or injuring circumflex
- Pacemaker complex right atrial appendage

Critical Errors
- Avoid placing an ablation line through the Sinus Tachycardia site at the right atrium. This can lead to an inability to generate an appropriate sinus tachycardia

298

response to normal exercise. This was a common complication of Maze-I procedure with 30% of patients unable to generate a heart rate above 100-110.

- Avoid transection of Bachmann's Bundle, both medial and superior to the roof lesion as this will delay the arrival of a sinus impulse from the RA to the LA.
- Avoid "Flutter Line" or "Isthmus Lesion" across the cavo-tricuspid isthmus (CTI) as this will result in the inability to develop an appropriate bradycardia when one is asleep.

Guidelines
2017 STS Guidelines on Surgery for Atrial Fibrillation
Adding AF surgery does not affect operative morbidity
- *Class Ia, Level B*

Adding AF surgery does not affect operative mortality
- *Class I, Level A*

2017 AATS Guidelines on Surgery for Atrial Fibrillation
Adding AF surgery does not affect operative morbidity
- *Class IIa, Levels A, B-R, B-NR*

Adding AF surgery *improves* operative mortality
- *Class I, Level A*

Suggested readings

- Philpott JM., et al. *Surgical Treatment of Atrial Fibrillation: A Comprehensive Guide to Performing the Cox Maze IV Procedure.* Academic Press, 2017.
- Badhwar V, Rankin JS, Ad N, Grau-Sepulveda M, Damiano RJ, Gillinov AM, McCarthy PM, Thourani VH, Suri RM, Jacobs JP, Cox, JL Surgical ablation of atrial fibrillation in the United States: Trends and Propensity Matched Outcomes. *Ann Thor Surg, (August)* 2017;104:493-500
- Barnett SD, Ad N. Surgical ablation as treatment for the elimination of atrial fibrillation: a meta-analysis. *Journal of Thoracic and Cardiovascular Surgery*, 2006 May;131(5):1029-35.
- Cullen MW, Stulak JM, Powell BD, White RD, Ammash NM, Nkomo VT. Left Atrial Appendage Patency at Cardioversion After Surgical Left Atrial Appendage Intervention. *Ann Thor Surg*, 2016;101(2):675-681.
- Forlani S, De Paulis R, Guerrieri WL, Greco R, Polisca P, Moscarelli M, Chiariello L. Conversion to sinus rhythm by ablation improves quality of life in patients submitted to mitral valve surgery. *Ann Thor Surg,* 2006;81(3):863-867
- Melo J, Santiago T, Aguiar C, Berglin E, Knaut M, Alfieri O, Benussi S, Sie H, Williams M, Hornero F, Marinelli G, Ridley P, Fulquet-Carreras E, Ferreira A. Surgery for atrial fibrillation in patients with mitral valve disease: Results at five years from the International Registry of Atrial Fibrillation Surgery. *J Thor Cardiovasc Surg,* 2008;135(4):863-869

47. TRICUSPID VALVE REGURGITATION
Emmanuel Moss, MD, and Robert A. Guyton, MD

Concept

- Indication for intervention on the tricuspid valve
- Preoperative considerations
- Choice of intervention - Repair vs. replace
- Valve choices - bioprosthesis vs. mechanical
- Critical steps of tricuspid valve repair and replacement
- Pitfalls and controversies

Chief complaint

"A 45-year-old man presents with a 6-month history of progressive fatigue, shortness of breath and lower extremity edema. Auscultation reveals a holosystolic ejection murmur at the left ventricular apex."

Differential

The clinical scenario mentioned is typical for congestive heart failure. The causes can be several (CAD, MR, MS, AS, etc.). The peripheral edema and murmur raise concern for tricuspid regurgitation. Other diagnoses to consider include: Cirrhosis, constrictive pericarditis, or restrictive cardiomyopathy.

History and physical

This patient may have valvular disease of any type but most likely has mitral or tricuspid regurgitation. Valvular disease can lead to symptoms of congestive heart failure. It is important to determine the onset and duration of her symptoms as well as the character (asthenia, fatigue, weakness, malaise, peripheral edema). Evaluate for signs of right heart failure (ascites, hepatosplenomegaly, pulsatile liver, peripheral edema, pleural effusions). Late findings include cachexia, wasting and jaundice. Atrial fibrillation is common. Look for evidence of coronary artery disease (chest pain, risk factors, etc).

If TR is high on the differential, then consider primary and secondary causes:

- *Primary (structural).* Congenital (e.g., Ebstein, AV canal/cushion defect), rheumatic disease (never isolated), endocarditis (IV drug use and Duke's criteria), myxomatous degeneration, endocarditis, iatrogenic (e.g., permanent pacemaker (PPM) lead, repetitive myocardial biopsies), carcinoid (see below for explanation), trauma (e.g., chordal rupture from anterior leaflet), valvular tumor.
- *Secondary (functional).* Most common form of TV dysfunction. Leaflets are normal. Caused by left sided lesion (e.g., mitral regurgitation), ischemic cardiomyopathy, dilated cardiomyopathy, cor pulmonale.

Tests

- *CXR*: cardiomegaly, enlarged RA/RV, pleural effusions.
- *TTE.* Transthoracic rather than transesophageal is particularly helpful for evaluating the tricuspid valve. It is used for diagnosis and decisions regarding management PREOPERATIVELY. For functional TR, intraoperative transesophageal echo is unreliable due to changes in vascular tone under general anesthesia, reducing the degree of regurgitation. For regurgitation, a jet that penetrates 2 cm into the RA is mild, 3-5 cm is moderate and systolic flow reversal of the hepatic or caval veins is severe. The grade is often reported as 1-mild, 2-moderate, 3-moderately severe, 4-severe. In addition, a jet radius greater than 9 mm, vena contracta > 0.7, ERO > 0.4 cm^2, or regurgitant volume 45 mL indicate severe regurgitation.

- Need to ask about the size of the annulus and the gradient. Annular size > 40 mm is a rough cut off for a valve that needs intervention. Mean gradient of 3-5 mmHg is considered severe. Also need to inquire on the character of the leaflets (tethered, thickened, prolapsed, flail).
- *TEE*. Important for getting more detailed information on the mitral valve. Should also assess pulmonary artery pressure (PAP), right ventricular (RV) function, presence of PFO or ASD (bubble test if there is a doubt), endocarditis (vegetations) or carcinoid lesions.
- *Catheterization*: evaluate for any coronary lesions. TR can be due to or result in RV failure. Obtain the cardiac index, LCWP, PAP, RA/RV end-diastolic pressure and CVP. Cardiac index may be unreliable in the setting of TR and you should rely on the EF for assessment of function. Absent X descent, prominent V wave, and ventricularization of RA tracing all *support tricuspid disease.*

Index scenario (additional information)
"Echocardiogam reveals a left ventricular ejection fraction of 45%, severe mitral regurgitation, moderate pulmonary artery hypertension, and moderate-severe tricuspid regurgitation with normal leaflets and a dilated annulus (45 mm)."

Treatment/management
This scenario addresses combined tricuspid and mitral valve disease. In addition to mitral valve (MV) repair or replacement, this patient meets criteria for tricuspid valve repair with an annuloplasty ring. This patient has several risk factors for persistent and progressive TR following mitral valve surgery. If the TV is deemed irreparable at the time of surgery, it is reasonable to consider replacement with a mechanical valve, depending on the patient's preference and other anticoagulation concerns. Although bioprostheses deteriorate at a slower rate in the tricuspid position, this patient will likely require a future intervention (whether surgical or transcatheter), while risk of thrombosis with bileaflet mechanical valve is greatly decreased compared to older models (ball-cag, tilting disk).

Indications for surgery: ACCF/AHA guidelines
- Class I
    - TV repair for severe TR in patients requiring MV surgery (level B).
- Class IIa
    - TV repair or replacement for severe, SYMPTOMATIC, primary TR (level C).
    - TV replacement is reasonable when not amenable to repair.
- Class IIb
    - Annuloplasty may be considered for less than severe TR in patients undergoing MV surgery when there is pulmonary hypertension or tricuspid annular dilation. (level C).
- Other suggested indications for concomitant repair (not AHA): End-systolic annular dimension > 40 mm or intraoperative measurement of anteroseptal to anteroposterior annulus > 70 mm (Dreyfus et al, 2005).
- *Endocarditis*. Not addressed in AHA guidelines. Generally accepted indications include: 1) severe TR with persistent sepsis, 2) vegetation > 15 mm, 3) persistent vegetation or sepsis despite med tx, 4) Recurrent pulmonary embolism.

Operative steps
- *Critical anatomy*: 3 leaflets (septal, posterior, anterior). Septal annulus relatively fixed, annulus dilates posteriorly > anteriorly. AV node contained in triangle of Koch (between coronary sinus, septal annulus, tendon of Todaro).

301

- Intraop TEE (assess valve function and dimensions, PFO), median sternotomy, aortic and bicaval cannulation with caval snares.
- *Cardioplegia*: cross clamp, antegrade +/- retrograde. For retrograde – after clamping, run antegrade, caval snares are tightened, right atriotomy, handheld retractor, purse string around coronary sinus, insert cannula and inflate balloon, pull back cannula until arrested by purse string (maximize distribution).
- Left sided lesions addressed first.
- Tricuspid valve can be addressed with the aorta clamped or the heart beating (PFO, if present, must be closed before releasing the cross clamp). Advantages of beating heart include assessment of iatrogenic conduction disturbances, reduce cross-clamp time. Concern with beating heart is ejection of air in the presence of an undetected interatrial communication and the added challenge of performing a precise annuloplasty on the beating heart.
- Oblique atriotomy directed posteriorly from appendage toward the right inferior pulmonary vein and inferior vena cava.
- On septal annulus, sutures are placed through the base of the septal leaflet to avoid damage to the AV node.

Annuloplasty techniques
- Ring annuloplasty
    - Interrupted mattress sutures leaving a gap at koch's triangle (roughly 1 cm from the anteroseptal commissure to midpoint on the septal leaflet. Be careful with the sutures near the anteropostero commisure. These can injure the RCA. Several rings available, with semi-rigid incomplete ring being the most commonly used (e.g., Edwards Classic, Edwards physio, MC3). Favored over flexible band.
    - *Methods of selecting ring size*: 1) Using sizer, measuring the septal leaflet and surface area of leaflet tissue arising from anterior pap muscle, or 2) 30-32 mm for female, 32-34 mm for male.
- *Suture annuloplasty (DeVega).* Simpler and faster, however, may have increased long-term risk of recurrence compared to rings. Both limbs of a pledgeted 2–0 Prolene running from anteroseptal commissure along the RV free wall portion of the annulus to the posteroseptal commissures.
- *Posterior leaflet plication (Kay).* Obliterates the posterior leaflet.

Replacement
- Preservation of native valve leaflets, similar to mitral valve.
- Sutures near the AV node placed through the septal leaflet.

Endocarditis
- Excise vegetations until healthy tissue. Close gaps primarily or with patch.
- Consider annuloplasty if valve competence is in question.
- Replace valve if extensive destruction.
- 2-stage replacement may be considered in IVDU (intravenous drug users), with normal RV function and PAP.

Intra-operative valve assessment. Fill RV with saline with a bulb syringe and assess coaptation. TEE to assess repair on CPB.

Potential questions/alternative scenarios
"What elements will influence your decision to address the TV in a patient undergoing mitral valve surgery?"

Decision to operate often a difficult clinical dilemma because improvement with repair of left-sided lesions remains unpredictable. In general, moderate to severe TR or any structural TR should be addressed concomitantly with left sided lesions. LV function, RV function, degree of pulmonary hypertension, tricuspid annulus size, and tricuspid valve morphology must all be assessed. The presence of preoperative right heart failure is a strong indication for addressing TR. Some advocate repair of even mild disease without risk factors for progression. If LV and RV function are near normal, the TV annulus is not dilated, pulmonary vascular resistance is low, and a good result is expected from MV repair, then progressive tricuspid regurgitation is less likely. When weaning from CPB, if TR persists and elevated RAP > LAP is encountered with an underfilled well-contracting LV, TV repair should be performed.

"What type of prosthesis would you use for TV replacement?"
Similar to mitral and aortic valve prosthetic valve planning, decision is based on age, anticoagulation considerations, and social issues. Incidence of valve thrombosis was considered prohibitive with older mechanical prostheses (ball-cage and tilting disk) but is not the case with bileaflet valves. However, bioprostheses have better freedom from structural valve deterioration than in mitral position, and unlike mechanical valves, they do not limit the implantation of a transvalvular PM lead in the future.

"Under what circumstances can TV excision without replacement be considered?"
In endocarditis and extensive destruction or an active IVDU. PAPs and RV must be near normal. Replacement can be performed months to years later. Early morality 12%, with hepatic failure frequently playing a role. Survival is 60% at 15 years, with 50% of patients having RV failure. Approach has fallen out of favor.

"When coming off pump following TV replacement, the RV dilates, CVP is high, and PAP decrease. How do you manage this?"
Routine checklist of possible causes of RV failure post CPB (metabolic, air embolism…) and TEE for anatomic assessment. Rule out RVOT obstruction due to redundant billowing of anterior leaflet tissue - If this is the case, central portion of anterior leaflet may be excised while maintaining chordal attachments. If ST changes are noted in the inferior leads, then consider RCA occlusion with the mattress sutures and perform a bypass to the right with vein. Even when all goes well after TVR, there may be an element of RV dysfunction which is treated in the ICU with inotropes (epinephrine or milrinone), fluid restriction, diuresis and pressors. Chemical unloading of the heart can be achieved with milrinone or nitroglycerin drip. An IABP can further help to unload a struggling RV in more severe cases and improve RCA perfusion. Note that you do not always have the luxury of Swan-Ganz monitoring after tricuspid valve surgery. It cannot be used if placing a mechanical valve. It is not ideal when placing a tissue valve. It can be used after a repair, but it would be best if it were manually inserted by the surgeon under direct visualization. This may factor into your selection process as well. A sick patient with poor EF may be better off with 1-2+ residual TR after a repair and a PA catheter for ICU management than no TR with a mechanical valve but no PA catheter.

"What are the risk factors for recurrence of TR following TV repair?"
No ring used, improper placement of the ring (usually by rotation), severity of baseline TR, residual TR at first operation, persistent pulmonary hypertension, residual left sided lesions, transvalvular PPM lead.

"What factors influence operative mortality in TV surgery?"
Preoperative functional class, ejection fraction, prior valve surgery, older age, excision without replacement.

"When should tricuspid valve repair be performed in patients who have undergone a previous mitral valve surgery?"

No consensus exists. Historically, operative mortality for reoperative TV surgery has been relatively high, making the benefit over medical therapy unclear. Waiting for the development of severe symptoms before TV repair in this setting has resulted in poor results, reinforcing the belief that this is a high-risk operation. Some now advocate early reintervention in mildly symptomatic patients, hoping to decrease operative risk. Effectiveness of this approach has not been proven.

"Coming of CPB you notice complete heart block (CHB)."
The sutures near the anteroseptal commissure can easily damage the AV node. This can also occur from radial force with the prosthetic valves. If both the mitral and tricuspid were replaced, then the chance of recovery is lower. Giving the patient time to recover in the ICU is reasonable but make sure that you have 2 sets of properly functioning ventricular pacing wires as well as a set of atrial wires. Eventually the patient may require an endocardial or epicardial permanent pacemaker. Endocardial pacers can be placed percutaneously into the atrium and through the coronary sinus to achieve ventricular conduction. If the coronary sinus cannot be cannulated, then worse case scenario they can traverse the repaired valve. If the patient had a tissue valve placed this can be harder but is still possible. Epicardial lead placement is another alternative and avoids a foreign object across the fresh repair/replacement. But you need to balance this decision with the risk of returning to the OR and be able to describe how you reoperate for an epicardial lead. If a mechanical valve is in place and you end up with heart block, then you will not be able to cross it with endocardial wires and the coronary sinus route or epicardial route may be needed ultimately.

"A patient with tricuspid valve endocarditis and a PPM for heart block undergoes a combined mitral/TV repair. How do you handle the pacer leads?"
The original wires should be removed in the setting of bacteremia and endocarditis. You have no way of knowing if it was the wires themselves that caused the infection or will seed a new infection. Some advocate debriding the wires or inspecting them, but the safest thing would be to remove them. Epicardial wires can be placed on the RV. Transvenous atrial wires can be placed later if needed. Place temporary wires as well since you will not be relying on the epicardial lead until it is connected, and a formal device check is performed. Be familiar with the procedure for epicardial lead placement (5-O prolene to fasten the RV lead, tunnel the lead through the left intercostal space a safe distance away from the mammary and out to an area in the skin where you make a subcutaneous pocket for the device.). If you are concerned about the degree of bacterial burden intraop and feel that the epicardial lead could get infected then you can wait a few days post op on antibiotics and place an endocardial lead through the coronary sinus, repaired valve or tissue valve.

"A patient with a prior history of brady syndrome and a PPM comes to the OR for a TVR."
Note that in the absence of endocarditis the wires can be left either around the sewing ring or through the valve itself accepting a slightly higher risk of recurrent TR. For a younger patient it may be worth placing the wire in the epicardial position since you would like to minimize the chance of recurrent TR. For a mechanical valve you will need to remove the wire and replace later or use an epicardial wire.

"After replacing the tricuspid valve, you feel the need to determine PAP and CI due to worsening hypotension."
You cannot float a swan in the setting of a mechanical valve, and it is not advised after a tissue valve. It can be done with caution in the setting of a repair. An alternative is to use the CVP with venous saturations and echo data to help guide your management. It can be placed through a tissue valve carefully if necessary.

"Coming of CPB you notice 2+ TR. The patient has extensive comorbidities, 4+ MR which you have just fixed and a low EF."
The management must weigh the risks of going back on CPB and arresting the heart against the risks of leaving behind residual TR. For this patient the most prudent course of action would be to leave the regurgitation alone. 2+ residual TR will rarely be a good reason to

304

replace the valve. The exception to this would be a younger patient with primary tricuspid disease and evidence of early right heart failure. For that patient you would want to remove as much of the regurgitant volume as possible.

"What is carcinoid valvular disease and how is the tricuspid valve managed with this disease process?"

Carcinoid tumors are serotonin-secreting tumors of the Kulchitsky cells of the GI tract.

They can metastasize to liver where serotonin and other vasoactive hormones are excreted, affecting the right sided cardiac valves and pulmonary bed. Carcinoid syndrome leads to focal or diffuse fibrous tissue deposits on the endocardium of valve cusps and cardiac chambers. White fibrous carcinoid plaques present on the ventricular side of the TV cusps cause adherence to the RV wall, preventing leaflet coaptation. Tricuspid valve replacement is required. Involvement of the pulmonic valve may necessitate its replacement as well. In the absence of an ASD or VSD, left sided heart valves are not affected due to inactivation by monoamine oxidase as it passes through the lungs.

Pearls/pitfalls

- Decision to intervene should be based on PREOPERATIVE TTE.
- Incomplete rings avoid suture placement near the triangle of Koch.
- For TV replacement, suture near AV node should be placed at base of septal leaflet, not in the annulus.
- Rule out PFO before performing TV repair with beating heart.
- Consider need for epicardial pacemaker lead at the time of surgery, particularly if implanting a mechanical valve.
- Risk of PPM following TV replacement is 6-10%, commonly following combined TV and MV procedures.

Suggested readings

- Bonow RO, Carabello BA, Kanu C, et al: ACC/AHA 2006 guidelines for the management of patients with valvular heart disease. *Circulation* 2006; 114:e84-e231.
- Chikwe J, Ayanwu AC. Surgical Strategies for Functional Tricuspid Regurgitation. *Semin Thoracic Surg* 2010;22:90-96.
- Dreyfus GD, Corbi PJ, Chan KM, Bahrami T: Secondary tricuspid regurgitation or dilatation: Which should be the criteria for surgical repair? *Ann Thorac Surg* 2005; 79:127-132.
- Duran CMG. Surgical Treatment of Tricuspid Valve Disease. Selke FW, del NIdo PJ, Swanson SJ (eds). Sabiston and Spencer - *Surgery of the Chest.* 2010; 1241-1258.

48. COMBINED CABG/VALVE
Mark Roeser, MD, and Ravi Ghanta, MD

Concept
- Indications for combined valve/coronary artery bypass grafting
- Preoperative considerations
- Critical steps in valve/coronary artery bypass grafting

Chief complaint
"A 64-year-old man with chronic exertional chest pain is referred to you with moderate aortic stenosis on a TTE obtained by his primary care physician. On follow up catheterization he is found to have 60% RCA stenosis, 80% LAD stenosis, and a 70% circumflex lesion."

Differential
Either the CAD or the aortic stenosis could be contributing to his symptoms.

History and physical
Ask and evaluate for evidence of syncope, angina, CHF, pulmonary edema, dyspnea, and other comorbidities which may factor into your decision regarding the aortic valve.

Tests
Careful review of the cath, echo, CXR, EKG and baseline labs. Catheterization and exercise testing can be used to clarify aortic valve stenosis.

Index scenario (additional information)
"Exercise testing shows a mean gradient of 45 mmHg with exercise. Review of the echo suggests a highly calcified aortic valve. He denies history of dyspnea or syncope."

Treatment/management
Indications for concomitant AVR in patients who require a CABG
- All patients with moderate to severe aortic stenosis
- All patients with moderately severe to severe aortic regurgitation
- Consider in patients with mild AS and moderate to severe calcification or rapidly progressing disease (decrease in AVA 0.3 cm^2 per year or increase in gradient 15-20 mmHg per year)
- Consider in patients with moderate AI

Indications for concomitant CABG in patients who require an AVR
- Any lesion > 70%
- LM lesion > 50%
- "reasonable" to consider bypassing lesions > 50% (LIMA for LAD)

In the above clinical scenario, the patient's symptoms are most likely due to the coronary disease, but he should also have the aortic valve replaced at the time of surgery. The data suggests that he will have a lower freedom from reintervention rate with this approach but not necessarily improved survival. Thus, you need to exercise judgement and balance the risks and benefits of an AVR with moderate AS in the setting of CABG. Frail, older patients with multiple comorbidities may benefit from an expeditious operation that addresses the CAD and leaves the moderate AS behind. On the other hand, a younger patient with few comorbidities will benefit from the decreased reintervention rate. You should also factor in the rate of progression of the aortic valve disease (see chapter on Aortic stenosis). Also, patients with moderate AS and low cardiac output should have the aortic valve replaced at the time of CABG to reduce afterload.

Potential questions/alternative scenarios
"A 58 year-old woman with history of moderate mitral stenosis secondary to rheumatic fever undergoes a cardiac catheterization for exertional chest pain. She is found to have an 80% lesion in the proximal LAD, 70% RCA and 60% OM2 not amenable to PCI."
Indications for concomitant mitral valve surgery in patients who require a CABG:

- *Mitral stenosis*: there are no uniform guidelines regarding mitral stenosis in the setting of a CABG but in general patients who require CABG should have the diseased mitral valve replaced if they meet criteria for an isolated MVR (refer to Mitral stenosis chapter) – i.e., moderate to severe MS with NYHA III-IV, asymptomatic with PAP > 60 mmHg, recurrent embolic events, new onset afib, or evidence of RV dysfunction. If a patient does not meet criteria for mitral replacement but has severe MS it is reasonable to replace. For moderate MS not meeting indications for MVR this is more controversial. The decision should factor in whether the patients coronary induced symptoms are potentially due to MS. You might also consider checking the catheterization to clarify the degree of mitral stenosis according to the Gorlin formula if there is a discordance between the echo and clinical presentation.

- *Gorlin formula*: valve area (cm^2) = CO / (HR x systolic ejection period (sec) x 44.3 x sq root mean gradient)

- *Structural mitral regurgitation*: severe or moderately severe mitral valve regurgitation secondary to structural valve degeneration (i.e., ruptured cord, leaflet prolapse, etc..) should undergo repair or replacement at the time of CABG. This would be an unusual presentation since most patients with dominant CAD and concomitant mitral regurgitation have ischemic MR. In the absence of a structural lesion assume ischemic MR (below).

- *In patients with ischemic (or "functional") mitral regurgitation*. Severe MR can get a ring annuloplasty repair or mitral valve replacement. Repair when feasible but replacement is acceptable with similar survival, especially for complex jets or sicker patients. Moderate MR is controversial. Patients may get either a ring annuloplasty, replacement or nothing (NIH trial ongoing). Addressing the MR may improve symptoms and decrease the chance of worsening MR. The decision depends on degree of symptoms attributable to the MR as well as comorbidities that make extra cross clamp time more hazardous.

Indications for concomitant CABG in patients who require mitral valve surgery:

- Any lesion > 70%
- LM lesion > 50%
- "reasonable" to consider bypassing lesions > 50% (LIMA for LAD)

In the above scenario, the patient needs to have her right sided heart pressures clarified. If she has moderate-severe pulmonary hypertension (PAP > 50 mmHg at rest or > 60 mmHg with exercise) then the mitral valve should be replaced. If she does not have pulmonary hypertension, new onset afib, right ventricular dysfunction, or embolic events then you should go back to the history and decide whether the moderate MS is more or less than likely to be contributing to her symptoms. Also factor in her comorbidities to see how well she will tolerate the extended cross clamp. In this scenario, exertional chest pain, as reported by the patient, is most consistent with coronary disease and is less likely to be from mitral disease. If she were older, frail with multiple comorbidities it would be reasonable to leave the mitral valve alone. On the other hand, if she could tolerate the extra operative time then MVR would remove the mitral disease as a potential source of her symptoms and source of postoperative problems. Thus, moderate stenosis should be left alone if unlikely to be involved in the patient's clinical presentation especially in the absence of an isolated indication for MVR. It can be considered if MS is borderline severe or likely to cause problems in the future in a good surgical candidate.

Combined aortic valve replacement/CABG
- Transesophageal echo (TEE).
- Median Sternotomy.
- LIMA + SVG procurement.
- Aortic and right atrial cannulation.
- Antegrade cardioplegia catheter. Retrograde cardioplegia catheter ideal (especially if tight proximal coronary lesions, significant LV hypertrophy, or significant AI).
- LV vent ideal but not required (institution/surgeon dependent).
- Aortic cross-clamp.
- *Cardioplegia.* It is important to appreciate that a CABG/AVR carries a higher mortality and is longer than any of the component procedures done in isolation. Cardioprotection for this case is critical and you must think through your protection strategy carefully before you start.
    - moderate - severe AI - retrograde induction and consider LV vent to avoid ventricular distension. Make sure the retrograde is in perfectly. Can try to give some through the antegrade but stop if distention occurs.
    - high grade proximal coronary lesions - antegrade is unlikely to be sufficient. Plan on antegrade, retrograde and direct cardioplegia down the vein grafts.
- Along these same lines, it is helpful to get to the distal anastomosis and particularly the right distal done ASAP. This will allow you to deliver extra cardioplegia directly down the coronary conduit and protect the RV. Do the same for the circumflex lesion.
- For the LAD you can do the LIMA to LAD and leave it clamped or do the LIMA to LAD following the AVR.
- Make sure you are administering a full dose of cardioplegia every 15-20 minutes.
- Size up the proximals with the heart distended.
- Complete the AVR and close the aortotomy.
- Proximal anastomosis.
- Wean from CPB.
- *Summary:* distals > AVR > proximals.

Operative sequence for mitral valve repair/replacement/CABG
- TEE.
- Median sternotomy.
- LIMA + SVG procurement.
- Aortic and bicaval cannulation.
- Aortic root vent, antegrade and retrograde cardioplegia.
- Distal anastomoses.
- Size up the proximals with the heart engorged.
- Left atrial vs. transseptal approach for mitral valve repair or replacement.
- Consider left atrial ablation +/- LA appendage ligation if concomitant atrial fibrillation prior to the mitral replacement due to the higher risk of AV rupture with manipulation of the heart (see chapter Afib/MVR for further details on management of concomitant AF).
- Mitral repair or replacement.

- Key concept is to perform the distal anastomosis first so that heart manipulation/lifting can be minimized after mitral valve replacement is performed. Additionally, performing distal first could facilitate additional cardioprotection down the grafts.
- Proximal anastomosis.
- *Summary*: distals > mitral repair/replacement > proximals.

Operative sequence for aortic and mitral valve surgeries plus CABG

- TEE.
- Aortic and bicaval cannulation with mild systemic hypothermia 32-34° C.
- This is definitely a longer operation. Systemic hypothermia and excellent cardioprotection increase the chances of getting through it safely.
- *Aortic*: root vent, antegrade and retrograde cardioplegia.
- Distal anastomoses and size up the proximals with the heart distended.
- Aortotomy and debride the aortic valve. The concept is to debride the aortic valve before performing mitral valve repair/replacement since debriding after a mitral valve repair/replacement can be problematic.
- Mitral valve replacement/repair via transseptal or left atrial exposure (do any afib procedures first)!
- AVR.
- Close the aortotomy and perform the proximals.
- Wean from CPB.
- *Summary*: distals > debride aortic valve > mitral > AVR > proximals.

Potential questions/alternative scenarios

"You have performed the CABG AVR but coming off CPB the CI is 1.7 and the heart function is decreased compared to baseline. You are on high doses of inotropes and vasopressors. The echo shows that the valve is well seated with no regurgitation and no significant gradient. The RCA appears to have flow in it by echo. There are no regional wall motion abnormalities. You assess the position of all your grafts which appear satisfactory and use a flow probe which reveals good flow in all the grafts. Your cross-clamp time was 2 hours long, but you had considerable difficulty with the position of the retrograde throughout the case. How should you proceed?"
These procedures are longer than usual. Cardioprotection must be carefully carried out. Note that if you perform the mitral via transeptal approach consider direct retrograde insertion into the coronary sinus. Perform the distals first and deliver cardioplegia directly down the distals. In this case the most likely diagnosis is cardiogenic shock from poor protection. You can rest the heart on full flow for 10-15 minutes (make sure the heart is completely decompressed) and see if you recover but ultimately it may be difficult to leave the OR without the aid of a IABP. If the shock persists or worsens in the ICU over the next 12 hours consider an angiogram to assess the grafts.

Pearls/pitfalls

- In general, combined procedures should be performed when indications for each procedure are met. For example, an AVR plus CABG can be performed if the patient meets the indications for AVR and meets the indications for CABG. When a patient however meets the surgical criteria for one cardiac operation (for example CABG), the threshold criteria for performing an additional procedure (for example AVR for moderate AS) maybe lowered after considering the patients overall state.
- Plan out your cardioprotection strategy carefully - plan on retrograde, antegrade and cardioplegia down the coronary conduits.
- General sequence is distals, aortotomy, MVR, AVR, proximals.
  - *CABG/AVR*: distals > AVR > proximals

309

- *CABG/MVR*: distals > MVR > proximals
  - *CABG/AVR/MVR*: distals > debride aortic valve > mitral > AVR > proximals
- Reasonable to bypass coronary lesions greater than 50% at the time of a valve operation; mandatory to bypass LM > 50% or any other reasonable target > 70%.

49. COMBINED AORTIC AND MITRAL VALVE DISEASE

Travis Abicht, MD, and Edwin McGee, MD

Adapted from 1st edition chapter written by *Alejandro E. Murillo-Berlioz, MD, and Carmelo A. Milano, MD*

Concept

- Indications for combined valve operation
- Preoperative considerations
- Intraoperative considerations
  - Sequence of operation
  - Myocardial protection
  - Valve choices
- Pitfalls
- Postoperative issues

Chief complaint

"A 75-year-old man is referred to your office after being diagnosed with a murmur heard by his primary care physician. He had a history of a febrile illness when he was younger. He has been increasingly lightheaded and short of breath with exertion to the point that he cannot walk a full block."

Differential

Given the patient's age, aortic stenosis is a concern. Other conditions that should be considered include mitral valve disease. Certainly, the patient could have a combination of aortic and mitral valve disease. Endocarditis is another possibility. As always, etiology such as ischemic heart disease and primary pulmonary issues should be ruled out.

History and physical

The history should focus on symptoms such as angina, syncope or congestive heart failure (CHF). Clarify the febrile illness. One should keep in mind any co-morbid conditions that may affect how treatment proceeds. The physical will emphasize vitals, neuro exam, edema, vascular exam, heart and lungs.

Tests

- *EKG*: Get a baseline EKG and consider prolonged EKG monitoring in patients who complain of palpitations or if there is a concern for paroxysmal atrial fibrillation. The presence of paroxysmal atrial fibrillation might indicate the need of ablation (pulmonary vein isolation or complete Cox-Maze).
- *Echo.* This is the most important piece of the puzzle in this scenario. The echocardiogram needs to be of high quality so that all valvular function can be adequately assessed. (Refer to technical note from chapter on Aortic Stenosis.) If there is any doubt of the findings or quality of the echo, then have it repeated by a cardiologist you trust or perform TEE. Other things to gain from the echo include the presence/absence of septal hypertrophy and annular sizes.
- *Cardiac catheterization*: rule out any concomitant coronary artery disease (CAD). Also, right heart catheterization will give insight into resultant pulmonary hypertension from MR/MS.
- *CXR +/- CT scan*: make sure there is no concomitant lung pathology. If there is evidence of calcified aorta, bicuspid aortic valve, or high-risk factors for atherosclerotic disease then get a CT.

Index scenario (additional information)

311

"It turns out that the patient had rheumatic fever as a teenager. He is otherwise healthy. His ejection fraction is 50%. He has what appears to be calcific aortic stenosis and rheumatic mitral stenosis by echo. A valve area of 0.7 cm² and a mean gradient of 45 mmHg were noted for the aortic valve, while a valve area of 1.5 cm² with thickened relatively immobile leaflets and moderate MR were noted for the mitral. TEE confirms these findings and shows a mean mitral gradient of 8 mmHg. Estimated PA systolic pressure was in the 40s. Right heart catheterization shows a PAP of 55 mmHg at rest. What are his options and what, if any, operation would you offer him?"

Treatment/management

This patient has severe aortic stenosis and moderate mitral stenosis. He is symptomatic with NYHA Class III. Operative choices include AVR with mitral valve repair or replacement versus AVR alone. The aortic stenosis meets indications for replacement (severe stenosis, symptomatic) and arguably the moderate mitral stenosis also meets indication for surgery (NYHA III, pulmonary hypertension). This presentation is typical of rheumatic heart disease and both valves can be affected with obstruction of flow. The procedure of choice for the mitral valve is replacement. Thus, a double valve replacement will provide the best results for this patient. The question of valve choice is also present. Given the patients age (75) he will be well-served by bioprosthetic valves in both positions. His freedom from structural valve deterioration (SVD) will be on the order of 85-90% at 10-15 years. Additionally, there are minimal thromboembolic and bleeding risks. If the patient were younger (< 60), then a mechanical valve would provide a lower rate of re-intervention (20-year freedom from re-intervention rate of 90%). Note if the patient had severe mitral stenosis and moderate AS then an AVR would still be advised. The reverse is not necessarily true. If moderate MS did not appear to be contributing to the patient's clinical presentation (normal PAP, minimal dyspnea, 2+ stenosis) then you might consider aborting the mitral procedure especially if the patient was high risk.

Operative steps
Combined aortic/mitral valve replacement
Goals – relieve obstruction/eliminate regurgitation, replace the valves, myocardial protection, prevent embolization.

- Large-bore IV access, arterial line, general endotracheal anesthesia (GETA), pulmonary artery catheter, foley.
- Intraoperative TEE to recheck valvular pathology and rule out any other unexpected pathology.
- Median sternotomy, elevate the right side of the pericardium, palpate the aorta for calcification. If there is any question of safety of cannulation site, then use the epiaortic ultrasound.
- Heparinize (400 mg/kg), central aortic cannulation, bi-caval cannulation, retrograde cardioplegia cannula. At ACT of 480 CPB can be initiated.
- Dissect Sondergard's groove.
- Insert antegrade cardioplegia catheter. Cross-clamp aorta and run antegrade cardioplegia for induction followed by retrograde. Intermittent doses of retrograde should be given throughout the operation. Delivery of cardioplegia into the coronary ostia with a handheld device should be considered if return of blood is poor during retrograde cardioplegia. If there is no return flow from the left ostia, then the retrograde catheter is likely not in place. An alternative at this point would be direct retrograde especially if if the approach to the mitral valve was trans-septal.
- *Aortotomy*: make sure that you know where the RCA is. Make aortotomy ~1 cm above the RCA and extend the incision a short distance toward the left and then extend the incision to the right, obliquely towards the middle of the noncoronary sinus.
- Inspect the aortic valve. Resect the leaflets along the annulus. Debride the calcium at this point (once the mitral valve has been replaced you run the risk of debriding your

mitral annular sutures).The conduction system is particularly at risk with a double valve procedure.

- An option that allows you to pressurize the left ventricle for testing the mitral valve after repair/replacement would be to do a simple running closure of the aortotomy at this point. Alternatively, a foley balloon catheter can be inflated in the LVOT to allow the LV to be pressurized during mitral valve testing.
- The most common approaches to the mitral valve are the left atrial approach and the trans-septal approach.
- For the left atrial approach: Make the left atriotomy in Sondergard's groove. Insert self-retaining mitral retractor (i.e., Cosgrove retractor). Inspect the mitral valve. In this instance, both the leaflets and subvalvular apparatus appear thickened.
- For the trans-septal approach: Make a right atriotomy and then incise the interatrial septum in the most posterior aspect towards the right. Anterior retraction of the left atrial septum results in excellent visualization of the mitral valve. The trans-septal incision is closer to the mitral valve than the left atriotomy incision. This procedure enables the assistant to see the mitral procedure and provide retraction. The trans-septal approach also provides a better visualization when there is fixation of the SVC and IVC.
- Simultaneous sizing of the mitral and aortic valves is possible. This helps to demonstrate the impact of the mitral prosthesis on aortic valve sizing.
- Perform a cord-sparing mitral valve replacement. Whether to excise any of the anterior or posterior leaflet is a personal/situational choice – you should do what you know and are comfortable doing. Keep in mind that it is hard to preserve thick cords and dividing the anterior leaflet is usually necessary in the setting of rheumatic disease. Take care near the posteromedial commissure. The conduction system is particularly at risk with a double valve procedure. Undersizing can result in patient-prosthetic mismatch, while oversizing can cause in failure to adequately seat the prosthetic valve and associated paravalvular leak.
- Place horizontal mattress sutures of 2-0 braided polyester with pledgets along annulus (inverting/everting is your choice but if the annulus is calcified, ventricular to atrial sutures are best).
- Pass the sutures through the valve ring. Seat the valve. Check the pledgets and then tie down the valve (beginning at the valve struts). Once the valve is tied down, remove the valve obturator. Remove your self-retaining retractor.
- Check for paravalvular leak by pressurizing the left ventricle with saline. If happy with results, then decompress the left ventricle and close the left atriotomy.
- If the initial aortotomy was closed, then reopen the aortotomy. Size your aortic valve.
- Place stay sutures at the commissures – this will help orient the valve. Place horizontal mattress sutures of braided 2-0 polyester with pledgets along the annulus.
- Pass the sutures through the valve ring and seat the valve.
- Check the pledgets, and both coronary ostia. Tie the valve in place. Irrigate and recheck the ostia. Close the aortotomy with a running non-absorbable monofilament suture.
- Transient complete heart block is common. Epicardial atrial and ventricular wires should be placed.
- Deair, and wean from CPB. Once off CPB, assess the valves with TEE.

Potential questions/alternative scenarios
"After separating from cardiopulmonary bypass, you note that the patient has a junctional bradycardia (ventricular escape in the 30's). What is a possible cause and how could you have potentially prevented this?"
As in operations for isolated mitral or aortic valve disease, the location of the conduction system needs to be kept in mind. For the mitral portion of the procedure, care should be taken

when placing annular sutures around the lateral aspect of A3. When replacing the aortic valve, care needs to be taken with annular sutures around the membranous septum (at the commissure of the right and non-coronary cusps). Furthermore, when replacing both valves, over sizing the valve could potentially cause compression of the conduction system between the new valves. In this scenario, assuming the valves were not oversized, the etiology of the conduction abnormality likely had to do with overly aggressive placement of annular sutures in aforementioned areas. Epicardial atrial and ventricular wires should be placed in all patients who undergo double valve replacement. Most patients will recover an intrinsic rhythm. The need for permanent pacemaker placement is ~5% for isolated valve surgery (with the risk being 3-fold higher for multiple valve surgery).

"You have trouble defibrillating coming off bypass and the post-bypass TEE shows lateral wall motion abnormality."
The important thing to remember in this situation is the intimate association of the circumflex with the mitral annulus. You have either distorted or injured the circumflex artery. In this scenario, you should re-heparinize immediately and go back on bypass. You will need your PA to get a length of vein adequate to bypass the circumflex. Take care when exposing the lateral wall as you now have a replaced mitral valve, and if you did any annular debridement, then you could potentially disrupt the AV groove. This scenario should be kept in mind for any mitral valve repair/replacement (refer to Mitral Valve Stenosis chapter for AV disruption).

"A 45-year-old otherwise healthy M (height: 5'10; Weight: 60 Kg) with a history of rheumatic fever presents with severe MS and severe AI. You perform a double valve replacement with mechanical prosthetics (AV size: 19 mm; MV size 33 mm). After coming of CPB, you notice blood pooling behind the heart. What happened?"
Keep in mind that when the heart is arrested, the mitral annulus can accommodate a larger prosthetic. Oversized mitral prosthetics can cause a LV rupture once the heart is contracting again after weaning CPB.

"A 19-year-old F presents with severe rheumatic MR and severe AS. The patient wishes to have children and therefore bioprosthetics are used. After replacing both valves and coming of CPB, anesthesia reports increased gradients across the LVOT. A strut of the mitral valve is noted to be protruding into the LVOT. What happened?"
It is imperative to verify that the struts of the mitral bioprosthetic are not encroached into the LVOT. Many prosthetic valves have markings that help avoid having struts directed into the LVOT. It's something to keep in mind when a de novo increased gradient at the LVOT is noted while using mitral a bioprosthetic. In this instance, re-replacement of the mitral valve may be required. Modifying the orientation of the bioprosthetic may avoid the LVOT obstruction. However, mitral replacement with a mechanical valve will eliminate LVOT obstruction.

"Your patient has severe aortic stenosis and severe mitral regurgitation. On induction, the patient arrests. Why did this happen and what are you going to do?"
On induction the SVR drops. Venous return decreases. This leads to decreased coronary flow and ventricular failure. The incidence of arrest on induction with these combined lesions is higher than that for isolated severe AS.

In treating this patient, the first step is to secure the airway. Ventilate the patient. CPR should be going on. Heparinize and have the patient prepped/draped while you are scrubbing. Perform emergent sternotomy. Perform aortic and venous cannulation. Initiate cardiopulmonary bypass. Proceed with AVR/MVR as above.

"On preoperative workup, the symptomatic patient has severe mitral regurgitation and an AVA of ~0.9 cm^2, but the gradient across the aortic valve is only 28 mmHg. How would you proceed?"
It is likely that there is low-gradient aortic stenosis in this situation. The calculation of AVA

314

is dependent upon measurements of the LVOT (which can be operator-dependent by echo). As such, if you do not trust the study then repeat it with a cardiologist whom you are confident. The patient may need a TEE to better define calcification of the valve or the measurements of the LVOT (which directly affect the measurement of the AVA). If after these repeat tests there is still discrepancy, then the patient can get stress testing (treadmill or dobutamine). This should confirm severe AS (keep in mind that patients with contractile reserve benefit more from AVR). Proceed with the operation as indicated from that point forward. Also note that even if the patient has moderate AS and meets an indication for mitral repair due to severe regurgitation then the aortic valve should be replaced.

"You have an 85-year-old otherwise healthy patient who has severe calcific aortic stenosis and 2+ mitral regurgitation. There are no mitral leaflet abnormalities noted. How would you proceed?"
This patient likely has functional mitral regurgitation that is accentuated by his/her severe aortic stenosis. The safest thing to do in this situation is the most expeditious operation possible. It is very likely that once the stenotic aortic valve has been replaced, then the mitral regurgitation will decrease to trace or mild– which in an 85-year-old patient can be medically managed without great fear of long-term complications. In other patients use the TEE to carefully delineate the mitral valve morphology and it may be worthwhile to "explore the valve" without necessarily committing to repair or replacement. If a definite structural abnormality is noted, then it may be repaired.

"A 65-year-old female presents with combined aortic insufficiency and mitral regurgitation. The AI is 3+ (moderately severe). She is short of breath with minimal exertion. Her EF is 45% and end diastolic volume is 7 cm^2. TEE confirms that the MR is severe."
For regurgitation, treat according to the dominant lesion and treat both if both are clearly contributing. In this case either the mitral or aortic could be contributing so both should be addressed by repair/replacement as deemed appropriate. If the MR were moderate (2+) then it is not indicated to repair/replace the valve. However, check the TEE and directly explore the valve if needed to rule out a structural lesion that is contributing to the regurgitation. If flail, chord rupture, or prolapse were noted you may be justified in repairing the valve if feasible, but rarely should you replace for moderate MR at the time of AVR. Conversely, if the aortic valve regurgitation were moderate and the mitral severe then treat the mitral valve and leave the aortic valve alone. Very rarely will moderate AI or moderate MR be the dominant lesion. Again, be sure to check the intraoperative TEE carefully to confirm that the lesions are indeed moderate and consider direct visual inspection if warranted.

Pearls/pitfalls
- When faced with combined valvular disease use TEE to confirm the degree of regurgitation or stenosis.
- Treat according to the dominant lesion.
- Once you are in the OR for at least one valve that meets surgical indication then replace all severely stenotic valves. In this setting, repair/replace all severe or moderately severe regurgitant valves (3-4+).
- The threshold for intervening on moderate aortic valve stenosis may be lowered in the setting of an MVR.
- Moderate aortic regurgitation (2+) does not necessarily require repair in the setting of an MVR but requires evaluation by intraoperative TEE and possibly direct inspection.
- Moderate mitral regurgitation (2+) does not necessarily require repair but requires evaluation by intraoperative TEE and possibly direct inspection depending on the TEE.
- Moderate mitral stenosis should be carefully evaluated with right heart catheterization and TEE. Replace the mitral in the setting of an AVR if there is evidence that it is contributing to the clinical picture (elevated PAP, NYHA III-IV, atrial fibrillation).
- Bioprosthetic valves are generally acceptable if patient > 60 years old.

- Remember that the order of replacement/repair is imperative: open aorta, excise leaflets, and debride annulus *prior* to performing mitral replacement/repair.
- Consider simultaneous sizing of aortic and mitral valves.
- Size the aortic valve *after* replacing the mitral valve.
- Take care not to oversize the mitral valve. This can lead to effective downsizing of the aortic valve and the possibility of having to use too small of an aortic valve (patient prosthesis mismatch).
- As in any mitral repair or replacement, take care when placing sutures in the mitral annulus around P2 or P3.—do not want to compromise the circumflex artery.
- After performing mitral valve replacement, avoid lifting the heart (see below).
- Bright red blood coming from behind the heart after coming off bypass—think AV dissociation. Do not lift the heart to examine. Go back on bypass, then determine where blood is coming from and repair as appropriate.
- Minimally invasive approaches for concomitant aortic and mitral valve surgery via right-sided mini thoracotomy are feasible with acceptable outcomes in centers with known experience in this area.
- See pearls/pitfalls in the chapters on aortic stenosis, mitral stenosis, mitral regurgitation

Suggested readings

- Bonow B. Tricuspid, Pulmonic and Multivalvular Disease. *Braunwald's Heart Disease—A textbook of Cardiovascular Medicine*, 9th ed. 2011.
- Gillinov AM, Blackstone EH, Cosgrove DM, et al. Mitral valve repair with aortic valve replacement is superior to double valve replacement. *J Thorac Cardiovasc Surg 2003*;125:1372-87.
- Carpentier A, Adams D, Filsoufi F. *Carpentier's Reconstructive Valve Surgery.* Section II, IV, V. 2010.
- Nishimura R, Grantham JA, Connolly HM, et al. Low-Output, Low-Gradient Aortic Stenosis in Patients With Depressed Left Ventricular Systolic Function: The Clinical Utility of the Dobutamine Challenge in the Catheterization Laboratory. *Circulation*. 2002;106:809-813.
- Gillinov AM, Gelijns AC, Parides MK, et al. Surgical ablation of atrial fibrillation during mitral-valve surgery. N Engl J Med. 2015;372(15):1399-409.
- Frank S, Pedro DN, Scott S. *Sabiston and Spencer Surgery of the Chest*, 9th ed. 2015
- Kirklin, Barratt-Boyes *Cardiac Surgery*, 4th ed. 2013
- Falk V, Baumgartner H, Bax JJ, et al. 2017 ESC/EACTS Guidelines for the management of valvular heart disease. Eur J Cardiothorac Surg. 2017;52(4):616-664.
- Nishimura RA, Otto CM, Bonow RO, et al. 2017 AHA/ACC Focused Update of the 2014 AHA/ACC Guideline for the Management of Patients With Valvular Heart Disease: A Report of the American College of Cardiology/American Heart Association Task Force on Clinical Practice Guidelines. Circulation. 2017;135(25):e1159-e1195.
- Lamelas J. Minimally invasive concomitant aortic and mitral valve surgery: the "Miami Method". Ann Cardiothorac Surg. 2015;4(1):33-7.
- Ando T, Takagi H, Briasoulis A, et al. A systematic review of reported cases of combined transcatheter aortic and mitral valve interventions. Catheter Cardiovasc Interv. 2018;91(1):124-134.

316

50. COMBINED CORONARY AND CAROTID PROCEDURES

Adnan Al Ayoubi, MD PhD, and Sharon Beth Larson, DO

Adapted from 1st edition chapter written by *Gabriel Loor, MD, and Douglas R. Johnston, MD*

Concept
- Identification of patients with carotid disease undergoing CABG
- Justify the sequence of interventions
- Perioperative strategies for stroke reduction

Chief complaint
"A 70-year-old man presents with a 2-month h/o chest pain to his local cardiologist. He recommends a stress test which is positive for myocardial ischemia. Cardiac catheterization shows the following lesions: 70% mid RCA, 80% mid circumflex and 60% proximal LAD. The patient had a transient ischemic attack (TIA) 1 month ago with no residual deficits. How would you proceed with evaluation and treatment?"

Differential
The patient has diagnosed coronary artery disease. The neurologic disease may be accounted for by embolic disease from arrhythmias or atherosclerotic disease in small or large vessels.

History and physical
The history for any patient undergoing open heart surgery should include a search for risk factors of carotid disease including prior strokes, peripheral vascular disease, coronary artery disease, age, prior carotid endarterectomy (CEA), smoking, diabetes, hypertension and family history. The physical exam should assess for any gross neurologic deficits, carotid bruits, arrhythmias or cardiac murmurs.

Tests
The patient in this scenario has risk factors for carotid disease (age, CAD and prior TIA) and should undergo a carotid duplex as well as a computed tomography (CT) scan of the head to evaluate for and characterize any new or old strokes. The ACCF/AHA issued in 2011 a class IIa recommendation for carotid artery duplex scanning in patients with high risk of concurrent carotid stenosis (age > 65, left main disease, PAD, history of stroke or TIA, hypertension, smoking or DM). An MRA or angiography may be considered for equivocal carotid lesions. It is important to document a complete preop neurologic exam in the event there are deficits postoperatively. The 2011 european peripheral artery disease guidelines recommend carotid duplex in patients ≥ 70 years old, or younger patients with history CVA, carotid bruit, multivessel CAD or PAD (class I, level of evidence C).

Index scenario (additional information)
"He has a history of hypertension and non-insulin dependent diabetes mellitus. He has a right carotid bruit and a duplex shows 70% right ICA stenosis. CT of the head showed no evidence of a prior stroke."

Treatment/management
Based on most recent guidelines, carotid revascularization is reasonable in CAD patients with neurologic symptoms secondary to substantial carotid stenosis (> 80%; class IIa recommendation, level of evidence C). In asymptomatic patients with severe carotid stenosis, carotid revascularization (regardless of chronology of repair) is safe and efficacious (class IIb recommendation, level of evidence C). These guidelines are based on large body of retrospective studies and expert consensus. Most experts agree that carotid revascularization is indicated if the lesion is symptomatic, bilateral, or both. There is no consensus regarding

the effectiveness or staging of prophylactic carotid revascularization in patients planned to undergo CABG.

The options for this man with symptomatic carotid disease (prior TIA) and multivessel symptomatic coronary disease include staged repair (CEA and then CABG) or reversed-staged repair (CABG then CEA) or a synchronous approach under one anesthetic. Meta-analysis has shown that the mortality and stroke rate are higher with a synchronous approach (death - 5% versus 3%; stroke - 6% versus 3%) and therefore should be avoided when possible. The risk of a myocardial infarction (MI) is higher with CEA followed by a CABG and the risk of stroke is higher for CABG followed by CEA. In general, the most symptomatic territories should be addressed first and in combination if both are equally severe. This patient has symptomatic carotid disease and symptomatic coronary disease thus he is at high risk of an MI with a CEA and a stroke with a CABG. The most prudent option would be a synchronous procedure.

If the carotid disease was symptomatic and his coronary disease was not as burdensome (no recent symptoms, chronic stable plaques, mostly < 70%) then it would be reasonable to proceed with the CEA followed in 4-6 weeks by CABG. MI is more common in this situation. If the carotid lesion was asymptomatic with no prior TIA or stroke then he should undergo a CABG followed by a CEA in 4-6 weeks. A severe carotid lesion (> 60% by angio or > 80% by duplex) that is asymptomatic is still grounds for a CEA either first or in combination depending on the severity and symptomatology of the coronary disease. The same goes for a 60-80% stenosis and contralateral occlusion.

Operative steps
- Supine position, arterial line, ETT, swan, cerebral oximetry for neuromonitoring.
- Alternative options for neuromonitoring include EEG, SSEP/MEP (somatosensory evoked potentials/motor evoked potentials), and transcranial Doppler.
- Prep and drape for both a CEA and CABG.
- Begin with the CEA while the leg vein is being harvested.
- Decide ahead of time what conduits to use, if any, and determine if an adequate length of vein is available for both the bypass and CEA. Vein patches may have increased tendency for aneurysmal dilation, many surgeons prefer using a prosthetic such as bovine or hemashield patch. Choice of patch is surgeon dependent. If eversion CEA is elected, no patch is required for closure.
- Oblique incision along the anterior border of the sternocleidomastoid muscle (SCM). Divide the facial vein.
- Dissect down to the carotid artery and expose the common, internal and external carotid. Take care not to injure the vagus during this dissection.
- Get proximal and distal control (external and internal) with vessel loops.
- Give 5000 - 10,000 units of heparin, clamp. Consider a shunt if the cerebral oximetry drops excessively or EEG changes. Open the artery from the proximal common carotid up to the internal carotid beyond the area of gross intimal disease.
- Dissect the plaque with a blunt dissector. Close with vein, bovine or hemashield patch if unable to close primary defect.
- Flush all vessels beginning with the external then the internal and finally the common carotid.
- Obtain hemostasis and pack the wound.
- Complete the vein harvest, median sternotomy, and mammary takedown. Carefully palpate the aorta given the risk for ascending calcification which may require axillary cannulation. Consider utilizing epiaortic ultrasound to place aortic cannula.
- General measures to reduce stroke risk would include keeping MAPs greater than 70 mmHg during bypass, avoiding excessive manipulation of the aorta and limiting cross clamp time and frequency (single clamp vs. double). Consider off-

pump CABG based on surgeon experience. After heparin has been reversed, ensure hemostasis in the neck and close over a drain.

"Postoperatively the patient has evidence of left sided upper extremity weakness."
A neuro exam should be performed as soon as possible following the combined approach. Any abnormalities warrant a head CT, neuro consultation and carotid duplex. Maintain a low threshold for returning to the operating room to explore the patch if there is any hint that the neurologic impairment is due to a structural issue with the patch.

"Postoperatively the patient develops a large neck hematoma with tracheal deviation."
If a neck hematoma develops and compromises the airway it should be opened immediately at the bedside or in the operating room if time permits. Always protect the airway with an endotracheal tube if the patient has already been extubated. After draining the hematoma, ensure hemostasis, irrigate and close over a drain.

Pearls/pitfalls

- Symptomatic coronary artery disease (worsening angina, NSTEMI, STEMI) requires coronary intervention urgently. If the patient has symptomatic carotid disease with at least moderate grade carotid stenosis (50% by duplex) then perform a CEA in the same setting. Carotid artery stenting in the same hospitalization/day may be performed prior to CABG. There are currently very limited data on the efficacy of this method.

- CEA should also be considered in the same setting if a patient who needs an urgent CABG has an asymptomatic carotid lesion > 60% by angio or > 80% by duplex. Same goes for a patient with 60-80% stenosis but contralateral occlusion.

- CEA can be safely delayed in patients undergoing CABG with mild or moderate grade lesions (< 80% duplex) who have not had a prior stroke or TIA.

- If the carotid disease is symptomatic and his coronary disease is not as burdensome (no recent symptoms, chronic stable plaques, mostly < 70%) then it would be reasonable to proceed with the CEA followed in 4-6 weeks by CABG.

Suggested readings

- Brott TG, Halperin JK, Abbara, S et al: 2011 SA/ACCF/AHA/AANN/AANS/ACR/ASNR/CNS/SAIP/SCAI/SIR/SNIS/SVM/SVS guideline on the management of patients with extracranial carotid and vertebral artery disease. A report of the American College of Cardiology Foundation/American Heart Association Task Force on Practice Guidelines, and the American Stroke Association, American Association of Neuroscience Nurses, American Association of Neurological Surgeons, American College of Radiology, American Society of Neuroradiology, Congress of Neurological Surgeons, Society of Atherosclerosis Imaging and Prevention, Society for Cardiovascular Angiography and Interventions, Society of Interventional Radiology, Society of NeuroInterventional Surgery, Society for Vascular Medicine, and Society for Vascular Surgery. *Circulation* 124:e54-e130, 2011.

- Naylor AR, Bown MJ. Stroke after cardiac surgery and its association with asymptomatic carotid disease: an updated systematic review and meta-analysis. Eur J Vasc Endovasc Surg 41:607-624, 2011

- Burger MA et al. Coronary bypass and carotid endarterectomy: does a combined approach increase risk of stroke? A meta-analysis. *Ann Thor Surg* 1999;68;14-20.

- Ouzounian M, LeMaire SA, Coselli JS. Chapter 73 Occlusive disease of the brachiocephalic vessels and management of simultaneous surgical carotid and coronary disease. Selke FW, del Nido PJ, Swanson SJ (eds). *Sabiston & Spencer Surgery of the Chest* 2016

- Kwon MH, Tolis Jr G, Sundt TM. Chapter 20 Myocardial revascularization with cardiopulmonary bypass. Cohn LH and Adams DH (eds). *Cardiac Surgery in the Adult* 2018

51. ENDOCARDITIS

Andrew M. Vekstein M.D., Brittany A. Zwischenberger M.D., Donald D. Glower M.D.

Adapted from 1ˢᵗ edition chapter written by *Katherine B. Harrington, MD, and Bruce A. Reitz, MD*

Concept

- Indications for surgical management of infective endocarditis
- Timing of surgical intervention
- Valve repair or replacement options
- Options for complex reconstruction

Chief complaint

"A 72-year-old man with diabetes presents with 2-3 days of low-grade fevers, weight loss, lethargy, and shortness of breath. About a week ago he completed treatment for a right knee infection with antibiotics. Preliminary blood cultures are growing gram positive cocci in 4 of 4 bottles. TTE shows moderate-severe aortic insufficiency (AI). How would you proceed with management?"

Differential

Endocarditis, bacteremia, structural valve disease, coronary disease, CHF

Definition and pathophysiology

- Infective endocarditis (IE) is infection of the endocardial surface of the heart, with the heart valves most commonly affected (mitral > aortic > tricuspid > pulmonary), and frequently, prosthetic valves. IE may also involve congenital heart lesions such as septal defects, patent ductus arteriosis, and coarctation of the aorta.
- The endocardial or valvular surface is damaged by turbulence, providing the substrate for the infective agent and a platelet/fibrin matrix to initiate colonization and persistence. Common risk factors include mitral valve prolapse, bicuspid aortic valve and rheumatic heart disease.

History and physical

The H&P should help establish the diagnosis, source, any adverse sequelae and stratify the patient for surgery if needed. *Establishing the diagnosis* - history of murmurs, structural heart disease, or immunosuppression. Social history focused on IV drug usage. Timing and duration of symptoms as well as any recent treatment. *Source* - inquire about infection (dental procedures, GI illnesses, recent invasive procedures). Inquire about recent skin/soft tissue infections or joint infections suggestive of septic arthritis. *Sequelae* - Evaluate for signs and symptoms of congestive heart failure, distal embolic phenomena, stroke/TIA. *Risk stratify* - other significant comorbidities, renal dysfunction, dialysis, diabetes, cardiopulmonary disease. Focused physical exam including vital signs, sequelae of possible neurologic emboli, murmurs, pulmonary congestion/edema, and endocarditis stigmata: Osler's nodes - painful nodules on hands and feet, Janeway lesions - small, flat, non-painful erythematous lesions on palms and soles, Roth's spots - pale retinal hemorrhages, and splinter hemorrhages in nails. Investigate all possible sources and whether source control has been achieved.

Tests

- *Blood cultures*: Follow-up speciation and full sensitivities. *Staph aureus* is now the most common causative organism, with other frequently identified organisms including *viridans* group strep, *enterococcus* and coagulase negative staph. If *strep bovis* is the causative organism, should get colonoscopy to rule out GI malignancy. If fungal infection, an ophthalmologic evaluation is required.

320

- *EKG:* obtain frequently to follow PR interval and look for the development of heart block, or evolving bundle branch block. This would indicate the development of annular abscess near the conduction system.
- *TEE:* Recommended as the first line study for all prosthetic valve endocarditis. Recommended in all cases of suspected endocarditis when the transthoracic echo is non-diagnostic or to further assess the severity of known endocarditis (i.e. annular abscess).
- *Coronary Angiography:* Follow guidelines for pre-operative evaluation prior to valve surgery (typically indicated for all females over 50 and all males over 40). Consider coronary CT angiography instead, especially if patient has no risk factors and left heart catheterization may cause embolization of known aortic valve vegetations. Forgo evaluation of the coronaries if patient requires emergent surgery.
- *Brain Imaging (CT or MRI):* Indicated for all patients with neurologic symptoms and may be considered to screen any asymptomatic patient with left-sided endocarditis for ischemic or hemorrhagic stroke.
- *Chest CT/CXR:* pulmonary infarcts or abscesses or prior to redo sternotomy.

Criteria for diagnosis of IE
- If there is no explicit clinical diagnosis of endocarditis, then the Duke criteria can be used. Duke criteria requires 2 major criteria, or 1 major and 3 minor, or 5 minor criteria for a "definite" diagnosis of IE.

Table 51-1. Modified Duke criteria for diagnosis of infective endocarditis.

Major criteria	Minor criteria
Microbiologic evidence of endocarditis - Typical organisms in 2 cultures - Atypical organisms in 2 cultures drawn at least 12 hours apart or in 3 of 4 cultures drawn at least an hour apart	Predisposition to endocarditis - Intravenous drug use - Prior prosthetic valve - Structural heart disease
Evidence of endocardial involvement on echo: - New valvular regurgitation - Abscess - Oscillating cardiac mass - Partial dehiscence of a prosthetic valve	Vascular phenomenon. - Systemic embolism - Septic pulmonary infarcts - Mycotic aneurysm - Janeway's lesions
	Immunologic phenomenon - Osler's nodes - Roth's spots - Glomerulonephritis

| Fever > 38° C |
| Microbiology finding not meeting major criteria |

"The TEE confirms moderate-severe AI and shows a 0.8 cm vegetation on the posterior leaflet of his mitral valve. Blood cultures are positive for methicillin sensitive staphylococcus aureus. He is otherwise hemodynamically stable."

Treatment/management

The decisions regarding surgical management of the patient with IE should be individualized, and requires consultation with the infectious disease physician, the cardiologist, and the cardiac surgeon. Appropriate antibiotic therapy based on blood culture data is the mainstay of IE therapy. If the patient is hemodynamically stable, serial blood cultures demonstrating blood sterilization after 48 hours of antibiotics is optimal (3 cultures drawn at least 24 hours apart) and may indicate effective treatment.

The patient in this scenario has two major criteria for endocarditis with septic arthritis as the most likely inciting event. He appears to have source control, and, with the severe AI, he meets criteria for surgical intervention. The following generalities can be made regarding timing of intervention for endocarditis:

Table 51-2. Indications for Surgery for IE (based on 2017 AHA/ACC Focused Update of the 2014 AHA/ACC Guideline for the Management of Patients with Valvular Heart Disease) with generally recommended timing.

Timing	Clinical Scenario
Emergent (next 12 hours)	- Valve dysfunction resulting in Class IV heart failure or cardiogenic shock (e.g. acute AI with early closure of MV or mitral leaflet or chordal rupture)
Urgent (next 12-48 hours)	- Valve dysfunction resulting in Class III heart failure - Heart block - Annular aortic abscess - Other destructive penetrating lesion (e.g. intra-cardiac fistula) - Mobile vegetation > 10mm
Early (next 3-7 days)	- Left-sided IE caused by S. aureus - Left-sided IE caused by fungal organisms - Persistent bacteremia or fevers >5-7 days after onset of appropriate antimicrobial therapy - Prosthetic valve endocarditis with persistence or recurrence of bacteremia - Multiple septic embolic phenomena
Delayed (1-4 weeks)	- Ischemic CVA (1-2 weeks) - Cerebral mycotic aneurysm (1-4 weeks) - Hemorrhagic CVA (3-4 weeks)

Prosthetic selection

If replacement is needed, valve choice can be discussed based on current guidelines, individual patient characteristics and preference. However, it is not until the valve is excised, debrided and inspected in the OR that the final decision regarding conduits can be made. There is no difference in reinfection risks between mechanical and bioprosthetic valves. In the presence of more extensive aortic annular involvement, abscess formation, or septal perforation, a tissue composite graft (homograft or xenograft) has been demonstrated to be a superior alternative.

After surgical correction, at least six weeks of appropriate antibiotic therapy is generally recommended but should be based on infectious disease consult recommendations.

Operative steps

- The most important operative goal for endocarditis is to *debride ALL grossly infected tissue.*
- The conduct of the operation is similar as that in standard aortic valve replacement and mitral valve replacement. See those chapters for detailed steps. However, surgical management of endocarditis requires a skillset to perform anything from a simple valve replacement to a valve and patch, double valve, root and even reconstruction of the fibrous skeleton of the heart.
- Sternotomy is the recommended incision for endocarditis
- Aortic cannulation, bicaval cannulation, with fastidious myocardial protection. For aortic insufficiency, a combination of antegrade, retrograde and/or direct ostial cardioplegia are necessary.
- Begin with the aortotomy above the STJ and inspect the aortic valve apparatus. Resect the aortic leaflets along with all infected tissue. Send for culture and pathology.
- To expose the mitral valve, left atriotomy or trans-septal approaches may be utilized. If additional visualization is necessary, extend incision to the superior dome of the left atrium.
- Repairing the mitral valve is reasonable if vegetation can be removed and there is no underlying damage to the valve apparatus. Avoid prosthetic bands or rings unless absolutely needed. If unable to be repaired, replace the valve. Close the left atrium.
- Re-examine the aortic valve and confirm that all infected tissue has been debrided. Usually replacement of the aortic valve is necessary, although repair is reasonable if vegetation can be removed and there is no underlying damage to the valve apparatus. Close the aortotomy.
- Consider opening bilateral pleural spaces. Wean from cardiopulmonary bypass. Be prepared to treat both septic (distributive) and cardiogenic shock with vasopressors and inotropes.

Potential questions/alternative scenarios

"There is an annular abscess at the right/non-coronary commissure."
If there is an abscess, it must be completely unroofed, and all grossly infected tissue debrided. The defect is then patched with autologous or bovine pericardium to exclude the abscess cavity from circulation. For a small abscess this patch will suffice. The right/non commissure is the site of the membranous septum, so there is high risk for VSD creation with aggressive debridement. This patient also has a high risk for conduction disturbance and pacemaker need. If the abscess is even more extensive and debridement of a large part of the annulus is needed, a homograft/xenograft root replacement may be the best option. The muscular annulus of the graft helps fill any tissue defects after extensive debridement. The graft is affixed to the annulus with multiple simple interrupted sutures or several running prolene sutures. The coronary buttons are reimplanted to the homograft/xenograft.

"Upon visualization the endocarditis appears to be confined to the P2 segment of his mitral valve."
Repair the mitral valve when possible. The infected segment can be removed with a triangular or quadrangular excision. Avoiding placement of a prosthetic valve in the mitral location is preferable in an infected setting, provided you can confidently excise all infected tissue. Any small focal holes in the mitral or aortic valves can be debrided and patched with autologous or bovine pericardium.

"After performing a left atriotomy for MV endocarditis, there appears to be an abscess extending into posterior mitral annulus."

323

Carefully debride all infected tissue and plan to reconstruct the posterior mitral annulus prior to valve replacement. If there is enough native tissue remaining, reinforce the posterior mitral annulus with interrupted figure-of-eight sutures from the LA to LV, creating a fold of tissue which can be used to secure the prosthetic valve. If more extensive debridement is necessary, reconstruction typically involves a crescent shaped pericardial patch sandwiching the LA and LV endocardium to re-create a posterior annulus, which is secured with interrupted pledgeted sutures.

Atrioventricular disruption is the most feared complication in patients with extensive mitral annular destruction. In this case, either of the above techniques could be used, or the annulus could be reconstructed with Teflon strips inside the LV and inside the LA with horizontal mattress sutures. If debridement or reconstruction potentially compromises the circumflex artery, empirically bypass the circumflex with vein graft.

"There is an abscess extending from the aortic root to the anterior mitral leaflet with complete disruption of the aorto-mitral curtain."

In patients with advanced endocarditis with abscess and destruction of the aorto-mitral fibrous skeleton (particularly in prosthetic valve endocarditis), you should be prepared to resect all infected tissue and proceed with reconstruction of the fibrous skeleton of the heart and double valve replacement (Commando Operation):

- An oblique aortotomy is performed and extended longitudinally into the aortic root in the non-coronary sinus.
- Debride all grossly infected tissue, which may include the aorto-mitral curtain, anterior leaflet of the mitral valve and dome of the left atrium.
- The mitral valve is replaced first. The horizontal pledgeted valve sutures are placed along the remaining annular tissue, which typically includes the posterior mitral annulus.
- A generous patch (typically bovine pericardium) is folded in half and sewn at its midpoint with running or horizontal pledgeted sutures to the remaining mitral valve sewing ring and anchored to medial and lateral fibrous trigones.
- The prosthetic aortic valve is secured to the native aortic valve annulus in the standard fashion with horizontal mattress sutures. At the annular defect, the prosthetic valve is secured to the patch with running or horizontal pledgeted suture to secure the valve cuff to the edge of patch.
- The lower fold of patch is folded over to close the dome of the left atrium. The upper half of the patch incorporated cephalad into the non-coronary sinus to close the aortotomy. The patch also allows for enlargement of the aortic root, if necessary.
- Alternatively, in cases with extensive aortic annular destruction, an aortic homograft may be used. The anterior mitral leaflet from the homograft can frequently be utilized instead of patch materials to reconstruct the fibrous skeleton and seat the mitral valve.

"His initial blood cultures are negative."

If the clinical suspicion of endocarditis is high, empiric antimicrobials should be started and continued in consultation with Infectious Disease team. Common causes of culture-negative endocarditis are the HACEK (*Haemophilus, Actinobacillus, Cardiobacterium, Eikenella,* and *Kingella*) and fungal organisms.

"Patient is found to have multiple embolic lesions on preoperative head CT."

The operative timing of patients with cerebral embolic lesions is controversial, but generally depends on overall patient status (hemodynamic stability, baseline frailty), etiology of stroke (ischemic vs hemorrhagic) and size of infarct. For ischemic strokes, some studies suggest waiting 1 week for infarcts less than 1cm and 2 weeks for infarcts larger than 1cm. For hemorrhagic strokes, consider waiting 3-4 weeks. However, timing must be considered in context of the patient's clinical status and risk profile. For patients with progressive heart failure, recurrent cerebral embolic events, sepsis or more virulent organisms on culture (e.g. Staph aureus), consider operating sooner. Multiple studies have suggested that, in patients with endocarditis and ischemic CVA, there is no increased risk of hemorrhagic conversion or in-hospital mortality when operating less than 7 days after CVA.

"A 50-year-old IV drug abuser is diagnosed with 3+TR and a 1 cm vegetation on the tricuspid valve. He also complains of worsening shortness of breath and lower extremity edema."

Early initiation of antibiotics and prompt surgical evaluation is key as these patients can rapidly decompensate with right sided heart failure and respiratory failure. Consider obtaining a TEE and right heart catheterization to evaluate right sided function and pressures. Usually medical management with antibiotics is sufficient. Surgical indications include failure of medical therapy, worsening TR, hemodynamic compromise (RV failure from TR), and recurrent pulmonary emboli with respiratory compromise. Surgical options depend upon the size of the lesion and extent of resection required, including:

- Simple vegectomy.
- *Valve repair/reconstruction*: May be considered in the case of limited debridement/resection of the tricuspid valve tissue. If the valve in incompetent after debridement of endocarditis, consider annuloplasty with prosthetic ring. Some surgeons prefer the DeVega annuloplasty technique (double ring of running mattress sutures from atrial to ventricular side of tricuspid annulus) to minimize prosthetic material. Small perforations or leaflet excisions can be repaired with pericardial patch. Triangular/quadrangular resections with ring annuloplasty may be considered.
- *Valve replacement*: mechanical versus bioprosthetic - no difference in overall survival. Bioprosthetic valve in the tricuspid position can be managed with aspirin only. Mechanical requires a high INR goal (> 3.0) due to the low pressure right sided system, however, may be more durable.
- *Valve excision without replacement*: If patient has a history of recurrent endocarditis, particularly in the context of IV drug use and nonadherence, with good RV and LV function, this may be considered as a lifesaving maneuver.

"A 68-year-old male undergoes a mini AVR for aortic stenosis and returns one month later with leaflet vegetations, fevers and chills."

Early PVE (< 2 months since original surgery) is often aggressive and most often requires intervention within 1-2 weeks of treatment. Any high-risk features such as paravalvular leak or other evidence of valve dehiscence require earlier intervention (24-48 hours). The principles of the operation are similar to those listed above. The prosthesis and all pledgets are removed and all infected tissue are debrided. Usually a homograft/xenograft is required.

For late PVE (> 2 months since original surgery), the indications for operation are similar to those for native valve endocarditis. Consider the patient specific factors and organism when planning early or late operation. For patients with recurrent endocarditis secondary to IV drug use, it is reasonable to consider prolonged course of antibiotics. Patients with more virulent organisms, such as Staph aureus, are less likely to improve with antibiotics alone. Fungal PVE is an indication for re-do surgery in an appropriate surgical candidate, as it will not resolve with medical therapy alone.

"After successful homograft aortic root replacement for endocarditis with root abscess, patient is found to be in complete heart block while weaning from cardiopulmonary bypass."

Although some patients may have transient CHB after cardioplegia, have a high index of suspicion of permanent heart block if the debridement or reconstruction disrupted the conduction system. Permanent atrial and ventricular epicardial pacing leads are preferred in patients with endocarditis, as these are less likely to become infected than transvenous leads.

325

- Surgical treatment of endocarditis is indicated with valvular lesions causing heart failure, conduction disturbance, annular or sub-annular abscess, fungal endocarditis, recurrent embolic phenomenon, or progressive prosthetic valve regurgitation.
- Debride all infected tissue, repair mitral and tricuspid valves when possible, replace aortic valves.
- Be prepared for anything with these procedures. Range of procedures can include simple AVR, homograft, mitral repair/replacement, double valve, double valve with reconstruction of the fibrous skeleton, and tricuspid repair/replacement.
- Prepare for postoperative heart block and both cardiogenic and septic shock.
- The patient usually receives at least six weeks of antibiotics postoperatively.

Suggested readings

- Pettersson GB, Coselli JS, Hussain ST, Griffin B, et al. 2016 The American Association for Thoracic Surgery (AATS) consensus guidelines: Surgical treatment of infective endocarditis: Executive summary. The Journal of Thoracic and Cardiovascular Surgery. 2017 Jun 1;153(6):1241–58.e29.
- Nishimura RA, Otto CM, Bonow RO, Carabello BA, Erwin JP, Fleisher LA, et al. 2017 AHA/ACC Focused Update of the 2014 AHA/ACC Guideline for the Management of Patients With Valvular Heart Disease: A Report of the American College of Cardiology/American Heart Association Task Force on Clinical Practice Guidelines. Journal of the American College of Cardiology. 2017 Jul 3;70(2):252–89.
- Pettersson GB, Hussain ST. Surgical Treatment of Aortic Valve Endocarditis. In: Cohn LH, Adams DH. *Cardiac Surgery in the Adult, 5th Edition.* McGraw-Hill; 2018.
- Pettersson GB, Hussain ST. Surgical Treatment of Mitral Valve Endocarditis. In: Cohn LH, Adams DH. *Cardiac Surgery in the Adult, 5th Edition.* McGraw-Hill; 2018.
- Fiedler AG, Lee LS, Chen FY, Cohn LH. Native and Prosthetic Valve Endocarditis. In Sellke FW, del Nido PJ, Swanson SJ. *Sabiston and Spencer: Surgery of the Chest, 9th Edition.* Elsevier, Inc; 2016.
- Moon MR, Miller DC, Moore KA, Oyer PE, Mitchell RS, Robbins RC, Stinson EB, Shumway NE, Reitz BA. Treatment of endocarditis with valve replacement: the question of tissue versus mechanical prosthesis. *Ann Thorac Surg.* 2001 Apr;71(4):1164-71.

52. CARDIAC TRAUMA

Mark Joseph, MD, and Andy C. Kiser, MD

Concept
- Management of penetrating cardiac trauma
- Preoperative considerations
- Operative strategies and choice of incision
- Pitfalls and alternative solutions

Chief complaint
"A 24-year-old man presents with a gunshot wound (GSW) to the chest. The patient is talking but confused, bedside sonography shows evidence of a pericardial effusion. The patient becomes increasingly agitated and hypotensive. What is the next step in management?"

Differential
Injury to the great vessels or heart.

History and physical
Proceed with standard ATLS workup and primary survey (ABCD's - secure airway, ventilation, IV access, fluid/blood resuscitation). Secondary survey - define the pattern of chest injury (anterior box - mid clavicular, notch to xiphoid = cardiac injury until proven otherwise; posterior box - between scapula = esophagus, aorta, airway; chest or thoracoabdominal = pulmonary, aortic, cardiac if transmediastinal, abdominal organs if thoracoabdominal). Quickly assess for other associated life-threatening injuries (head trauma, GCS), order chest x ray, auscultate for breath sounds, prepare for a thoracostomy tube insertion on the side of the injury, review the echo, and send labs. CT scans should be performed on hemodynamically stable patients only and is warranted if the CXR shows a widened mediastinum. Sonography can determine the presence of pericardial fluid, physical examination may reveal Beck's triad (muffled heart sounds, jugular venous distention, and hypotension) or Kussmaul's sign (jugular venous distention with inspiration) indicating pericardial tamponade. Should the patient decompensate and lose their pulse an emergent left anterolateral thoracotomy becomes part of the primary survey (see below).

Tests
- *CXR*: evaluate widened mediastinum.
- *FAST (focused assessment with sonography for trauma)*: evaluate pericardial fluid and other potential injuries.
- *Echocardiography (the gold standard)*: can be used to further delineate valves, pericardial effusions, RV compression, tamponade physiology and foreign bodies/missiles within the myocardium or cardiac chambers.
- *CT scan*: may be helpful to identify additional injuries (abdominal) if patient is stable, but in general not helpful unless a vascular injury is suspected.

Index scenario (additional information)
"FAST revealed pericardial fluid with a wide mediastinum on CXR. The patient became pulseless. You performed an antero-lateral thoracotomy and found a hole in the left ventricle."

Treatment/management
On arrival, nearly half of patients with cardiac injury may are hemodynamically stable and then suddenly deteriorate. Unstable patients may respond to fluid resuscitation, but arrest is always eminent. Establishing an airway with appropriate ventilation and large bore IV access

are critical. If the patient responds to fluids, its usually transient but does provide the clinician time to formulate a plan. The main branch point in the treatment algorithm is to discern whether a patient is stable (or nearly stable) or unstable (or pulseless). Stable patients can get a CXR, echo, labs, access, and chest tube if warranted. If a pericardial effusion is present assume a cardiac injury has occurred and plan to get to the OR immediately. A subxiphoid pericardiocentesis may help buy time if the patient needs other critical preoperative information (i.e., a head CT in the setting of severe head trauma). But in general penetrating and isolated chest trauma with an effusion requires a trip to the OR for a median sternotomy. If the patient with penetrating trauma arrests in transit to the ED (within 20 minutes) or in the trauma bay then an ED thoracotomy (left anterior thoracotomy) is warranted to evacuate the tamponade, open cardiac massage and identify/control the injury if possible. If the patient is in the OR, a median sternotomy is acceptable for penetrating wounds. As with all trauma patients, be sure to prep from the patient's chin to ankles in the event there's a need to harvest the saphenous vein for a coronary artery injury. Otherwise a bilateral trans-sternal anterolateral thoracotomy ("clam shell") provides excellent exposure to the mediastinum and pleural spaces (see below).

Operative steps

ED thoracotomy

- Have airway secured, NGT in place (helps to locate the esophagus), IV access.
- Small towel roll under the left chest, prep and drape expeditiously.
- Perform left anterior thoracotomy in approximately the 5th intercostal space (below the nipple) down to the bone (antero-lateral exposure).
- Chest retractor.
- Open the pericardium longitudinally. Stay above the phrenic nerve.
- Identify, bluntly dissect and clamp the descending aorta to optimize perfusion to the heart.
- During the left anterior thoracotomy if the source of bleeding is not immediately identified and left ventricular injury suspected, inflow may be reduced by manually occluding the left hilum. Left ventricular injuries can be temporarily managed with a finger or occlusion using a foley catheter balloon.
- If the patient is stabilized, then proceed to the operating room for definitive management. The types of injuries that may be encountered and the operation required may be highly variable. Epicardial lacerations may undergo simple closure with prolene sutures. Coronary artery injuries may require ligation and distal bypass with vein. An intraop TEE will reveal valvular injuries that may require debridement and repair/replacement. Aortic injuries are treated like ruptures and may require anything from simple suture ligation to circulatory arrest and aortic graft placement.
- In stable patients with a pericardial effusion and suspected cardiac injury, skip the ED thoracotomy and proceed to the OR for median sternotomy +/- CPB.

Potential questions/alternative scenarios

"You wean off bypass and the echo shows new localized anterolateral wall motion abnormalities and the patient is started on high dose inotropic support."
Strongly consider a coronary artery injury in the region of your repair and bypass the appropriate vessel.

"You open the chest and identify a right atrial injury."
Right atrial injuries can usually be controlled with a clamp and do not necessitate the need for CPB. A series of clamps can be used to approximate long injuries. Suture closure can be performed under the clamps. The repair can usually be performed with pledgeted suture. Caution should be given to avoid tearing the atrium with traction. Similarly, superior caval injuries can sometimes be repaired without institution of bypass. The benefit of avoiding CPB is the avoidance of heparin in a patient with multisystem trauma (i.e., heparin would not be

328

ideal in the setting of a GSW to the abdomen, head or extremity). On the other hand, if you are reasonably certain you have an isolated chest trauma involving vascular structures and or lung parenchyma then CPB and arresting the heart gives you the best chance of a successful and hemostatic repair.

"You notice both right atrial and ventricular injury?"

Injuries from gunshot wounds can damage all chambers of the heart. The friability of the tissue, injury location, and hemodynamic instability may necessitate CPB. Injuries that involve multiple chambers require thorough investigation to rule out valvular or septal injury. Direct visualization of the bullets path and intraoperative echo are invaluable. Trans cardiac injuries imply a path from one chamber to the next and the potential for an intracardiac injury. CPB and cardiac arrest with cardiotomy are necessary. If the injury is small, use horizontal pledgeted mattress sutures. Larger defects, however, require reconstruction using pericardium. Posterior cardiac injuries can be visualized by elevating the heart out of the pericardium while on CPB. Injuries to the coronary sinus should be ligated as a patch repair is very difficult in a heart that is already friable. Still, a patch can be considered for reinforcement. If reasonable hemostasis is achieved but the patient is spiraling into a coagulopathy then you can always pack and leave the chest open until coags normalize.

"A stab wound has caused a laceration to the distal LAD?"

Coronary artery injuries require CPB and may require coronary bypass using a conduit. Vein conduit is most appropriate in an emergent situation. Distal coronary artery injuries, especially beyond the distal third of the vessel, may only require ligation. However, if there is salvageable ventricular dysfunction, then the vessel should be bypassed. Cardiac injuries in proximity but without direct injury to the coronary artery may require repair without compromising coronary flow. Passing the pledgeted sutures through the myocardium behind the coronary allows repair without compromising coronary patency.

Pearls/pitfalls

- In a patient with penetrating trauma who is pulseless within 20 min of arriving to the ED or in the ED, an anterolateral thoracotomy with release of tamponade, open cardiac massage and cross clamping the aorta is the procedure of choice.
- Cardiac injuries in proximity to coronary arteries can be managed with horizontal mattress sutures going under the vessel as to avoid occlusion or injury to the artery. If artery is injured, then bypass should be considered.
- Complex injuries to the heart and other blood vessels should be treated in order of most life-threatening first followed by other injuries such as intracardiac or valvular injuries.

Suggested readings

- Ascnsio JA, Stewart BM, Murray JA, et al: Penetrating cardiac injuries. *Surg Clin North Am* 1996;76:685.
- Thourani VH, Feliciano DV, Cooper WA, et al: Penetrating cardiac trauma at an urban trauma center: a 22-year perspective. *Am Surg* 1999;65:811.
- Ivatury RR, Rohman M, Steichen FM, et al: Penetrating cardiac injuries: twenty-year experience. *Am J Surg* 1987;53:310.
- Wall Jr. MJ, Mattox KL, Chen C, et al: Acute management of complex cardiac injuries. *J Trauma* 1997;42:905.

53. Type A Aortic Dissection

Heidi Reich, MD, and Dominic Emerson, MD

Adapted from 1st edition chapter written by *Armin Kiankhooy, MD, and Ravi Ghanta, MD*

Concept

- Diagnosis and management of acute type A dissection
- Operative techniques and potential pitfalls
- Postoperative management

Chief complaint

"A 63-year-old man presents to the emergency room with sudden onset of severe tearing chest and back pain."

Differential

This presentation warrants a high index of suspicion for acute aortic dissection. Up to 30% of patients with acute aortic dissection are initially thought to have another diagnosis. Two-thirds of all patients with aortic dissection present with involvement of the ascending aorta (Stanford type A) and one-third present with isolated involvement of the descending aorta (type B). Differential includes acute aortic syndromes (aortic dissection, intramural hematoma, and penetrating aortic ulcer), acute coronary syndrome, aortic aneurysm, acute aortic insufficiency, pulmonary embolism, pericarditis, and musculoskeletal pain.

History and physical

A focused history elicits the quality (ripping, migrating), location (mid-sternum or interscapular), and chronicity of the pain, as well as signs of malperfusion, i.e., stroke, paraplegia, abdominal pain, anuria/oliguria, and claudication. Family history of aortic dissection or aneurysm should be assessed. On exam, hypertension, hypotension, and a pulse differential or deficit may be apparent. Presence of a blowing, diastolic, decrescendo murmur at the left 3rd intercostal space suggests aortic regurgitation. Tamponade physiology, with characteristic JVD, pulsus paradoxus, and pericardial friction rub, suggests aortic rupture. Neurologic assessment, abdominal exam, and pulse exam should be clearly documented prior to surgery.

Pathophysiology

Medial degeneration, leading to compromised aortic wall structural integrity, intimal tear, and propagation of the intimal flap, is associated with development of aortic dissection. Hypertension is the key mechanical force contributing to dissection. The tear is typically > 50% of the circumference and usually occurs along the right anterior aspect of the ascending aorta and circumferentially spirals around the arch and into the descending thoracic and abdominal aorta on the left and posteriorly. Approximately 10% of the time, the dissection propagates retrograde to involve the coronary ostia. Forty percent of patients with acute type A aortic dissection die immediately. Thereafter, mortality is 1-2% per hour in the first 48 hours and, without surgical intervention, up to 90% at 30 days. If rupture does not occur, weakening of the outer media and adventitia results in aneurysmal dilatation. Early mortality results from 1) aortic rupture with or without pericardial tamponade, 2) acute aortic insufficiency and congestive heart failure, 3) acute myocardial infarction due to coronary involvement, and 4) stroke due to arch vessel involvement. Urgent surgery converts a 90% mortality risk to at least a 70-80% probability of survival.

Risk factors

The most frequent risk factor is hypertension. Other risk factors include connective tissue disorders, personal or family history of aortic aneurysm or dissection, aortic valve disease, pregnancy, recent aortic manipulation (catheter-based or surgical), and stimulant use.

Tests

- *Labs*: Establish baseline lab values (CMP, CBC, Coags). No ideal screening lab test exists for acute aortic dissection. D-dimer below 500 ng/mL has been proposed as an exclusionary test, but reduced sensitivity of D-dimer limits its reliability in certain scenarios, such as short-segment or subacute dissections.

- *EKG*: Ischemic changes, ranging from non-specific ST/T wave changes to ST-segment elevation, result from hypotension, coronary ostial involvement (most commonly inferior wall ischemia in RCA distribution), and pre-existing coronary artery disease. Initial misdiagnosis of acute coronary syndrome is common.

- *CXR*: Classic findings include widened mediastinum and pleural effusion, but over 20% of acute type A dissections present with normal mediastinal and aortic contour.

- *CT angiography*: Diagnostic study of choice due to widespread availability and high sensitivity/specificity. Delineates proximal and distal flap extent, aortic root and arch involvement, associated aneurysms, and pericardial effusion. An ECG-gated CT of the entire aorta, neck to pelvis through the femoral vessels, is ideal.

- *TEE*: Preferred diagnostic study for unstable patients and can be performed on-table in the operating room. Identifies the intimal tear, true and false lumens, aortic valve characteristics, aortic insufficiency, proximal coronary involvement, and pericardial effusion.

- If clinical suspicion is high and initial aortic imaging is negative, a second imaging study (CT, TEE, or MRI) should be performed.

Index scenario (additional information)
"This patient has < 24 hours of pain and CT angiography reveals a type A dissection. There is no aortic root or arch involvement. How would you like to proceed?"

Treatment/management
This patient meets the criteria for acute type A aortic dissection *without arch or root involvement*. Surgery is indicated to prevent life-threatening complications including aortic rupture. The goal is to prevent death and irreversible end-organ damage. Pre-operative anti-impulse (dp/dt) treatment with short-acting beta-blockers (goal HR ≤ 60) and peripheral vasodilators ("permissive hypotension" and goal SBP 90-120 mmHg) is critical and reduces transmural aortic wall stress and sheer stress. Pain control is also important. The presence of type A aortic dissection is an indication for immediate repair. Only minor delays for CT imaging in a stable patient can be justified. Hemodynamic instability demands immediate surgery. Focal neurologic deficits mandate a head CT. Relative contraindication to surgical repair include coma or dense neurologic deficits, age over 80 years, and significant comorbidities. For the most part type A dissections will be operative without delay.

Operative steps
Acute type A dissection repair
The primary goals of surgery are to save the life of the patient and, when feasible, to provide more definitive treatment to reduce the need for future aortic surgical interventions. The extent of aorta requiring replacement depends on the location and extent of the tear and aneurysm. The most common operation is supracoronary replacement of the ascending aorta and hemi-arch replacement. Considerations regarding the extent of surgery include patient age, comorbidities, clinical stability, presence of malperfusion, and extent of the aortic dissection.

- Anesthesia & monitoring
  - General endotracheal anesthesia with central venous access, PA catheter, arterial lines (right +/- left radial and femoral), TEE, and bladder and esophageal temperature probes.

331

- Neurologic monitoring with electroencephalography and near-infrared cerebral oximetry.
- Neck, chest, abdomen, and bilateral lower extremities are prepped and draped widely.

- Cannulation Strategies
  - *Arterial Cannulation:* It is crucial to achieve arterial cannulation of the true lumen. If high line pressures are encountered, this may be the result of false lumen cannulation. Stop the pump and obtain arterial cannulation at a different site.
  - Right axillary artery: Prior to opening the chest, an 8-10mm graft is sewn end-to-side to the right axillary artery exposed infraclavicular or in the deltopectoral groove. Avoid in presence of axillary extension of the dissection. Disadvantages include additional time required for exposure and risk of axillary dissection.
  - Ascending aorta: Direct cannulation of the ascending aorta is performed using Seldinger technique under TEE guidance to ensure true lumen cannulation. This strategy remains controversial.
  - Femoral artery: Preoperative CT and pulse exam delineate if the femoral artery is perfused by the true lumen. Femoral cannulation is desirable due to ease of rapid access, which makes femoral cannulation a reasonable option for unstable patients. Disadvantages include the risk of differentially pressurizing the false lumen and resultant malperfusion. Arterial flow is switched to the aortic graft sidearm after circulatory arrest to ensure true lumen perfusion while rewarming.
  - *Venous cannulation*: Bicaval or dual-stage venous cannulation are used depending on whether retrograde cerebral perfusion is planned.
- Initiate CPB and begin systemic cooling with ice placed around the patient's head. A retrograde cardioplegia cannula and LV vent are inserted. Monitor closely for LV distension.
- During cooling, perform proximal dissection. When the heart fibrillates, carefully cross clamp the mid-ascending aorta, monitoring for distal malperfusion, and divide the aorta. Administer retrograde cardioplegia with or without direct ostial antegrade cardioplegia. Inspect aortic root and aortic valve. Perform as much proximal work (see below) as able while cooling.
- Cool to below 20° C with electrocerebral silence or empirically for at least 45 minutes, place the patient in Trendelenburg and initiate circulatory arrest. Administer selective antegrade or retrograde cerebral perfusion (see Circulatory Arrest chapter for details). Circulatory arrest times not exceeding 30-45 minutes with deep hypothermia are considered safe.
- Perform an open distal anastomosis under circulatory arrest. This ensures true lumen perfusion, facilitates inspection of the arch for intimal tears or other pathology that would change the planned operation, and allows the cross-clamp site to be resected. The distal extent of resection (ascending aortic replacement, hemiarch, total arch) depends on the location and extent of the intimal tear, as well as surgeon and center experience. The goal, at minimum, is to completely resect the intimal tear and replace the ascending aorta. The false lumen is obliterated, and the distal anastomosis is reinforced with strips of felt and pledgeted sutures. Resume cardiopulmonary bypass with central perfusion by switching arterial cannulation to the graft sidearm if using direct aortic or femoral cannulation initially, deair, and clamp the graft.
- Prior to the proximal anastomosis, confirm the root and coronaries are not involved. If the sinotubular junction is involved, reapproximate the dissected layers between internal and external strips of felt ("sandwich technique"). Trim the Dacron tube graft to an

appropriate length and perform the proximal anastomosis. Wean bypass, deair, aggressively correct coagulopathy, and decannulate.

Potential questions/alternative scenarios

"The patient's CT angiography demonstrates a type A aortic dissection with arch vessel involvement. How would you proceed?"

Hemiarch replacement is often sufficient to completely resect the intimal tear, exclude the false lumen, and re-establish arch vessel perfusion. Under circulatory arrest, the resection is extended as a tongue along the concavity of the arch. Tears in the arch can be oversewn. More extensive resection is warranted for arch rupture and large arch aneurysms (> 5.5 cm). Alternatively, total arch repair with frozen elephant trunk can be performed with reimplantation of the arch vessels individually using a trifurcated graft or as a Carrel patch.

"The patient has an unknown connective tissue disorder and CT angiography reveals the aforementioned findings as well as a widened aortic root. TEE demonstrates additional findings of retrograde propagation involving the aortic root and severe aortic regurgitation. How would you proceed?"

Patients with aortic dissection, particularly if under the age of 40 years, should be evaluated for underlying connective tissue disorders, including Marfan syndrome, Loeys-Dietz syndrome, and Turner syndrome (female patients only), as well as non-syndromic connective tissue disorders or annuloaortic ectasia. When connective tissue disorders are known or suspected, replacement of the entire aortic root is indicated. Options include root replacement with a mechanical valved conduit or handsewn pericardial composite root and coronary reimplantation (modified Bentall), or in experienced centers only a modified David procedure. Yacoub-type repairs should be avoided. Future reinterventions are most frequently due to failure to replace the entire root, failure to replace the entire ascending aorta, or aneurysm of the aortic wall at the coronary artery button.

In the absence of a known or suspected connective tissue disorder, if the regurgitation is secondary to commissural detachment and the valve leaflets appear normal, commissural resuspension with pledgeted sutures and closure of the proximal false lumen can be performed. This will often provide adequate repair with a competent aortic valve and allows the sinuses to be preserved.

"The initial CT angiography demonstrates intramural hematoma involving the ascending aorta." Would this change your surgical management?"

The spectrum of acute aortic syndromes includes aortic dissection, intramural hematoma (IMH), and penetrating aortic ulcer. The hallmarks of IMH are the absence of an intimal tear and absence of false lumen flow. While 10% of IMH will resolve, the majority will not and may convert to a classic dissection or the aorta may enlarge and rupture. Generally, IMH in the ascending aorta is considered equivalent to full proximal dissection and should be treated alike. Select patients with aortic diameter (including hematoma) < 5 cm, IMH thickness < 1 cm, and no pericardial effusion may be managed expectantly. Repeat imaging is obtained within 48 hours of presentation to assess for progression.

"Upon opening the aorta, you are surprised to find that this patient has dissection of both coronary ostia. How would you address the coronary dissections?"

Coronary malperfusion in type A dissection may result from obstruction of the coronary ostia by the intimal flap or dissection of the coronary ostia. Compromise of the RCA is more frequent than the left. The surgical approach must ensure adequate myocardial protection reliant upon retrograde cardioplegia and the extent of the coronary dissection dictates the extent of the repair. Local repair techniques include mobilization of coronary buttons and reapproximating the dissected layers, which is reserved for dissection that reaches the coronary ostium without tear of the coronary itself. If the coronary itself is dissected and not amenable to repair, bypass or interposition with saphenous vein is performed.

"The patient demonstrates a decrease in the femoral pressure after initiation of bypass."

333

Distal malperfusion is caused in most cases by false lumen compression on the true lumen. Most likely, either the femoral arterial line is in the false lumen or the arterial cannula is in the false lumen. To clarify the later check the radial pressure reading. If it is normal, then the femoral line is unreliable or a regional malperfusion event has occurred due to a distal re-entry tear. If the radial line is dampened, then stop the pump and switch to arterial cannulation at another site. Due to re-entry tears in the dissection flap and changes in distal flow dynamics it is possible to have malperfusion events during initiation of CPB, cross clamping, or after circulatory arrest.

"The patient complains of severe abdominal pain. CTA demonstrates occlusion of the SMA by the false lumen. How would you proceed?"
Malperfusion in type A dissection results from severe true lumen compression, branch vessel involvement, or both. Prompt recognition of myocardial, cerebral, iliofemoral, renal, mesenteric, innominate or spinal malperfusion is crucial. Distal malperfusion associated with a type A dissection will often resolve by re-establishing flow to the true lumen. If there is a question of the integrity of the bowel, a laparotomy should be performed at the time of dissection repair. Percutaneous fenestration, true lumen stenting, and branch vessel stenting may be indicated. Of note, iliofemoral malperfusion generally requires additional revascularization with axillofemoral or femorofemoral bypass and a low threshold for fasciotomies. After the operation, distal complications can be monitored through clinical examination, CT scan, and duplex as needed.

"The patient is unable to move his left upper and lower extremities. How would you proceed?"
For patients with type A dissection, treatment strategies when a neurologic deficit is noted on presentation present a dilemma. Comatose patients or those with dense neurologic deficits have poor prognosis, but patients with less severe deficits have similar outcomes to patients who present neurologically intact. Paraplegia is not an absolute contraindication to surgery and may reflect a hemispheric infarct or spinal cord malperfusion. Surgical repair of the type A dissection is warranted.

"A 63-year-old male patient undergoes a CT chest for evaluation of a solitary lung nodule. Incidentally a 5.6 cm ascending aortic aneurysm is noticed with signs of chronic dissection. How would you like to proceed?"
Chronic type A dissection is uncommon (4-31%), as most patients do not spontaneously heal acute type A dissections, but when they present in the chronic phase they usually present asymptomatically as an incidental finding. Surgery is indicated for symptomatic patients, large associated aneurysm, eccentric expansion, rapid expansion (> 1 cm per year), or aortic insufficiency. Operative mortality for chronic type A dissection ranges 4-17%, with a 4% risk of stroke. Rate of reoperation if native aortic valve preserved is 20%. Annual imaging follow-up with CT or MRI is recommended.

Operative steps are like acute type A dissection; however, the rate of native aortic valve preservation is less due to the chronicity of the disease. The distal false lumen is intentionally not obliterated, as many distal vascular beds may dependent on false lumen flow. A staged elephant trunk procedure is required in rare instances when the chronic type A dissection with aneurysm dilation extends from the ascending aorta through the arch and into the descending thoracic aorta.

Long-term management
- After type A dissection surgical repair, most patients on follow-up reveal distal false lumen perfusion. This places patients at risk for aneurysmal dilatation and potential rupture. Therefore, blood pressure control (< 120 mmHg) is critical to prevent late death from rupture and chronic dissection.
- CT or MR imaging of the aorta, plus TTE, prior to discharge and at 1, 3, 6- and 12-months post dissection is recommended, with annual imaging thereafter if stable.

- The majority (60-70%) of patients are free from reoperation at 10 years, however routine echocardiographic monitoring of the aortic valve and diagnostic imaging of the aortic diameter are still warranted. The rate of reintervention may be much higher in young patients and patients with connective tissue disorders: 70 - 90% at 10 years.

Pearls/pitfalls
- High index of suspicion
- Diagnosis with CT angiography
- Be comfortable describing alternative cannulation
- Open distal anastomosis under circulatory arrest
- Hemiarch most common repair (full arch rarely needed)
- Resuspend commissures, if possible, to preserve the native valve
- Replace the root if known connective tissue disorder
- Permissive hypotension preoperatively with strict dp/dt control pre/post-op
- Monitor for malperfusion

Suggested readings
- Hiratzka LF, et al. 2010 CCF/ AHA/ AATS/ ACR/ ASA/ SCA/ SCAI/ SIR/ STS/ SVM Guidelines for the Diagnosis and Management of Patients With Thoracic Aortic Disease. Circulation. 2010;121:e266-e369.
- Hussain ST and Svensson LG. Acute Type A Dissection Repair. In: Stanger OH, et al. (Eds). Surgical Management of Aortic Pathology: Current Fundamentals for the Clinical Management of Aortic Disease. 2019:837-83.
- Desai ND and Bavaria JE. Chapter 58: Aortic Dissection. In: Kaiser LR, Kron IL, Spray TL (Eds). Mastery of Cardiothoracic Surgery, 3rd ed. Philadelphia, PA: Lippincott Williams & Wilkins, 2014: 563-74.

54. Type B aortic dissection

Katherine B. Harrington, MD, and Michael P. Fischbein, MD, PhD

Concept

- Presentation and classification of aortic dissections
- Initial treatment
- Medical versus surgical therapy
- Operative steps for repair

Chief complaint

"A 56 year-old man presents to the ED with sharp, tearing back pain. CT scan shows an aortic dissection extending from just distal to the left subclavian artery to the aortic bifurcation."

Differential

The diagnosis, aortic dissection, is already known. The dissection must be classified into Type A vs. Type B, acute vs. chronic, and complicated vs. uncomplicated. Dissections are considered "acute" in the first 14 days after development of symptoms. After 14 days dissections are considered "chronic" as patients typically stabilize after this time and are managed under a different algorithm.

There are several anatomic classification schemes for describing aortic dissections. The Stanford system considers all dissections which involve the ascending aorta, i.e., the aorta proximal to the right innominate artery, to be Type A, and those which involve only the descending aorta, i.e., everything distal to the left subclavian, to be Type B dissections. The Debakey classification classifies dissections into three groups. Type I and II include the ascending aorta. In Type I it propagates at least to the aortic arch and often further distally, while Type II is confined to the ascending aorta. Type III originates in the descending aorta is further broken down into Type IIIa (descending thoracic aorta only) and Type IIIb (extending into abdominal aorta).

"Complicated" dissections are those with persistent pain, thoracoabdominal malperfusion (spinal, visceral, and extremity), impending rupture, or other life-threatening complications. The majority of Type B dissections are "uncomplicated."

History and physical

The most common presenting symptom is abrupt onset, sharp, severe, chest or back pain. Patients tend to be significantly hypertensive when they present. Most patients have a history of long-standing hypertension. Social history should query amphetamine or cocaine use, both risk factors for dissection. A brief skeletal exam should assess for connective tissue disorders, especially in younger patients. A very thorough vascular exam should be documented. Pulse deficits are present in approximately 10% of patients.

Tests

- *Initial CXR*: mediastinal widening or abnormal aortic contour in 56% of patients.
- *Laboratory*: serum creatinine, liver function tests, and lactate (evaluate for renal or visceral malperfusion).
- *Diagnostic procedures*: computed tomographic angiographic scanning (CTA), transesophageal echocardiography, and magnetic resonance angiography. Study interpretation should include dissection classification, extent, primary intimal tear (PIT) location, and presence/absence organ malperfusion. Further information can also be acquired for possible endovascular stent graft insertion including the dimensions of descending aorta, size of true and false lumen, arch branch vessel anatomy, potential landing zones, and femoral/iliac dimensions for access.

"Upon further questioning the patient's pain started this morning. He continues to have severe pain even after his blood pressure is brought to appropriate levels and is requiring a large amount of narcotics."

Treatment/management
As soon as acute aortic dissection is suspected, emergency medical therapy should be initiated and continued while the diagnostic procedures are performed. Medical treatment includes reduction of mean, peak, and rate of rise in arterial pressure (dP/dt) with both an intravenous (a) B-Blocker (esmolol, labetolol) and (b) vasodilator (nipride). Parenteral calcium channel antagonists, like diltiazem or nifedipine, that lower arterial blood pressure and left ventricular dP/dt can also be used.

For Type B dissections medical treatment results in equal if not better results than surgical repair. Current registry studies show medical management carries a 30-day mortality between 9-16% while surgical management yields an operative mortality of 27-32%, biased by the more complicated patients receiving intervention. Comparative retrospective studies which attempted to match risk adjusted cohorts have shown that long-term survival, as well as freedom from late aortic reintervention, is similar for both medically and surgically treated patients.

Currently, a "complication-specific" approach is recommended, reserving surgical or endovascular intervention on the descending aorta for those with complicated dissections. Other conditions that should prompt consideration of early intervention include extensive aortic arch involvement, expectations of poor medical compliance, and underlying connective tissue disorders.

After determining that an intervention is required, the surgeon must decide between an open versus endovascular approach. Endovascular stent grafts should be considered in patients who are older, poor operative risks (renal failure, COPD, poor cardiac function, acidotic from malperfusion), and have favorable anatomy. Younger patients, good surgical candidates, patients with connective tissue diseases, and patients with unfavorable endovascular stent graft anatomy receive a central aortic operation.

Operative steps
Goals – patients with acute Type B aortic dissection is graft replacement of a limited segment of the descending thoracic aorta, hopefully including the site of the PIT, to restore flow to the true lumen and obliterate flow to the false lumen.

- After insertion of a double-lumen endobronchial tube, and often a lumbar intrathecal catheter for cerebrospinal fluid drainage, patients with acute Type B dissections are explored through a left posterolateral thoracotomy through the third or fourth intercostal space, providing access to the transverse arch and proximal descending aorta. Alternatively, a second entry point into the 7th intercostal space may provide access to the distal thoracic aorta.
- Full cardiopulmonary bypass with antegrade perfusion is preferred. Arterial cannulation strategies include the following: perfusion into the arch, left subclavian artery, left common carotid artery, right subclavian artery, left ventricular apex and across the aortic valve, or femoral artery (perfuse true lumen). Venous return can be accomplished with central venous cannulation via the femoral vein or retrograde cannulation through the main pulmonary artery.
- Hypothermic circulatory arrest is utilized to perform an open proximal anastomosis. Most Type B dissection tears originate at the origin of the subclavian artery; clamping between the left common carotid and left subclavian arteries may be utilized, but frequently results in insufficient length for a proximal anastomosis. If left ventricular distension occurs during systemic cooling and subsequent ventricular fibrillation, the

left heart may need to be decompressed with a vent via the left superior pulmonary vein or left ventricular apex. During hypothermic circulatory arrest, myocardial protection is from systemic hypothermia only.

- The phrenic and vagus nerves are identified and dissected free from the transverse arch, with special attention paid to the recurrent laryngeal nerve near the ligamentum and along the posterior proximal aortic neck. The transverse arch, proximal descending thoracic aorta, left subclavian artery, and distal aortic anastomotic site are circumferentially dissected.

- The primary goal is to replace only a short segment of aorta to redirect flow into the true lumen. This strategy allows one to stay above T7 and therefore prevents the need to re-implant intercostal arteries.

- When the goal hypothermic temperature is achieved (18-22° C core temperature), the pump is turned off, and the proximal descending aorta opened. An appropriately sized woven double velour Dacron graft is selected and sewn proximally to undissected aorta with an open technique taking care to excise the entire PIT. If the dissection extends into the arch (retrograde from the PIT), incorporate both the aortic intima and adventitia while performing the anastomosis to obliterate the false lumen. The left subclavian artery may need to be individually reimplanted if the PIT is very close or proximal to the left subclavian artery. Carefully identify the recurrent laryngeal nerve along the proximal aortic neck, especially while transecting the aorta along the posterior wall (common site of nerve injury while performing proximal anatomosis).

- Resume arterial flow to the head and heart slowly (about 500-700 mL/hr) either through the axillary or a perfusion cannula inserted directly into the graft. Replace the cross clamp on the graft after taking care to evacuate any air trapped in the heart or ascending aorta.

- Proximal intercostals arteries (above T7) are oversewn to eliminate steal of blood from the spinal cord.

- The distal anastomosis is also performed with an open technique under circulatory arrest, taking care to incorporate both aortic layers and obliterate the false lumen. Distally, intima and adventitia may occasionally be reapproximated with a Teflon felt media or adventitial bolster. Proximal cross-clamp is released, air is evacuated both proximally and distally prior to tying the sutures, and both anastomoses checked for hemostasis. Systemic rewarming is commenced approximately 10 minutes after reperfusion to allow oxygen debt reversal. After warming to 35-36° C, CPB is discontinued. Transesophageal echo should be used to assure perfusion of the true lumen at the level of the diaphragm.

Potential questions/alternative scenarios

"Post-operatively the patient has a rising lactate and creatinine…"
Visceral malperfusion postoperatively should be monitored with urine output and serial lactates/ABGs. Malperfusion results when a dissection compromises blood flow to end-organs and occurs in approximately 21% of dissections. Two pathophysiological mechanisms of malperfusion are commonly described: dynamic and static branch malperfusion. Dynamic branch compromise is the more common mechanism of malperfusion (80%) and occurs when the true lumen is narrowed or compressed due to the majority of flow occurring in the false lumen- this should be alleviated by open repair. Static branch malperfusion occurs when the dissection flap or intimal tear extends into a branch vessel ostium, leading to mechanical obstruction of flow from the intimal intussusception. This may be treated percutaneously with balloon septal fenestration and uncovered stenting in collaboration with an interventional radiologist.

"The patient wakes up and is not able to move his/her legs."
Paraplegia is a significant risk of any descending thoracic aortic repair (both open and endovascular). Dissection patients have an increased risk, although short segment replacement mitigates this somewhat. Patients with prexisting AAA repair have a higher risk.

Pre-operative lumbar drain placement is commonly done, but not required. If it was not done pre-operatively in this patient, it needs to be placed now. If pre-existing, the amount of drainage should be increased and every effort should be made to get the ICP to less than 10, if not as low as possible. However, caution should be used in draining more than 20 mL per hour due to the risk of subdural hemorrhage. MAP should be increased to > 80-90 mmHg with neosynephrine or vasopressin to increase spinal cord perfusion pressure. Several adjunct strategies, such as a naloxone drip may be used, but no data support its benefit. There is no benefit to high dose steroid treatment.

"A similar patient presents but there is no visible flap, just hematoma within the wall of descending thoracic aorta."
Intramural hematomas (IMH) and penetrating aortic ulcers (PAU) are pathological variants of the classic aortic dissection. Importantly, in contrast to the dissection, neither IMH nor PAU has blood flow down a false lumen. IMH likely results following aortic vasa vasorum rupture, causing hemorrhage into the aortic media. PAU originates from an intimal lesion (ruptured atherosclerotic plaque) that penetrates the aortic media and results in a variable amount of IMH. IMH is treated similarly to a dissection. Emergent anti-impulse therapy should be initiated.

"A patient with a previously uncomplicated Type B dissection several years ago returns with pain and a descending thoracic aorta that has now grown to 7 cm."
All patients with acute Type B dissections should have serial CT scans at 3 months, 6 months, and then yearly to monitor for aneursymal development of the dissection. Surgical intervention for chronic Type B dissections may be considered for both symptomatic patients (pain, mesenteric ischemia) and asymptomatic patients (rapidly expanding or > 6 cm aneurysmal aortic dissections). The techniques utilized are identical to those for an acute Type B dissection, although the extent of resection is usually greater (remove all enlarged aorta) (Refer to descending aneurysm section). Importantly, prior to performing the distal anastomosis, a "tongue" of chronic dissection flap is excised from the aorta- a "flap septectomy," allowing blood flow into both true and false lumens distally (visceral or iliac arteries may originate from either true or false lumens). Surgical resections distal to T-7 may require reimplantation of large intercostal arteries to avoid spinal cord ischemia.

Pearls/pitfalls

- Type B dissections involve the descending aorta. Current management for acute dissections involves aggressive anti-impulse blood pressure therapy with a beta blocker and vasodilator.
- Surgical or endovascular management is generally reserved for "complicated" dissections: those with persistent pain, refractory hypertension, thoracoabdominal malperfusion (spinal, visceral, and extremity), impending rupture, or other life-threatening complications.
- Endovascular stent grafting is reserved for elderly or non-operative candidates. Younger patients or those with connective tissue disorder should receive an open central aortic operation, if indicated.
- The goal of surgical treatment is graft replacement of a *short segment* of the descending thoracic aorta, including the site of the PIT, to restore flow to the true lumen and obliterate flow to the false lumen.
- Circulatory arrest with axillary cannulation is the simplest way to deal with the proximal and distal anastamosis.

Suggested readings

- Hagan PG, Nienaber CA, Isselbacher EM et al. The International Registry of Acute Aortic Dissection (IRAD): new insights into an old disease. *JAMA* 2000 February 16;283(7):897-903.

- Umana JP, Lai DT, Mitchell RS et al. Is medical therapy still the optimal treatment strategy for patients with acute Type B aortic dissections? *J Thorac Cardiovasc Surg* 2002 November;124(5):896-910.

- Suzuki T, Mehta RH, Ince H et al. Clinical profiles and outcomes of acute Type B aortic dissection in the current era: lessons from the International Registry of Aortic Dissection (IRAD). *Circulation* 2003 September 9;108 Suppl 1:II312-II317.

- Ehrlich MP, Dumfarth J, Schoder M et al. Midterm results after endovascular treatment of acute, complicated Type B aortic dissection. *Ann Thorac Surg* 2010 November;90(5): 1444-8.

55. IATROGENIC AORTIC DISSECTION
Vakhtang Tchantchaleishvili, MD, and Peter A. Knight, MD

Concept
- Predisposing risks
- Timely recognition of iatrogenic aortic dissection
- Delayed iatrogenic aortic dissection
- Critical operative steps
- Complications of iatrogenic aortic dissection
- Pearls/pitfalls

Chief complaint
"A 68 year-old man is brought to the OR for a CABG. Shortly after placement of the arterial cannula in the ascending aorta, the perfusionist notes a high line pressure with the test transfusion and a purple colored hematoma begins to form."

Differential
Iatrogenic aortic dissection from cannulation should always remain high on the differential in this scenario because early recognition and therapy can be life saving. Adventitial hematoma is another possibility but would not explain the high line pressure and you are entitled to check a TEE immediately either way. Non-functioning or misplaced aortic cannula is possible but should be a diagnosis of exclusion.

History and physical
Prompt evaluation of cannula site to look for adventitial discoloration. Check systemic blood pressure.

Tests
Immediate transesophageal echocardiography is needed even if you suspect a simple hematoma. TEE can demonstrate an intimal tear in the ascending aorta at the cannulation site with a dissection flap that may extend proximally and or distally

Index scenario (additional information)
"The patient has three-vessel disease for which he is undergoing a CABG. Preoperative CT scan showed a normal aorta with no aneurysm. You just placed an arterial cannula in the ascending aorta. Shortly afterwards there was an increase in arterial line pressure and the purple hematoma has now involved the entire ascending aorta. The patient is hypotensive with MAPs at 50. There are no ST changes and the pericardium appears unchanged. The TEE demonstrates a flap in the ascending aorta. How do you proceed?"

Treatment/management
The patient has an iatrogenic aortic dissection from arterial cannulation. Aortic dissection occurs in 0.01-0.09% of all ascending aortic cannulations. The following factors seem to be associated with iatrogenic aortic dissection: dilated ascending aorta, atherosclerosis, older age and high blood pressure at the time of dissection. In most cases, aortic dissection occurs at the start of the procedure, however it may occur hours or even days after the cardiac procedure. When recognized early, survival ranges 66-85%. When discovered in a delayed fashion the survival drops to 50%. Prompt action is needed to maintain perfusion and limit the dissection. This includes pharmacologic control of hypotension and operative repair of the dissection. Step #1 is to stop perfusing through the cannula and treat hypotension as you normally would with volume and pressors as needed using the central line. Remember that in this scenario you discovered the dissection very early. You have time. You will not tamponade because the pericardium is opened. You are unlikely to rupture. The most likely "serious" thing that could be giving you severe hypotension is myocardial ischemia from a dissected coronary or

potentially acute AI. You need to secure an alternative cannulation site relatively quickly and hopefully you have time to make it the axillary. The femoral is the second option. Finally, you have the ascending aorta with a percutaneous and TEE guided approach to ensure cannulation of the true lumen (learn your cannulas and have a sense of how you would do this). After/during the initial resuscitation, the first option is the best, but you may be forced down an alternative pathway if the patient is crashing despite best medical therapy.

Operative steps

- Remove the cannula and tie down purse string sutures.
- Obtain right axillary access with a graft or alternative access as discussed above.
- Have the anesthesiologist assess the degree of dissection as well as the presence of AI and LV dysfunction. (LV distention is a sign of retrograde dissection and new onset AI.)
- If the dissection was appreciated once you started flowing on CPB then stop flowing, remove the arterial cannula and use the venous line as a volume line as needed.
- Otherwise, obtain venous access; institution specific - single RA cannula versus bicaval depending on your mode of cerebral protection (i.e., antegrade cerebral versus retrograde cerebral).
- Place your retrograde coronary sinus catheter and make space in the AP window for a cross-clamp.
- Begin cooling to 18° C.
- Be prepared to clamp and arrest if the heart distends and fibrillates.
- The benefit of an LV vent for treating distention and fibrillation would be in a situation where you could not physically clamp the aorta as in a porcelain aorta or extremely distended aorta which is rarely the case.
- Do not place a root vent.
- Arrest the heart with retrograde and vent the root by making your aortotomy above the STJ. Antegrade coronary perfusion can be used if needed only if the integrity of the coronaries is not at all in question. If they are and the retro is inadequate, place bicaval snares, open the atrium and place the retrograde direct.
- Refer to standard aortic dissection repair chapter but in short, do your proximal work on the valve as needed (resuspension versus replacement), circ arrest, brain perfusion of choice, hemiarch repair (some might consider an ascending depending on how clearly localized the tear is and how aneurysmal the distal ascending is), deair and resume full flow, perform the proximal and place a root vent.
- Once the graft is constructed, perform your distal anastomoses followed by the proximals off the graft as usual. The one caveat is that if the coronary was dissected then you should suspect that your distal coronary anatomy may have been altered. For instance, if the left main is dissected then make sure you graft the distal LAD and OM, if the right was dissected graft the PDA. Dissected coronaries can be difficult to reimplant and distal perfusion will be uncertain unless an angio is done.

Potential questions/alternative scenarios

"During cooling the heart begins to over distend."

This is not uncommon and reflects valve incompetence. You must prepare for this prior to initiating bypass so be sure to have room to clamp and access to arrest. The easiest venting strategy is an aortotomy but an LV vent is used as safe practice in many institutions. The main benefit of the LV vent is in improving exposure during the proximal valve work (see above).

"Dissection diagnosed at the end of operation by routine transesophageal echocardiography evaluation."

This can occur from removal of the cross clamp under pressure, the proximal anastomosis or an unrecognized tear from the antegrade or proximal cannulation. Re-heparinize, axillary cannulation and follow the steps addressed above.

"In addition to dissection at the cannula site, TEE demonstrates 3+ AI but the leaflets appear intact. The patient had only trivial AI preoperatively. How do you proceed?"
Repair aortic dissection as outlined in the operative steps above. Resuspend the aortic valve as long as the leaflets are clearly preserved, and the anatomy is such that the resuspension will realign you with the center of coaptation. Reevaluate the valve function with the TEE postoperatively. 1-2+ may be acceptable in most situations but be prepared for the possibility of 3-4+.

"You complete a CABG. In the CVICU, shortly after the operation, the patient develops signs of myocardial ischemia and unexplained hemodynamic instability. What is your next step?"
Differential diagnoses include graft dysfunction and thrombosis, reperfusion injury, coronary artery embolus, iatrogenic aortic dissection. Obtain STAT chest X-ray, EKG, and transthoracic echocardiography; if non diagnostic get TEE. If a dissection is present return to the OR for a dissection repair as outlined above.

"Your patient is three years status post CABG. He had a chest CT done for workup of a cough and was found to have an ascending aortic dissection. What is the most likely explanation?"
Chronic dissection that developed as a result of the prior cardiac operation. While this patient is asymptomatic and the aorta is non-aneurysmal, a chronic ascending dissection has the potential to cause valvular incompetence, chest pain, dilation of the aorta or even rupture, all of which are indications for surgery. Careful follow up with echo and CT imaging is needed but surgery is not warranted unless any of the indications are met.

"During a mini-thoracotomy for mitral valve surgery, resistance is noted while threading the wire for antegrade arterial access. You remove the wire and do an angio through the sheath and discover a dissection that appears to extend up towards the infrarenal aorta."
Abort the procedure. Check a TEE to rule out an ascending component. Check a post op CT. Treat the patient medically for a Type B dissection for as long as possible (> 4-6 weeks) prior to returning to the OR and performing the mitral repair with central cannulation.

"You complete a CABG on a patient with an EF of 20% with a balloon pump that was placed preoperatively. In the ICU he loses his RLE pulse. The patient is on minimal inotropic support."
The differential includes embolic disease, localized thrombosis/dissection/mechanical occlusion from the sheath, or a descending aortic dissection from the IABP. Assuming the patient does not need the IABP the best initial therapy is to remove it and follow the vascular exam. Vascular duplex maybe helpful. If ischemia persists, check a CTA of the chest abdomen and pelvis with lower extremity runoff. If a Type B dissection is discovered with persistent evidence of limb ischemia, then go the OR emergently for a Fem-Fem bypass using inflow from the non-dissected limb.

Pearls/pitfalls
- Ascending aortic dilatation, known atherosclerosis, older age, and high blood pressure are risk factors for iatrogenic aortic dissection.
- Mostly common they present at the beginning of the operation, although they may present in a delayed fashion after cardiac surgery.
- Immediately discontinue use of the offending cannula. Let anesthesia resuscitate while you switch to axillary cannulation.
- Know alternative cannulating strategies if needed and know the conduct of a dissection repair as this may come up in several different cardiac surgical scenarios.

343

Suggested readings

- Januzzi JL, Sabatine MS, Eagle KA, et al. Iatrogenic aortic dissection. *Am J Cardiol.* 2002 Mar 1;89(5):623-6.

- Fleck T et al. Intraoperative iatrogenic Type A aortic dissection and perioperative outcome. *Interact Cardiovasc Thorac Surg.* 2006 Feb;5(1):11-4.

56. AORTIC ROOT ANEURYSM

Muhammad Aftab, MD, Ismael de Armas, MD, and Faisal G. Bakaeen, MD, FACS

Concept
- Clinical Presentation of aortic root aneurysms
- Diagnostic modalities
- Indications for surgery and choice of conduit
- Technique of aortic root replacement
- Complications
- Follow up

Chief complaint
"A 44-year-old man is referred to you by his cardiologist for the evaluation of severe aortic regurgitation and enlarged aortic root after presenting with a 1-month history of increasing shortness of breath and cough. How would you proceed with work up and management?"

Differential
Usually patients with aortic root aneurysm are asymptomatic and the condition is diagnosed during the workup of other disease processes or it could cause symptoms such as pulmonary congestion that can masquerade as respiratory in origin. Symptoms such as shortness of breath and chest pain should also raise concern for pneumonia, dissection, aneurysmal disease, pulmonary embolism, or MI.

History and physical
A focused history should attempt to elicit any symptoms relevant to the aneurysm or aortic regurgitation such as chest pain, back pain or shortness of breath. Significant history of bleeding diathesis or significant dental pathology e.g., caries, infection is also important in preparation and planning for surgery. Ask for history/family history of Marfan disease, other connective tissue disorders or aneurysms. Evaluate for the risk factors of aneurysm formation and progression such as hypertension, atherosclerosis, and smoking. Physical examination of patient with un-ruptured aortic root aneurysms is often unremarkable. Nonetheless, check lungs for evidence of pulmonary edema, listen for murmurs and evaluate distal pulses. One may discover findings such as a water-hammer pulse with wide pulse pressure and low diastolic pressure and a decrescendo diastolic murmur. AAA is present in 10-20% of patients with atherosclerotic ascending aortic aneurysm. Patients with Marfan syndrome have characteristic features including thin, tall stature, lax joints, ectopia lentis and high arched palate. Also evaluate for the phenotypic features of Loeys-Dietz syndrome such as blue sclera, hypotelorism, bifid uvula, malar flattening, retrognathia, translucent skin with visible veins and arachnodactyly.

Tests
- *CXR*: prominent right mediastinal border. Aortic valve and aortic root calcifications (lateral projection).
- *EKG*. Usually there will be no EKG abnormality specific to aortic root aneurysm. However, left ventricular volume overload from aortic regurgitation is supported by increased QRS complex voltage (best seen in the chest leads) and prominent septal depolarization reflected by Q waves in leads V4 to V6.
- *Echocardiogram*. TEE is the imaging modality of choice. Accurate visualization of aortic root and ascending aorta is imperative. It is also important to determine if the aortic valve is bileaflet, since this may influence when to surgically intervene. Carefully evaluate valve anatomy to determine whether the valve repair is feasible. For

aortic root measurements, the widest diameter, typically at the mid-sinus level should be used.

- *Computed tomography angiography (CTA).* Most common imaging to study the aorta. Ability to image the entire aorta including lumen, wall, branch vessels, arch, periaortic regions and distal aorta with 3-dimensional data. EKG gated imaging helps to eliminate motion artifact at the aortic root and helps assess coronary arteries, aortic valve morphology and function. While the widest diameter is typically at the mid sinus level, measurements should be taken at all four levels including annulus, sinotubular junction, mid sinus and ascending aorta. Limitation includes risk of contrast-induced nephropathy.

- *Magnetic resonance imaging (MRI).* A valuable imaging modality for diagnosis of thoracic aortic diseases in stable patients with sensitivities and specificities comparable to CT and TEE. A preferred imaging modality for patients requiring repeat imaging for the follow-up of aortic pathology without exposing them to radiation and iodinated contrast agents.

- *Cardiac catheterization.* Considerations should be given to perform cardiac catheterization to rule out presence of coronary artery disease in patients greater than 40. Make sure to define the ostial anatomy and look for anomalies such as a left from the right, right from left, or separate circumflex and LAD orifices.

Index scenario (additional information)

"He is a 6-foot-tall, thin gentleman with a significant smoking history and worsening dyspnea on exertion. He is noted to have a holo diastolic murmur radiating towards the apex. His CXR revealed a prominent right mediastinal border. On echocardiogram he is noticed to have gross aortic root dilatation, a trileaflet non-stenotic aortic valve with severe aortic valve regurgitation, mild mitral regurgitation and moderately dilated LV. His aortic root diameter is 7.2 cm (mid sinus) on CT scan and tapers down to normal size at the mid ascending."

Treatment/management

Criteria for surgical intervention of an ascending aortic aneurysm includes:

- Sporadic (5.5 to 6.0 cm)
- Connective tissue disorder (4.5 to 5.0 cm)
- Bicuspid aortic valve (5.0 to 5.5 cm)

The surgical procedure to be performed on an aortic root aneurysm will be dictated by the status of the aortic valve and the condition of the patient. If the aortic valve is structurally normal a valve sparing procedure is becoming a popular treatment choice at experienced centers. When choosing the valved conduit consideration should be given to the patients' age, life expectancy, underlying disease condition, comorbidities, lifestyle, preference, risk of bleeding from anticoagulation, risk of possible reoperation and finally surgeons experience. Aortic root replacement using a graft and mechanical valve (composite or separate) is recommended for younger patients (age < 60 years) with no contraindication to anticoagulation or patients of any age requiring anticoagulation for other indication such as pulmonary thromboembolism, atrial fibrillation or mechanical valve in other valvular position. Advantages include long term durability and relatively ease of implantation compared to other root replacement options. Complications are related to thromboembolic events and anticoagulation.

When tissue valve is desired during aortic root replacement, a stented bovine or porcine bioprosthetic valve is hand sewn to a tube graft to make a composite biological valve graft conduit. Bioprosthetic grafts are recommended in patients older than 65 years of age with the benefit of freedom from anticoagulation as well as better durability in elderly patients. Bioprosthetic valved graft conduit may also be used in patients of any age with medical or personal contraindication to anticoagulation.

For the David procedure (valve sparing root replacement) the aortic valve is preserved by reimplanting it inside the Dacron tube graft. This is possible in almost 30% of patients requiring aortic root replacement. This is ideal in patients with root dilatation, AI and structurally normal valves.

The stentless composite porcine aortic root grafts such as Freestyle (Medtronic, Inc., Minneapolis, MN), Prima plus (Edwards Life Sciences, Irvine, CA) and Toronto Root (St. Jude, Minneapolis, MN) are alternate options for biological root replacement. The most commonly used graft is Freestyle porcine root. This option is recommended in patients older than 65 years with no risk factor for thromboembolic conditions, thus offering them freedom from anticoagulation. Benefits over the tissue valve may include enhanced durability, superior hemodynamics, and less patient prosthesis mismatch. Homografts may be considered for endocarditis and a Ross is an option for very young patients < 40-year-old who do not want anticoagulation.

Operative steps
Aortic root replacement
- Wide prep and drape in case the femoral vessels and or right axillary artery are necessary for cannulation. Median sternotomy and pericardial dissection carefully palpate the aorta for calcifications. The distal ascending aorta at the location free of disease is the preferred access for arterial cannulation. Other option is the axillary or femoral artery. In general, a dual stage atriocaval cannula through the right atrial appendage is the preferred method for venous drainage, unless the aortic aneurysm is large enough to preclude the access of the right atrium for cannula placement. In this case the right femoral vein becomes an option for venous cannulation.

- A large aortic aneurysm abutting the sternum, redo aneurysm or evidence of contained rupture are situations where one may consider being on pump through the axillary and femoral vein prior to the sternotomy. A surgeon should be prepared to go on emergent cardiopulmonary bypass by femoral arterial and venous cannulation in a patient who becomes hemodynamically unstable (due to rupture or tamponade).

- Prior to initiating CPB, have the necessary exposure and access for retrograde cardioplegia and cross clamping since a patient with severe AI may very well fibrillate with CPB. Initiate CPB with moderate hypothermia, +/- LV vent through right superior pulmonary vein (RSPV). Cardioplegia is delivered in an antegrade fashion into aortic root if there is no aortic regurgitation or directly into each coronary ostium as well as retrograde cardioplegia into the coronary sinus.

- Ascending aorta is transected 3 to 4 cm above the sinotubular junction. Aortic valve is inspected for possible preservation otherwise leaflets are excised, and annulus is debrided if necessary.

- Orientation of right and left coronary arteries and their height above the annulus is noted for coronary reimplantation. The coronary arteries are dissected free from the root with few millimeters of aortic wall as coronaries buttons and are adequately but carefully mobilized to allow for tension free implantation into the root graft.

Mechanical composite valve graft (CVG) conduit
- After excising the aortic leaflets and debridement of aortic annulus, mechanical valve sizers are used to choose appropriate CVG. The valve and conduit can also be sewn as separate entities if desired. Pledgeted horizontal mattress non-absorbable sutures are used to implant the valved conduit with the rigid sewing cuff in an intra-annular position. These sutures are placed across the annulus from the aorta to LVOT and then across the sewing ring of CVG. CVG is seated and sutures are tied. Coronary arteries are then reimplanted. A round opening is made in the tube graft using an ophthalmic cautery device. Coronary artery buttons are sutured to the opening with continuous 5-0 prolene sutures starting with the left and finishing with the right coronary implantation

347

without tension or kinking. If the aortic tissue is friable a ring of felt may be used to reinforce the anastomosis.

Bioprosthetic composite stented valved graft (CVG) conduit

- Bioprosthetic valve sizers are used to select the valve required. Usually a tube graft of size 3 to 5 mm larger than the valve is chosen. The hand sewn composite valve graft conduit is then sewn to the annulus using the same technique as described for mechanical CVG conduit implantation.

Valve sparing aortic root replacement

- Aorta is transected just beyond the aneurysmal dilatation. Aortic root is first dissected circumferentially down to the lowest point of aortic annulus. All three aortic sinuses of valsalva are excised, leaving a 5 mm aortic wall rim around the valve leaflets. Multiple interrupted horizontal mattress 2-0 Ticron sutures are placed from inside to outside the LVOT just below the aortic valve. Sutures are placed in a single horizontal plane along the fibrous portion of LVOT and below the nadir of the valve leaflets and commissural structures. Care should be taken to avoid injury to the conduction system in the membranous septum and the number of sutures in this area could be minimized because this is not the haemostatic suture line. A Dacron tube graft with diameter equal to double the average leaflet height is selected. This is typically 26-28 mm for women and 28-30 mm for men. Previously placed sutures through LVOT are passed through the graft and tied on outside of the graft. Sutures are spaced symmetrically along the muscular interventricular septum and correspondingly closer on the Dacron graft in the fibrous portion of LVOT thus correcting the annular dilatation. Fibrous portion of LOVT is the location where dilatation occurs in patients with connective tissue syndromes. The Dacron graft is trimmed 2-3 cm above the commissures, which are then pulled vertically and suspended to the graft using 4-0 pledgeted mattress prolene sutures. Now the valve, which sits entirely inside the graft, is re-implanted to the graft using 4-0 prolene sutures in running fashion along the residual sinus tissue. Coronary buttons are then reimplanted to their respective sinuses. Aortic cusps are inspected for coaptation and any leaflet prolapse is corrected if necessary. Neoaortic sinuses are created by plicating 2-3 mm of graft material in each sinus at the level of commissure by placing figure of eight 5-0 prolene suture. Alternatively, a commercially available graft with the sinuses of valsalva can also be used. Intraoperative aortic valve competence can be evaluated by clamping the distal end of graft and injecting cardioplegia under pressure. Absence of ventricular distension suggests no more than trace aortic insufficiency. Distal anastomosis is then performed to distal ascending aorta.

Stentless aortic root xenograft

- The implantation technique of aortic root xenograft is similar to that described for CVG replacement with few technical considerations. After excising the aortic valve leaflets the size of aortic annulus is measured. The bioprosthesis selected may be of the same size or 2 mm larger than aortic annulus. The coronary anatomy of porcine aortic root differs from the human root as the coronary ostia of porcine root are relatively closer to each other (90-110° apart) compared to humans (120-140° apart). To place the prosthesis in an anatomical position relative to the coronaries it is usually rotated 120° such that the porcine non-coronary sinus will be used for reimplantation of either right or left coronary artery. It is also very critical to attach the left coronary artery perfectly to its corresponding sinus, avoiding any kinking which may result into postoperative coronary insufficiency. The inflow suture cuff of the bioprosthesis is attached to the aortic valve annulus using either continuous or interrupted horizontal mattress sutures. The suture line can be further reinforced with either Teflon felt or strip of autologous pericardium.
- After completion of aortic root replacement using your procedure of choice systemic rewarming is started. The heart is deaired with TEE guidance and a warm shot of

348

cardioplegia is typically given before removing the cross clamp. That final shot of cardioplegia can help detect significant bleeding along suture lines and test for valve competence. The cross clamp is removed, an aortic vent is placed. Temporary pacing wires are placed, and the LV vent could be removed if there is no ventricular distension and the cardiac contractility is resumed. Lung ventilation is started.

Potential questions/alternative scenarios

"You just finished replacing the aortic root and while deairing, you notice > 1 mm ST elevation in the inferior leads (II, III, and AVF). How would you manage that?"

Postoperative coronary insufficiency is the most dreaded complication. Although it is not a common complication after aortic root replacement, it is often caused by the kinking and changes in the orientation of the proximal RCA. This can be prevented by careful sizing with the heart engorged, meticulous technique of coronary implantation and ensuring that coronary ostia are properly aligned. It is suspected in the situation of difficulty in coming off cardiopulmonary bypass, new regional wall motion abnormality, arrhythmias, new EKG changes and unexplained right ventricular failure in the presence of non-obstructed coronaries. This can also be caused by inadequate myocardial protection, coronary air embolism, and protamine or transfusion related reaction. An early decision to bypass the involved artery with the saphenous vein graft is crucial.

"You complete a valve sparing root replacement and discover 3+ AI."

If this occurs you must be prepared to go back on CPB, arrest the heart, resect the valve and replace with a mechanical or bioprosthetic valve.

"When coming off CPB you notice persistent blood coming from behind the proximal anastomosis."

This can be a serious condition that is difficult to fix. One should anticipate that the etiology is bleeding from the root. The other possibility is bleeding from the LCA suture line. Manipulating the graft and placing sutures posteriorly in a blinded fashion is not advisable. The most prudent course of action is to pack the root with sponges or mild topical agents and wait. Do not give protamine until you have reasonable hemostasis. Eventually remove the packing and check. If it is persistent and the source is not clear, then go back on CPB and address. One may even have to re-arrest to adequately achieve hemostasis and potentially replace the root. An alternative in a patient who will not withstand a second cross clamp at that point in time is to pack, give heparin and, if needed, leave the chest open with a planned second look after reversing all coagulation factors. If you need to replace the root, you might consider a homograft or xenograft which may offer better hemostasis for friable tissues.

"How do you follow these patients?"

Blood pressure control and anticoagulation management requires a close postoperative follow up. Scheduling of post-operative CT or MRI is required to assess the growth of non-resected aorta and to evaluate for possible aneurysm formation. CT scan or MRI of the aorta is reasonable at 1, 3, 6, and 12 months and, if stable, annually thereafter so that any threatening enlargement can be detected in a timely fashion.

"How would you manage this patient if he is asymptomatic and aortic root diameter is 3.5 cm?"

There is no medical therapy which will treat the underlying condition resulting into aortic root dilatation or aneurysm. Guidelines for the medical treatment of patients with aortic aneurysms include strict control of hypertension, optimization of lipid profile, smoking cessation, and risk factor modifications for the atherosclerosis.

"What are the Genetic syndromes and familial conditions associated with aortic root aneurysms and how do they affect treatment and management?"

The genetic syndromes associated with aortic root aneurysms are Marfan syndrome, Loeys-Dietz Syndrome, Ehlers-Danlos Syndrome and familial thoracic aortic aneurysm and dissection syndrome (FTAAD). Bicuspid aortic valve patients are also known to have associated aneurysmal disease. Patients with these conditions should undergo elective operation at smaller diameters (4.0 to 5.0 cm depending on the condition) to avoid acute dissection or rupture.

- *Marfan syndrome* – Symptomatic aneurysm, asymptomatic with of diameter > 5.0 cm, Asymptomatic with diameter < 5.0 cm with family history of aortic dissection at < 5.0 cm, rapidly expanding > 0.5 cm/year, Aortic diameter > 4.0 cm in Marfan women desiring pregnancy (Class IIA, Level of evidence C).

- *Loeys-Dietz syndrome* - Aortic diameter ≥ 4.2 cm by transesophageal echocardiogram (internal diameter) or 4.4 to 4.6 cm or greater by computed tomographic imaging and/or magnetic resonance imaging (external diameter), Class IIA, *Level of Evidence: C.*

- *Bicuspid Aortic Valve* - Symptomatic aneurysm, Asymptomatic aneurysm with diameter > 5.0 cm or diameter > 4.5 cm in patients undergoing aortic valve repair or replacement (Class I, level of evidence C).

"You are doing a redo aortic root replacement and you find it very difficult to dissect the tissue around the aortic root especially posteriorly. What are its implications and your options?"
This implies that mobilization of coronary arteries will be difficult or even dangerous. One option is the Cabrol technique which involves coronary reimplantation by placement of 8-10 mm interposition tube graft to each coronary ostium and then side to side anastomosis to the main aortic graft. Alternate option includes the direct implantation of right coronary button, which is usually easier to mobilize, and reimplantation of left coronary artery using an interposition graft between left coronary ostium and aortic graft (Hemi-Cabrol).

Pearls/pitfalls

- Criteria for surgical intervention includes: sporadic (5.5 to 6.0 cm), connective tissue disorder (4.5 to 5.0 cm), bicuspid aortic valve (5.0 to 5.5 cm).

- When presented with an aortic root aneurysm decide whether it needs to be resected or not.

- Decide what type of root replacement technique is ideal and which one you are the most comfortable describing.

- Make sure the preoperative workup is complete including risk assessment distal aortic imaging and cardiac catheterization.

- Recognize potential complications and solutions of root replacement.

Suggested readings

- Yuh DD, Vricella LA, Baumgartner VA (eds). *The Johns Hopkins Manual of Cardiothoracic Surgery.* 1st ed. New York, NY: McGraw Hill; 2007:585-606.

- Khonsari S, Sintek CF. *Cardiac Surgery: Safeguards and Pitfalls in Operative Technique.* 4th ed.Philadelphia, PA: Lippincott Williams & Wilkins; 2008.

- Franco KL and Thorani VH (eds). *Cardiothoracic Surgery Review.* 1st ed. Philadelphia, PA: Lippincott Williams & Wilkins;2012:315-327.

- Hiratzka LF, Bakris GL, Beckman JA, et al. 2010. ACCF/AHA/AATS/ACR/ASA/SCA/SCAI/SIR/STS/SVM Guidelines for the Diagnosis and Management of Patients with Thoracic Aortic Disease. *J Am Coll Cardiol.* 2010;55:e27-e129.

- Bonow RO, Carabello BA, Chatterjee K, et al. ACC/AHA 2006 Guidelines for the Management of Patients with Valvular Heart Disease: a Report of the American College of Cardiology/American Heart Association Task Force on Practice Guidelines (writing committee to revise the 1998 Guidelines for the Management of Patients With Valvular Heart Disease). *Circulation.* 2006;114:e84-231.

57. Ascending Aortic Aneurysm

Leora Yarboro, MD, and John A. Kern, MD

Chief complaint
"A 58-year-old man presents to clinic for evaluation of incidentally noted ascending aortic aneurysm (5.8 cm) and aortic stenosis."

Differential
In this case there is little else in the differential. However, it is important to personally review the films to confirm the measurements of the aorta as well as the extent of involvement (i.e., root–transverse arch). Obtain any previous studies to determine rate of growth. Rule out chronic dissection.

History and physical
Many patients with ascending aortic aneurysms are asymptomatic. However, in your history be sure to ask about any chest pain, dyspnea, embolic events and ask about commonly associated conditions including: atherosclerosis, bicuspid aortic valve, family history, connective tissue disorders (Marfan's syndrome, Loeys-Dietz, Ehlers-Danlos) and inflammatory conditions. Perform complete cardiovascular, pulmonary, and neurologic exams.

Pathophysiology
Aortic aneurysms can arise in the setting of connective tissue disorders, bicuspid valve disease or in an otherwise normal tri-leaflet valve (degenerative). The natural history of aortic aneurysms is to continue to dilate over time due to forces imposed in accordance with the Law of Laplace Tension = Pressure x Radius. Although some aneurysms stay remarkably stable over time. Risk of rupture and dissection are directly related to the diameter of the aneurysm with significant increase in mortality for ascending aneurysms > 6 cm.

Connective tissue disorders
Recommendations are covered under the chapter on Aortic Root Aneurysms but here are a few additional details:

Patients with connective tissue disorders typically present at a younger age and have higher risk of rupture at smaller diameters. Most centers recommend surgical intervention for ascending aortic aneurysm associated with connective tissue disorders at 4.5-5.0 cm.

- *Marfan's syndrome*
  - Autosomal dominant, prevalence 1/5000, mutation in gene on chromosome 15 encodes fibrillin-1. Phenotype is highly variable. Major diagnostic criteria include: positive family history of Marfan's, pectus excavatum and/or arm span - height ratio > 1.05. Mitral insufficiency can also be associated with Marfan's syndrome. Without surgery most

- patients with Marfan's die in their third decade from complications of aortic root aneurysm. There is data to suggest that patients with Marfan's syndrome should be on beta-blockers and angiotensin receptor blockers to reduce the rate of growth of aneurysms.

- *Loeys-Dietz*
  - Mutation in TGF-B receptor. Patients may have hypertelorism, bifid uvula, and arterial tortuosity. Dissection can occur in children. May consider surgery for adults if aortic root > 4.4 cm (by CT) or descending thoracic aorta > 5 cm. For children, consider surgery when aortic root z-score is > 3 or expansion greater than 0.5 cm/yr.

- *Ehlers-Danlos syndrome*
  - Autosomal inherited disorder of connective tissue COL3a1 gene encodes Type III collagen. Present with arterial or visceral rupture. Any surgery in this population carries increased risk—as such no formal guidelines exist for operative intervention.

Degenerative (sporadic) ascending aortic aneurysms

Occur in the setting of tri-leaflet aortic valve in patients without connective tissue disorders. May be associated with family history, hypertension, smoking and/or atherosclerosis. Aneurysms tend to grow at a rate of 0.1 cm/yr. Serial imaging is important in this population either with echo or CT scan. Growth rate > 1 cm/year or diameter > 5.5 cm in a patient with acceptable surgical risk is an indication for surgery.

Infectious/inflammatory aortic aneurysms

Syphilis destroys muscular and elastic fibers of media. Once commonly associated with ascending aneurysms, now less prevalent since improved antibiotic therapy.

Aneurysms associated with aortic dissection

Patients with previous dissection may have continued dilation of the ascending aorta. There is a faster growth rate and associated rate of rupture when compared to degenerative aneurysms.

Tests

- *Contrasted CT scan or MRA*: to evaluate the extent of the aneurysm including the carotids. You should know preoperatively whether a root or arch replacement is necessary. The CT scan should include abdomen and pelvis if femoral cannulation is considered. Carefully evaluate CT or MRA to see if aneurysm is abutting the sternum. This may increase risk of rupture during sternotomy.

- *Echocardiogram*: is also important in preoperative evaluation with special attention to valve disease and overall cardiac function. This study is limited and may be used to follow root aneurysms but should not be the sole study for operative planning for an ascending aneurysm.

- *Cardiac catheterization*: to evaluate coronary vessel disease.

- *Pulmonary function tests (PFTs)*. Aneurysmal disease is more common in smokers with COPD. PFTs are not always essential but may help to determine perioperative risk.

- *Labs*: CBC, CHEM, Coagulations studies, Type and cross.

Index scenario (additional information)

"The patient has no family history of aneurysmal disease. He has no symptoms. His CT shows an isolated mid ascending aneurysm with no effacement of the sinotubular junction. The aneurysm tapers down to 4 cm proximal to the innominate artery. The AV mean gradient is 45 mmHg."

Treatment/management

If the patient meets criteria for intervention, a thorough preoperative assessment is warranted. This patient needs an aortic valve replacement and ascending repair above the sinotubular junction. Imaging and preoperative assessment should proceed as discussed above. The patients systolic blood pressure should be kept between 90 and 110 mmHg.

Operative steps
The procedural steps will vary depending on the extent of the aneurysm and whether the aortic valve needs to be replaced.

Normal aortic valve, no root or arch involvement

- *Perioperative monitors.* PA catheter, cerebral oximetry, Foley catheter with temperature probe, transesophageal echo, and arterial line.
- *Cannulation.* Central cannulation can be used for an isolated ascending aortic aneurysm if there is enough room to cannulate and clamp beyond the dilated portion. This is usually accomplished with a high cannulation in the arch. These purse strings need to be very secure. Consider pledgeted purse strings. An alternative is to axillary cannulate.
- *Cardioprotection.* Antegrade and retrograde cardioplegia lines are placed as well as a left ventricular vent. A left ventricular vent can be omitted if there is no significant aortic insufficiency (be able to describe alternate methods of decompressing the left ventricle in the case of fibrillation). Cool to 34° C.
- *Dissection.* Transect ascending aortic aneurysm at midpoint. Extend proximally leaving enough room to safely do the anastomosis above the coronary ostia. Distally leave a rim of aorta to sew to before the clamp.
- *Graft.* Impregnated Dacron graft and 4-0 prolene suture to perform anastomosis. Felt may be used to reinforce aorta if tissue is felt to be of poor quality or connective tissue disorder. Remember not to leave the graft too long as it may kink when the heart fills. Perform the distal anastomosis first with running 4-O prolene suture. Then you may clamp the graft and check the back side for hemostasis. Then pack and perform the proximal anastomosis in a running fashion. Place root vent in the graft prior to cross clamp removal and turn off vents while performing the distal anastomosis to aid in deairing.
- Postoperatively maintain tight blood pressure control. Discharge on beta-blocker, ARB and statin.

Expected outcomes

- Known complications from aortic surgery include bleeding (2.4-11% requiring reoperation) neurologic injury (1.9-5%). Reports of perioperative mortality range from 1.7%-17.1%.

Potential questions/alternative scenarios
"Not enough room to cannulate and cross clamp distally."
Plan for axillary or femoral cannulation. If still not able to clamp with adequate sewing cuff, then may need circulatory arrest (see arch aneurysm chapter).

"Graft is kinked when heart fills."
It can be easy to overestimate the amount of graft necessary. You can try to plicate the graft along the lesser curve. You may need to cross clamp and arrest the heart in order to remove a portion of the graft and sew graft to graft.

"Aortic dissection occurs with cannulation."
Potential complication of untreated aneurysms and can occur during cannulation of the aneurysm. Be prepared to discuss alternate cannulation strategies, cooling protocols and repair (see dissection chapter).

"Patient has left ventricular distension once commencing bypass."
Significant aortic insufficiency may be present. You should have a sense that this may happen preoperatively. Be prepared to clamp and arrest the heart with retrograde. In the acute setting if you do not yet have an antegrade vent in place, you can decompress the heart by transecting the aorta. You can then deliver direct coronary cardioplegia. You can also decompress the heart via an LV vent if you have one in place. If the valve is not competent it should be replaced.

"Patient has a bicuspid aortic valve with mean gradient of 48 mmHg, shortness of breath and a 4.7 cm ascending aneurysm."
Bicuspid aortic valve disease occurs in 1-2% of the population. Males 4:1. Most have 3 sinuses and 2 cusps (fusion of the right and left cusps). Dominant circumflex circulation with small right coronary. At risk for premature degenerative changes in the media of aortic root and ascending aorta. Consider ascending aorta replacement if performing aortic valve replacement in bicuspid aortic valve and ascending aorta > 4.5 cm.

"The aorta ruptures during the median sternotomy."
For a presumed rupture you need to ensure you have sufficient help available in the room. Place towel clamps to close the sternum. Ask anesthesia to get PRBC in the room. Let perfusion know of impending need for cannulation. Do not try and fix or dissect out the rupture at this time since this will only make the tear worse. For the most part, towel clamps on the sternum can provide reasonable tamponade. Dissect out the femoral artery, give heparin, place your retractor attempt to tamponade the ruptured area if possible, with manual compression while you gain venous access by direct puncture and cannulation of the right atrium. Place a basket sucker in the field for drainage into the CPB reservoir. Start cooling in the event you need circulatory arrest. Once you are stable on bypass try to clamp the aorta above the rupture and arrest the heart. Now continue with your resection and repair. Place your retrograde coronary sinus cannula and LV vent if needed. Note that for aneurysms that are at risk of rupture or closely abutting the sternum it may be best to perform your sternotomy with the heart on bypass through the axillary and groin. If there is a very high chance of entering the vessel you might even cool to 18° C for circulatory arrest if needed prior to sternotomy.

Pearls/pitfalls
- Surgical intervention for ascending aneurysm > 5.5 cm diameter.
- Consider surgery for ascending aneurysm > 5 cm in patients with bicuspid aortic valve or 4.5 cm for connective tissue disorder.
- Aneurysms tend to grow at a rate of 0.1 cm/yr. Growth rate > 0.5 cm/year or diameter > 5.5 cm in a patient with acceptable surgical risk is an indication for surgery.
- Make sure to look for root or arch involvement prior to surgery.

Suggested readings
- Elefteriades JA. Natural history of thoracic aortic aneurysms: indications for surgery, and surgical versus nonsurgical risks. *Ann Thorac Surg.* 2002 Nov;74(5):S1877-80.

354

58. Arch Aneurysms

John F. Lazar, MD, and Peter A. Knight, MD

Concept

- Indications
- Preoperative assessment
- Operative management (Hemiarch/total arch/elephant trunk)
- Circulatory arrest
- Brain protection options
- Chronic dissection

Chief complaint

"A 57-year-old man with known aortic diastolic murmur presents to your clinic after complaining to his PCP that he has increased shortness of breath. After a full work up, including chest CT and an echo he is found to have moderate aortic insufficiency and an ascending aortic aneurysm extending to the proximal arch of 5.5 cm in size."

Differential

Aortic insufficiency with ascending/arch aneurysm, aortic dissection, coronary artery disease.

History and physical

Most patients with aortic aneurysms are asymptomatic and are discovered incidentally. Of those who present with symptoms, 25-75% present with chest pain (usually anterior chest). Acute pain generally implies impending rupture or dissection. Hoarseness of the voice implies stretching or damage to the recurrent laryngeal nerve. Risk factors include smoking, hypertension, atherosclerosis, personal history of chronic aneurysms or previous repair, bicuspid aortic valves, trauma, and genetic disorders such as Marfan and Ehlers-Danlos syndromes. The physical exam is often unremarkable. A diastolic murmur will be heard if dilation of aortic annulus results in AI.

If a thoracic aneurysm is diagnosed, a thorough vascular examination should follow looking for any peripheral vascular disease, carotid disease, and sequelae of distal embolization. It is also important to document a thorough neurologic exam to establish baseline clinical status in the event of changes postoperatively. Abdominal aortic aneurysms are present in 10 to 20% of patients with atherosclerotic involvement of an ascending aortic aneurysm.

Tests

- *EKG*: may be completely normal; if AI is present may have LV enlargement; assess for ischemic coronary changes.
- *CXR*: may be the first test to detect a silent aneurysm. An enlarged ascending aorta produces a convex contour of right superior mediastinum.
- *CTA*: is the test of choice for assessing the aortic aneurysm and provides rapid and precise evaluation of the root, ascending and arch. CT scanning detects areas of calcification, and accurately identifies dissections and mural thrombus. Axial measurements should be taken perpendicular to the line of flow. The entire thoracic and abdominal aorta should be scanned. The main disadvantage of CT scans is the need for contrast solution for optimal resolution, which may be contraindicated in those patients with renal insufficiency or a history of a dye allergy.
- *MRI/MRA*: effective means of assessing the aorta but is more suitable for those who cannot tolerate CTA dye and in a non-urgent setting.
- *ECHO*. TTE is good for evaluating the valves and ascending aorta but gives little information on the arch. Echo can also be used to corroborate aortic dimensions found

by either CTA or MRI/MRA. TEE is done in the operating room and can help rule out Type A dissections.

- *Cardiac catheterization.* Rule out coronary artery disease in patients undergoing aneurysm repair prior to surgery. May be omitted safely in females of age < 35 and males < 40 with no cardiac risk factors.

Index scenario (additional information)
"Patient has no past medical or surgical history. He takes no medications. He used to smoke a pack a day for 20 years but quit 7 years ago. His father died suddenly in his 50's from a ruptured aneurysm but the rest of his family is still alive and well. Other than being overweight and having a 3/6 diastolic murmur in the right parasternal position his physical exam is completely benign. The aneurysm extends into the proximal arch but tapers to normal size by mid-distal arch. The root is not dilated. The echo shows normal function, 3+ AI and a normal root. How would you like to proceed?"

Treatment/management

This patient has symptomatic AI which requires intervention as well as a 5.5 cm uncomplicated ascending/arch aneurysm that requires repair. In general, 5.5 cm is a safe cutoff for interventions on the arch. 5 cm is the threshold for Marfans, Ehlers-Danlos or bicuspid aortic valve, while even lower thresholds may be used for Loeys-Dietz (4.5 cm). Symptomatic aneurysms of any size require surgical intervention. Asymptomatic aneurysms should be addressed at the time of surgery for aortic valve procedures if the size is at least 4.5 cm and the patient is a reasonably good candidate. Finally, a growth rate of > 0.5 cm/yr justifies repair in asymptomatic patients with aneurysms less than 5.5 cm.

Additional preoperative testing

- Patients with poor pulmonary function should have spirometry and room air arterial blood gases.
- Smoking cessation, antibiotic treatment of chronic bronchitis, and chest physiotherapy may prove beneficial in elective situations.
- Severe carotid disease is a risk factor for stroke during aortic operations. Patients > 65 should have duplex imaging of their carotids pre-operatively or any patient with h/o TIA or bruits.
- Abdominal aortic aneurysms occur in 10 to 20% of patients with ascending aortic aneurysms and should be investigated.
- Head CT to ensure an intact Circle of Willis.

Operative steps

There are a few different ways to approach aortic arch aneurysm repairs. The main decision is whether to perform a hemiarch, total arch or elephant trunk. This decision depends almost exclusively on the distal extent of the aneurysm. Usually you can be well prepared for either intervention ahead of time based on the CT scan, but things may get altered in the OR. All of these cases require circulatory arrest. Right axillary cannulation is safe for all of these. Retrograde brain perfusion through the SVC is reasonable for an uncomplicated hemiarch but the more advanced the procedure becomes the more likely that antegrade brain protection will be needed. The operative details that follow all assume axillary artery cannulation with antegrade brain perfusion (see below for details of circulatory arrest).

- LBIV, arterial line in left arm and leg, general endotracheal anesthesia, pulmonary artery catheter, foley.
- temp probe in the bladder, nasopharynx and venous perfusate.
- *Brain monitoring*: EEG, Bispectral index (BIS).
- Check the intraoperative TEE for AI and aortic dimensions.
- Dissect right axillary artery (or right femoral artery for arterial cannulation).

356

- Median sternotomy, pericardial stay sutures, inspect aorta.
- Heparin 400 mg/kg, arterial cannulation, 2 stage venous cannula or bicaval if retrograde brain perfusion, retrograde coronary cannula; once ACT is 480 initiate CPB, +/-LV vent through right superior pulmonary vein.
- Commence cooling while you mobilize the distal ascending aorta and proximal arch and dissect out the great vessels.
- Clamp and arrest with antegrade/retro/direct coronary.
- Once the patient is at 18-20° C and the EEG is silent, give a dose of cardioplegia, position the patient in Trendelenburg and pack the head in ice. +/- pentobarbital and mannitol given.
- CPB is turned off.

Hemiarch

- The aorta is transected longitudinally along the ascending aneurysm and inspected proximally and distally.
- Ascending aorta is transected along the lesser curve to create a cuff extending from the base of the innominate artery on the right to approximately mid arch or 1 cm proximal to the ligamentum arteriosum and the recurrent laryngeal nerve. The further you transect the more difficult the anastomosis becomes.
- Clamp the right innominate and initiate antegrade brain perfusion at 500 mL/min (or 10-15 cc/kg) with a mean pressure of 40-60 mmHg. Check for backflow through the left CCA. If not then place a coronary perfusion catheter up the LCCA and Y it into the antegrade perfusion circuit at a similar flow rate.
- Size the aorta with freestyle sizers to determine the aortic graft diameter required.
- The distal graft is beveled and anastomosed to the aorta with a continuous 3-0 or 4-0 polypropylene suture (a cuff of Teflon felt or strip of pericardium can be used outside the aorta for friable tissue).
- Once the anastomosis is complete, remove the clamp on the right innominate, gradually resume systemic flow while deairing the graft, clamp the graft and check the back wall carefully for hemostasis.
- Begin rewarming at approximately 1° C/5 min until 36° C.
- This completes the hemiarch – the remainder of the procedure is dictated by the proximal pathology.

Total arch

- Indicated when the aneurysm extends into the mid arch. Need to decide if head vessels are aneurysmal and need reconstruction. If not, the head vessels can be fashioned to the graft as an island.
- While cooling dissect out the arch and head vessels (may need an expanding incision into the neck). Prepare the appropriate graft. The limbs to the innominate and head vessels/LSCA are typically 12 and 8 mm respectively. Trifurcated grafts are available, or any combination of bifurcated or single limb grafts can be sewn individually to the respective vessels.
- Once the circulation is arrested, transect the proximal arch vessels and the aorta along the lesser curve up to the level of the distal arch which is often beyond the LSCA. Clamp the LCCA if too much blood return obscures your view. Note that if the LSCA is too deep in the chest for a feasible anastomosis it can be ligated. The distal anastomosis can then be done proximal to the LSCA which can be bypassed at a future date or off pump at the end of the case, prior to protamine.
- Usually a bifurcated graft to the R innominate and the left CCA is sewn first and then clamped to allow antegrade brain flow through both head vessels. If reimplanting the LSCA it is sewn next. Then the distal anastomosis and finally the appropriate graft to

357

graft anastomoses. Trifurcated grafts may decrease the number of anastomoses. Whatever the method, stick to what you know best.

- Note that if the proximal arch vessels can be preserved then you may be able to sew them into the graft collectively as an island.
- Deair, clamp the graft, resume systemic flow and complete your proximal work or proximal anastomosis. A graft extension may be required to avoid kinking if an ascending is being performed as well.

Elephant trunk

- Indicated for distal arch or isthmus involvement.
- Follow the same steps as in the total arch except instead of an end-to-end anastomosis between the distal aorta and distal graft the distal 5-10 cm of the graft needs to be invaginated within the aorta and then sutured into place.
- On completion of the suture line, the graft is everted, and the head vessels are sewn into the graft with a running prolene as an island.
- The graft is de-aired, clamped and hemostasis is assessed. The proximal work is completed.
- The trunk can later be incorporated into the reconstruction of the descending aorta either by open or endovascular techniques.

Circulatory arrest

- At 18° C cerebral metabolism and oxygen consumption are 17 to 40% of normothermia. Measure temperatures at the bladder, nasopharyngeal and venous perfusate. Monitor brain with EEG or BIS. Most investigators report increased mortality and adverse neurologic outcomes after 40 to 65 minutes of circulatory arrest. Most surgeons try to keep the period of arrest at less than 40 minutes if the operation allows. Consider antegrade brain perfusion for procedures lasting > 30 minute.

Brain protection options

- Antegrade brain perfusion: Line pressure is monitored. The head vessels are collectively perfused with cold blood between 10-18° C and at approximate flows of 10-15 mL/kg/min. Perfusion pressures are restricted to 40 to 60 mmHg which can be difficult to monitor unless you have a left radial arterial line. Most go off of either weight-based flows or a flat rate of 500 mL/min.
- Retrograde cerebral perfusion (RCP): During RCP the SVC is snared and perfused at blood pressures not exceeding 25-30 mmHg that is monitored via CVP, temperatures between 8 and 18°C, and flows between 250 and 400 mL/min. In theory RCP has the added benefit of flushing atherosclerotic material and air from the brachiocephalic vessels while keeping the brain cool.

Potential questions/alternative scenarios

"A stable patient with occasional chest pain is referred to you for evaluation of a chronic Type I dissection with a 5.7 cm aneurysm involving the ascending and proximal arch."
This patient has a symptomatic dissection and aneurysmal disease both of which require treatment. The operation proceeds very much like that of a Type A dissection with circulatory arrest and an open distal anastomosis. In this case the aneurysm involves the proximal arch and thus requires a hemiarch configuration as described above. If the aneurysm proceeded more distally, a total arch or even elephant trunk may be necessary. The only technical difference in the setting of dissected head vessels is that these vessels must be anastomosed directly in an end-end fashion to the tube graft limbs rather than an island for a total arch or elephant trunk. Also, the chronic dissection flaps should be fenestrated or resected as far as possible.

358

"On the preoperative imaging you notice an aberrant left vertebral artery on a patient who was being worked up for a total arch replacement due to an isolated arch aneurysm."

On occasion the left vertebral artery (LVA) will exit the arch directly. This requires duplex US evaluation of the right vertebral artery (RVA) to ensure patency and antegrade flow. With a patent normal RVA, the LVA can be temporarily occluded during selective cerebral perfusion and reimplanted during patient rewarming. Three options have been used: 1.) direct reimplantation of the LVA into the left common carotid artery 2.) attachment of a portion of reverse saphenous vein to the vertebral artery 3.) anastomosis to the arch graft or the left subclavian limb of the trifurcated graft. A very small LVA (< 2 mm) with a patent RVA may be ligated.

"You are called to evaluate a patient with a known arch and descending aneurysm who is complaining of excruciating chest pain. Workup for MI is negative and there is no evidence of dissection. However, there is some periaortic density concerning for a contained early rupture."

The issue here is that an elephant trunk would normally be the ideal procedure for this patient, but it does not allow for a distal seal until the completion elephant trunk is performed. This patient needs a complete procedure involving the arch and descending thoracic aorta. A hemi-clamshell incision or "thoracosternotomy" extended into left 4th ICS allows adequate exposure for both the standard cannulation techniques and the distal repair. An elephant trunk-like strategy can still be used with the graft invaginated through the isthmus and anastomosed distally to the descending aorta. The head vessels would be sewn as an island unless they were aneurysmal.

"You are presented with an 86-year-old relatively healthy female with a 6.5 cm ascending aneurysm which tapers to 4.5 cm at the proximal arch. She has no familial genetic syndromes."

Elderly patients do not tolerate circulatory arrest as well as their younger counterparts. They have a higher risk of stroke and heart failure. The 4.5 cm proximal arch does not necessarily have to be addressed in this setting. The arterial cannula can be placed high on the arch with carefully placed pledgeted cannulation sutures and the clamp can be beveled proximal to the cannula and along the lesser curve. Alternatively, the axillary can be cannulated if it proves too hazardous to cannulate high on the arch. An isolated ascending replacement can then be performed without circulatory arrest.

Pearls/pitfalls

- Clarify whether the patient does or does not have an indication for repair of the aneurysm.
- Clarify the location and extent and decide whether it needs a hemiarch, total arch, or elephant trunk.
- Consider whether a hemiclamshell is needed to definitively address the arch and descending in a single setting (usually only in the case of rupture).
- Decide on your cannulation strategy and brain protection strategy.
- Know the sequence of arch anastomosis depending the type of graft you are using. Also know the sequence of de-airing and removal of clamps.

Suggested readings

- Brinster DR, Rizzo RJ, and Bolman RM. Ascending aortic aneurysms. Cohn LH (ed). *Cardiac Surgery in the Adult.* New York: McGraw-Hill Medical. 2008:1223-1250.
- Spielvogel D, Mathur MN, and Griepp RB. Aneurysms of the aortic arch. Cohn LH (ed). *Cardiac Surgery in the Adult.* New York: McGraw-Hill Medical. 2008:1251-1276.

- Caffarelli AD, Van der Starre PJ, and Mitchell RS. Ascending and arch aneurysms of the aorta. Yu DD et al. (eds). *The Johns Hopkins Manual of Cardiothoracic Surgery.* New York: McGraw-Hill Medical Pub. 2007:663-700.

59. DESCENDING AORTIC ANEURYSMS

Patrick Vining, MD and Joel Corvera MD

Adapted from 1st edition chapter written by *David Griffin, MD, and Stephen Bailey, MD*

Concepts

- Pathophysiology/classification (isolated descending vs. thoracoabdominal)
- Indications for repair
- Open versus endovascular approaches
- Considerations for thoracoabdominal aneurysms
- Pitfalls/Pearls

Chief complaint

"A 75-year-old woman with a history of hypertension, Chronic Obstructive Pulmonary Disease (COPD) and Marfan syndrome is referred to you after her primary care physician obtained a CXR during a recent COPD exacerbation finding an enlarged descending aorta. After recovering from her COPD exacerbation, she is referred to you for evaluation and further management if warranted."

Differential

Isolated descending thoracic aortic aneurysm, Extent Type I/III aneurysm, type B Dissection (acute/chronic) with associated aneurysm, thoracic or thoracoabdominal aortic aneurysm, mediastinal mass

History and physical

Approximately 50% of descending aortic aneurysms (DAA) are found incidentally. Most common symptoms attributed to DAA are pain from expansion or erosion into the spine. Pain is described as sharp or stabbing usually between the scapulae. Acute severe pain may signal dissection or rupture. Enlargement may cause compression of the mediastinal structures causing hoarseness (recurrent laryngeal nerve impingement), dyspnea (airway obstruction) or dysphagia (esophageal compression). Occasionally, evidence of distal embolization such as trash foot may be present. Pathophysiology is generally related to degenerative disease of the media or prior Type B dissection. Less commonly, infections or connective tissue disorders (particularly in young patients or those with a family history of Marfan, Ehlers-Danlos or Loeys-Dietz syndromes) may also result in aneurysmal degeneration of the descending aorta.

Always perform a complete history and physical exam focusing on potential symptoms such as pain or evidence of malperfusion, risk factors including hypertension, tobacco abuse, steroid use as well as personal history of aortic dissection or family history of connective tissue disease or aortic problems. Evaluation should also include an ocular exam of the sclera and lens, as well as examination for arachnodactyly or other stigmata of Marfan syndrome, particularly in young patients. A complete baseline neurologic exam should be performed if a patient undergoes surgical intervention and develops postoperative neurological change. It is also important to perform a complete examination of radial and femoral pulses for symmetry. Operative risk should also be documented, with specific focus on high-risk comorbidities, including diabetes, renal disease, pulmonary and cardiac conditions, and vasculopathy).

Tests

The justification for these imaging modalities is discussed in other chapters devoted to aneurysmal disease. Essentially the goal of imaging is to clarify the anatomical features of the aneurysm, determine other cardiovascular problems that may be surgical (i.e. valve incompetence, coronary stenoses) and risk stratification.

- CTA of the chest, abdomen and pelvis with intravenous contrast
- Labs including hemogram, chemistries and coagulation studies

361

- Carotid duplex
- EKG/echocardiography/coronary angiography
- PFTs

Index scenario (additional information)

"A careful history and physical reveals no evidence of pain, malperfusion or distal embolization. She is not on oxygen or steroids currently for her COPD. She has not smoked for several years but has a 60-pack year history. Her PFTs show a mild obstructive defect but her DLCO is preserved. She has no symptoms to suggest myocardial ischemia. She is on a low dose ACE inhibitor for her hypertension. You obtained a CTA which demonstrates a 6.5 cm fusiform descending aneurysm. It begins 3 cm distal to the left subclavian artery (LSCA) and tapers to 4 cm above the aortic hiatus. How would you proceed with managing this patient?"

Treatment/management

Isolated DAAs occur between the takeoff of the LSCA and the aortic hiatus/suprarenal aorta. This differs from a thoracoabdominal aneurysm (TAA) which, by definition, extends to the abdominal aorta near the level of the celiac artery. Management for both entities depends on whether the aneurysm is symptomatic, rapidly enlarging, or meets established size criteria for intervention. Symptomatic aneurysms require urgent or emergent repair by either endovascular or open approach.

AHA/ACC recommendations for aortic disease should guide decision making. For all patients, strict control of blood pressure (<140/90 in patients without diabetes, 130/80 in patients with diabetes or chronic kidney disease), optimization of lipid profile, and smoking cessation are Class I recommendations. A beta blocker with either an ACE inhibitor or ARB can be used for blood pressure optimization, with ARB preferred in Marfan syndrome (Class IIa). Statins should be used with a goal LDL of less than 70 mg/dL in patients with coronary artery disease (Class IIa). In patients with asymptomatic thoracic aneurysms, surgical repair should be considered at a diameter of greater than 5.5 cm or growth of 0.5 cm per year, with a cutoff of 5 cm in patients with Marfan or other connective tissue disease, bicuspid aortic valve, or familial aortic aneurysm and dissection (Class I). In symptomatic patients with suggestion of expanding aneurysm, prompt surgical intervention should be considered. In patients with degenerative thoracoabdominal aneurysms, saccular aneurysms, or postop pseudoaneurysms, an endovascular stent can be considered at 5.5 cm (Class I). If stent options are limited and surgical morbidity is elevated, surgery should be considered at 6 cm (Class I). Additionally, in patients with evidence of end-organ ischemia or significant visceral artery stenosis, additional revascularization should be performed (Class I). In patients with unstable coronary syndrome and significant coronary artery disease revascularization should be performed prior to endovascular or surgical intervention (Class I), but in patients with stable CAD, preoperative revascularization is not well-established (Class IIb).

Elective repair in appropriate candidates should be undertaken following evaluation of cardiopulmonary function and operative risk. In this patient, COPD exacerbations place her at increased risk of respiratory complications and should be discussed with the patient. Either operative or endovascular repairs are reasonable options anatomically. Given her pulmonary disease a stent graft would be ideal. However, given that she has a connective tissue disorder, an open surgical procedure may provide the best long-term outcome and avoid secondary procedures. In general, DAA may be best treated with open repair if the anatomy is not favorable for standard endovascular repair, in the setting of connective tissue disease, and in chronic aortic dissection given that the patient's risk profile for open surgery is reasonable.

Operative steps

Open repair of isolated DAA

- Spinal drainage is placed the day of or prior to surgery. The patient is placed in right lateral decubitus position with the hips flexed back to expose the femoral vessels.

- Double lumen endotracheal intubation is required. Single lung ventilation of the right lung is established to deflate the left lung. Invasive cardiac monitoring including central venous catheters and pulmonary artery catheters are placed.

- Radial and femoral arterial lines are placed. The radial line serves to indicate the pressure generated by the heart's contraction on partial bypass while the femoral line indicates the pressure generated by the pump. The goal is to achieve a similar mean arterial pressure in both lines. If the upper extremity pressure is high, partial bypass flows can be increased to empty the left atrium and increase flow to the lower body. If the upper extremity pressure is low, partial bypass flow is reduced to allow the left side of the heart to fill and increase output to the upper body.

- Left posterolateral thoracotomy through the 4th, 5th, or 6th interspace is made. The exact interspace for entry is determined by the location of the aneurysm. A rib below or above may be partially resected to improve exposure of the aneurysm.

- The inferior pulmonary ligament is divided, and the lung retracted medially.

- *Proximal control.* The distal arch and left subclavian artery are identified and dissected proximally. The vagus, recurrent, and phrenic nerves are identified and preserved. Tacking sutures on the soft tissue can help to reflect the nerves gently out of the operative field. The ductus remnant is divided if needed. In some cases, the vagus nerve may be ligated distally to prevent traction injuries to the recurrent branch, but this strategy is avoided unless necessary.

- *Distal control.* The distal extent of the aneurysm is identified. The descending aorta is dissected free taking care to avoid the thoracic duct and esophagus.

- It is most convenient to cannulate the left inferior pulmonary vein for venous drainage (i.e. circuit inflow) and the descending aorta below the aneurysm for distal arterial perfusion (i.e. outflow). The left atrial appendage and the left femoral artery are also acceptable alternative sites for cannulation. Left heart bypass (LHB) with moderate hypothermia (32° C) is begun after systemic heparinization (150 U/kg Heparin). When compared with simple-cross clamping, various studies have shown that LHB has a lower mortality rate. In conjunction with mild hypothermia, LHB is an effective means of maintaining organ and spinal cord perfusion and myocardial protection.

- *Proximal anastomosis.* Ideally, the cross clamp is placed distal to the takeoff of the left subclavian artery. A second clamp is placed a few centimeters distal to the first. The aorta is opened between the clamps and the proximal anastomosis is fashioned with a running polypropylene suture and a properly sized dacron graft. Teflon reinforcement can be used if needed. A rim of proximal aorta should be carefully separated from the esophagus to avoid esophageal injury. The proximal clamp is moved onto the graft and hemostasis of the suture line is achieved.

- *Intercostal ligation/reimplantation.* The distal descending aorta is then clamped, and the thoracic aneurysm incised longitudinally. Any upper thoracic intercostal branches (above T8) are suture ligated from within the aorta to prevent "steal" from the spinal cord. Intercostal arteries from T8-L1 can be incorporated into the proximal graft as a patch with running polypropylene to improve spinal cord perfusion. The proximal clamp is replaced on the graft distal to the patch to assess hemostasis.

- *Distal anastomosis.* The distal anastomosis is fashioned with a running polypropylene suture, the graft is de-aired, clamps are removed, and hemostasis is ensured. The patient is weaned off bypass, decannulation is conducted, and heparin is reversed.

- *Immediate postoperative care.* The patient's mean blood pressure is maintained above 80 mmHg. If spinal cord ischemia is suspected or the patient is high risk for this complication, the mean arterial pressure should be maintained above 100 mmHg. Coagulopathy should be corrected, and chest drain output closely monitored. Urine output is assessed hourly as a surrogate of end-organ perfusion. Cardiac preload is optimized, and inotropic support can be used to maintain an appropriate cardiac index.

- *Alternative sequence.* An alternative and efficient approach is to clamp the aorta proximal and distal to the aneurysm, with the longitudinal incisional along the

363

aneurysmal aorta. The incision is beveled at the distal end of the aorta proximal to the distal clamp to preserve the intercostal arteries below T8. The distal graft is beveled, and the distal anastomosis closed. The graft is then clamped, allowing reperfusion of the intercostal arteries, hemostasis ensured, and the proximal anastomosis closed.

Other perfusion techniques to repair descending thoracic aortic aneurysm or dissection include using full cardiopulmonary bypass with or without deep hypothermia and circulatory arrest. However, the perfusion technique chosen should be predicated upon the institutional and the surgeon experience.

Potential questions/alternative scenarios
"A 75-year-old woman with a history of COPD, diabetes and malnutrition presents with an isolated asymptomatic descending aortic aneurysm 6.0 cm in diameter. She has no history of dissection or connective tissue disorder."

Endovascular repair

- Appropriate candidates are screened with a CTA to evaluate potential access sites, the tortuosity and calcification of the vascular system, and the relationship of the aneurysm to the arch and visceral vessels. The proximal and distal landing zones, the size(s) of the endovascular device(s), the device-side access vessel, the imaging-side access vessel and the need for branch revascularization needs to be determined *prior* to the start of the procedure. The operative plan is 80% of the procedure. The remaining 20% of the procedure is execution.

- A lumbar drain should be placed if coverage of the descending aorta is greater than 180 mm or the patient has had prior thoracic or abdominal aortic repair.

- Vascular access is obtained either through the common femoral arteries using ultrasound guidance or by an open retroperitoneal approach to the common iliac arteries. The access arteries should be chosen according to inner luminal diameter of the vessel in comparison to the outer diameter of the endovascular device or sheath. Close attention should be made to the tortuosity and calcification of the vessel, prior placement of endovascular devices and other arterial pathology including chronic dissection or aneurysm with thrombus.

- If the external iliac and common femoral arteries are not suitable access vessels, a 10 mm dacron graft may be sewn to the common iliac artery through an open retroperitoneal exposure. A stiff guidewire is advanced in the aortic root, past the proximal landing zone using fluoroscopy (and intravascular ultrasound in the setting of chronic aortic dissection) and deflected off the aortic valve. An angiographic catheter is typically placed from the contralateral femoral artery.

- A commercially available endovascular aortic graft is deployed according to the manufacturer's instructions for use. Most endovascular devices can address a range of aortic sizes from 18 mm to 42 mm. Proximal or distal landing zone smaller than 16 mm or larger than 42 mm are not suitable for endovascular repair.

- A landing zone of at least 20 mm of uninvolved, non-tapered, healthy aorta is needed at the proximal and distal landing zones to reduce the risk of a Type I endoleak.

- The left subclavian artery may be covered in the proximal landing zone (zone 2), however may require revascularization with a left common carotid to left subclavian artery bypass if there is increased risk of spinal cord ischemia or posterior circulation stroke (i.e. dominant left vertebral artery).

- The graft is typically oversized by 10-20% to ensure an adequate seal.

- A completion angiogram is obtained. Endoleaks should be assessed. Typically, type II endoleak from intercostal arteries do not need intervention. Type II endoleak from the left subclavian artery will require embolization and occlusion of the left subclavian artery origin.

- Balloon molding of the device or extension grafts are applied in the presence of a type I endoleak.

"A 68-year-old male with a history of HTN and an MI in the past presents with a 7 cm aneurysm beginning distal to the LSCA and extending to the infrarenal abdominal aorta."

This patient has a Crawford Type II thoracoabdominal aneurysm (I - proximal descending aorta to proximal abdominal, II - proximal descending to infrarenal aorta, III - distal descending, below T6, to infrarenal aorta, IV - distal descending aorta below the diaphragm to the infrarenal aorta, V- distal thoracic to suprarenal aorta). These almost always require surgical intervention as described above with a few modifications:

- *Incision*: posterolateral thoracotomy exposure is obtained extending inferiorly towards the umbilicus. The 5th ICS is entered, the 6th rib can be removed or shingled. The exact incision can be adjusted to the proximal and distal extent of the aneurysm. The retroperitoneum is entered through the abdominal incision and the costal margin is divided. The diaphragm is incised circumferentially leaving a 2 cm cuff along the chest wall, rendering the retroperitoneum and left chest a single cavity. An Omni or Bookwalter retractor stabilizes the exposure. The aorta and involved visceral and intercostal branches are identified and exposed carefully. Proximal and distal control of the aneurysm is established, and preparations are made to initiate bypass.

- LHB is initiated and proximal clamps are placed. The proximal anastomosis and intercostal reimplantation proceeds as described above.

- *Visceral reimplantation*: the distal aortic clamp is moved to the infrarenal aorta and the visceral aorta is opened. Balloon-tipped catheters connected to the arterial line of the bypass circuit can be introduced into the orifices of the visceral arteries to perfuse blood and limit ischemia time. Alternatively, a cold saline preservation solution can be administered to the renal arteries. Typically, the celiac, superior mesenteric and right renal arteries can be sutured as a large Carrell patch to the thoracoabdominal graft. The graft is clamped distal to the new anastomosis and hemostasis is addressed. The left renal artery can be reimplanted as a separate Carrell patch. There are a variety of ways to revascularize the visceral vessels, including the use of branched surgical grafts. The different visceral revascularization techniques employed are usually determined by the aortic pathology, institutional and surgeon experience.

- *Lumbar arteries* are typically oversewn, however may be selectively reimplanted if thought to be important in maintaining spinal cord perfusion avoiding spinal cord ischemia.

- *Distal anastomosis*. the clamp on the infrarenal aorta is placed at the aortic bifurcation and the final anastomosis is performed. Occasionally a bifurcated graft may need to be used to create anastomoses to the bilateral common iliac arteries.

As for DAAs, the TAAA can be repaired using other perfusion techniques as well. Full cardiopulmonary bypass with or without deep hypothermia and circulatory arrest are other well described techniques. Institutional and surgeon experience should dictate the technique used for elective thoracoabdominal aneurysm repair.

"A similar patient with a Type II thoracoabdominal aorta presents with a ruptured aneurysm."

Aggressive upfront resuscitation is required however the systolic blood pressure should be maintained less than 100 mmHg. Placement of spinal drain should not be done preoperatively in the interest of time, though one should be placed postoperatively. The simplest and most versatile perfusion strategy is femoral venous and arterial cannulation
for full cardiopulmonary bypass. All steps are performed as discussed above with an emphasis on gaining immediate proximal and distal control of the ruptured aorta with cross clamps. In this emergent scenario, it is unnecessary to replace the entire aneurysmal aorta if there is reasonably normal appearing and sized distal aorta to sew. The patient can return for a follow up operation later after recovery from emergent intervention. If the rupture is in the abdominal aorta, then it may suffice to start with the abdominal exposure as you would for a

AAA and clamp the supraceliac aorta. If the aorta is too aneurysmal in this area, then extend the exposure to the left chest through the costal margin to obtain proximal control.

"Postoperatively the patient is unable to move his legs."

Differential includes ischemic injury from the clamp period, embolic disease, spinal hematoma, central stroke or increased local spinal cord pressure. If the spinal cord injury is thought to be ischemic, it is important to optimize spinal cord perfusion through collateral pathways. Ensure the spinal drain is working well and maintain the CSF pressure no greater than 10 cm H2O. Improve the systemic MAP to > 100 mmHg, using vasopressor agents with avoidance of hypotensive episodes. Transfuse packed red blood cells to obtain a hemoglobin level of 10 g/dL to increase oxygen delivery. Optimize cardiac output with inotropic agents. Risk of paralysis is significant after 30 minutes of cross clamping during "cut and sew procedures." Using mild hypothermia with LHB and deep hypothermia techniques, the risk of spinal cord ischemia is less. Reimplantation of intercostal arteries from T8 to L1 seems to reduce the risk of paraplegia, including delayed paraplegia. If spinal hematoma/central stroke is suspected, a head CT and/or MRI of the spinal cord should be performed. To rule out embolic disease-causing lower extremity ischemia, assess the distal pulses. If intact, limb ischemia caused by large emboli are unlikely to account for neurological symptoms.

"Postoperatively the patient has a bloody bowel movement."

Differential includes ischemia and reperfusion injury to the bowel after mesenteric vessels reimplantation or failure to reimplant a significantly sized inferior mesenteric artery. A 30-60 min window is a safe time frame for clamping and re-implanting the visceral vessels. Prior to reimplantation, the visceral circulation is supported by LHB and distal aortic perfusion. Embolic disease resulting from showering to the mesenteric vessels may also result in ischemia. If suspected, an emergent general surgery consult must be obtained. Antibiotics should be started, and optimization of cardiac output and oxygen delivery maintained. Colonoscopy and possibly exploratory laparotomy should be performed if transmural necrosis is suspected.

"Postoperatively the patient stops making urine and her creatinine triples."

If the renal vessels are reimplanted or bypassed, a 30-60 min ischemic time under LHB support with mild hypothermia and the use of cold preservation solution is usually well tolerated. Optimization of the patient's cardiac output and systemic blood pressure in the ICU is essential. If the central venous and pulmonary artery pressures are optimized and the patient is still oliguric it may ultimately be necessary to challenge the patient with diuretics and consider renal replacement therapy, if indicated.

"Following a technically successful repair, her left hemidiaphragm is persistently elevated and she remains ventilated on the third postoperative day. What is the suspected problem and work up?"

A left phrenic nerve injury is suspected. Ventilator weaning proceeds as able. Fluoroscopy (Sniff Test) can confirm paradoxical motion of the affected diaphragm. Early enteral nutrition should be initiated. Surgical plication, either via open or thoracoscopic means is considered if patient is unable to wean from the ventilator. A tracheostomy may be considered as well.

"She is extubated on the first postoperative day and is noted to have a hoarse voice."

A recurrent laryngeal nerve injury is suspected. ENT evaluation and direct laryngoscopy is warranted. A trial of conservative measures including vocal exercises, regulated diet, and aspiration precautions should be attempted. If there is no aspiration, there is a chance that this represents paresis rather than paralysis and conservative measures may suffice. Medialization of the paralyzed cord can improve voice quality and is often done after demonstrating no improvement with voice therapy after 6 months.

"You placed a covered stent in the descending aneurysm and partially occluded the origin of the left subclavian artery to obtain fixation. Postoperatively, the ipsilateral hand is cold, and she reports paresthesias."

Unfortunately, there is inadequate collateral circulation to the left subclavian system that was not apparent on preoperative evaluation. The extremity should be revascularized either with a carotid to subclavian bypass or subclavian transposition immediately.

"The patient has high output milky secretion from the left chest tube on POD 2."
Refer to "Chylothorax" chapter under "General Thoracic Surgery."

"Preoperatively the patient is found to have a 6.5 cm aneurysm of the arch extending down to the celiac vessels. The patient notes both chest and abdominal pain that wakes her up from sleep."
This discussion assumes that you need to address both the arch and descending component in the same setting. Indications for this include evidence of contained rupture or severe symptoms in which waiting for a staged repair is not ideal. If a staged repair is reasonable, it is usually the better option. Replacement of the transverse arch and placement of either a surgical elephant trunk graft or frozen elephant trunk endograft through a median sternotomy can be reasonable first stage options, followed by open descending aortic or thoracoabdominal aortic repair after 2-3 months of recovery. A two-staged procedure may decrease the risk of paraplegia.

If you must address the proximal and distal components in a single stage and the aneurysm is unable to be clamped between the LCCA and LSCA, deep hypothermia and circulatory arrest is required. In the standard right lateral decubitus and thoracoabdominal exposure, left femoral venous and arterial cannulation can achieve full cardiopulmonary bypass. Venous cannulation is usually performed with transesophageal echo guidance to ensure that the guidewire is safely placed in the right atrium. A long venous cannula should be positioned in the right atrium or with the distal tip in the superior vena cava. Additional arterial cannulation sites can include the transverse arch or descending aorta. Additional venous cannulations sites can include the left atrium or main pulmonary artery. Left ventricular distension must be avoided during the period of hypothermic fibrillation and an apical left ventricular decompression catheter is needed. An alternative for aneurysms completely contained within the chest is a clamshell incision. This exposure allows standard ascending aortic and right atrial venous cannulation and myocardial protection strategies as well as axillary arterial cannulation.

"The patient has a chronic Type B aortic dissection with a 7 cm Crawford Type I aneurysm."
The repair proceeds similarly to the thoracoabdominal repairs described above with a few exceptions. Care must be taken to preserve distal perfusion and that the arterial cannula is placed in non-dissected femoral artery and perfusion is directed to the true lumen. The proximal anastomosis should be performed to non-dissected aorta, ideally. Often, a cross clamp must be placed between the L CCA and the L SCA in the arch. The distal flap should be fenestrated to ensure perfusion to both true and false lumen. The intercostal arteries are usually patent and may originate from either the true or false lumen. The intercostals in the vicinity of T8 to L1 should be inspected for reimplantation to reduce the risk of spinal cord ischemia. Bypasses to aortic branch vessels should provide flow to both true and false lumens.

Pearls/pitfalls
- Asymptomatic TAA > 6.0 cm should be surgically addressed.
- Thoracic endograft repair is appropriate for patients with isolated thoracic DAAs with 20 mm landing zones proximally and distally. Patients with multiple comorbidities and who cannot tolerate open repair may be best suited for thoracic endograft repair. Patients with connective tissue disorders, either genetically triggered or familial, may be best suited to open repair if the surgical risk is reasonable. Thoracic endografts

should be oversized by no more than 20% and less than 10% for blunt traumatic aortic injury.

- Thoracic and thoracoabdominal repairs require a thoracotomy dictated by the proximal extent of disease. Distal retroperitoneal exposure is needed for abdominal involvement.

- *Alternative cannulation strategies.* In general, LHB is instituted by drainage from the left atrial appendage or left inferior pulmonary vein with descending aortic or femoral artery perfusion. Femoral artery and vein cannulation allow full cardiopulmonary bypass, allows for systemic cooling if needed and is the most expeditious if a rupture is present.

- *Principles of thoracic or thoracoabdominal repairs include*: appropriate proximal and distal aortic exposure, LHB for distal aortic perfusion during proximal aortic reconstruction, separation of the aorta from the esophagus during the proximal aortic anastomosis, ligation/reimplantation of intercostals, sequential distal clamping of the graft after reimplantation and reperfusion of intercostals and visceral arteries.

- In the setting of diffuse aortic enlargement, repair is generally staged with the symptomatic segment addressed first. If the "mega-aorta syndrome" is asymptomatic, the proximal segment typically is addressed first. A surgical elephant trunk or frozen elephant trunk thoracic endograft can facilitate the second stage repair.

Suggested readings

- Descending and Thoracoabdominal Aneurysms. Cohn LH. *Cardiac Surgery in the Adult*, 3rd Edition. 2008.

- Descending Thoracic and Thoracoabdominal Aortic Surgery. *Sabiston and Spencer - Surgery of the Chest 8th Edition*. 2010.

- Coady et al. "Surgical Management of descending thoracic aortic disease: Open and endovascular approaches: A scientific statement from the American Heart Association." *Circulation*. 2010; 121:2780-2804.

60. HYPERTROPHIC OBSTRUCTIVE CARDIOMYOPATHY

Muhammad F. Masood, MD, and Vinay Badhwar, MD

Concept

- Establishing the diagnosis as primary entity or in conjunction with aortic stenosis
- Indications for operation and preoperative planning
- Anatomic landmarks and extent of myomectomy
- Role of surgical treatment of the mitral valve in the setting of left ventricular outflow tract obstruction (LVOTO)

Chief complaint

"A 30-year-old previously healthy man has presented to you with a complaint of 6 months of progressive worsening shortness of breath and left sided chest pain that is exacerbated with exercise and relieved by rest. He usually runs 5 miles twice a week but now can only run 1 mile. His symptoms however are relieved by rest. He states his older brother died suddenly at age 35. Patient is apprehensive about what is going on?"

Differential

Hypertrophic obstructive cardiomyopathy (HOCM), arrhythmogenic right ventricular dysplasia (ARVD), Wolff-Parkinson-White (WPW) syndrome, long QT syndrome, and Brugada syndrome are the most common causes of sudden cardiac death in young healthy/athletic individuals. The progressive nature of this patient's symptoms without syncope is suggestive of HOCM.

History and physical

Focused history to elicit symptoms of angina, dizziness, or dyspnea, which are often exacerbated with exercise. Diuretic or vasodilator therapy, used to treat presumed congestive heart failure, will often exacerbate symptoms. Family history of sudden cardiac death in young first degree relative is important. Focused examination to elicit a systolic ejection murmur and premature ventricular contractions (PVC) is essential. Increased murmur intensity with valsalva and notation of a brisk bisferens pulse can often hint towards HOCM instead of aortic stenosis.

Tests

- *EKG.* Left ventricular strain pattern, large T-waves in precordial leads, frequent PVCs.
- *Echocardiogram*: to evaluate level and degree of left ventricular outflow obstruction (LVOTO), degree of systolic anterior motion of mitral valve (SAM), and determine if cavitary hypertrophy is diffuse as in HOCM or asymmetric and focal as can be associated with aortic stenosis or hypertension.
- *Gradients*: diagnosis defined by peak instantaneous LV outflow tract gradient (not mean gradient).
  - a. Basal (resting) gradient: > 30 mmHg
  - b. Provocative gradients: with stress valsalva or amyl nitrite > 30 mmHg
  - c. Intervention is considered when gradient is > 50 mmHg
- *Septum.* Septal hypertrophy of > 15 mm is helpful in identifying HOCM. Other abnormalities causing ventricular and septal hypertrophy must be ruled out, e.g., HTN, aortic stenosis. Asymmetric septal hypertrophy is noted when the hypertrophy is focused and limited to the outflow tract septum. Wall thickness of > 30 mm in HOCM patients has a strong correlation with sudden cardiac death (SCD).
- *Mitral Valve.* Systolic anterior motion of mitral valve (SAM) – due to the Venturi effect of blood ejecting from LV, resulting in outflow obstruction by the anterior mitral

leaflet which may often be associated with secondary mitral regurgitation. SAM may often involve the body of the anterior leaflet. In some cases, this may be limited to just the subvalvular structures, which may be referred to as chordal SAM.

- *Chamber size and function.* Athletic hearts can have 13-15 mm LV thickness with normal relaxation and chamber dilation. In HOCM, ejection fraction is supra-normal and if LV dilation occurs it often represents advanced heart failure.

- Exercise echo is performed in asymptomatic patients with gradients of < 50 mmHg.

  - *Angiography.* Brockenbrough–Braunwald–Morrow sign occurs following a PVC in HOCM where the LV pressure on the aortic tracing is much greater than prior to the PVC due to more time for LV filling.

  - *Cardiac MRI:* can be adjunctive to echocardiography if available. In many experienced centers it can be the diagnostic and primary tool for following HOCM patients.

Index scenario (additional information)

"This young patient does not have CHF. He does have apical heave and a systolic murmur. EKG demonstrates paroxysmal atrial flutter. Echo reveals peak instantaneous LVOT gradient of 60 mmHg with septal thickness of 27 mm and left ventricular outflow tract obstruction due to SAM. His coronary angiogram was normal. What are his treatment options?"

Treatment/management

This patient meets criteria for treatment. His options are medical, interventional, or surgical. His symptoms of angina and dyspnea are caused by outflow obstruction, subendocardial ischemia and SAM with potential MR. His atrial dysrhythmia is further decreasing his LV filling and cardiac output thus making his symptoms worse. Medical therapy may be used to relieve symptoms. Initial pharmacotherapy is with beta blockers for rate control to optimize LV filling. For patients that cannot tolerate beta blockade, non-dihydropiridine calcium channel blockers such as verapamil may be used. In this case, attempts at medical or electrical cardioversion of atrial fibrillation should be considered to optimize LV filling and relieve symptoms. Disopyramide can be used if symptoms persist. Diuretic use should be very judicious and only in setting of marked volume overload as they could worsen the LVOTO.

"Patient was started on a low dose beta blocker but was not able to tolerate it due to bradycardia. Treatment with disopyramide was started, however, 4 months later he developed dry mouth, blurred vision and constipation."

Although utilization of medications for symptomatic control is often attempted first, adverse side-effects or persistent symptoms would prompt options to mechanically relieve the LVOTO. While surgical myectomy is often considered first line for symptomatic patients who fail medical therapy, other options include alcohol septal ablation, ventricular pacing, or even cardiac transplantation.

Septal myectomy is indicated in symptomatic patients who fail conservative medical therapy. Patients with septal thickness of > 30 mm have an increased risk of SCD and long standing LVOT obstruction leads to heart failure. Excellent 5 and 10-year survival of 96% and 83% has been demonstrated with < 1% peri operative mortality. Care should be taken with the anterior mitral leaflet and degree of SAM as this may influence the degree of myectomy. If MR is present it is often improved with myectomy alone although sometimes you may need to address the valve.

Operative steps
Trans-aortic septal myectomy
Goals – relieve LVOTO, improve hemodynamics and symptoms.

- Establish invasive monitoring. Arterial line, central venous catheter, PA catheter, foley.
- *Intra operative TEE*: re-evaluate septal thickness, gradients, mitral valve pathology to include degree of anterior leaflet involvement (body of leaflet vs. chordal SAM only), degree of MR severity, presence of anterior leaflet calcification or posterior leaflet excess. The concomitant presence of myxomatous mitral disease or excess posterior mitral leaflet tissue may point to the necessity to address the mitral valve or highlight a potential pitfall in isolated septal myomectomy. The intraoperative TEE interpretation will be a key point for planning the operative approach.
- Sternotomy and pericardial marsupialization. Administer heparin. Standard aortic cannulation, but bicaval venous cannulation is recommended. If mitral valve pathology is identified or if after septal myectomy any need arises to address the mitral or septum, it will be easier to address with bicaval cannulation and this will show important foresight in your operative planning.
- Myocardial protection is critical. Antegrade and retrograde recommended (thick ventricle may need both routes for myocardial protection). LV vent through right superior pulmonary vein (RSPV). Myocardial septal temperature probe can be considered.
- A low transverse aortotomy with extension into the non-coronary sinus is performed. Exposure of the aortic valve and sub-aortic septum can be performed with sutures if needed (careful not to damage leaflets), or a Ross retractor in certain cases. Sub-aortic septum may be transiently exposed additionally by a gentle push on the free wall of right ventricle.
- *Extended myectomy*. Using #11 scalpel on long handle, an incision is made below the nadir of right coronary sinus and a parallel incision below the left coronary commissure is made and connected 3 mm below the aortic annulus. The area between the two incisions is cut as a trough, towards the base of the anterior papillary muscle. This incision provides a myectomy length of 7 cm. Extreme care is taken not to allow muscle tissue to drop in the ventricle; one way is to place a traction suture (a pledgetted 4-0 prolene for example) prior to commencing your resection. The landmarks of importance are the anterior leaflet of the mitral valve, the membranous ventricular septum and the aortic leaflets; all of which could be damaged as part of the myomectomy.
- Close aortotomy and re-animate. Ventricular ectopy is common, and one should be prepared for chemical or electrical defibrillation. Wean bypass, fill the heart (restrict venous drainage and stop RSPV vent). Evaluate using TEE: LVOT velocity, gradient, presence/absence of VSD, SAM or MR. If an obstructive concern is raised, come off bypass but remain cannulated and volume load. Repeat myectomy is recommended if the gradient is > 10-15 mmHg. You can challenge the patient intraoperatively with a vasodilator to look for SAM when tachycardic.
- Once successful myomectomy is performed, decannulate and close in the standard fashion.
- Postoperatively avoid tachycardia and keep volume loaded.

Potential questions/alternative scenarios

"Patient is apprehensive about surgical intervention and would like to consider catheter-based therapies."

Ventricular pacing has been used in some patients to activate the septum before the LV free wall in an asynchronous manner to reduce the LV outflow tract gradient. The benefit of pacing remains controversial with perceived benefits being limited.

Alcohol septal ablation involves injecting alcohol into septal perforators of the left anterior descending coronary artery to create what amounts to a controlled myocardial infarction of the outflow tract septum. It has been shown to improve symptoms in experienced hands, but the outcome can be highly variable based on center experience.

371

It is associated with relatively higher incidence of mortality (1.5% as opposed to 1%). Morbidity can be significant: 11% pacemaker rate due to permanent heart block, 1.8% risk of coronary artery dissection, 2.2% rate of ventricular fibrillation, 1.1% risk of stroke, with 6% patients requiring repeat ablation and 2% requiring surgical myectomy. Patients with multiple co-morbidities with high or prohibitive surgical risk may be offered this therapy. In addition, catheter-based septal ablation does not address the potential need for concomitant treatment of mitral valve or coronary pathology and therefore cannot be offered to this group of patients.

"Before incision is made, on table TEE demonstrates presence of mild to moderate mitral regurgitation."
Evaluation of the mitral valve is of paramount importance. The principle mechanism of symptomatic LVOTO is from SAM so it is expected that the mitral valve will be involved and that in many cases MR will exist. Deciding how much of the MR is from SAM and how much may be related to primary mitral pathology is the key question here. Ask about the relationship between the posterior mitral leaflet (PML) and anterior mitral leaflet (AML) in terms of length or excess leaflet tissue or the presence of primary mitral pathology such as ruptured chordae, clear myxomatous degeneration or annular dilation. If you have excess PML height, anticipate the potential need to add an adjunctive PML treatment to decrease PML height. This may require concomitant repair (sliding valvuloplasty) or low-profile mitral replacement based on the comfort of the surgeon and the discussion with the patient preoperatively.

Presuming mild to moderate MR as stated in the question it is likely that there is not major valvular pathology and that the SAM (likely chordal SAM) will likely resolve with therapeutic septal myomectomy. If no significant primary valve pathology exists that predisposes to SAM, over 85% of cases will demonstrate resolution of regurgitation and will not require additional mitral valve interventions.

"Patient post-operative day 2 after septal myectomy is having increasing oxygen requirements. A new harsh holosystolic systolic murmur is heard. PA systolic pressures have increased from 35 to 55 mmHg."
The importance of this question is to ascertain if these findings are due to SAM or a rarer complication of post myectomy, VSD. Evaluate if the patient had received diuretics or vasodilators or if the patient was in atrial fibrillation, all of which could decrease LV preload, recurrence of SAM and MR that could explain the above symptoms. These would be readily treatable with volume loading, restoration of sinus rhythm and medical therapy. However, as the question specifically notes a "new harsh holosystolic murmur" this is likely due to a postoperative VSD. Focused physical exam should demonstrate the above-mentioned murmur, precordial heave and elevated CVP manifested by jugular venous distension. Diagnostic confirmation may be obtained by transthoracic or transesophageal echocardiography or by a PA catheter to document a step-up in oxygen saturation between the proximal and distal ports. Imaging to establish the location and size of the VSD will be imperative to determine treatment and surgical therapy. Once confirming the diagnosis and location, plan return to OR with TEE to re-evaluate VSD, septum, mitral valve and presence or absence of a new wall motion abnormality. Following sternal re-entry and bicaval cannulation, a right atriotomy is then performed and the tricuspid valve exposed. The membranous septum is exposed below the septal leaflet of the triscupid valve. Repair is then performed using autologous pericardium or a GoreTex patch. Avoid primary suture repair in these cases due to tissue friability. It is important to identify that there is not a mid-ventricular defect by preoperative imaging as your operative approach will need to be tailored to assure coverage and repair appropriately.

Pearls/pitfalls

- Septal myectomy in HOCM is the best, most effective and proven approach to change the course of heart failure by relieving obstruction at LVOT.
- *Classic Morrow's technique for myectomy.* Using #11 blade, incision is made below the nadir of right coronary and resection of 3 cm of sub aortic muscle is performed. Extended myectomy is a long 7 cm resection up to the LV apex and often the treatment of choice of true HOCM.
- Vasoconstrictors (i.e., phenylephrine or vasopressin) are used for acute hypotension. Positive inotropy, vasodilators and diuretics should be avoided.
- Mitral valve replacement is no longer commonly performed as the first line surgical therapy of HOCM. Septal myectomy usually corrects the MR and SAM when there is no major concomitant mitral pathology. Mitral valve repair is performed with the goal of reduction of PML height when clear myxomatous degeneration exists or ruptured chordae is revealed. If repair is contemplated, be sure to place a large ring following repair and consider concomitant septal myomectomy. In the setting of severe mitral pathology, a low-profile prosthetic replacement with/without myomectomy is a safe strategy.
- Aggressive treatment of pre or post-operative atrial fibrillation is of key importance.
- Routine septal myectomy for sub-valvular hypertrophy at time of aortic valve replacement for severe aortic stenosis is not yet a universally accepted treatment recommendation. The diagnosis of asymmetric septal hypertrophy is made by preoperative TEE or catheterization to document non-valvular LVOT sub-valvular gradients. The scenario may be one of a diagnosis of aortic stenosis, but normal aortic leaflets are noted. If asymmetric septal hypertrophy is identified in the absence of HOCM, septal myectomy can be performed to improve symptoms of heart failure.
- Genetic testing (GT) is not used for establishing a diagnosis of HOCM, but rather for screening potential family members once a diagnosis is made. It may also be useful in predicting the progression or complications of HOCM.

Suggested readings

- Gersh BJ, et al. 2011 ACCF/AHA guideline for the diagnosis and treatment of hypertrophic cardiomyopathy. A report of the American College of Cardiology Foundation/American Heart Association Task Force on Practice Guidelines. *J Thorac Cardiovasc Surg* 2011;142;e153-e203.
- Brown ML and Schaff HV. Surgical management of obstructive hypertrophic cardiomyopathy: the gold standard. *Expert Review of Cardiovascular Therapy* June 2008 p715-725.
- Di Tommaso L, Stassano P, Mannacio V, et al. Asymmetric septal hypertrophy in patients with severe aortic stenosis: The usefulness of associated septal myectomy. *J Thorac Cardiovasc Surg* 2012 Feb epub p1-5.
- Bonde P, Yuh D. Surgical management of hypertrophic obstructive cardiomyopathy. Yuh D, Vricella LA, and Baumgartner WA (eds). *Johns Hopkins manual of cardiothoracic surgery* 2007.

61. CARDIAC TUMORS

Muhammad F. Masood, MD, and Vinay Badhwar, MD

Concept

- Identification of cardiac tumor as a differential diagnosis
- Knowledge of sub-types of cardiac tumors, their prognosis and treatment
- *Operative strategy*: cannulation, tumor handling and reconstruction of chamber walls

Chief complaint

"You are evaluating a 45-year-old woman who presents with a 3-week history of fatigue and feeling unwell. She reports a syncopal episode 2 weeks ago. Over last week she has experienced progressive worsening shortness of breath (SOB), both during exertion and lying down. She is admitted to the hospital due to SOB and currently is on 4 liters of oxygen via nasal cannula."

Differential

Endocarditis with mitral or multi-valvular involvement, cardiomyopathy with arrhythmias, aortic stenosis, regurgitation or pulmonary pathology. Given presumed new onset and symptoms regardless of position or activity, this would be concerning for an obstructive pathology such as a myxoma.

History and physical

Focused history to elicit risk factors for infective endocarditis (recent dental visit), risk factors for acute cardiomyopathy (recent viral illness, peri-partum state, alcohol abuse, history of coronary artery disease, family history of sudden death or cardiomyopathy), or additional history consistent with myxoma such as prior history of myxoma, fever, cachexia, hemoptysis or new tachycardia. Physical examination for signs of left sided involvement or obstruction include peripheral embolic phenomenon (limb, renal, cerebrovascular, ischemic bowel), pulmonary edema, arrhythmia, systolic murmur, diastolic murmur ("tumor plop"), and conjunctival pallor consistent with anemia. Right sided involvement may manifest with pulmonary emboli or tricuspid obstruction and related signs of jugular venous distension, peripheral edema or ascites. Ask about pulmonary pathology as well including asthma or COPD.

Tests

- *CXR*. Chamber obstruction can be seen either as enlarged cardiac silhouette or increased pulmonary vascular markings or pulmonary edema/effusions.
- *EKG*. Non-specific commonly, however may show bundle branch block, complete heart block or arrhythmias.
- *Lab*: anemia common, elevated CRP and ESR common but non-specific.
- *Echocardiogram*: transthoracic or transesophageal (preferred) echocardiogram is often diagnostic for cardiac tumor, particularly myxoma.
  - *Evaluate*: tumor size, extent, mobility, stalk, degree of obstruction, chamber and wall involvement, and proximity to valvular/electrical intracardiac structures to plan therapy.
- *Cardiac catheterization*. Coronary artery evaluation should be considered if procedural embolization risk is minimal. Beneficial in evaluation of ventricular involvement of malignant tumors (blush) or existence of concomitant coronary disease.
- Cardiac CT or MRI is performed to evaluate tumor burden, wall penetration and relation to extracardiac structures. Also of benefit to ascertain consistency of mass (i.e., solid, lipomatous, hemorrhagic).
- Focused imaging important for peripheral emboli for co-morbid risk stratification based on symptoms (neuro, peripheral vascular, pulmonary, GI).

"This patient does have significant SOB on high supplemental oxygen, and some necrosis of tip of left fingers. CXR shows increased pulmonary markings and enlarged cardiac silhouette of left heart border. EKG is nonspecific. TEE shows EF of 50%, 4 cm, mobile, left atrial septal mass, producing intermittent obstruction to mitral valve orifice. Pulmonary artery pressures are half systemic. All head CT scans are negative. How would you like to manage this clinical process?"

Treatment/management

This patient is demonstrating signs of left atrial enlargement, pulmonary hypertension and obstructive heart failure due to the tumor in the left atrium causing diastolic mitral orifice inflow obstruction. Digital necrosis represents distal embolization. Myxoma is the most common cardiac tumor and presents most commonly with signs and symptoms of cardiac chamber obstruction followed by tumor embolization. Some patients present with prodromal symptoms of fatigue, fever, cachexia, anemia, and malaise. Complete surgical excision including a minimum of 5 mm circumferential atrial septal excision with the stalk is the mainstay of the treatment with associated rare recurrences. Preoperative critical assessment of all cardiac chambers is necessary to rule out presence of additional tumor burden, myocardial wall involvement or extracardiac involvement (TEE, Cardiac MRI if available).

Operative steps

Goals – adequate exposure, minimal cardiac manipulation prior to aortic cross clamp, complete excision of mass along with a minimum of 5 mm cuff of normal tissue and reconstruction of cardiac chamber, often using an atrial septal patch.

- *Invasive monitoring*: arterial line and central venous access. Careful consideration of jugular PA and CV catheters should be done in cases of right sided tumors to prevent tumor embolization.
- Intra operative TEE is essential to re-evaluate tumor size, mobility, extent, cardiac chamber involvement, degree of obstruction and plan excision and conduct of operation.
- Standard midline sternotomy, marsupialization pericardium and heparinize.
- It is important for minimal to no cardiac manipulation until aortic cross-clamp is applied.
- Standard aortic cannulation.
- *Bicaval venous cannulation*. In the case of right sided tumors, cannulate high on SVC and low on IVC. Snare cavae in preparation for complete cardiopulmonary bypass (CPB). Likely avoid pre-clamp retrograde in case right sided involvement or risk of embolization with intracardiac pre-bypass manipulation.
- Vent the left ventricle through aortic root. Do not use right superior pulmonary vein (RSPV) vent especially in case of left sided tumors as it risks tumor embolization.
- Myocardial protection can be achieved utilizing only antegrade cardioplegia as these patients are often young and do not have coronary artery disease or myocardial hypertrophy.
- Systemic cooling is often not necessary for left atrial myxoma excision.
- Commence CPB, cross-clamp and arrest. Mobilize SVC and IVC.
- Options for exposure for a left atrial myxoma are bi-atrial or right atrial approaches.
  - *Right atrial*: snare cavae and make standard right atriotomy and exposure with retraction sutures. You can often detect the stalk penetrance of the left sided myxoma by the visual thickening of the septum. Incise atrial septum lateral to suspected location with an 11 blade then very carefully extend after directly visualizing tumor to assure avoidance or manipulation of the tumor or stalk. Perform wide local excision of atrial septum by a minimum of 5 mm circumferentially around tumor mass and stalk. Remove involved atrial

septum and mass in toto and send to pathology. Aggressively inspect entire left atrium, atrial appendage, mitral valve and even left ventricle for any residual tumor burden, residual tissue or damage to mitral leaflet (that may require repair). Irrigate clean and patch septal defect with patch (Gore-Tex or autologous pericardium).

- Another option for complex tumors is a bi-atrial approach. This can either be done with separate left and right atriotomies to gain exposure or a bi-atrial incision from the RSPV vestibule extended over to right atrium to attain biatrial approach. This approach can be helpful but does carry with it a slight increase risk for postoperative arrhythmias.

- Be wary of tumor fragmentation and utilize outside suction during tumor excision. Following excision, aggressively irrigate and suction the cardiac chamber.

- Following excision check for residual ASD or VSD as appropriate and valvular integrity.

- Avoid primary closure of defect. Close right atrium with 4-0 or 5-0 prolene.

- De-air through root vent, wean CPB. Once off bypass re-evaluation of all cardiac chambers with TEE is important to rule out any ASD or VSD, new mitral or tricuspid insufficiency.

- Heart block is relatively uncommon, but placement of atrial and ventricular wires can prevent post operative complications from transient rhythm abnormalities. Reverse heparin, place drainage tubes and proceed with closure.

Potential questions/alternative scenarios

"Patient arrests on induction of anesthesia."
Loss of vasomotor tone can lead to drop in preload to the left atrium leading to tumor potentially obstructing mitral inflow causing low to no cardiac output, lack of coronary perfusion pressure and shock. ACLS protocols to be followed. Once secure airway is confirmed and presuming that arrest/shock does not reverse after catecholamine administration and CPR while prepping, then perform immediate midline sternotomy, heparinize and place on CPB.

Following sternotomy simultaneous with heparinizing, open pericardium and proceed with rapid cannulation of aorta and right atrium (provided known isolated LA myxoma). If there is foreknowledge of bi-atrial involvement, central aortic and isolated SVC partial or peripheral venous drainage can be initially established. Once CPB and full circulation is established then can change to bi-caval cannulation and proceed as above.

"An atrial septal defect is seen after coming off bypass."
Attempt to determine the size and location of the defect by TEE in order to plan management. Only if tiny leak is noted conservative post-protamine approach may be adequate. However, this is often an iatrogenic error and will likely require surgical correction. Resume bi-caval CPB, open the right atrial incision, and assess defect size, atrial septal wall and tissue integrity. If the sutures have pulled through (particularly if you tried to close it primarily the first time), use a pericardial patch closure. Small defect due to improper suture technique can be closed by reinforcement sutures provided healthy surrounding atrial tissue.

"Tumor is in right atrium causing obstructive symptoms, ascites, and hepatomegaly."
Pre-operative assessment of tumor location and extent is of critical importance. Along with TEE, CT/MRI or even venography may be helpful to evaluate the extent of caval involvement. During operative set up, it is imperative to use TEE to best guide venous cannulation. For extensive caval involvement, the patient may need right internal jugular (IJ) and femoral venous cannulation. Often the tumor and its atrial base can be readily excised via a right atriotomy. Rarely those with SVC or IVC extension may either have to be managed by extending the atriotomy onto the SVC (laterally to avoid the SA node) or onto the intrapericardial IVC facilitated by peripheral venous cannulation or, very rarely, facilitated by

a brief period of hypothermic circulatory arrest to assure full resection. Always assess all chambers, protect the tricuspid valve while excising the tumor, and be careful to avoid the AV node in Triangle of Koch (Boundaries - Tendon of Todaro, Septal leaflet and coronary sinus).

"Tumor is high in SVC and has embolized to PA."

This patient's cannulation and operative conduct strategy is the key point here. Central aortic and peripheral venous cannulation will be best. Femoral venous multi-stage cannula would be most helpful brought up to just before the RA-IVC junction (i.e., biomedicus 21 or 25 F multi-stage venous). Upper drainage will depend on the imaged extent of the SVC involvement. Though right IJ cannulation is often preferred and commonly used for minimally invasive surgery (i.e., percutaneous use of a 15F biomedicus arterial cannula), given the nature of the extent in question, this may need to be in the left IJ or subclavian for venous access to assure avoidance of tumor mass. Preoperative central venous access would likely be best in the contralateral subclavian. High SVC mobilization above the azygous will be important and proximal snaring as appropriate. Clamp, antegrade cardioplegic arrest is achieved. Once on total CPB and snared, if no documented left sided involvement, a small RSPV vent will be helpful. These tumors can often be excised via a right atriotomy with extension laterally on the SVC to avoid the SA node. Be sure to inspect the RV and RV outflow tract from the right atrium to look for tumor. A separate pulmonary arteriotomy can be used to extract the tumor embolus. Rarely, if visualization is difficult or if emboli are diffuse, a brief period of hypothermic arrest may facilitate full removal of tumor burden from the distal PA.

"Ventricular myxoma"

A rarer entity, right or left ventricular involvement is often first related to an intra-atrial myxoma and secondary extension below the AV valve in the ventricular outflow tract. These can be approached via the outflow tract or via the AV valve. For myxoma arising from the base of the papillary muscle or within chordae of the AV valve, the surgical approach will involve repair or replacement of the valve. Full inspection of the ventricular chamber along with the atrial chamber is important but ventriculotomy is often avoided.

"Small pedunculated mobile density attached to the aortic valve is seen during pre-op ECHO for coronary artery bypass graft (CABG). Patient has had no fevers, no history of intravenous drug use and no indwelling venous catheters. Patient has had a normal dental exam."

This small density seen on pre op ECHO is most likely Papillary Fibroelastoma. These are benign tumors that are most commonly incidental findings. Due to their embolic potential, they are excised when diagnosed, particularly during a concomitant cardiac operation. This patient should undergo an on-pump CABG along with transverse aortotomy and primary excision. The fibroelastoma often arises from valvular endocardium at the coaptation zone of the leaflet. Resection is often performed with full leaflet and annular preservation as there is usually a small stalk that can be amputated flush with the leaflet without incurring any leaflet damage. The aortotomy is closed in the standard manner and the proximal anastomoses are performed.

Pearls/pitfalls

- Benign tumors comprise 80% of cases and prognosis is good with surgical excision. They include cardiac myxoma as the most common followed by lipoma then fibroelastoma. Papillary fibroelastoma arise from valvular endocardium and have equal distribution among heart valves. Surgical strategies for complete resection of myxomas are important to mitigate recurrence.
- Malignant tumors comprise up to 20% of cases. They are primarily sarcomas and present often below age 50. They include rhabdomyosarcomas, angiosarcomas, fibrosarcomas, myxosarcoma, and liposarcomas. Long term survival is poor.

377

- Surgical strategies for cardiac tumor require careful thought on cannulation, prevention of intraoperative tumor embolization by avoiding over manipulation prior to cross clamp, operative exposure often involving more than one chamber, surgical excision and tension free repair. Obstruction of cardiac output, chamber extension/embolization, and heart block are common pitfalls that should be thoughtfully prepared for.

Suggested readings

- Centofanti P, Di Rosa E, Deorsola L, et al. Primary cardiac tumors: early and late results of surgical treatment in 91 patients. Ann Thorac Surg 1999;68:1236-1241.
- Bireta C, Popov AF, Schotola H, et al. Carney-complex: multiple resections of recurrent cardiac myxoma. J Cardiothorac Surg 2011;6:12.
- Benign Cardiac Tumors: A Review. Reardon MJ et al. Methodist Debakey Cardiovasc J 2010 Jul-Sept;6:20-6.
- Blackmon SH and Reardon MJ. Cardiac Neoplasms. Lawrence Cohn (ed). Cardiac Surgery in the Adult 2012.

62. OPERATIVE MANAGEMENT OF PULMONARY EMBOLISM
Emily Downs, MD, and Gorav Ailawadi, MD

Concept
- Diagnosis of pulmonary embolism
- Indications for surgical embolectomy
- Surgical technique
- Chronic pulmonary embolus and management

Chief complaint
"You are called to see a 47-year-old woman with a recent diagnosis of localized pancreatic cancer who presented to the emergency department with a 1-week history of progressive fatigue and dyspnea on exertion. She appears short of breath, heart rate is 116 beats/min, blood pressure is 100/66, oxygen saturation is 88% on room air. CT chest with pulmonary arteriography shows a large embolus nearly occluding the right pulmonary artery."

Differential
The diagnosis of pulmonary embolism (PE) is established from the history and high index of suspicion. A PE protocol CT with contrast during the pulmonary phase (CTPA) is diagnostic. Extent of pulmonary and hemodynamic compromise is important in determining management.

History and physical
Key points include contributing factors to thrombosis, determining clinical status and extent of hemodynamic instability. Determine patients risk profile for invasive therapeutic options such as surgery or thrombolytic therapy. Thrombosis risks are summarized by Virchow's triad: venous stasis, endothelial injury, and hypercoagulability. History should evaluate:
- *Venous stasis*: recent immobility due to travel, illness, surgery, prolonged bedrest.
- Endothelial injury from surgery, trauma, venous access procedures.
- Hypercoagulable state associated with malignancy, inherited thrombophilia, use of medications (oral contraception) or history of thrombosis.

Hemodynamic stability is evaluated with close attention to signs of shock and right heart strain. Thrombolysis with tissue plasminogen activator (several formulations available) may be considered but must rule out absolute contraindications. Ask patients about history of stroke, intracranial tumors, or recent trauma or surgery.

Tests
- *EKG*: most common finding is tachycardia; may have T-wave abnormalities, right bundle branch pattern, atrial arrhythmias, S1Q3T3 (S wave in I, Q wave in III, inverted T wave in III—not common but highly specific).
- *Echocardiogram*. Transthoracic study done at bedside can detect signs of PE but cannot image the pulmonary arteries directly: evaluate for right heart strain (dilation, septal flattening), overall function, intra-atrial thrombus. Transesophageal study (TEE) can directly image the pulmonary arteries and atria.
- *Pulmonary angiography*: may be used to further evaluate clot extent and location.
- CTPA is the diagnostic test of choice for pulmonary embolism.

Stratification of early risk of death from PE
- *Low-risk PE*. Embolus identified without presence of shock/hypotension, RV dysfunction, or myocardial injury (positive troponin). Low-molecular weight

heparin, unfractionated heparin infusion, or fondaparinux treatment with transition to long term oral anticoagulation.

- *Intermediate-risk PE.* Embolus present with RV dysfunction and/or myocardial injury, but without shock or hypotension. Options include unfractionated heparin infusion, low-molecular weight heparin or fondaparinux treatment, with transition to long term oral anticoagulation.
- *High-risk PE.* Presence of hemodynamic compromise (shock or hypotension) and RV dysfunction. Heparin infusion with thrombolysis or embolectomy. Risk of imminent death is ~10%, 30-day risk is ~30%.

Regardless of the risk stratification of a pulmonary embolism, it is critical to recognize this condition and initiate anticoagulation promptly. In the case of high-risk embolism, aggressive management and intensive observation is warranted. Survival rate decreases sharply if a patient requires cardiopulmonary resuscitation (CPR). In one study, patients who required CPR demonstrated mortality of 57% compared with 12% in patients who never required CPR.

Index scenario (additional information)
"Heparin infusion is initiated immediately. Echocardiogram is obtained and shows moderate dilation of the right ventricle with floating thrombus in the right atrium. The patient's clinical condition deteriorates shortly after the study is obtained: Blood pressure 78/52, heart rate 132/min, increasing dyspnea with oxygen saturations of 84% on 100% O2 by nonrebreather mask. What are the options for management?"

Treatment/management
Hemodynamic compromise automatically classifies this as a high-risk pulmonary embolism and intervention is indicated. The recommended treatment is heparin infusion plus thrombolysis or embolectomy. Systemic administration of thrombolytic agent reduces the risk of death in patients with acute PE exhibiting signs of shock, but there is a significant risk of bleeding. Absolute contraindications to systemic thrombolysis include:

1. *Stroke.* Any history of hemorrhagic stroke or stroke of unknown origin, ischemic stroke in the past six months.
2. Central nervous system neoplasm.
3. *Past three weeks*: major trauma, surgery, or head injury.

Additionally, approximately 8% of patients who receive thrombolysis fail this treatment and continue to experience hemodynamic instability with persistent clot burden. In hemodynamically compromised patients with absolute contraindications to thrombolysis or a failed attempt at systemic thrombolysis, surgical intervention should be considered. Patients who have already experienced a code event (pulseless electrical activity or other arrhythmia) have higher mortality rates than those who are hemodynamically unstable but have not experienced PEA. This has led some to advocate more aggressive approach to hemodynamically unstable patients with PE, and even consideration of surgical intervention for intermediate-risk patients without hypotension but already with right ventricular dysfunction and significant clot burden if there is a contraindication to early thrombolysis.

Catheter-based embolectomy has been used in place of surgical intervention in unstable patients with contraindication to systemic thrombolysis or failed attempt at systemic thrombolysis. At centers where this technique is available, it may be used as an alternative to open surgical procedure, but some concern remains that catheter-based technique may cause fragmentation of proximal clot and showering to more distal arteries. This approach is highly dependent on the skill of the operator.

Another approach in the case of significant hemodynamic compromise and poor oxygenation is to utilize extracorporeal membrane oxygenation (ECMO) via peripheral cannulation. This provides support while heparin therapy takes place and may be a viable alternative for poor surgical candidates or those whose burden of clot requires more time for resolution. It may be used as a backup for catheter-based embolectomy. ECMO does not fully unload the RV and thus it will help with systemic perfusion, but myocardial injury may persist until the clot burden is relieved.

Surgical embolectomy has been described in the literature with varying success rates, though there is little data comparing this strategy to medical management. A series of 47 patients by Leacche et al describes prompt surgical intervention in patients with large clot burden and contraindications to thrombolysis or failure of medical therapy. Operative mortality was 6% and 1-year survival was 86% for this series.

Operative steps

Goals – remove clot from pulmonary arteries, remove clot in transit in the right atrium, explore smaller segmental arteries to remove more distal clot.

- Large-bore IV access, arterial line, general endotracheal anesthesia, TEE probe in place, foley catheter.
- Evaluate extent of clot with TEE, examine right atrium and ventricle for clot in transit, evaluate for patent foramen ovale (PFO) as clot has been documented extruding through PFO during embolectomy. Some centers also use epicardial echo to locate emboli and determine cannulation sites.
- Median sternotomy, pericardial stay sutures.
- Heparinization, cannulation for cardiopulmonary bypass with attention to locations of emboli visualized on TEE.
- Normothermia if the thrombus is known to be in the main trunk of the PA. If more extensive thrombectomy is anticipated, cool patient depending on plan for circulatory arrest. Cardiac arrest is generally not necessary unless repair of PFO or ASD is needed.
- Longitudinal arteriotomy incision of main pulmonary artery (PA), may extend transversely onto right or left PA, some also perform arteriotomy of the right PA between the ascending aorta and the superior vena cava if preop evaluation indicated presence of clot accessible from this location.
- Removal of clot with suction and gallbladder stone forceps. Intermittent reduction in bypass flow aids visualization of emboli. In some cases, with extensive clot distally in branch pulmonary arteries, circulatory arrest may be required to create a bloodless field. Prepare for this ahead of time.
- Removal of distal clot—methods vary; may use a choledochoscope to visualize distal clot, also reports of opening pleura and using gentle lung massage to evacuate clot (careful as this may cause pulmonary hemorrhage; not all centers advocate entering the pleura for this purpose).
- IVC filter placement within 24 hours of surgery if not placed intraoperatively. Some centers report using right atrial purse-string cannulation site to place the IVC filter after performing the embolectomy.

Table 57-1. Summary of treatment options for high-risk pulmonary embolism.

	Systemic thrombolysis	Catheter-based technique	Surgical embolectomy
Patient candidates	Poor operative candidates; no contraindications to thrombolysisv	Poor operative candidates, proximal clot accessible via catheter, contraindication to systemic thrombolysis	Patients with high-risk emboli, significant proximal clot burden, contraindication to thrombolysis

381

Mortality rate*	7-30%	10-20%	14-27%
Major risks	Bleeding, failure of treatment in 8% with persistent clot burden	Distal showering of clot, damage to vessels from mechanical thrombectomy	Risks associated with bypass, sequelae of distal clot burden

* Mortality rate for acute massive pulmonary embolism with any management strategy is approximately 30% at one month after diagnosis.

Potential questions/alternative scenarios

"Chronic pulmonary embolism and pulmonary hypertension: A 58-year-old man presents to clinic with chief complaint of progressive shortness of breath. Three years ago, he underwent hip surgery complicated by a large pulmonary embolus postoperatively and was treated with thrombolysis. He recovered from this event but over the past several months has had increasing dyspnea. Echocardiogram demonstrates pulmonary artery pressure of 64 mmHg. What are the next diagnostic steps?"

The patient presents with symptoms and echocardiogram findings consistent with chronic thromboembolic pulmonary hypertension (CTEPH). Approximately 1-5% of patients who experience acute pulmonary embolism go on to develop this complication, presenting with vague dyspnea and fatigue after initially recovering from the acute embolic event. Further workup includes pulmonary angiography to assess the location of the vasculopathy causing pulmonary hypertension. Right heart catheterization provides helpful hemodynamic information, but wedge pressures may be difficult to obtain due to irregular contour of pulmonary arteries. Pulmonary function testing should be used to evaluate coexisting obstructive or restrictive lung disease, which if severe would steer away from surgical intervention.

If a patient is evaluated and felt to be a good candidate for surgery for CTEPH, there are some key differences between the surgical procedure for acute massive pulmonary embolus versus CTEPH. For patients with chronic disease, the intervention is a pulmonary artery endarterectomy with removal of thickened scar-like tissue from the vessel intima, in addition to removal of the gross thrombus which characterizes the procedure for acute PE. Pulmonary endarterectomy is performed under hypothermia with intermittent circulatory arrest to facilitate thorough removal of intraluminal fibrinous material and optimally reduce pulmonary hypertension. This procedure has a mortality rate of 4-7% when performed at high-volume centers.

"TEE performed just prior to pulmonary endarterectomy for CTEPH demonstrates moderate to severe tricuspid regurgitation. How should this be addressed?"

Many patients with CTEPH will exhibit some degree of tricuspid regurgitation. In general, once the pulmonary arterial pressure is reduced and the right ventricle is unloaded, the valvular insufficiency resolves. One option is to wean bypass support and evaluate valve function after the embolic burden is relieved, then repair the valve if regurgitation warrants this. Consider repair for severe tricuspid regurge with structural damage to the tricuspid valve or annular dilation (> 40 mm).

"72 hours after pulmonary endarterectomy the patient is noted to have a diffuse opacity in the right middle and lower lobes."

Reperfusion syndrome occurs in 8-10 percent of patients after endarterectomy. Treatment is mainly supportive with ventilation and pressors as needed. Patients should be diuresed and FiO2 should be weaned. Rarely inhaled NO or ECMO are required. The syndrome tends to resolve after 7-10 days.

Pearls/pitfalls

- Diagnosis of PE with hemodynamic instability (shock, signs of RV dysfunction), contraindication to thrombolysis or failure of initial attempt at thrombolysis—consider surgical embolectomy.
- Chronic thromboembolic pulmonary hypertension—thorough endarterectomy can help reduce pulmonary hypertension and symptoms.
- Tricuspid regurgitation with CTEPH—repair usually not needed; regurgitation decreases as right ventricle remodels postoperatively.

Suggested readings

- Leacche M et al. Modern surgical treatment of massive pulmonary embolism: Results in 47 consecutive patients after rapid diagnosis and aggressive surgical approach. *Journal of Thoracic and Cardiovascular Surgery* 2005; 129: 1018-1023.
- Madani MM, Jamieson SW. Pulmonary Endarterectomy for Chronic Thromboembolic Disease. *Operative Techniques in Thoracic and Cardiovascular Surgery.* 2006; 264-274.

63. PERICARDIAL DISEASE/PERICARDIECTOMY

Vakhtang Tchantchaleishvili, MD, and Peter A. Knight, MD

Concept
- Causes of chronic pericardial disease
- Pathophysiology, physical findings and diagnostic workup
- Operative indication
- Critical operative steps
- Alternative scenarios
- Pearls/pitfalls

Chief complaint
"A 67-year-old man who was treated for stage II thymoma, including thymectomy done two years ago by you returns with fatigue, dyspnea on exertion, and peripheral edema."

Differential
Radiation-induced chronic pericarditis, congestive heart failure, restrictive cardiomyopathy, recurrence of malignancy

History and physical
Inquire about duration, progression and severity of symptoms. Inquire about dyspnea at rest or orthopnea. Ask about risk factors for constrictive pericarditis such as history of acute pericarditis, infections, renal failure, lupus, rheumatoid arthritis, radiation, prior MI, trauma or cardiac surgery. On physical examination, look for evidence of decreased atrial filling and elevated RV diastolic pressure - jugular venous distention, hepatomegaly, peripheral edema, ascites, decreased breath sounds (effusions) and pericardial knock (early rapid ventricular filling with elevated pressures during diastole - "S3").

Tests
Purpose of these tests are to confirm the diagnosis of constrictive pericardial disease and differentiate it from restrictive myocardial disease. The later is treated by transplantation and not pericardial stripping. The CT scan/MRI/echo showing pathology of the surrounding pericardium often gives the most valuable information for making this distinction. The physiology of constrictive pericarditis becomes evident on cardiac catheterization, echo or physical exam. The primary problem is decreased atrial and ventricular compliance. This "stiffness" results in higher atrial pressures with rapid filling of the ventricle during diastole. The stiff ventricles give off an audible S3 during diastole. On cardiac catheterization the ventricular pressure readings show a classic square root sign (rise in ventricular pressure at end diastole). During inspiration the preferential inflow to the right heart over the left is met with increased RV stiffness leading to the classic bowing of the RV to the LV seen on echo. This discordance shows up on catheter derived pressure tracings.

- *CXR*: pericardial calcification (40%) or signs of compression.
- *CT scan or MRI*: (90% sensitivity) helpful in visualizing thickened and/or calcified pericardium.
- *EKG*: non-specific ST-T changes.
- *Echo*: constrictive physiology = bowing of the interventricular septum to the left with inspiration, thickened pericardium.
- *Cardiac catheterization pressure readings suggestive of constrictive pericarditis*: square root sign, RV end diastolic pressure greater than ⅓ of the RV systolic pressure, equalization of pressures across the atria during diastole, equalization of pressures across the ventricles during end diastole (except during inspiration).

- *Distinguishing features of restrictive disease*: small or normal size heart, reduced LV function, pulmonary and hepatic congestion, prominent x and y descents on atrial pressure readings. If diagnosis is still in doubt, endomyocardial biopsy or ultimately mini- exploratory thoracotomy with inspection of the pericardium. BNP levels are not elevated with constrictive pericardial disease, but may be significantly increased with restrictive cardiomyopathy.

Index scenario (additional information)

"The patient had radiation in addition to thymectomy. His fatigue and dyspnea on exertion has been going on for several months. Recently he developed peripheral edema. Jugular venous distension is noted. On physical exam, there is systolic retraction and a pericardial knock. CXR demonstrates pericardial calcification. There are nonspecific ST-T changes on EKG. Right and left heart catheterization shows a square root sign, elevated RV end diastolic pressures with equalization of right and left atrial pressures during diastole. How do you proceed?"

Treatment/management

The patient has a radiation-induced chronic constrictive pericarditis. The basis of the disease is formation of pericardial scar from a wide range of pathologic processes (infectious, postoperative, therapeutic radiation), which results in compromised filling of the ventricles and leads to venous congestion and low cardiac output. Surgery is curative for constrictive pericarditis, thus the diagnosis in the setting of symptoms is a general indication for pericardial stripping. As mentioned, it is imperative to differentiate constrictive pericardial disease from restrictive cardiomyopathy which, despite similar clinical presentation, is not an indication for pericardial stripping. Notably in some cases like radiation-induced heart disease, there may be a concurrent presence of both conditions. If only minimally symptomatic from constrictive pericardial disease, patients with serious concomitant disease may forgo surgery. Although surgery improves or alleviates symptoms in vast majority of patients, long term survival is diminished in patients with radiation induced constrictive pericarditis.

Operative steps

Goals – excise the pericardium from phrenic nerve to phrenic nerve anteriorly, diaphragm, AV groove and around the entrance of caval/pulmonary veins posteriorly.

- Median sternotomy is used most commonly, however some surgeons prefer a thoracotomy approach.
- You can begin the dissection on the right, but cardiopulmonary bypass is often needed for resection of the left sided heart structures.
- After developing a plane on the left side of the heart and freeing up the diaphragm it helps to retract the heart towards the right in order to dissect out the left sided pulmonary veins. Release as much as you can posteriorly along the AV groove but be careful not to injure the esophagus. Check for the TEE probe and stay clear of it.
- The lack of surgical plane can lead to significant blood loss, epicardial coronary vessels and major venous structures are at risk of damage during the dissection (refer to chapter on Venous injuries).
- Complete pericardial resection may not always be possible, especially in cases of radiation induced pericardial disease and small islands of pericardium can be left behind especially over the coronaries.

Potential questions/alternative scenarios

"You begin dissecting the right atrium and start getting small tears that you are able to oversew. You've lost nearly 500 mL from the atrial dissection alone and still do not have it well exposed. You experience too much hypotension to perform the left sided dissection safely. What is your cannulation strategy?"

385

Always have your cannulation strategy in mind prior to starting a pericardiectomy. Bypass is not always necessary, and it is hard to predict when it is. In this case, keep manual pressure over the atrial tear while you work on getting aortic access for cannulation. Once the aorta is exposed heparinize, cannulate the aorta and cannulate the atrium through the tear. Once the procedure is complete, switch to bicaval cannulation and repair the tear with a patch if needed. If you cannot expose the aorta and cannot control the tear with manual pressure then heparinize, dissect out the groin and cannulate the femoral vessels. These procedures can be difficult. Have blood available and the groins well marked prior to starting. Having the groin vessels exposed is not an unreasonable approach if you anticipate a particularly hazardous dissection.

"The patient was found to have constrictive pericardial disease. He has some fatigue but minimally decreased exercise tolerance, and no edema. He also has advanced COPD, chronic renal insufficiency, and a history of stroke with residual deficits. How would you proceed?"
Given patient's serious concomitant disease, the operation can be delayed until more significant symptoms develop from his pericardial disease.

"The patient who is status post CABG 6 weeks ago presents to your clinic for postoperative follow-up. He has a significant dyspnea. His exercise tolerance, which initially improved after the surgery, has been worsening again. How do you proceed?"
Perform a physical exam, EKG, chest X-ray, and echo.

"Your workup demonstrated constrictive pericarditis. You take the patient to OR for pericardiectomy, however during the operation you enter one of the bypass grafts. How do you proceed?"
Go on cardiopulmonary bypass, be aware of the territory the graft supplies and its significance. Check the EKG and hemodynamics for changes. Depending on the extent of the injury and hemodynamics you could give partial dose heparin, clamp the graft and do a primary repair. Alternatively, you can do an interposition graft with vein or go on CPB, arrest the heart and do a completely new bypass.

"The patient has a remote history of lymphoma. His workup shows constrictive pericardial disease. You take him to the operating room and find large implants on the pericardium which were not visualized on preoperative imaging. How would you proceed?"
Remove a diagnostic sample of the pericardium and send for frozen pathology.

"Frozen pathology results are concerning for malignancy."
Abort the operation and refer the patient to oncologist.

Pearls/pitfalls

- Early clinical symptoms of constrictive pericarditis include dyspnea, fatigue, decreased exercise tolerance. Late symptoms include peripheral edema, hepatic congestion and ascites. May see "square root sign" on cardiac catheterization.

- Physical examination can reveal jugular venous distention, peripheral edema, and pericardial knock.

- With diagnostic tests, look for for constrictive physiology on echocardiography, thickened and/or calcified pericardium on CT/MRI, equal end-diastolic pressures in heart chambers on cardiac catheterization.

- Pericardial stripping is curative and either completely alleviates or significantly reduces the symptoms.

- Median sternotomy is the most commonly used operative approach, however a thoracotomy can be used as well.

- Cardiopulmonary bypass is not necessary but may be needed. Thus, OR with cardiopulmonary bypass capability is preferred and have cannulation options in mind ahead of time.
- The lack of surgical plane can lead to significant bleeding, epicardial coronary vessels are at risk of damage as are major venous structures (see chapter on Venous injuries).
- Long term survival is diminished in patients with radiation induced constrictive pericarditis.

Suggested readings

- Cho YH, Schaff HV. Surgery for pericardial disease. *Heart Fail Rev*. 2012 Aug 15.
- Napolitano G, Pressacco J, Paquet E. Imaging features of constrictive pericarditis: beyond pericardial thickening. *Can Assoc Radiol J*. 2009 Feb;60(1):40-6.
- Leya FS, Arab D, Joyal D, et al. The efficacy of brain natriuretic peptide levels in differentiating constrictive pericarditis from restrictive cardiomyopathy. *J Am Coll Cardiol*. 2005 Jun 7;45(11):1900-2.

64. ACUTE SHOCK – MECHANICAL CIRCULATORY SUPPORT

Daniel Ryan Ziazadeh, MD, Clauden Louis, MD, Sunil Prasad, MD

Concept
- Short term MCS
    - ○ Cannulation options
    - ○ Patient selection
- Clinical Trials (MOMENTUM & ENDURANCE)
- INTERMACS
- Pitfalls that arise in of the above steps

AMBIOMED BVS 5000
This was the very first FDA device that was approved for use in the management of cardiogenic shock in the early 1990s. It is a pneumatically driven, pulsatile, extracorporeal, asynchronous ventricular assist device capable of providing cardiac outputs of 5 L/min to 6 L/min via univentricular or biventricular support.

Thoratec pVAD

The Thoratec pVAD is a pneumatically driven peripheral ventricular assist device that is designed to provide left, right, or biventricular support for short to medium term recovery

Centrimag
Similar to the pVAD, the Centrimag pump is also made by Thoratec. This short term paracorporeal device is magnetically levitated and can be used to provide left, right, and biventricular short-term support and can be attached to a membrane oxygenator for ECMO. In contrast to early generation short term devices, the Centrimag's non-pulsatile continuous flow design mitigates several side effects that hampered its predecessors including hemolysis, thrombosis, inflammatory activation, and heat.

Tandem Heart

The Tandem Heart is another percutaneous ventricular assist device that can be used for left and right, but not biventricular support. In the LVAD configuration, the Tandem Heart uses a unique left atrial to femoral artery bypass system via a trans-septal cannula from the RA into the LA via the femoral vein.

Chief complaint
"A 56-year-old male presents to the Emergency Department with an anterolateral STEMI and is taken emergently to the Cath Lab for intervention. His hemodynamics decline during the time it takes to get to the Cath Lab. During interventional access he has an episode of ventricular fibrillation which is successfully defibrillated. He remains persistently hypotensive and you are consulted for emergent placement of VA ECMO."

Differential
Cardiogenic shock

History and physical
Any patient requiring mechanical circulatory support needs to have a comprehensive systems-based history and physical to identify history of stroke, renal disease, coronary lesions, respiratory problems, bleeding disorders, or peripheral vascular disease. Often, this cannot be performed prior to initiation of mechanical circulatory support, however it is important to determine their neurological status or last known well.

- Biochemical Profile (CMP, LFTs)
- CBC
- Cardiac Enzymes (Troponin, CK, LDH)
- ABG (Base Deficit)
- Lactate (Serial Arterial)
- BNP
- ECHO (TTE/TEE) to evaluate for Tamponade, Wall Rupture, Septal Defect, Ejection Fraction
- CXR (Interstitial edema, Kerley B lines, cardiomegaly, bilateral effusions)
- Coronary Angiography (Assess coronary vasculature to evaluate need for revascularization)
- EKG (evaluate for STEMI, NSTEMI, life threatening arrhythmia)
- Swan-Ganz catheterization

These tests allow for rapid diagnosis, identification of critical lesions that require immediate intervention, help guide resuscitation, and supportive therapies.

Index scenario (additional information)
"The patient has a normal neurological exam prior to entering the Cath Lab. Norepinephrine is immediately started, but the patient remains with refractory hypotension. Radial access is obtained for catheterization and diagnostic angiography demonstrates critical LM stenosis extending to the proximal LAD/LCX bifurcation. ABG demonstrates an arterial lactate of 6."

Treatment/management
This patient will require initiation of mechanical circulatory support in the setting of cardiogenic shock. While Interventional Cardiology is performing PCI, femoral groin access should be obtained for tandem placement of venous and arterial cannulas and initiation of VA-ECMO. In the event of a cardiac arrest, one team member can perform compressions, while anesthesia manages the airway. Another option in this scenario may include devices such as Impella.

Placing an individual on VA ECMO provides a bridge to definitive intervention. Patients in shock lack the oxygen carrying capacity of the heart to meet the demands of the body. The patient's MAP should be kept at the upper range of normal to ensure adequate perfusion pressure to the end organs (renal, hepatic, and brain). ECMO RPMs should be titrated to allow for full support when initially placed with a goal cardiac index of 2.2 - 2.4 if at possible.

While other support therapies such as IABP may help reduce afterload, increase coronary perfusion pressure and augment blood pressure, they do not deliver direct cardiac output to end organs. The patient in this scenario has likely suffered significant myocardial injury. Emergent revascularization with PCI will be beneficial in the long term to provide the myocardium with more oxygen carrying capacity, but in the short term myocardial stunning, hibernation, or infarction has ensued to the point that the heart is unable to provide sufficient cardiac output.

Contraindications
Relative
- DNR
- Severe neurological event

- Known PVD (distal aortic thrombus and severe aorta-iliac disease are specific to femoral access)

ACLS

- Secure the airway
- Assess for bilateral breath sounds
- Maximize circulation via compression, fluids, inotropes

Cannulation

- Determine access (Femoral, Central, Axillary).
- Use ultrasound guidance if immediately available to avoid access complications.
- For groin access, palpate the femoral artery for a pulse if present.
- Alternatives include groin cut down for direct visualization and arterial cannula purse string sutures to aid in repair at time of ECMO explant.
- If access to instruments are not available, perform a blind stick. Often, a femoral pulse is not present in cardiogenic shock. Make sure to mark appropriate anatomy (inguinal ligament) to avoid a high stick.
- Once intraluminal access is obtained, pass a flexible J-tip guidewire into the artery and vein.
- Access ipsilateral Superficial Femoral Artery via antegrade stick for placement of 6F reperfusion catheter & 15F or larger arterial ECMO cannula.
- Give Heparin
- Sequentially dilate the vessel via Seldinger technique.
- Insert minimum 15F arterial and 25F venous ECMO cannulas and flush with heparinized saline and clamp with tubing clamps.
- Always attempt to use the smallest size catheter for adequate cardiac output for a given BSA.
- Connect ECMO tubing in air-free manner. If saline is unavailable for de-airing, can use blood by carefully loosening tube clamps.
- Y in 6F reperfusion catheter to arterial ECMO cannula. De-air via stopcock.
- Check your lines to ensure no air bubbles. Release tubing clamps and initiate ECMO.
- Alternative venous cannulas include central right atrial, right internal jugular, subclavian vein.

Initiation

- Check your ACT and make sure you are > 250.
- Ensure there is no obstruction in the pump.
- Specify your temperature.

Maintenance

- Check for pulsatility.
- If chugging occurs, add volume.
- Maintain MAPs (usually 65-75 mmHg) – use inotropes or fluids as needed.
- Flow is usually 4.4-4.5 L/min, which is equal about Cardiac Index of 2 in most patients with 15F arterial cannula. Flow increases to 5.8L with a 17F arterial cannula.
- Assess perfusion via arterial blood gas, lactate, venous saturation, urine output.
- Increase or decrease Sweep to modulate pCO_2.
- Cooling to mild hypothermia (32-34°C) may allow a decrease of flow and MAPs when needed.

- Check ECHO - heart should be fairly full, CVP and PAP should be normal or slightly elevated.
- Check sats, ABG, oxygenation, visual inspection of arterial blood - should be bright red and there should be no clots in the circuit).
- Check Doppler signals specifically DP/PT in the ipsilateral limb of the arterial ECMO cannula to evaluate for critical limb ischemia.
- For Axillary/Subclavian cannulation, place pulse oximetry and radial arterial line to assess perfusion to the ipsilateral arm.
- There are a variety of roller or centrifugal ECMO pumps that can be used. We prefer centrifugal (Centrimag, Rotaflow, CardioHelp, and Sarns) pumps as they are non-occlusive, provide passive displacement, and have less hemolysis.

The patient determines the course of VA ECMO. Goal is to maximize the mechanical flow of the machine at full RPMs to wean vasopressors and inotropes as able.

Potential questions/alternative scenarios

"After initiation of VA ECMO, arterial lactate begins to normalize. You obtain an ECHO and notice that the LV appears severely hypokinetic and distended. EF is estimated at ~5%. What do you do?"

The ventricle is not decompressed, and the heart is barely ejecting. Strong consideration should be made for an LV vent. Initial management should include maximizing drainage of the ECMO circuit. Evaluate for any signs of pulmonary edema or severe mitral regurgitation as the heart may not be able to overcome the regurgitant volume from the atrium. Medical optimization via inotropes should be attempted first. A mechanical circulatory vent such as an Impella can be placed across the LVOT and Aortic Valve to decompress the ventricle but be careful and watch out for signs of hemolysis. Alternatively, trans-septal atrial puncture can be performed, by going up the femoral vein into the IVC across the right atrium and into the left atrium to facilitate placement of a TandemHeart Cannula. Passive venting can also be achieved with an 8F suction catheter trans-apically across the aortic valve.

"Four days later, repeat ECHO shows significantly improved LV EF 50% compatible with myocardial recovery. The patient is hemodynamically stable and has developed a pulsatile waveform with MAP >65. What do you do?"

Weaning from ECMO

In general, you need to be warm, have pulsatility, stable rhythm and be ventilating in order to come off ECMO.

- Confirm that myocardial and hemodynamic recovery has occurred as assessed by echocardiography (LV EF >25%, Aortic VTI >10cm, TDSa >6 vm/s)
- Slowly wean speeds to decrease flow 0.5L/30 mins
- Ensure patient is stable on minimal ECMO support (flow 2L/min)
- Evaluate for resolution of metabolic disturbances (afebrile/euvolemic)
- Confirm pulsatile waveform for >24 hours
- Ensure MAPs acceptable (>65mmHg) in absence of pressor/inotrope
- Confirm acceptable pulmonary function (clear CXR, PaO2 >100mmHg with FiO2 21%)
- Wean sweep and adjust ventilator settings to maintain proper ventilation if still intubated

Profile 1: Critical cardiogenic shock
Life-threatening hypotension despite rapidly escalating inotropic support, critical organ hypoperfusion, often confirmed by worsening acidosis vs lactate levels.

Profile 2: Progressive decline

391

Declining function despite intravenous inotropic support, may be manifest by worsening renal function, nutritional depletion, inability to restore volume balance "Sliding on inotropes." Also describes declining status in patients unable to tolerate inotropic therapy.

Profile 3: Stable, inotrope dependent
Stable blood pressure, organ function, nutrition, and symptoms on continuous intravenous inotropic support (or a temporary circulatory support device or both) but demonstrating repeated failure to wean from support due to recurrent symptomatic hypotension or renal dysfunction "Dependent stability."

Profile 4: Resting symptoms
Stable close to normal volume status but experiences daily symptoms of congestion at rest or during ADL. Doses of diuretics generally fluctuate. More intensive management and surveillance strategies should be considered, which may in some cases reveal poor compliance that would compromise outcomes with any therapy.

Profile 5: Exertion intolerant
Comfortable at rest and with ADL but unable to engage in any other activity, living predominantly within the house. Patients are comfortable at rest without congestive symptoms, but may have underlying refractory elevated volume status, often with renal dysfunction. If underlying nutritional status and organ function are marginal, patient may be more at risk than INTERMACS 4, and require definitive intervention.

Profile 6: Exertion limited
Without evidence of fluid overload; comfortable at rest; fatigues after the first few minutes of any meaningful activity. Attribution to cardiac limitation requires careful measurement of peak oxygen consumption, in some cases with hemodynamic monitoring to confirm severity of cardiac impairment.

Profile 7: Advanced NYHA III
Without current or recent episodes of unstable fluid balance, living comfortably with meaningful activity limited to mild physical exertion.

There is no single metric used to determine whether a patient is suitable for discontinuation from ECMO, rather it is a combination of clinical, radiographic, laboratory, and hemodynamic factors. Once the decision has been made to discontinue ECMO, venous return to the right heart will increase as ECMO flows decrease. The left heart will compensate if myocardial recovery has occurred and offset any effects from a reduction in ECMO flows. The patient should be decannulated as quickly as possible to avoid risk of complications as the number of days on VA ECMO increases. The cardiovascular surgery team should be mobilized to the operating room or interventional suite to remove the cannulas via open cut down or with percutaneous closure devices. If the patient is still intubated, transesophageal echocardiography should be used to monitor cardiac function in real time. Electrolytes and volume status should be optimized. Inotropes can be restarted as needed to assist with cardiac output post decannulation. Serial arterial blood gases can be drawn to monitor for any cardiopulmonary dysfunction.

Potential questions/alternative scenarios
"40 y.o. female with no previous past medical history who endorses fatigue and dyspnea on exertion that has progressively worsened over the last several months however has not sought previous care. She does not have children however does endorse a history of a tubal pregnancy requiring surgery several months ago. She undergoes an echocardiogram this admission with global hypokinesis and EF to 15%. She is brought to the cardiac cath lab for further evaluation and management of her heart failure with consideration for advanced therapies. Her coronary cath is nonrevealing and her bedside hemodynamics display a CVP of 17, CI of 1.2, and SvO2 of 40%. Additionally, she has decreased urine output and elevated LFTs. While in the cardiac catheterization lab, angiographic

evaluation of her femoral arteries reveals 4 mm femoral vessel and her BSA is 2.1." What support would you recommend, and concerns do you have if any?

Several therapeutics exist from chemical to mechanical. Given her very limited cardiac function and cardiogenic shock state, chemical therapeutics alone may not be suffice. She should be considered for a mechanical support of which several modalities and routes of administration exist. Coronary augmented perfusion alone will not improve her state thus IABP is not considered. Given the size of her vessels she is unable to be supported by Impella CP (14Fr sheath) and ultimately Cardiac surgery should be considered for surgical placement of Impella device with cutdown for proximal and distal vessel control. Also, placement in the axillary vessel allows for ambulation as oppose to the immobility that follows placement in the femoral vessels. In this patient given the current devices at the time of writing of this text she can be considered for Impella 5.0 placement (or 5.5) through a tunneled right axillary approach with graft.

"Should she be considered for peripheral VA ECMO of the lower extremities?"

For the same reason the Impella will not be placed in the femoral vessels VA-ECMO should not be considered at this site. The arterial cannula for this patient should be a 15 French cannula or 17 French optimally based on her BSA, but her femoral vessels are disproportionally smaller. The 15 French cannula has a 5 mm outer diameter. There is likely a combination of her vessels being clamped down in her shock state as well as small vessels intrinsic to this patient. Although vessels are much more compliant in younger patients that older/calcified vessels issues with distal perfusion will remain with small vessels.

Pearls/pitfalls

- Always use ultrasound if available, vessel injury is devastating to the shock patient
- *Always place distal reperfusion catheter in ipsilateral superficial femoral artery as, limb loss increases mortality of the patient to near 100% in some series*
- If possible, artery and vein in contralateral leg, however in the emergent settings access whatever vessels you can
- 15 Fr arterial and 25 Fr venous are nearly universal sizes for the adult.

Suggested readings

- John R, Long JW, Massey HT. Outcomes of a multicenter trial of the Levitronix CentriMag ventricular assist system for short-term circulatory support. *The Journal of Thoracic and Cardiovascular Surgery,* 2011:*141*(4), 932–939.
- Sultan I, Kilic A, Kilic A. Short-Term Circulatory and Right Ventricle Support in Cardiogenic Shock: Extracorporeal Membrane Oxygenation, Tandem Heart, CentriMag, and Impella. *Heart Failure Clinics*, 2018:*14*(4), 579–583.
- Deshpande A, Kar B, Paniagua D. Tandem Heart, percutaneous left ventricular assist device treatment for severe refractory cardiogenic shock: The Debakey VA experience. *Journal of the American College of Cardiology,* 2014:*63*(12), A1854.
- Kar B, Adkins LE, Civitello AB. Clinical experience with the Tandem Heart percutaneous ventricular assist device. *Texas Heart Institute Journal,* 2006:*33*(2), 111–115.
- Kurihara C, Kawabori M, Critsinelis A. Impact of Tandem Heart Use for Heart Failure Patients as a Bridged to Long-term Continuous Flow Left Ventricular Assist Devices. *The Journal of Heart and Lung Transplantation,* 2018:*37*(4), S321–S322.

65. Durable Support – Mechanical Circulatory Support

Clauden Louis, MD, Daniel Ryan Ziazadeh, MD, Igor Gosev, MD

Concept
- Identifying LVAD malfunctions, common errors and troubleshooting techniques
- Post-operative concerns (right heart post procedure, pump pocket infection)

Terms
Bridge to Transplant (BTT):
Bridge to Decision (BTD):
Destination Therapy (DT): Refers to implantation of a VAD or TAH as a definitive device for end-stage heart failure.

Durable Support (Long Term MCS)
Ventricular assist devices take over the function of the damaged ventricle in order to re-establish normal hemodynamics and end-organ blood flow. Unloading of the native heart and correcting the underlying cause of myopathy can optimize conditions for cardiac recovery. While some patients may overcome the initial injury and sequelae of acute cardiogenic shock, those without evidence of meaningful myocardial recovery should be considered for durable support either as bridge to transplantation or destination therapy. While heart transplantation remains the most successful and desirable long-term option, organ scarcity prevents ~50% of patients on the waitlist from receiving an organ. Waitlist mortalities are institution dependent but range from 15-47% at one year. Some patients are also not candidates for transplantation making durable mechanical support devices important in maximizing survival and minimizing morbidity.

Like short term devices, they can support the right, left or both ventricles. They can be implanted through a full median sternotomy, mini upper hemi-sternotomy, or bilateral thoracotomies. For LV support, an inflow cannula is attached to the LV apex and the outflow cannula is tunneled and anastomosed to the ascending aorta, thereby bypassing the LVOT and the aortic valve. For RV support, the inflow cannula is attached to the RA or RV while the outflow cannula terminates in the pulmonary artery.

Thoratec pVAD/IVAD

The Thoratec pVAD was one of the 1st generation durable support devices available. Similar to its use in acute shock, it is indicated for use as bridge to transplantation (BTT) and bridge to recovery (BTR) and can provide uni or biventricular support. Similarly, the IVAD functions in the same manner of the pVAD, but its smaller size makes it suitable for intracorporeal support. It has also been approved for BTT and BTR. For more information, see above.

Novacor

The Novacor LVAD was another 1st generation pulsatile, intracorporeal device that was designed for durable cardiac support. It was the first VAD to provide more than four years of continuous circulatory support without pump replacement. With over 20 years of clinical use, primary device failure has remained rare with no deaths attributed to its failure. The INTREPID trial studied its feasibility as a device for BTT with a remarkable 78% survival to transplantation, which led to its approval for BTT in 1998. It shares similarities with the original HeartMate I, with an electric, dual pusher plate and pump housing constructed of polyurethane with inflow and outflow grafts containing porcine bioprosthetic valves. It featured the same external drive line system and portable power pack used in current LVADs. The device required systemic anticoagulation to prevent thromboembolism with target INR of 3.0 to 3.5.

HeartMate II™, Abbott, IL, USA

Axial flow LVAD designed for durable cardiac support. The REMATCH trial was groundbreaking and demonstrated for the first time that a durable device (the pulsatile HeartMate XVE) could have a dramatic survival advantage (53% vs 25%) at one year

394

compared to maximum medical therapy. As technology evolved, the second-generation HeartMate II offered advantages given its smaller, continuous axial flow design. It featured an inflow and outflow cannula without valves and eliminated the reservoir necessary in pulsatile pumps. It was approved for BTT after a study demonstrated that 42% of heart transplant candidates supported via HeartMate II underwent HT within the 6 months of support, with an overall 1-year survival of 68%. In the landmark HEARTMATE II trial, the HeartMate II significantly improved the probability of survival free from stroke and device failure at 2 years as compared with the HeartMate XVE. To date, more HeartMate II's have been implanted than any other device.

HeartWare®, Medtronic, MN, USA

Heartware also known as (HVAD) is a continuous flow centrifugal left ventricular assist device. As a small pump it allows for the intrapericardial implantation as well as lesser invasive approaches and particularly suitable for the bride-to-transplant cohort.

Advance BTT Trial was a multi-center (30), 140-patient, prospective trial designed to evaluate the HVAD® System as a bridge to heart transplantation for patients with end-stage heart failure. Endurance DT trial was a prospective, randomized, multi-center, non-inferiority clinical trial to evaluate the use of the HVAD® System in advanced heart failure patients for destination therapeutics.

HeartMate 3™, Abbott, IL, USA

Centrifugal flow LVAD designed for durable cardiac support. Landmark clinical trial that sought to answer the question of whether a new magnetically levitated centrifugal pump (HM3) was both non-inferior and superior to an axial flow pump (HM II) regarding reoperation for device malfunction or disabling stroke at six months after implantation. Previous trials including REMATCH and HEARTMATE II demonstrated that in patients with advanced heart failure refractory to medical management, left ventricular assist device (LVAD) placement was effective in providing temporary support as a bridge to heart transplantation and improved survival and quality of life in patients who were not eligible for transplantation (destination therapy).

Each subsequent iteration of LVAD technology has improved, beginning with first generation axial flow pump to the second-generation centrifugal flow pump, which lead to fewer mechanical failures and strokes. However, the second generation was particularly susceptible to pump thrombosis that often necessitate emergent reoperation. The HM3 improved on the first axial flow design by including a magnetically levitate pump with wider blood flow channels and asynchronous pulsatility. The MOMENTUM 3 final analysis at two years demonstrated a 14.6% absolute reduction in pump thrombosis rates in HM3 vs HM II, which coincided with a 15.4% absolute reduction in reoperation rates for device malfunction. The study met its primary endpoint of 12% absolute increase in patients implanted with HM3 who were alive and free of disabling stroke or reoperation to replace or remove a malfunctioning device at 2 years.

Chief Complaint

"A 55-year-old male with severe non-ischemic cardiomyopathy (NICM) and end stage systolic and diastolic congestive heart failure presents to the heart failure clinic with worsening symptoms and is found to have NYHA Class 4 symptoms and Stage D failure. After being presented in multidisciplinary heart failure conference, he is planned for LVAD implantation as destination therapy for INTERMACS Profile 4. Discuss your pre-operative workup."

Evaluation of patients for destination therapy VAD therapy should include a complete and systematic workup equivalent to evaluation for cardiac transplantation. This workup includes:

- Cardiac Catheterization (LHC + RHC) depending on presence of previous imaging and renal function
- Echo Complete TTE or TEE if imaging limited
- CT Chest – Non-contrast
- CTA Coronary Protocol with 3D Reconstruction if greater than 6 months from prior CABG

- Draw surveillance blood cultures, obtain MRSA swab up to 72 hours pre-op
  - UA with Reflex obtained *only* in symptomatic patients
- ID consultation should be obtained for any patient currently on antibiotics
- Remove and replace old central lines to minimize line related infections
- Operative notes from prior Cardiac Surgery should be obtained and reviewed
- Psychosocial evaluation is necessary whether for bridge-to-transplant or destination therapy

Medication Guideline:
- Hold SQ heparin products 48 hours pre-implant;
- Hold IV anticoagulation drips 6 hours pre-implant
- Consider stopping Amiodarone if clinically indicated
- Primary sternotomy INR < 2.0 / Redo stereotomy INR < 1.5
- Anti-platelet
  - Stop clopidogrel (Plavix) 5 days priors to surgery
  - Stop ticagrelor (Brilinta) 7 days prior to surgery
  - Bridging agents to be determined on case by case basis
- *Hold oral heart failure agents 72 hours preoperatively:*
  - ACEI/ARBs cause vasoplegia intraoperatively
  - Hold long acting beta blockers (Carvedilol/Bisoprolol/Toprol XL)

Operative Steps

Describe the operative procedure for LVAD implantation:

The patient is brought in the operating room and placed in supine position. He is placed under general anesthesia with care to monitor very closely hemodynamics. The patient is prepped and draped in the appropriate fashion for open heart surgery although it is important to avoid a belly button towel. Appropriate invasive monitoring lines are placed including arterial line, PA catheter and a TEE probe.

A standard sternotomy incision is performed. Alternatively, for bilateral minimally invasive thoracotomy (left 5th interspace at the inframammary crease and right 2nd parasternal interspace). The retractor placed, pericardium opened, stay sutures placed. Full dose IV heparin is given to the patient to maintain an ACT of greater than 480 seconds. Standard aorto-right atrial cannulation is performed, and cardiopulmonary bypass is initiated. Normothermia is maintained and cardioplegic arrest is avoided.

A circular ventriculotomy is made in the left ventricular apex. The LV is inspected for thrombus. Obstructing trabeculations removed and sewing ring secured to the left ventricle with interrupted pledgeted sutures (using the core then saw technique). (Alternatively, one can saw then core.) Also, the sutures can be placed in the LV apex prior to making the ventriculotomy. The outflow graft is connected to the LVAD and the anti-rotation clip is placed to lock the graft from rotating. The pump is then connected to the sewing ring and locked in place. The bend relief is then secured in place and the outflow graft inspected for twisting.

The driveline is then tunneled to the premarked location and connected to the controller. The outflow graft is measured and cut to the appropriate length with a 60-degree bevel. A partially occluding clamp is placed on the right side of the ascending aorta and longitudinal aortotomy performed. The outflow graft is then anastomosed to the aorta with prolene suture. The graft is clamped, the aorta is unclamped and the graft deaired typically by sticking it multiple times with a small (24-26g) needle.

The patient is placed in steep Trendelenburg position and aggressively de-aired with a venting needle in the outflow graft. Flow is gradually increased on the LVAD and weaned the patient off bypass successfully on the first attempt without problems. Right ventricular function is assessed. Post-implant evaluation by TEE evaluates for PFO and septum midline positioning with the LVAD at appropriate RPM.

Protamine is started. The bypass cannulas removed. Hemostasis acquired. Chest tubes placed and multiple layers of suture in the skin and liquid adhesive applied. The driveline exit site

396

closed with suture and then anchored with prolene suture. The driveline exit site was covered with dry gauze and occlusive dressing.

"What is your anticoagulation strategy for Continuous Flow LVADs post operatively?"

- The goal is to prevent thromboembolism and minimize bleeding. Start heparin drip when bleeding <50 cc/hour and after the chest has been closed. Our institution favors starting without a bolus and at a reduced dose (~10u/kg/hr). Most of these patients have some level of end organ dysfunction and the initial PTTs can be quite high.
- Target INR should be between 2-3 once bleeding is no longer an immediate postoperative concern. Oral anticoagulation with VKA antagonist (Warfarin) is started.
- Plavix can be restarted 48 hours post implant for patients with existing stent
- Compared to previous pump devices, HM 3 LVAD has shown to be more resistant to pump thrombosis and tolerate less strict anticoagulation thus a standardized regimen does not exist currently

"What is your strategy for removing tubes and wires post operatively?"

- Pleural and mediastinal tubes can be pulled while on heparin or warfarin
- Temporary pacing wires should be pulled when INR<1.9
  - ○ If on heparin, pause the heparin gtt for 2 hours immediately before and after wire removal
- Some institutions do not routinely use epicardial pacing wires after LVAD placement.

Index scenario (additional information)

What if during your preoperative workup, the patient's echocardiography reveals moderate to severe aortic valvular insufficiency.

Valvular regurgitation in the setting of LVAD placement poses a problem as this physiology compromises LVAD efficiency. In the setting of aortic regurgitation, the LVAD recirculates regurgitant blood decreasing cardiac output. Patients with aortic insufficiency experience a reduced survival versus patients without as noted by Topkara et al 2018. Consensus reports favor concurrent repair/replacement of aortic valve for aortic insufficiency greater than mild. Severe mitral and/or tricuspid regurgitation is a matter of debate although some find it reasonable on case by case bases dependent on patient risk factors and implantation status of destination versus bridge therapeutics.

Alternative Scenarios

Following uneventful LVAD placement, the patient was placed in steep Trendelenburg position and aggressively de-aired with a venting needle in the outflow graft. You gradually increase the flow on the LVAD and attempt to wean the patient off bypass. You notice there is an increase in right sided filling pressures, and you are unable to successfully wean from bypass. The anesthesia monitor shows the following values: CVP 24, PCWP 14, PA 40/17, and SvO2 45%. What is the next step in your management?

There is significant concern for RV failure. Start by evaluating the right ventricular function on post-implant TEE. Check for PFO and confirm the septum is midline. It is estimated that RV failure occurs in 20-50% of patients after LVAD implantation, and it remains a common cause of instability, morbidity and mortality. Preoperative risk factors for post-LVAD RV failure include female gender, non-ischemic cardiomyopathy, and the need for preoperative support with mechanical ventilation, intra-aortic balloon pump, or temporary mechanical circulatory support.

Of note, patients without pulmonary hypertension are more likely to develop RV failure as these patients have inadequate RV contractility to overcome an acute increase in pulmonary vascular resistance (PVR). Strategies for dealing with post-LVAD RV issues include pulmonary vasodilators (inhaled nitric oxide or veletri) and/or the addition of a lusitrope (milrinone). Finally, if the patient remains in significant RV failure, mechanical circulatory support options (ECMO vs. RVAD) can be employed.

Index scenario (additional information)

After an uneventful post-operative recovery, the patient is seen in clinic six weeks later where he is found to have blood pressures with MAP 120-130 mmHg. He does not have significant peripheral edema or LVAD alarms or concerns. How would you optimize his hemodynamics?

The goal of LVAD therapy is to utilize the pump to unload the left ventricle, by setting the speed such that it will provide a pulse pressure of 10-20mmHg. Pharmacologic therapy is used to decrease afterload and blood pressure, which optimizes pump flow. Non-invasive blood pressure cuffs alone are inaccurate as there is no pulsatile flow. A doppler probe should be used to accurately obtain blood pressure measurements.

Hypertension:

MAP should be between 70-80 mmHg with Doppler assistance. MAP <90mmHg may be acceptable based on the clinical situation. When a peripheral pulse is palpable, the target systolic BP is ~120 mmHg. It is reasonable to decrease systolic targets to 110 mmHg in asymptomatic patients.

Index scenario (additional information)

Patient has done well with his left ventricular assist device (LVAD) now s/p 12 months since implantation. He currently takes ASA 325mg and Warfarin with INR goal between 2-3. He now presents with a 5-day history of worsening malaise and fatigue. He describes recurrent bowel movements which have progressively darkened in color. His examination is concerning for sinus tachycardia and blood pressure with MAP 60 with intermittent suction events. His hematocrit is now 18. What is the concern and next step in the management of this patient?

The patient's presentation is concerning for a gastrointestinal bleed, which is a common complication after LVAD implantation. The bleeding is thought to be caused by altered blood flow patterns from continuous flow. Loss of pulsatile perfusion is implicated in intestinal hyperperfusion, distention of the submucosal venous plexus, and acquired von Willebrand factor deficiencies.

Evaluation of the patient should begin with a full history and physical exam. Evaluate and auscultate the LVAD to check for any suction or PI events. Obtain a CMP, CBC, and PT/INR to ensure the patient's anticoagulation is not supratheraptuic. In the setting of life-threatening GI bleed, anticoagulation should be held and the patient should be started on IV Protonix. Gastroenterology should be consulted for endoscopic evaluation. Due to alterations in blood flow, patients will often have evidence of angiodysplasia and arteriovenous malformations. After correcting any underlying coagulopathy, a significant portion of LVAD patient with GI bleed will self-resolve. Should these patients remain refractory, an upper and lower endoscopy should be performed to cauterize or clip any active bleed.

If patients are intolerant to anticoagulation secondary to recurrent life-threatening GI bleeds, then antiplatelet and anticoagulation may need to be held indefinitely. A risk/benefit discussion should be had given increase risk for pump thrombosis and exchange. New data has shown that cessation of anticoagulation for bleeding in HM3 is safe.

Reversal for Elevated INR:
- FFP for INR reversal for urgent procedures
- INR trend for elective procedures
- Factor 4 prothrombin (K-centra) for life threatening bleeding per attending and institution

GIB Readmit:

For patients with recurrent GIB concerning for AVM, more aggressive therapeutics can be added for each occurrence. Danazol has been shown to decrease GI bleed rehospitalization and pRBC transfusion
- 1st GIB: Resume warfarin and anti-platelet agent once H/H is stable following conservative therapy
- 2nd GIB: Start danazol low dose twice daily in addition to warfarin and anti-platelet agent

- 3rd **GIB:** Increase danazol to medium dosing twice daily, hold anti-platelet agents and consider lowering INR goal.

Index scenario (additional information)

After holding anticoagulation for 3 months, your patient returns to clinic without recurrent GI bleeding. On routine physical, your patient appears to be slightly jaundiced. Routine labs demonstrate elevated indirect bilirubin, mildly elevated LDH, and anemia. What is the likely cause of your patient's findings?

Hemolysis is a common complication of LVAD therapy and is associated with device malfunction. In severe cases, thrombosis can occur, and the device may need to be exchanged. The etiology of hemolysis is unclear but thought to be a result of destruction of red blood cells secondary to mechanical shear stress, flow acceleration, and abnormal blood device interactions.

INTERMACS further stratifies hemolysis as major and minor.

- **Minor Hemolysis:** A serum lactate dehydrogenase (LDH) level greater than 2.5x normal after the first 72 hours post-implant *in the absence of clinical symptoms* or findings of hemolysis or abnormal pump function.
- **Major Hemolysis:** A serum LDH level greater than 2.5x normal after the first 72 hours post-implant and *associated with clinical symptoms* or findings of hemolysis or abnormal pump function.
    - Hemoglobinuria
    - Anemia
    - Hyperbilirubinemia (total bilirubin > 2)
    - Pump malfunction and/or abnormal pump parameters

Guideline:
- LDH should be monitored monthly
- *For patients with minor hemolysis*, defined as a LDH >2.5x normal:
    - Optimize pump speed and blood pressure
    - Evaluate patient volume status, consider decrease diuretics
    - Review of INRs for time in therapeutic range
    - If above criteria controlled, consider INR goal adjustment to 3-3.5, continue current anti-platelet dosing
- *For patients with major hemolysis* or *new onset heart failure symptoms obtain:*
    - LDH, CBC, INR, CMP
    - VAD interrogation for alarms, PI events, power spikes
    - TTE or TEE with RAMP to check pump function
    - Consider CTA with 3d reconstruction if ECHO is unremarkable
    - Ensure optimal anticoagulation
    - CXR for evidence of pulmonary edema.
    - Blood cultures to rule out bacteremia

Treatment Guideline
- Optimize fluid status based on patient exam and renal function
- Optimize pump speed with RAMP ECHO and/or right heart catheterization
- **If patient have findings of hemolysis in the presence of therapeutic INR, add unfractionated Heparin**
    - Continue warfarin if INR <3.
    - When aPTT in therapeutic range, check Unfractionated Heparin and anti-Xa level.
    - Monitor patients for internal bleeding while on high dose anticoagulation.
- If hemodynamically unstable, utilize inotropes as required to maintain CI, organ perfusion

Treatment Options for Unresolved Hemolysis

1. Consideration for UNOS listing upgrade and urgent transplantation
2. Pump exchange if patient is a surgical candidate
3. Pump explant for patients with positive LVAD wean study
4. Consider thrombolytics in patients who are *not* surgical candidates

Potential Questions / Alternative Scenarios

Your patient is now 3 years s/p implantation and had been doing relatively well. He presents after 1 week of dyspnea on exertion, dark color urine over the past 48 hours. VAD interrogation demonstrates decreased pump flow and increased pump power over the last 72 hours. What is your concern and the next step in management?

The patient is presenting with signs and symptoms concerning for pump thrombosis. The incidence of continuous axial flow LVAD pump thrombosis during the first year after implantation in the current era is 5-12%. Patients may present with pronounced heart failure symptoms such as increased shortness of breath, ascites, or extremity edema. Pump alarms may or may not sound.

The patient should be admitted to the hospital and lactate dehydrogenase levels, INR, ECHO, and CTA Chest should be obtained. The VAD coordinator should be called and the device should be thoroughly interrogated. An ECHO can support the diagnosis of pump thrombosis with findings of a dilated left ventricle, opening of the aortic valve with every heartbeat, and worsening mitral regurgitation. A pulsatile waveform would indicate increased ventricular ejection and decreased ventricular decompression by the pump. A right heart catheterization can also reveal elevated filling pressures and a low cardiac index. CTA would show no contrast opacifying in the outflow graft and retrograde filling of the LVAD from the ascending aorta.

Medical therapy should be tailored to the patient's heart failure symptoms with appropriate inotropes, diuresis, and oxygen. It is important to arrest propagation of the clot with heparin gtt and to lyse it via intraventricular thrombolysis. With timely diagnosis and adequate treatment most cases will resolve, but pump exchange must be considered if initial measures fail. Several etiologies exist as to the cause such as pump position, pump migration and subtherapeutic anticoagulation. Bark pigment in the urine is an early sign of hemolysis and/or pump thrombosis.

LVAD thrombosis requires aggressive treatment and ultimately may require pump exchange. Transplant list priority is increased while with LVAD thrombosis. Is treated aggressively with medical therapy including IV antiplatelet therapy plus heparin or bivalirudin prior to consideration of LVAD exchange.

Potential questions/alternative scenarios

Workup confirms pump thrombosis and the patient is scheduled to undergo pump exchange. Immediately after redo-sternotomy, massive bleeding is noted at the xiphoid. What are the best next steps in management?

There is significant concern for outflow graft compromise. Immediately pack the chest, turn the device off, maximize inotropic support, maximize volume infusion, emergently establish femoral cardiopulmonary bypass, insert pump suckers, cool the patient to 18C, and initiate circulatory arrest. Entrance into the outflow graft is a feared and dramatic complication of re-operation for LVAD explant. A rapid institution of a defined series of events will help to prevent death from exsanguination. Axial flow pumps do not have valves, therefore turning the device off allows for retrograde flow through the device. Ejection of the native heart will create forward flow through the aorta, but also retrograde flow through the outflow graft. A concerted effort by anesthesia to improve forward flow (by maximizing inotropes and administering volume) will improve mean arterial pressure but will also impose a fair amount of afterload on the pulmonary circulation by acutely increasing LVEDP. Turning the device off and administering inotropes is the first step, but only a temporary solution. Since the graft is presumably adherent to the chest wall, packing the chest and binding it together with perforating towel clips may reduce the blood loss. Groin bypass is rapidly established, and the patient cooled towards 18C. The safest method is to cool for a full twenty minutes and arrest the circulation. The outflow graft must be identified and clamped on both sides of the graftotomy, since there is bidirectional flow. If the sternum is almost completely divided there is inclination to go after the graft without circulatory arrest. The problem with this intervention is the possibility of widening the aperture and exsanguinations before definitive control is obtained. A short period of circulatory arrest is generally well tolerated, and the patient may be rewarmed after control of the graft is obtained. The downside is the increased likelihood of pulmonary congestion from the acute increase in LVEDP.

Suggested readings
1. Bhatia, A, Juricek, C, Uriel et al: Increased Risk of Bleeding in Left Ventricular Assist Device Patients Treated with Enoxaprin as Bridge to Therapeutic INR. Asaio J. 2017 May.
2. Jennings, Shullo et al: Assessing Anticoagulation Practice Patterns in Patients on Durable MCS Devices: An International Survey. Asaio J. 2016 Jan-Feb;62(1): 28-32.
3. Saeed, Jorde et al: Antiplatelet Therapy and Adverse Hematologic Events during HMII support. CircHeartFailure 2016;9.
4. Momentum 3 Medical Management Working Group Recommendations. Chairs: Uriel, Horstmanshof, Naka. 1-20-2017.
5. HeartMate II Left Ventricular Assist System Instructions for Use: Thoratec Corporation, 2014.
6. HeartMate III Left Ventricular Assist System Instructions for Use: Thoratec Corporation, 2015
7. HeartWare Left Ventricular Assist System Instructions for Use: HeartWare Corporation, 2014.
8. Bennett MK, Adatya S. Blood pressure management in mechanical circulatory support. J Thorac Dis 2015;7(12):2125-2128.
9. Nir Uriel (University of Chicago), Douglas Horstmanshof (Integris Baptist Medical Center), Yoshifumi Naka (Columbia University). MOMENTUM 3 Medical Management Working Group Recommendations 1/20/2017]
10. Maltais S, Kilic A, Nathan S, Keebler M, Emani S, Ransom J et al. Prevention of HeartMate II pump thrombosis through clinical management: The prevent multi-center study. J Heart Lung Transplant. 2016.
11. Maltais S, Kilic A, et al. PREVENtion of HeartMate II Pump Thrombosis Through Clinical Management: The PREVENT multi-center study. J Heart Lung Transplant, 36 (2017) pp. 1-12.
12. Intermacs Manual of Operations, Version 5.0. Adverse event definitions 2/4/16
13. Katz J, Jensen B, Kirklin J, et al. A multicenter analysis of clinical hemolysis in patients supported with durable, long-term left ventricular assist device therapy. J Heart Lung Transplant, 34 (2015) pp. 701-709.
14. Kirklin JK, Naftel DC, Kormos RL, et al. Interagency Registry for Mechanically Assisted Circulatory Support (INTERMACS) analysis of pump thrombosis in the HeartMate II left ventricular assist device. J Heart Lung Transplant 33 (2014), pp, 12-22.
15. Whitson B, Eckman P, et al. Hemolysis, Pump Thrombus, and Neurologic Events in CFLVAD Recipients. Ann Thorac Surgery 97 (2014), pp. 2097–103.
16. Feldman D, et al. The 2013 International Society for Heart and Lung Transplantation Guidelines for mechanical Circulatory Support: Executive Summary. J Heart Lung Transplant, 32 (2013), pp. 157-187.
17. Goldstein DJ, John R, Salerno C et al. Algorithm for the diagnosis and management of suspected pump thrombus. J Heart Lung Transplant. 2013; 32:667-70.
18. Schroder J, Milano C. Is is time to get more aggressive with aortic valve insufficiency during LVAD implantation? JACC 2018; 6(11):961-913

66. CARDIAC TRANSPLANTATION

Taylor Kantor, MD, John M. Trahanas, MD, Francis D. Pagani, MD, PhD

Concept

- Patient selection and preoperative evaluation
- Combined organ transplantation
- DCD (donor after cardiac death vs. DBD (donor after brain death) transplantation
- Operative technique
- Postoperative care
- Infection, rejection, and chronic complications
- Cardiac retransplantation
- Potential questions/alternative scenarios
- Pearls/pitfalls

Chief complaint

"A 59-year-old male with end-stage, symptomatic heart failure (HF) is referred for heart transplantation."

Patient selection

Patient selection for cardiac transplantation involves a multidisciplinary committee to ensure appropriate allocation of organ resources. Inclusion and exclusion criteria do differ slightly amongst different centers; however, all centers aim to treat patients with end-stage cardiac disease refractory to alternative therapies who have the potential to resume a relatively normal quality of life.

Heart transplantation is indicated for advanced heart failure that is refractory to guideline directed medical therapy and the patient has an anticipated annual mortality of approximately 15 to 20% or greater. All alternative therapies and support should be utilized with documented evidence of failure or lack of candidacy prior to listing for cardiac transplantation. Common etiologies for systolic heart failure with reduced left ventricular ejection fraction (HFrEF) include ischemic heart disease (i.e., history of coronary disease) or non-ischemic heart disease such as idiopathic dilated cardiomyopathy from genetic or familial causes. Etiologies of heart failure with preserved ejection fraction (HFpEF) such as hypertrophic cardiomyopathy or amyloidosis may also lead to heart transplantation.

Similar to other transplantation protocols, cardiac transplant recipients should have no medical contraindications, no active source of infection, negative workup for malignancy, be actively participating in their medical care while following their medication regimens and have a good support system in place to aid through the pre- and post-operative transplant process. These restrictions for candidacy are in place due to the strict allocation of organ donations due to the limited resources. Common prognostic criteria to predict disease severity are below with EF and reduced VO_{2max} being the most important indicators:

- Low ejection fraction (<20%)

- Reduced VO_2max (<14 mL/kg/min or less than 50% of predicted)

- Ventricular arrhythmias

- High PCWP (>25 mmHg)

402

- Hyponatremia (Na <130)

- BNP (>5000)

Absolute contraindications for heart transplantation include advanced age (> 65 to 75 years of age depending on institution), fixed pulmonary hypertension (PVR > 4-6 Woods units), and systemic illness or disease such as neoplasms, immune compromise by HIV that is not adequately managed with antiviral therapy, active multisystem diseases such as SLE or sarcoid, and other irreversible end-organ dysfunction not amenable to co-transplantation. Relative contraindications include recent malignancy, moderate to severe COPD with an FEV_1 generally less than 50% of predicted, recent PE, diabetes resulting in end-organ damage with retinopathy, nephropathy or hemoglobin A1c > 7 to 8 gm/dl, PAD with evidence of claudication or non-healing ulcer, CVD, active peptic ulcer disease, diverticulitis, severe obesity (BMI greater than 38 to 40), severe osteoporosis, history of non-compliance, significant neurocognitive dysfunction, poor psychosocial support, and active substance abuse.

Preoperative evaluation – Recipient

Any patient referred for cardiac transplantation must have a comprehensive, systems-based examination with history and physical identifying past medical, surgical, social and family history. A psychiatric assessment should also be performed, and social work should be involved to determine adequate social and financial support. Additional evaluation includes routine hematologic and biochemical laboratory testing.

For cardiac assessment, a dedicated heart failure team should assist with preoperative evaluation. Standard evaluations include ECG, Holter monitor to assess for ventricular arrhythmias, echocardiography, and cardiopulmonary exercise testing to evaluate functional capacity. A well-established inverse relationship exists between VO_{2max} and heart failure mortality, thus making cardiopulmonary exercise testing the cornerstone of evaluation of heart failure prognosis. Right heart catheterization should also be performed to evaluate heart failure severity and presence of pulmonary hypertension (PH). Left heart catheterization w/ coronary angiography, PET scan, or cardiac MRI may also be useful in determining candidacy for revascularization and confirm the likely etiology of the heart failure. For patients in which the cause of heart failure is unknown, an endomyocardial biopsy should be performed.

Upon heart transplant listing, patient urgency for heart transplantation is established by a 6-tier allocation system provided by the United Network for Organ Sharing (UNOS). The current heart transplant allocation system went in effect October 2018 and is provided below:

- Status 1: patients on VA ECMO support, non-dischargeable biventricular support devices, or mechanical support with life-threatening ventricular arrhythmias.
- Status 2: non-dischargeable LVAD, persistent or recurrent VT or VF, mechanical support w/ malfunction, or patients requiring percutaneous endovascular mechanical support or IABP. Also, for TAH, BiVAD, RVAD, or VAD patient's with a single ventricle.
- Status 3: LVAD < 30 days, requiring multiple inotropes and hemodynamic monitoring, mechanical support with hemolysis, thrombosis, RHF, device infection, mucosal bleeding, or aortic insufficiency, VA ECMO >7 days, non-dischargeable LVAD >14 days, percutaneous mechanical support >14 days, or IABP >14 days.
- Status 4: Dischargeable LVAD >30 days, inotropes w/o hemodynamic monitoring, CHD, ischemic heart disease w/ intractable angina, amyloidosis, hypertrophic, or restrictive cardiomyopathy, heart re-transplant.
- Status 5: On waitlist for heart and second organ.
- Status 6: All other candidates suitable for transplant.

- Status 7: Inactive due to change in condition.

Preoperative evaluation – Donor

Organ donors undergo a three-phase screening regimen to determine potential for cardiac donation. Primary screening is undertaken by an organ procurement agency and includes routine laboratory data and demographics. Secondary screening is undertaken by a cardiac team to determine candidacy for donation as well as the necessary hemodynamic support until time of procurement. Donor selection criteria include the following:

- Normal biventricular function and normal valve function

- Minimal left ventricular hypertrophy, generally a septal wall thickness less than 1.2cm

- Donor to recipient weight ratio of 0.7

- Age <50-60. Donors aged 40 or older or who have 3 or more risk factors for CAD, or history of cocaine use should have a coronary angiogram.

- Absence of prolonged cardiac arrest or hypotension, preexisting cardiac disease, severe chest trauma, sepsis, malignancy, positive viral serologies (HIV, HepB, or HepC) [Note: many institutions have recently established programs to accept HepC+ donors with use of antiviral therapy post-transplant to eradicate post-transplant viremia]

- <50% lesion in two or more coronary arteries is a contraindication to donation

The final screening is undertaken at time of procurement. Procurement surgeons will proceed with donor cardiectomy if no evidence of cardiac dysfunction is present. Of note, some centers participate in expanded donor criteria due to the heart donor shortage that exists. By expanding the donor pool to apply marginal donors to marginal recipients, more heart transplants can take place. Criteria include older donors, decreased height ratio of donor:recipient, donors w/ CAD, mild LV dysfunction, positive viral serologies, or history of cocaine abuse but not IV drug abuse.

Combined Organ Transplantation

In patients with end-stage heart failure with other end-organ dysfunction, sole cardiac transplantation should not be performed. However, these patients may benefit from multiorgan transplantation. The most common combined organ transplants are for patients with end-stage HF and renal failure who undergo combined heart-kidney transplantation. Prior to consideration for heart-kidney transplantation, the patient should receive maximal medical therapy to determine reversibility of the renal dysfunction. However, patient's with modest kidney impairment may also benefit from combined heart-kidney transplantation due to the risk of further renal injury both intra-operatively and via calcineurin inhibitors as part of the post-operative immunosuppression therapy. Additionally, some studies have shown there are fever episodes of cardiac allograft rejection and cardiac allograft vasculopathy with combined heart-kidney transplantation.

Patients with end-stage HF and end-stage lung disease may benefit from combined heart-lung transplantation. The most common indication is for patients with congenital heart disease with Eisenmenger syndrome, but the procedure is also performed in patients with diseases such as idiopathic pulmonary arterial hypertension (IPAH) or cystic fibrosis (CF) causing right heart failure (RHF), and patients with cardiomyopathy leading to chronic lung disease. (See Ch.20: Lung Transplantation for additional details on selection for single and double lung transplantation)

Combined heart-liver transplantation is a potential option for patients with end-stage HF symptoms and cirrhosis. However, this procedure is not commonly performed, and candidates must be selected very carefully due to the number of comorbidities generally involved and the risk of operating on cirrhotic patients. The most common indications include amyloidosis, hepatitis C-associated cirrhosis, hemochromatosis, and congestive hepatopathy leading to cirrhosis.

DCD vs. DBD Heart Transplant
While DBD donors remain more common, the first DCD heart transplants were performed in the United States in late 2019. Outside of the U.S., centers in England and Australia have shown outcomes after DCD heart transplants that are equivalent to those of brain-dead donors. The procurement of a DCD heart requires a postmortem assessment of the heart using a normothermic perfusion system such as the Transmedics OCS, or in situ normothermic regional perfusion.

Index scenario (additional information)
"The patient is a 47-year-old male with a history of ischemic cardiomyopathy with reduced EF of 10%. He is currently on mechanical support with LVAD therapy for bridge to transplant. He is admitted to the ICU with hematuria, elevated pump power, decreased pulse index, and evidence of pump thrombosis.

The patient is upgraded from Status 4 to Status 2. Within days, an offer is accepted for DBD heart transplantation."

Operative steps
Donor (DBD)

- Communication and coordination with implant team and other procurement teams at every step is key!
- Median sternotomy
- Open pericardium and create pericardial well
- Inspect heart, taking note of contractile function, coronary calcification, any distention, contusion or injury, and congenital anatomic abnormalities
- If acceptable communicate that to implant team and determine need for explant delay
- Dissect and isolate aorta, SVC, and IVC. If lungs will be harvested develop inter-atrial groove
- Control SVC superior to azygos with tie, clamp, or Rommel
- Ligate and divide azygos
- Heparinize (250 to 300 u/kg)
- Place cardioplegia cannula into ascending aorta
- Occlude SVC, vent the left heart (place yankour), incise IVC, cross clamp aorta, initiate cold preservative solution, place ice slush in the field
- Continuously check that aortic root pressure adequate and heart not distended
- Complete division of IVC just above pericardial reflection
- Divide SVC, aortic arch vessels, main PA at level of the bifurcation
- Divide pulmonary veins at level of pericardium (or if lungs are being procured create left atrial cuff around orifices of pulmonary veins)
- Pack in three sterile bags with preservation solution and ice slush, or use commercially available perfusion system
- Upon arrival at the implant center on back table, divide posterior left atrium to create cuff. Close a PFO if it exists. Close the left atrial appendage if it was used to vent

Donor (DCD)

- For DCD donor, sternotomy must be rapid but controlled.
- Insert canula in right atrium to vent the heart and collect blood for perfusate. No preservation solution for any organ should be infused prior to collecting 1.5L of blood to prime normothermic perfusion device.
- Then, cardioplegia cannula placed in ascending aorta, cross clamp applied, and flush begins.
- The left atrial appendage is amputated to vent the left side of the heart and ice slush put on the field.
- The remainder of the donor explant is similar to a DBD procurement, except that the heart is placed on a normothermic perfusion device for preservation and evaluation.

Recipient Explant
- If recipient is a re-do sternotomy, expose or place sheaths in femoral vessels for rapid cannulation in the event of cardiac injury during re-entry sternotomy
- Sternotomy is performed and the superior and inferior vena cava are dissected, and snares are placed around them.
- The ascending aorta is cannulated as well as the cavae, and bypass is established
- If the recipient is a redo sternotomy the SVC, IVC, and ascending aorta should be exposed early so that cannulation can be performed to facilitate the remainder of the explant
- IF a ventricular assist device exists the outflow graft is dissected free and should be clamped just before the initiation of bypass. After bypass is initiated the apex of the heart and the device should be dissected free. Over aggressive manipulation prior to bypass should be avoided to minimize the risk of entraining air or dislodging clot.
- A cross clamp is applied, and the aorta and pulmonary artery are transected just above the valves
- The SVC and IVC are transected at their junction with the right atrium, and the swan-ganz catheter removed from the heart and preserved for replacement in the donor.
- If a bi-atrial anastomosis is planned, the RA is divided to create a cuff including SVC and IVC but eliminating the recipient right atrial appendage. The inter-atrial septum is divided to open the left atrium and create the LA cuff
- Any permanent pacing leads are placed on tension and divided
- The dome of the left atrium is incised, and a left atrial cuff created
- The recipient heart is then removed
- The driveline is removed from the field, but the remainder is not removed from the sub cutaneous tissues until after the chest is closed as this is a contaminated field.

Donor Implant (Bi-Caval Technique)
- The bicaval technique better preserves normal atrial morphology, sinus node, and valvular function, and is associated with shorter hospital stay and rate of pacermaker placement.
- The donor heart should be brought onto the field and the vessel lengths assessed and trimmed. Cardioplegia should be administered prior to beginning the implant
- Steroids are administered
- Implantation starts with the left atrium using a long arm 3-0 polypropylene suture. A left ventricular vent should be placed via the right superior pulmonary vein. The suture line is begun at the left superior pulmonary vein of the recipient which is aligned with the base of the donor left atrial appendage
- The subsequent order of anastomosis may vary depending on surgeon preference, but typically procedes LA, then PA, followed by aorta, IVC and SVC
- The PA catheter should be replaced prior the completion of the PA anastamosis

406

- If there is a long ischemic time, the left atrium and aorta can be completed and the cross clamp removed, with the right sided anastomoses completed with the heart perfused.
- With all anastomosis it is imperative to assess size discrepancy and correct while sewing, as well to size the length appropriately to prevent kinking (some redundancy in the aortic anastomosis may be desired to facilitate hemostasis of back wall).
- The SVC anastamsois is especially prone to narrowing and should be performed with many small bites or triangulated with stay sutures.
- The heart is de-aired, and the cross clamp is removed and the donor heart re-perfused. Atrial pacing or isoproterenol should be used to keep the donor heart rate 100-120 to prevent RV distention.
- Bypass is weaned, and the recipient is decannulated. Any pre-existing pacemaker or ICD generator should be removed prior to closing the chest. After closing the chest, the driveline is removed at the skin

Donor Implant (Bi-Atrial Technique)

- This is the original technique popularized by Shumway and Lower.
- The left atrial anastomosis is completed with the front wall sewed to the inter-atrial septum
- The donor heart is then prepped for the right atrial anastomosis by incising the donor from the base of the IVC up onto the right atrial appendage, thus preserving the donor sinoatrial node. The right atrial anastomosis is then completed with the back wall sewn to the inter-atrial septum.
- The PA and aortic anastomoses are completed in the standard fashion as above.

Postoperative care
Care of the post-transplant patient is similar to any post cardiomyotomy patient.

- Depletion of myocardial catecholamine stores in donor hearts, and vasoplegia in patients who previously had continuous flow durable left ventricular assist devices may lead to a prolonged need for high dose catecholamines in the post-operative period.
- Severe primary graft dysfunction refractory to pharmacologic therapy may necessitate mechanical support. Pulmonary vasodilators may be useful for right heart failure, which remains the leading cause of early mortality.
- Arrhythmias should warrant further investigation to rule out cardiac ischemia, rejection, or infection.

Infections, Rejection, and Chronic Complications
Hyperacute rejection is rare due to screening for preformed antibiodies. It manifests as a mottled graft within minutes to hours of implantation.

Most rejection episodes in heart transplants are represented by cellular rejection. Acute rejection may occur in the first 6 months after transplant and is typically asymptomatic, but may present with low grade fever, malaise, arrhythmias, and heart failure. Heart transplant recipients are frequently monitored for this complication via right heart biopsy. Biopsy typically occurs every 7-10 days for the first few months and then the interval is extended. Rejection is graded in severity according to a standardized ISHLT Grading scheme with Grade 0R being no rejection, and Grade 3R indicating severe rejection. Most episodes are effectively treated with steroids.

Antibody-mediated rejection is less common but occurs within the first year and may manifest as hemodynamic instability requiring inotropic support. Plasmapheresis, steroids, heparin, and IgG may be required. Chronic low-grade vascular rejection may play a role in the development of allograft coronary artery disease.

Despite preventative measures, post-transplant infection is common. Hospital acquired organisms such as *Pseudomonas* and *Staphylococcus* occur as they do with any surgical patient. CMV infection has considerable morbidity as it may be associated with precipitating acute rejection and post-transplant lymphoproliferative disease. Fungal infections such as candidiasis may occur frequently, and more dangerous fungal infections such as aspergillus and mucormycosis have been known to occur in these immunocompromised hosts. Protozoa such as *Pneumocystis carinii* and *Toxoplasma gondii* may also infect heart transplant recipients.

Cardiac allograft vasculopathy (CAV) is a diffuse intimal proliferation causing diffuse luminal stenosis of the coronary arteries. It is the leading cause of death after the first year and is present in 40-50% of recipients by 5 years. Eventually this process may lead to silent myocardial ischemia and decline of allograft function. Given the diffuse nature of the process, angioplasty and stenting are ineffective, and only the only treatment is retransplantation.

Hypertension, hyperlipidemia, renal dysfunction, and malignancy are also common common long-term complications of heart transplantation.

Cardiac Re-transplantation
Cardiac transplantation is a seldom performed operation accounting for approximately 2-3% of all cardiac transplants yearly. Primary indications include hyperacute/acute graft failure, cardiac allograft vasculopathy, and refractory acute rejection. For patients who need early re-transplantation, overall one-year survival is lower than that of primary cardiac transplant recipients; however, the survival is near equivalent for patients requiring re-transplantation after 2 or more years. Age is a significant factor as each decade increases likelihood of graft failure at one year by approximately 20%. Patients bridged to transplant also do considerably worse, speculatively due to immune activation and increased inflammatory response, most notably in patients undergoing bridging via ECMO. Careful selection of patients to undergo re-transplantation can result in favorable outcomes.

Potential questions/alternative scenarios
"A 35-year-old male patient with ischemic heart failure undergoes a heart transplant. His intraoperative course had no complications and he was transferred to the ICU on low inotropic and vasopresser support. Within hours, his inotropic support drastically increases, and bedside echo shows an EF of 5% w/ a diffusely edematous allograft. What is the primary concern?"

The primary concern would be that the patient is undergoing hyperacute allograft rejection. Today, this is rare due to the screening of ABO blood typing and PRA screening. Hyperacute rejection occurs within minutes to hours and results in immediate heart failure due to antibody deposition with interstitial hemorrhage and edema. This must be treated emergently with plasmapheresis, IVIG, and initiation of mechanical support usually with VA ECMO. Re-transplantation is the only salvage therapy but is generally not recommended due to the high mortality.

"A 42-year-old female underwent heart transplantation approximately 6 months ago. Recently, she has been experiencing intermittent fevers, occasional feeling of palpitations, reduced exercise tolerance, and lower extremity edema. What diagnostic procedure should be performed?"

The patient is exhibiting symptoms which may be consistent with acute allograft rejection. With today's current immunosuppression regimens, patients with acute allograft rejection often go undetected sometimes until late in the disease process as symptoms can be

408

very mild. Routine right ventricular endomyocardial biopsies are the gold standard for diagnosis. Most institutions have biopsies performed within the first

two weeks of surgery with the patient undergoing subsequent biopsies every 3-6 months. Any suspicion of rejection warrants additional endomyocardial biopsies. Grade of rejection is based on histologic parameters and will help to determine if the patient needs alteration of immunosuppression regimen or may require re-transplantation. Corticosteroids are the main supplements used to curtail rejection.

"A 37-year-old female with previous ischemic cardiomyopathy s/p heart transplantation over one year ago is seen in clinic for increased dyspnea on exertion and reduced exercise tolerance. The patient undergoes stress testing which is positive. A LHC is performed and shows diffuse stenosis of all major vessels and peripheral pruning. What is the most likely diagnosis?"

This patient is exhibiting signs and symptoms of cardiac allograft vasculopathy or CAV. This is a rapid and progressive form of diffuse atherosclerosis characterized by intimal proliferation rather than atherosclerotic plaques. It is in fact the leading cause of death in the first year after transplant and the limiting factor to long-term survival in transplant recipients. Clinical diagnosis can be difficult to make due to denervation of the heart and the absence of typical chest pain. For this, LHC's are performed routinely, usually annually, for the first several years after transplant. Everolimus and sirolimus have been shown to possibly inhibit the severity of CAV, however, once it occurs, the only form of treatment is re-transplantation. These patients are not candidates for coronary revascularization procedures.

"A 45-year-old male underwent a cardiac transplant and is now POD5. He has had a relatively uneventful post-operative course, however, becomes acutely bradycardic to the 30's with a drop-in blood pressure. Atropine is emergently administered but has no effect. What could be the possible cause?"

A transplanted heart has altered physiology as the heart was denervated during transplantation. This alters the heart's response to certain therapeutic interventions and physiologic conditions. For example, the transplanted heart relies on circulating catecholamines rather than direct sympathetic stimulation during episodes of stress such as hypovolemia, hypoxia, or anemia and results in a delayed tachycardia response. In addition, vasovagal maneuvers such as carotid sinus massage and Valsalva, or therapeutic interventions with anticholinergics, such as atropine, are no longer effective.

"A 47-year-old male underwent cardiac transplantation one week ago and is scheduled to undergo his first trans-jugular biospy. The interventionalist notes that the jugular vein is very full and easy to access, but has difficulty passing the biopsy catheter into the heart. What could be the cause?"

The SVC anastomosis is relatively narrow in caliber and is notoriously easy to narrow or purse-string if not sewed with proper technique. This may manifest as difficulty accessing the heart from the neck vessels for post-transplant biopsy. Severe cases may resemble SVC syndrome with facial flushing and edema and require revision of the SVC anastomosis.

"A 59-year-old female with a history of ischemic cardiomyopathy and a left ventricular assist device is in the operating room awaiting arrival of a donor heart. The heart is dissected free of adhesions, aorto-bicaval bypass instituted, and the LVAD turned off. Despite vacuum assisted drainage, the heart remains full and the perfusionist notes difficulty maintaining an adequate mean arterial pressure. What did the surgeon forget?"

As an LVAD is designed for continuous forward flow, the outflow grafts do not contain a valve to prevent reverse flow, and for this reason must be clamped when the device is turned off. If not, a large circular shunt will be established in which aortic blood can return to the left side of the heart causing distention and poor forward flow. The outflow graft must be handled carefully, as catastrophic arterial bleeding can occur if injured, especially if injured on re-entry with the sternal saw. This may require emergent bypass and circulatory arrest to repair.

- No irreversible steps should be taken during recipient explant until the donor heart has arrived safely
- Care must be taken during construction of left atrial anastomosis to properly align IVC and SVC
- The LV should be vented to prevent accumulation of pulmonary vein effluent which may warm donor heart prior to reperfusion
- Great vessels and vena cavae should be trimmed to proper length to avoid kinking

Suggested readings

- Cohn LH, Adams DH. Heart Transplantation. Chapter 60. Shemin RJ, Deng M. Cardiac Surgery in the Adult. 5th Edition. 2018.
- Messer S, Page A, Axell R, Berman M, Hernandez-Sanchez J, Colah S, et al. Outcome after heart transplantation from donation after circulatory-determined death donors. J Heart Lung Transplant. 2017 Dec;36(12):1311–8.
- Sharma A, Peltz M, Wait MA, Ring SW, Mathur A, Jessen ME, et al. The conduct of thoracic organ procurement. Asian Cardiovasc Thorac Ann. 2020;28(3):158–67.
- Cheng A, Slaughter MS. Heart transplantation. J Thorac Dis. 2014;6(8):1105-1109. doi:10.3978/j.issn.2072-1439.2014.07.37

Jessica G.Y. Luc, MD, Christopher C. Cheung, MD, Jamil Bashir, MD

Concept

- Overview of the cardiac conduction system
- Epicardial pacing
- Transvenous pacing
- Transcutaneous pacing
- Pacing modes
- Pacemaker troubleshooting
- Potential questions / scenarios

Cardiac Conduction System

Normal cardiac activity originates at the sinoatrial (SA) node, located in the superior right atrium and near the junction with the superior vena cava. Cells in the SA node has intrinsic automaticity to generate a spontaneous action potential, resulting in a cyclical depolarization and repolarization and forming the basis of intrinsic cardiac electrical activity. Following depolarization, the electrical impulse spreads across both atria, arriving at the atrioventricular (AV) node. The AV node, located within the triangle of Koch (delineated by coronary sinus, tendon of Todaro, and tricuspid valve septal leaflet), serves as an important "gatekeeper" regulating depolarization of the ventricle. Following depolarization of the AV node, the electrical impulse enters the His-Purkinje system to depolarize the ventricles. The His-Purkinje network branches into the left and right bundle branches, allowing for rapid synchronized conduction of the electrical impulse down to ventricular muscle.

Disease can occur at any point along the cardiac conduction system. Typically, pathology associated with the SA node can result in sinus node dysfunction or commonly termed "sick sinus syndrome," leading to resulting sinus bradycardia or pauses. Pathology in atrial tissue can result in ectopic atrial beats (i.e. premature atrial complexes), atrial flutter and fibrillation. Prior instrumentation of the atrium may lead to scar formation, providing the substrate for re-entry for atrial flutter. Pathology at the level of the AV node can result in the non-conduction of atrial or sinus impulses to the His-Purkinje system, commonly resulting in progressive conduction block. Pathology in the infra-Hisian conduction system manifests as intraventricular conduction block, or right or left bundle branch block, frequently associated with cardiomyopathy and leading to dyssynchronous contraction of the ventricle. Disease in ventricular myocardium, frequently arising from progressive cardiomyopathies or infarction, can result in scar formation and re-entry circuits and forming the substrate for ventricular arrhythmias.

Options for Pacing/Pacemaker Implantation

A. Epicardial Pacing

Pacing Wire Insertion

Temporary epicardial pacing wires are often utilized to allow temporary pacing after cardiac surgery to treat temporary rhythm disturbances. Depending on surgeon preference, some prefer not to place pacing wires in patients with no evidence of bradycardia or heart block immediately after cardiopulmonary bypass to avoid bleeding complications. However, if a patient is bradycardic, has low cardiac output, heart block or has undergone valvular surgery, a minimum of ventricular wires should be considered. Epicardial wires are manufactured with a small needle on one end. This is used to embed the wire in the myocardium, after which the needle is cut off. Some wires are coiled to assist fixation; others can be clipped or loosely sutured in place. A larger straight needle on the other end of the wire is used to penetrate the body wall, bringing the wire to the surface. The lead should be sufficiently well anchored in the myocardium to avoid premature dislodgement, while still allowing eventual removal by gentle traction.

Epicardial wires can be placed on the epicardium prior to closing the chest during open heart surgery. Atrial wires are placed on the right atrium typically away from the SA node. Ventricular wires can be placed anywhere on the right ventricle. Most surgeons seek out exposed muscle for best threshold and sensing and place them just under the epicardium. The wires should be tested intraoperatively to confirm capture and threshold while there is still an opportunity for repositioning. Both sets of wires are then brought out to the skin by passing them directly lateral to the xiphisternum, taking care to not traverse the plane of the sternum to avoid entrapment upon sternal closure, and are then sutured and secured in place.

Temporary Pacing Wire Removal
When the patient is no longer bradycardic or has evidence of conduction system disease, usually by postoperative day 3, temporary epicardial pacing wires can be removed. It is safest to be done during daytime hours in case of bleeding complications. Patients who are anticoagulated should have their INR<2.0 and heparin should be discontinued for three hours prior to pacing wire removal. Platelet counts should be above 100,000 and the patient should not hypertensive. The patient should be in a recumbent position.

Vitals should be taken prior to wire removal. The wires are mobilized from the skin edge and with gentle traction, the wires can be pulled out smoothly one at a time. If resistance is encountered upon attempt to remove the wires, the wires can be pulled taut and cut flush to the skin. Following pacing wire removal, the patient should remain on telemetry, in bed in a recumbent position with vitals taken every 15 minutes to monitor for hypotension for 45 minutes. If hypotension or arrhythmias develop, one should retain a low index for suspicion of tamponade and appropriate measures taken.

B. Permanent Epicardial Pacemaker Leads
Permanent epicardial pacemaker leads can also be implanted in patients with an expected pacemaker requirement, such as those with known underlying conduction disease or a prior indication for permanent pacemaker. In addition, patients with severe cardiomyopathy requiring cardiac resynchronization pacing may also benefit from synchronized pacing of the left ventricle. In such cases, pacemaker leads can be implanted transvenously (in the coronary sinus) or through an epicardial approach. The ideal place for the left ventricular lead is basal, just anterior and inferior to the left atrial appendage where there is visible muscle between the obtuse marginal artery branches. Furthermore, permanent epicardial leads would be the desired option for patients with complicated vascular access (e.g. venous thrombosis, congenital anatomical variations, prosthetic tricuspid valve, prior failed transvenous pacing implantations) or active bloodstream infection in which the placement of transvenous leads may be contraindicated. Steroid eluting bipolar button leads have the best long-term outcomes.

C. Transvenous pacing
Most patients who require temporary or permanent pacing will receive transvenous pacing, either through the insertion of a temporary pacing wire or implantation of permanent pacemaker leads. Further, some Swan-Ganz catheters have a port for a pacing wire. Risk factors for requiring permanent pacing after cardiac surgery include age, preoperative bundle branch block and conduction system disease, valvular surgery, prolonged cardiopulmonary bypass, transcatheter aortic valve implantation and suboptimal intraoperative myocardial protection.

Temporary transvenous pacing wires
Temporary transvenous pacing wires are typically inserted at the bedside in patients requiring urgent ventricular pacing due to bradycardia or ventricular pauses. The temporary pacing wires are typically advanced through a single lumen sheath in the internal jugular vein or femoral veins and directed towards the right ventricle. It is important to insert a sheath that is

412

large enough to fit the pacing wire, but not too large as it will result in bleeding around the wire itself. Transvenous pacing wires can be both rigid tip (inserted under fluoroscopic guidance) or balloon-tip (fluoroscopic guidance not necessary).

When using the balloon-tip pacing wire, it is common to test the balloon prior to insertion. Once the balloon is deflated, it can be connected to the pacing box and the balloon tip advanced into the single-lumen sheath. Once the balloon tip is sufficiently within the body (past the end of the sheath, approximately 10 cm), the balloon can be re-inflated and locked. The catheter should be carefully advanced while observing cardiac telemetry for demonstration of ventricular capture. It is common to see pacing spikes on telemetry, but the absence of ventricular capture, demonstrate that the pacing wire is not in the correct position.

As the balloon is gradually advanced, ventricular capture will become evident on cardiac telemetry. At this point, the balloon can be deflated, and the ventricular capture threshold checked. Positioning of the temporary pacing wire should also be evaluated by chest radiography. Fluoroscopy can be used to facilitate any temporary pacemaker insertion if necessary.

Permanent transvenous pacemaker
Permanent transvenous pacemakers are the most common cardiac devices implanted in patients requiring long-term pacing support. Pacemaker leads are typically inserted in the cephalic vein using a cut-down approach which has literature proven lowest complication rate and best lead longevity, or in the axillary or subclavian veins through needle puncture and fluoroscopic guidance (Seldinger technique). Access can be performed on either the left or right side. Once the vein is cannulated, the pacemaker leads can be advanced (typically through a sheath in the case of the axillary or subclavian vein access) into the superior vena cava and into the heart.

Permanent pacemaker leads can be advanced and fixated into atrial and ventricular tissue, and into the coronary sinus for cardiac resynchronization devices. Permanent pacemaker leads typically use an active fixation mechanism with a screw-in tip. Passive fixation leads are used less frequently than active fixation leads due to the greater ease of site selection, ease of extraction and position stability. Once in position, the pacemaker leads are tested to ensure appropriate capture thresholds, sensed atrial/ventricular amplitudes, and lead impedances. The pacemaker leads are then carefully sutured into place without dislodging or pulling back the pacemaker lead. Finally, the pacemaker leads are connected to the device and placed in the pocket and closed. Ensuring that the lead is very securely fixed at the exit site will prevent dislodgement.

Intra-operative and post-operative complications of permanent pacemaker implantation include:
1. Pneumothorax
2. Arterial injury
3. Acute pocket hematoma
4. Pericardial effusion
5. Tricuspid leaflet dysfunction/valve regurgitation associated with pacemaker lead
6. Venous thrombosis +/- superior vena cava syndrome
7. Cardiac implantable electronic device infection (can present with sepsis, endocarditis, pocket infection, lead erosion)

D. Transcutaneous pacing
Transcutaneous pacing is frequently considered in situations when patients are asystolic or significant bradycardic resulting in cardiac arrest. Transcutaneous pacing pads connected to the pacing/defibrillation system are applied to the patient, typically in the anterior/precordial and lateral/apical positions. The pacing rate and output is dialed into the pacing system. Transcutaneous pacing should be avoided in conscious patients, as transcutaneous stimulation can be associated with significant discomfort.

3. Pacing Modes

Pacing settings are classified using the Heart Rhythm Society / British Pacing and Electrophysiology Group Generic Code (the NBG Code) as follows:

I	II	III	IV	V
Chamber paced	Chamber sensed	Response to sensing	Rate modulation	Multisite pacing
O = none	O = none	O = none	O = none	O = none
A = atrium	A = atrium	T = triggered	R = rate modulation	A = atrium
V = ventricle	V = ventricle	I = inhibited		V = ventricle
D = dual (atrial and ventricular)	D = dual (atrial and ventricular)	D = dual (triggered and inhibited)		D = dual (atrial and ventricular)

Pacing modes:

I	II	III	Description	Indication
A	O	O	Asynchronous atrial pacing	Sinus bradycardia
A	A	I	Demand atrial pacing	Sinus bradycardia, junctional bradycardia
V	O	O	Asynchronous ventricular pacing	No ventricular rhythm, cautery
V	V	I	Demand ventricular pacing	Heart block
D	O	O	Asynchronous dual pacing	No ventricular rhythm, cautery
D	V	I	AV sequential, ventricular demand pacing	Suitable for most bradyarrhythmias
D	D	D	AV sequential, dual chamber demand	Heart block
D	D	DR	AV sequential, dual chamber demand with rate responsiveness	Combination sinus node dysfunction and heart block

Typical pacemaker settings:

Atrial and ventricular output	10-20mA
PR interval / AV delay	150 ms (20-300 ms) or 'auto', determined by rate
Lower rate limit ('rate')	40 (backup); 60-100 (pacing)
Atrial overdrive stimulation	Up to 500 ppm
Atrial sensitivity	0.5 mV (0.4-1.2mV)
Ventricular sensitivity	2.5 mV (0.8-5mV)
Post-ventricular atrial refractory period	250 ms or 'auto', determined by rate

Figure 1: Simplified decision tree approach to setting the pacing mode

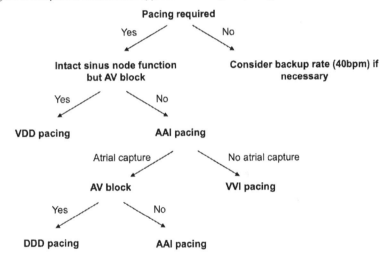

Pacing Definitions
1. Sensitivity = minimum amplitude that the pacemaker is able to sense. A lower number corresponds to a greater sensitivity. For example, if the pacemaker senses or "sees" an electrical impulse of 5 mV, but the sensitivity is set at 6 mV, it will not "detect" the impulse. The sensitivity will need to be lowered to detect the electrical impulse.
   a. To check sensitivity in temporary epicardial or transvenous pacing boxes:
      i. Set pacemaker rate below the patients' native rate
      ii. Place in VVI, AAI or DDD modes (i.e. intrinsic cardiac activity should inhibit the pacemaker)
      iii. Slowly increase sensitivity threshold until the sense indicator stops flashing

415

      iv.   Check that pacing is occurring asynchronously in the chamber being tested

2. Pacing threshold = minimum output required for pacing capture. A higher number corresponds to a higher capture threshold. For example, if the pacemaker paces with an output of 1 mA but is unable to capture the ventricle, the pacing threshold is higher than 1 mA, and the pacing output will need to be increased until ventricular capture is demonstrated.

    a.   To check pacing threshold in temporary epicardial or transvenous pacing boxes:

        i.   Gradually decrease the output until there is no longer pacing capture. Before doing so, ensure that the patient is not dependent.

        ii.   Following loss of capture (simultaneously evident on cardiac telemetry), increase the pacing output back to the capture threshold. Typically, the pacing output is set at approximately 2-5 times the capture threshold to ensure reliable capture.

The above steps can be performed with pacing boxes connected to temporary epicardial and transvenous pacing wires. Evaluating sensitivity and capture threshold in permanent pacemakers requires the use of a programmer.

Pacemaker Troubleshooting

For all issues with pacing, one should see and assess the patient to ensure hemodynamic stability. A systematic approach is essential and can include the following:

1. Review rhythm strip and 12 lead ECG
2. Check integrity of circuit (start at patient -> pacing box): lead placement, polarity, integrity, tightly connected to correct port of pacing box (atrial/ventricular), battery, settings
3. Check mode
4. Check rate
5. Check capture threshold (find threshold and double it for safety)
6. Check sensitivity (normal = 2-5mV) – changes with position
7. Fixes: change patient position, reverse bipolar pacing leads, convert to unipolar pacing, replace pacing equipment, try high-output pacer or return to operating room for reinsertion of epicardial wires or transvenous pacemaker implantation
8. Back up plan in emergency: transcutaneous or transvenous pacing, atropine, adrenaline, isoprenaline, ephedrine, correction of electrolytes or underlying metabolic issues such as severe acidosis

Common Issues with Pacing/Pacemakers

The following is a summary of common issues and potential complications that may arise with the use of temporary epicardial pacing wires:

A. *Failure to pace*

Failure to pace occurs when there is no electrical output at the pacing wire tip when the pacing mode set requires output. Failure to pace is distinguished from failure to capture by the absence of pacing spikes in ECG at a heart rate less than the minimum heart rate set on the pacemaker.

Differential: (from easiest to hardest to fix)

1. Pacing output may be too low -> correct by turning up the pacing output
2. Leads or contacts faulty -> check all connections yourself, swap pacing wires between ports, change pacing cable
3. Box battery may be low -> check box battery and if necessary, change batteries
4. Pacing wires not in contact with myocardium
5. Pacing wires short-circuiting

Treatment if patient hemodynamically unstable:

416

1. External pacing pads
2. Insert transvenous pacing wires

B. Failure to capture
Failure to capture is when there is electrical output at the pacemaker wire tips, as confirmed by visible pacing spikes on ECG, which fail to cause a depolarization and cardiac contraction. Failure of cardiac contraction can be confirmed by an absent cardiac impulse on arterial pressure waveform or pulse oximeter waveform.

Differential
1. Pacing output may be too low -> correct by turning up the pacing output
2. Pacing wires have been dislodged or in contact with area of high threshold -> try to reposition or change pacing wires
   a. Differential for increased threshold:
      i. Myocardial ischemia
      ii. Electrolyte imbalance (e.g., hyperkalemic, acidosis)
      iii. Post defibrillation
      iv. Medications (e.g., beta blockers, calcium channel blockers, antiarrhythmics)

Treatment if patient hemodynamically unstable:
1. External pacing pads (transcutaneous pacing), or;
2. Insert transvenous pacing wires

C. High threshold
A high threshold occurs when a high amount of energy is required to achieve myocardial capture. In temporary pacing wires, this can be a result of lead dislodgement and may raise concern of further dislodgement or failure to capture. In permanent pacemakers, this can also be a sign of lead dislodgement (and associated complications), lead integrity (i.e. lead fracture), and may also influence battery life if the threshold remains persistently high.

Differential:
1. Pacing wire dislodgement or in contact with an area of scar or high threshold
2. Metabolic and pharmacologic considerations (i.e. myocardial ischemia, electrolyte imbalance, post-defibrillation, medications)
3. Hematoma
4. Edema
5. Scarring

Treatment:
1. Consider transvenous wires if threshold >10mA in a pacing-dependent patient

D. Oversensing
Oversensing occurs when the pacemaker "senses" too much- for example, if the pacemaker senses T waves, or double-counts the QRS complex, this can result in inappropriate inhibition of pacing. This is particularly relevant in pacemaker dependent patients, as it can lead to excessive bradycardia or pauses.

Treatment:
1. Increase sensing threshold
2. Change modes

E. Diaphragmatic pacing
Differential:
1. Proximity of phrenic nerve with lead.
2. Incorrectly positioned lead (cardiac vein, myocardial perforation, migration)
3. High stimulation amplitude

Treatment:
1. Reduce output
2. Use ventricular pacing (rather than atrial pacing), given that atrial wires are often closer to the phrenic nerve.
3. Reposition of pacing wires

F. Retained wire
Generally temporary epicardial pacing wires can be removed postoperatively with gentle traction. However, if resistance to traction occurs, the pacing wire can be cut flush with the skin so that the residual wire retracts into the tissue.

Complications with retained epicardial pacing wires include:
1. Localized cutaneous abscess or fistula
2. Distant migration of the temporary epicardial pacing wires
3. Infective endocarditis (theoretical risk)
4. Contraindication to MRI

G. Pericardial effusion or tamponade after transvenous pacing wire/pacemaker insertion
The development of a pericardial effusion or tamponade after transvenous pacing wire/pacemaker insertion can occur if there is perforation secondary to the pacing wire. This can occur in either the right atrium or right ventricle, as both are thin-walled structures.

Clinical findings:
1. Chest discomfort, shortness of breath or evidence of pericarditis
2. Progressive hypotension and tachycardia
3. Elevated jugular venous pressure and pulsus paradoxus
4. Muffled heart sounds and pericardial rub

Diagnosis:
1. Physical signs
2. Chest x-ray: enlarged cardiac silhouette
3. Echocardiography: pericardial fluid with right ventricular diastolic collapse
4. CT scan of the chest with contrast (if patient is hemodynamically stable): examine for lead positioning and contrast extravasation which would suggest of lead perforation
5. Pacemaker interrogation: if pacemaker functions well, it is unlikely that the lead has perforated

Treatment:
Importantly, the pacing wire/pacemaker lead should not be immediately removed, as it may be "plugging the hole" and preventing further development of a pericardial effusion or tamponade. It should be removed under close observation, typically in the surgical OR.
1. IV access, telemetry, monitors (blood pressure, heart rate, oxygen saturation)
2. Volume resuscitation
3. Aspiration / Drainage: Pericardiocentesis, correcting coagulation and await 3-4 days for the hole to scar down and thrombose. Following this, lead repositioning should then be attempted.

H. Pericardial effusion or Tamponade after temporary epicardial pacing wire removal

Clinical findings:
1. Progressive hypotension and tachycardia
2. Elevated jugular venous pressure and pulsus paradoxus
3. Muffled heart sounds and pericardial rub
4. Decreased urine output

418

Diagnosis:
    6.   Physical signs
    7.   Chest x-ray: enlarged cardiac silhouette
    8.   Echocardiography: pericardial fluid with right ventricular diastolic collapse

Treatment:
    4.   IV access, telemetry, monitors (blood pressure, heart rate, oxygen saturation)
    5.   Volume resuscitation
    6.   Aspiration / Drainage: Pericardiocentesis, subxiphoid pericardial window or urgent resternotomy

Potential questions / scenarios

What is the difference between an intrinsic left bundle branch block and a paced rhythm?

The major difference is that the QRS will almost always be negative in V5-V6 with a paced rhythm.

What does it mean if my patient develops a new right bundle branch block during pacing after implantation of a permanent transvenous pacemaker?

A typical paced QRS morphology from a right ventricular lead resembles a left bundle-branch block morphology (with minor differences). However, the finding of a right bundle branch block morphology, or tall R-wave in V1, suggests left-sided pacing. This can occur if the right ventricular lead is advanced inadvertently into the coronary sinus, or the right ventricular lead is advanced through a patent foramen ovale / atrial septal defect into the left ventricle. Pacing wires in the coronary sinus are typically used for cardiac resynchronization pacing but should not be used routinely as a surrogate for right ventricular pacing, as the wire itself may dislodge and have important implications for pacemaker-dependent patients (sudden loss of capture). Pacing wires in the left ventricle due to a patent foramen ovale / atrial septal defect will also substantially increase the risk for stroke or systemic embolism. In both cases, the pacing wire will capture the left ventricle and should be repositioned.

What is the effect of paced rhythms on an ECG's ability to detect an acute myocardial infarction?

As with an intrinsic left bundle branch block, ventricular pacing results in depolarization and repolarization abnormalities that can confound the ECG's ability to detect an acute myocardial infarction. The Sgarbossa criteria is frequently referenced as a method to identify an acute myocardial infarction in patients with intrinsic left bundle branch block. Although the Sgarbossa criteria was not validated with paced QRS morphologies, it is sometimes extrapolated to patients with paced QRS morphologies. However, the Sgarbossa criteria itself is specific but not sensitive for acute myocardial infarction with concordant ST elevation >1mm having the highest specificity for acute myocardial infarction in paced rhythms. However, the absence of these findings does not rule out an acute myocardial infarction.

Postoperative patient from cardiac surgery with cardiac arrest. A code blue is called. What do you do?

Ensure adequate IV access. Assess the rhythm. The Society of Thoracic Surgeons protocol for resuscitation of patients who arrest after cardiac surgery should be followed if the patient is <10 days after surgery. For patients beyond day 10, the protocol should still be followed but a senior clinician should decide whether resternotomy is indicated. Briefly, for the following scenarios:
    1.   Ventricular fibrillation or tachycardia -> DC shock x 3 should be attempted after which basic life support should be initiated and amiodarone 300mg should be given by central venous line. The team should prepare for emergency resternotomy and continue CPR with single DC shock every 2 minutes until resternotomy.
    2.   Asystole or severe bradycardia -> if pacing wires available, external pacing should be attempted. If external pacing fails, the team should continue CPR until emergency resternotomy.

3. Pulseless electrical activity -> if the patient is paced, turn off pacing to exclude underlying ventricular fibrillation. If ventricular fibrillation, resort to ventricular fibrillation pathway. If pulseless electrical activity, the team should continue CPR until emergency resternotomy.

During this time, epinephrine should not be given unless a senior physician advises for it. If an intra-aortic balloon pump is in place, change it to pressure trigger. Examine for reversible causes for cardiac arrest including hypovolemia, hypoxia, acidosis, hypo-/hyperkalemia, hypothermia, tension pneumothorax, cardiac tamponade, pulmonary thrombosis, coronary thrombosis and toxins as per Advanced Cardiovascular Life Support algorithm.

You are called to see a patient post-permanent transvenous pacemaker insertion with a pericardial effusion with concern for ventricular lead perforation. What do you do?
Go and assess the patient. If patient is hemodynamically unstable, bedside echocardiogram can demonstrate tamponade physiology and the patient should undergo urgent pericardiocentesis or be taken immediately to the operating room. If the patient is hemodynamically stable, one should obtain a 12-lead ECG and chest x-ray to evaluate for changes in lead position. A CT scan of the chest with contrast may also be helpful when looking for lead migration or perforation with contrast extravasation. If the echocardiogram does not demonstrate tamponade physiology and the pacemaker interrogation demonstrates that the pacemaker is functioning well, then the pericardial effusion is likely due to microperforation during lead insertion and can be treated conservatively if not large.

If the patient is pacing dependent and electrocautery will be used, this can result in inappropriate inhibition of the pacemaker due to sensing of the noise from the electrocautery. Inappropriate inhibition can result in excessive bradycardia or pauses, particularly in pacemaker-dependent patients. In such cases, the pacemaker can be programmed to AOO, VOO or DOO depending on whether there is an intact atrioventricular conduction. This should be re-evaluated or re-programmed as soon as electrocautery is not needed. Another option is to place a magnet over the generator for the pacemaker- a magnet will cause the pacemaker to default to an asynchronous mode (e.g. VOO or DOO).
Utilization of bipolar cautery is preferred with short duration cautery bursts <5s allowing for >5s between bursts when using monopolar electrocautery is recommended. In addition, the electrosurgical receiving plate should be positioned so that the current pathway does not pass through or near the pacemaker. Backup equipment for urgent transcutaneous pacing, defibrillation or cardioversion should be prepared. These steps would be especially important if the surgical site is above the hip.

Do patients with permanent transvenous pacemakers or epicardial leads require endocarditis antibiotic prophylaxis for procedures?
Patients with pacemakers or defibrillators are considered negligible risk and do not require endocarditis antibiotic prophylaxis prior to procedures.

My patient has a permanent transvenous pacemaker and requires an MRI. What do I do?
The concern with MRI is that the induced currents during imaging can lead to risk of arrhythmia induction, capture threshold changes, lead dislodgement and device damage. If the patient is pacemaker dependent and the pacemaker is MRI conditional, it means that the specific MRI environment with the device with specified conditions of use does not pose a known hazard. However, many devices have an "MRI-mode" that should be turned on prior to undergoing the MRI, and most devices should be checked before and after the MRI is performed to ensure of no unanticipated programming changes.

Patients with non-MRI compatible devices include those with device/lead manufacturer mismatch, or those with simply non-compatible devices. In rare circumstances, these patients can also undergo MRI with close monitoring and a collaborative effort with radiologists. Finally, MRI is contraindicated in patients with a new pacemaker implantation (within 4-6 weeks) as this may cause dislodgement of the leads, even in MRI compatible devices. In such cases, the MRI is typically deferred until after the waiting/recovery period. However, if there are any concerns, an appropriate consultation should be obtained to determine if imaging would be reasonable.

Suggested Readings

- Reade MC. Temporary epicardial pacing after cardiac surgery: a practical review Part 1: General considerations in the management of epicardial pacing. doi:10.1111/j.1365-2044.2007.04950.x
- Reade MC. Temporary epicardial pacing after cardiac surgery: a practical review Part 2: Selection of epicardial pacing modes and troubleshooting. doi:10.1111/j.1365-2044.2007.04951.x
- Shaikhrezai K, Khorsandi M, Patronis M, Prasad S. Is it safe to cut pacing wires flush with the skin instead of removing them? 2012. doi:10.1093/icvts/ivs39
- Society of Thoracic Surgeons Task Force on Resuscitation After Cardiac Surgery T, Dunning J, Levine FRCS A, et al. The Society of Thoracic Surgeons Expert Consensus for the Resuscitation of Patients Who Arrest After Cardiac Surgery The Society of Thoracic Surgeons Task Force on Resuscitation After Cardiac Surgery*. 2017. doi:10.1016/j.athoracsur.2016.10.033
- Madhavan M, Mulpuru SK, McLeod CJ, Cha YM, Friedman PA. Advances and Future Directions in Cardiac Pacemakers: Part 2 of a 2-Part Series. J Am Coll Cardiol. 2017;69(2):211-235. doi:10.1016/j.jacc.2016.10.06
- Mulpuru SK, Madhavan M, Mcleod CJ, Cha Y-M, Friedman PA. The Present and Future State-of-The-Art Review Cardiac Pacemakers: Function, Troubleshooting, and Management Part 1 of a 2-Part Series A Brief History of Cardiac Pacing.; 2017.
- Chakravarthy M, Prabhakumar D, George A. Anaesthetic consideration in patients with cardiac implantable electronic devices scheduled for surgery. Indian J Anaesth. 2017;61(9):736-743. doi:10.4103/ija.IJA_346_17

68. MINIMALLY INVASIVE CARDIAC SURGERY

Clauden Louis, MD., Daniel Ryan Ziazadeh, MD and Peter A. Knight, MD

Concept

Minimally invasive cardiac surgery, although a very broad statement for the purposes of this chapter, describes a variety of less invasive heart surgery operations that are performed through incisions that are substantially smaller and less traumatic than the standard full sternotomy. Specialized handheld and robotic instruments are used to project the dexterity of the surgeon's hands through these small incisions.

Minimally invasive surgery is attractive to patients and surgeons for many reasons including smaller scars, shorter hospital stays, less pain, less bleeding and earlier recovery. While the absolute risk of morbidity and mortality are comparable to conventional surgery, significant differences do exist. Numerous studies and meta-analyses have shown key postoperative events favor minimally invasive approaches during mitral valve surgery including less pain, decreased bleeding, lower transfusion requirements, shorter ICU length of stay, decreased ventilator dependence, and shorter overall hospital length of stay. However, these benefits come at the expense of longer total operative, cross-clamp times and sometimes higher costs.

While other chapters of this book are devoted to the index operations described below, this chapter will provide a brief overview and non-exhaustive discussion of various minimally invasive procedures. We will review safe methods for cannulation, various cardiopulmonary bypass strategies, the selection process for these procedures, and various tips and tricks.

Minimally Invasive Aortic Valve Replacement

- Procedure can be performed via right anterior thoracotomy, usually at the 2nd intercostal space or via various hemisternotomy techniques including "J-Type", "T-Type" or upper hemisternotomy (other variations include smaller skin incision however with full sternotomy)
- Central arterial cannulation is favored via the ascending aorta; however, a vast majority perform arterial cutdown as peripheral arterial cannulation
- Venous cannulation can be performed centrally via the right atrium or peripherally via percutaneous common femoral vein approach
  - This decision is typically based on accessibly of the right atrium for cannulation
- Liberal use of pericardial stay sutures helps to expose and mobilize the aorta laterally prior to cross clamp
- It is important to have normal biventricular function when starting out in practice as the aortic cross clamp time will likely be longer
- Various myocardial protection strategies can be employed including fibrillatory arrest via systemic cooling, high potassium cardioplegia solutions such as HTK or Del Nido
- In cases of severe aortic insufficiency, a retrograde cardioplegia catheter can be placed along with left ventricular sump via the right superior pulmonary vein

Minimally Invasive Mitral Valve Repair/Replacement

- Procedure can be performed by right lateral thoracotomy, at the anterior axillary line and 4th intercostal space or robotically via 4 or 5 ports
- Lateral thoracotomy provides a direct view of the mitral valve that easily rivals even the best visualization of the annulus obtained by full sternotomy
- To facilitate additional exposure and a 3D thoracoscopic camera is used by writer's institution for all cases. This allows the entire room to see a every step of the repair or replacement.

- Through the side arm of the camera port, the operative field is flooded with CO_2 throughout the case to facilitate pneumothorax and deairing of the heart
- Peripheral cannulation is favored using either percutaneous or cutdown exposure of the femoral vessels; right internal jugular venous cannula can be added if SVC drainage is inadequate
- Once bypass has been established, a pericardiotomy is performed 5-8cm medial and parallel to the phrenic nerve
- A cross clamp is applied, however if an endoclamp is available, it can be considered due to its ease of use, ability to deliver cardioplegia, and decluttering the operative field
- Bilateral radial or brachial arterial lines and cerebral oximeters should be placed to evaluate for limb and neuro ischemia in the setting of endoclamp migration and covering of the arch vessels
- This procedure is amenable to single dose cardioplegia administration in an antegrade fashion
- An intrathoracic self-retaining left atrial retractor is used to expose the mitral valve

Minimally Invasive Tricuspid Repair/Replacement
- Other right heart operations including Mini-ASD and Mini-Myxoma excision will follow this same approach
- Procedure can be performed using the same exposure for mitral valve repair via right lateral thoracotomy, at the anterior axillary line 4th interspace, providing excellent exposure to the right atrium
- One noticeable difference is the need for bicaval cannulation either in the form of an additional SVC cannula via the right internal jugular vein or a single femoral bicaval cannula with vacuum assist
- Peripheral cannulation is favored using either percutaneous or cutdown exposure of the femoral vessels; pursestring sutures should be placed prior to seldinger cannulation to control the vessels. Axillary cannulation can be performed for patients with severe peripheral vascular disease.
- If concomitant mitral valve surgery is needed, then the mitral valve procedure should be performed first via Waterstons groove (Saundergaard). While not routinely performed, a transseptal approach can be used.

Minimally Invasive Bentall
- The success of the right mini thoracotomy approach for aortic valve surgery can translate into improved outcomes in select patients requiring aortic root replacement.
- The author's institution preferentially performs these procedures via right parasternal thoracotomy via 2nd intercostal space.
- We select patients with ascending aortic root or hemiarch pathology only. Patients need to have normal biventricular ventricular function. The maximum age of patients considered is 75. Patients require normal cerebral circulation and minimal peripheral vascular disease. Severe atherosclerosis is a relative contraindication. The author's do not recommend this approach as a redo operation.
- Cross clamp times of up to 150 minutes is acceptable in this approach.
- We recommend sufficient experience be acquired using the video assisted right mini-thoracotomy approach for aortic valve replacement prior to the initiation of a mini-thoracotomy Bentall program.
- Alternative approach is via upper hemisternotomy with T off to the right 3rd or 4th interspace.
- The author's institution performs femoral vessel cutdown and pursestring suture placement prior to Seldinger cannulation to control the vessels.

Minimally Invasive MAZE

- Procedure can be performed by right anterior axillary line 4th interspace or midway sternal notch and xiphoid. Should this be performed with concomitant mitral valve surgery, the right anterior axillary line, lateral thoracotomy, provides a direct view of the valve.
- Peripheral cannulation is preferred. The author's institution performs femoral vessel cutdown and pursestring prior to seldinger cannulation to control the vessel should bypass be required.
- Minimally invasive pitfalls include accessing posterior left atrium and the left atrial appendage
- Typically minimally invasive mitral valve setup
- See chapter 46 regarding additional MAZE procedure details

Minimally Invasive Coronary Artery Bypass Graft
- Left sided anterolateral wall revascularization
- Exposure is typically via the 4th intercostal space
- Novel techniques exist such as being combined with off-pump or PCI for hybrid for patients given varying comorbidities or concern
  - o Examples include: calcified aorta, poor LVEF, severe PVD, severe COPD, renal failure, coagulopathy, patients with transfusion issues, i.e., Jehovah's witness.
- There are many variations of minimally invasive CABG, some of which the same meaning however many of them robotic, many of them can be performed off-pump as well
  - o **TECAB** - Totally endoscopic coronary artery bypass
    - IMA takedown and coronary anastomosis done completely endoscopic
    - Can use "partial" lung ventilation
    - Can provide long length LAD
  - o **MIDCAB** - Minimally Invasive Direct Coronary Artery Bypass
    - Best for 1-2 vessel CAD using IMAs and/or PCI for hybrid with coronary anastomosis via mini-thoracotomy
    - May require "single" lung ventilation
    - Exposure may limit LAD length
- **Other Terminologies**
  - o **Robotic MIDCAB**- Robotic Minimally Invasive Direct Coronary Artery Bypass
  - o **PACAB/PortCAB** - Port-Access Coronary Artery Bypass
  - o **endoACAB**- Endoscopic Atraumatic Coronary Artery Bypass
  - o **MINICAB**- Mini-thoracotomy Coronary Artery Bypass
  - o **RCABG**- Robotic Coronary Artery Bypass Grafting
- **Placement of ports in Robotic CABG**
  - o Triangulation with camera at 4th/5th space, and two additional ports 2nd/3rd and 6th/7th anterior axillary lines with at least palm spacing between each
- Various retrospective studies have shown similar perioperative and mid-term quality outcomes amongst the various treatment strategies with minor differences in cost

	Off Pump Open CABG	TECAB	MIDCAB	HYBRID
Lesions	Multivessel	Left Sided	Isolated LAD	Multivessel
CPB	No	No	No	No
Blood Products	Less	Few	Few	Few
LOS	Long	Short	Short	Short

Pain	Yes	Less	Yes	Yes
Recovery Time	Long	Short	Short	Short
Stroke	Equivocal	Less	Less	Less

Minimally Invasive Ventricular Assist Device
- As current generations of centrifugal continuous flow LVADs have decreased in size, minimally invasive surgical approaches have become more feasible.
- Traditional paracorporeal ventricular assists devices such as the CentriMag pump have been combined with ECMO for patients in acute cardiogenic shock and eliminate the need for sternotomy and cardiopulmonary bypass, with decreased blood product utilization and bleeding events. The authors' institution employs this configuration for patients in acute cardiogenic shock.
- Intracorporeal ventricular assist devices have also begun to be implanted in a more minimally invasive fashion. The LATERAL trial demonstrated that implantation of the HVAD system via left lateral thoracotomy for the inflow and either right anterior thoracotomy or upper hemi sternotomy for the outflow was a safe and effective alternative to median sternotomy in selected patients intended for a bridge to transplant.
- The benefits of minimally invasive intracorporeal VAD implantation has also been demonstrated in the HeartMate 3 using a complete sternal sparing approach with a significantly decreased incidence of RV failure, fewer blood transfusion products, and shorter length of stay compared to traditional sternotomy.
- Standard preoperative evaluation as for traditional sternotomy should be performed. Abnormalities found on preoperative imaging including intracardiac thrombus, valvular pathology, and PFO are relative, but not absolute contraindications to this approach.
- The operative approach is described below:
  - Two surgeons should work in tandem
  - An incision inferior to the left inframammary crease at the 5th or 6th intercostal space will provide excellent exposure to the LV apex
  - The authors' favor our standard minimally invasive aortic valve exposure for the outflow graft by making an incision in the right anterior 2nd intercostal space at the midclavicular line
  - Both on and off pump techniques can be employed
    - A combination of Magnesium, Lidocaine, and Adenosine can be employed to decrease arrhythmia issues as the time of ventricular coring
  - For on-pump techniques, the authors' favor central aortic cannulation and peripheral femoral venous cannulation
- This complete sternal sparing technique is especially beneficial in the bridge to transplant patients, where the sternum is spared for future heart transplantation.

Robotic Cardiac Surgery
- Many of the above procedures can be done robotically with some variation to location and port placement and extent of robotic use for some, most or all portions.
- Benefits include decreased pain, more rapid return to work, diminished blood loss and reduced length of hospitalization when compared with a traditional sternotomy.
- For mitral valve surgery, studies have shown equivalent long-term mortality and freedom from recurrent mitral regurgitation compared to traditional sternotomy and other minimally invasive techniques.

425

- Additional surgical procedures include CABG, Mitral Valve, Tricuspid Valve, Aortic Valve, Atrial Fibrillation, Pericardiectomy, HoCM, Lead placement and limited experience in Congenital

Cannulation Strategies
- Central Aortic
  - Preferred when possible for aortic valve cases
  - Can be performed for both upper hemi-sternotomy and right anterior thoracotomy
  - Pericardials bring the aorta closer to the incision
  - The aorta is typically cannulated by Seldinger technique
  - May sometimes hinder exposure of operative field
  - Following CT imaging, some centers use hemisternotomy for leftward aorta and right anterior thoracotomy for midline aorta as a right anterior thoracotomy on a very leftward aorta may have increase difficulty
- Femoral Artery
  - Preferred for mitral and tricuspid valve cases
  - Provides retrograde perfusion
  - Use of the Endo-Clamp Occlusion Balloon declutters the operating field and allows for administration of cardioplegia by ascending aortic positioning to provide antegrade cardioplegia and root vent, must carefully position so arch vessel perfusion is not compromised with migration
  - Small vessels may require Dacron graft anastomosis
  - Must be mindful of distal limb ischemia, although this usually occurs without sequela during short operations
  - Percutaneous cannulation is amenable to percutaneous closure devices however cutdown allows for definitive access and control of the vessel(s)
- Axillary Artery
  - Provides antegrade perfusion at a peripheral site
  - Dacron graft anastomosis can provide for easy decannulation and allows for bidirectional flow
    - Right upper extremity ischemia is rare due to the abundance of collateral vessels
- Femoral Vein
  - Percutaneous femoral venous cannula with ultrasound guidance should be placed at the level of the SVC/RA junction under TEE bicaval view
    - Relative contraindication is the presence of IVC filter or known IVC occlusion
  - After decannulation percutaneously, 20-minute manual pressure following skin suture (figure eight or "U" suture) will tamponade the venostomy and provide hemostasis given ow pressure flow
- Internal Jugular Vein
  - Seldinger technique by ultrasound guidance
  - After decannulation percutaneously, acquire hemostasis by skin suture (figure eight or "U" suture)
- Central Venous (SVC)
  - For right atrial isolation the SVC can be cannulated.
  - The cannula preferentially can be tunneled through an additional tunnel incision to avoid clutter. This incision can later be used for chest tube.

Clinical Scenario
A 53-year-old male presents to the structural valve clinic with known bicuspid aortic valve and severe aortic insufficiency. Echocardiogram reveals a moderately dilated left ventricle with a mildly reduced left ventricle ejection fraction. His ascending aorta measures 4.7cm

426

and has grown 0.6cm from his last imaging a year ago. His cardiologist has discussed less invasive approaches and the patient is adamant that he does not want his "chest cracked". What is your plan and approach for this patient?

Differential
Aortic Stenosis, Bicuspid Aortic Valve, Ascending Aortic Aneurysm, Congenital Aortopathy

History and Physical
Any patient who is being evaluated for minimally invasive Cardiac Surgery needs to have a comprehensive system-based history and physical to identify standard STS risk factors including but not limited to history of stroke, renal disease, coronary lesions, respiratory problems, bleeding disorders, or peripheral vascular disease. The patient should be evaluated for minimally invasive Bentall procedure.

Absolute Contraindications
- Extensive atherosclerotic plaque
- Severe aortoiliac disease
- Porcelain aorta
- Severe chronic obstructive lung disease
- Need for concomitant coronary artery bypass grafting

Relative Contraindications
- Obesity
- Severe Pectus Excavatum
- Previous Right Thoracotomy
- Breast augmentation
- Multiple repair/concomitant procedures
- Insufficient experience with right anterior thoracotomy approach
- Poor LV (will not tolerate longer clamp time)
- Severe scoliosis with leftward mediastinal shift

Tests
- Biochemical Profile (CMP, LFTs)
- CBC
- ECHO (TTE/TEE)
- CXR
- Coronary Angiography
- EKG (Baseline)
- RHC if concern for pulmonary hypertension
- CT Chest/Abdomen/Pelvis with IV contrast if possible
- Pulmonary Function Tests
- Carotid Duplex Imaging

Index scenario (additional information)
"Preoperative workup demonstrates that the patient is an appropriate candidate for minimally invasive surgery. Genetic testing reveals no evidence of congenital aortopathy. The patient is consented for minimally invasive Bentall procedure. What are the operative steps?"
The patient is intubated via single lumen endotracheal tube. Anesthesia lines and TEE monitoring is placed after induction. The patient is prepped from above the clavicles to the knees bilaterally. A 5 cm incision for planned right anterior thoracotomy at the second intercostal space. The pectoralis muscle is spread to expose the intercostal muscles. The right pleural space is entered lateral to the right internal thoracic artery (RITA). The RITA is then ligated with ties and clips. A laparotomy pad is placed in the chest to compress the lung. A

427

soft tissue wound protector and a mini intercostal retractor expose the mediastinum. A small 5mm incision is made for the camera port in the second interspace lateral to the main incision. Carbon dioxide is infused to reduce the risk of retained intracardiac air.

The pericardium is opened and extended toward the pericardial reflection to the aorta. Pericardial stay sutures are placed. A right femoral artery and vein cutdown is performed. The femoral artery and vein are cannulated via Seldinger technique. 25F venous cannula is positioned over wire into the SVC with TEE guidance. 18F arterial cannula is advanced over wire that has positioned in the descending thoracic aorta under TEE guidance. Cardiopulmonary bypass with vacuum assist is initiated and the patient is cooled to 18*C.
An LV sump is placed in the right superior pulmonary vein to vent the left ventricle. Through the wound a fogarty cross clamp is applied. An antegrade cardioplegia needle is inserted and the aorta is cross clamped with a combination of adenosine and 2 liters of HTK cardioplegia solution to enable approximately 2 hours of cross clamp time.

The cardioplegia needle is removed and the aortotomy is made through the needle insertion site. The aorta is transected and retracted cephalad with silk suture. Commissural stay sutures are placed. The leaflets are excised, and the annulus is debrided and sized. Once cooled to 18*C, the patient is placed in Trendelenburg and circulatory arrest is commenced with cerebral oximetry monitoring. The cross clamp is removed, and the remaining segment of ascending aorta is resected up to the level of the innominate artery. Valsalva graft is used, and the distal anastomosis is completed using 4-0 propylene. The head vessels, arch, and graft are then de-aired, and the aortic graft is clamped. CPB is then re-established and warming is commenced.

The root is then exposed, and the remaining portion of the aorta and sinuses are resected. We construct the coronary buttons and retract them using stay sutures. The inflow suture line is created using 2-0 non-absorbable braided sutures. The valve is seated and secured with titanium fasteners. Coronary holes are fashioned in the graft with scissors. The left main coronary anastomosis is then completed with 5-0 polypropylene followed by the right main. The graft to graft anastomosis is completed in a running fashion using 4-0 propylene and de-airing is performed. Glue is used on all the anastomoses. The left ventricle and ascending aorta are de-aired, and the cross clamp is removed at low flow. The anesthesiologist uses TEE to meticulously evaluate appropriate de-airing, ventricular function, and prosthetic valve function. CPB is then discontinued. The second rib is then secured to the sternum with FiberWire. Intercostal nerve blocks are performed under direct visualization with bupivacaine (0.25%) with epinephrine. The femoral vessels are decannulated and purse string sutures are tied down. Distal pulses are checked, two drains are placed, and the wound is closed in layers.

Potential alternative scenarios
The same patient is taken to the operating room for the above index procedure. Cannulation is performed peripherally via the right femoral vein and centrally via the ascending aorta. On initiation of bypass, the arterial line pressure is in excess of 350 mmHg and the arterial pump flow is 1 L/minute. What is your concern and next best step?
Quickly evaluate the arterial line for kinks or extrinsic compression, the depth of the arterial cannula in the aorta, visually inspect the aorta, and evaluate with TEE for findings of aortic dissection. If TEE confirms the diagnosis of aortic dissection, prompt termination of bypass is crucial to successful management of this severe complication. Alternate arterial cannulation should be performed via the femoral or axillary artery and continue systemic cooling to 18*C to achieve deep hypothermic circulatory arrest. Plan for replacement of the ascending aorta and proximal arch if appropriate. The aortic valve is replaced once arch reconstruction is complete while rewarming.

Potential questions/alternative scenarios

428

A 49-year-old male with history of percutaneous PDA ligation and bicuspid aortic valve with severe aortic insufficiency is scheduled for aortic valve replacement. He vehemently refuses a mechanical valve because he wants to avoid life-long anticoagulation. Following right thoracotomy for aortic valve replacement, a large right atrium is viewed, obscuring the aorta. What additional maneuvers can be done to improve exposure.

For the right thoracotomy, additional pericardial stay sutures are necessary to lateralize the aorta and improve exposure. One can also disarticulate an additional rib involving the same 2nd intercostal space or consider going on bypass to empty right heart.

What is your cardioprotection strategy?

Retrograde cardioplegia may be very difficult from the right thoracotomy incision. Antegrade cardioplegia at the root in the setting of severe aortic insufficiency is not a good idea as well. Ostial perfusion using handheld cannula and cooling is more appropriate in this setting.

Following implantation of the bioprosthetic valve you attempt to re-dose cardioplegia by ostial catheters however you can no longer see the left or right coronary ostium. What is the next step in the management of this patient?

There is great concern that should the procedure continue as planned, this patient may have coronary ischemia due to obstruction of the coronary ostium. One must avoid compromise of the coronary artery by being sure the annular sutures are well below the coronary artery and the valve is seated on the annulus. In the scenario above, the first step is to probe with right angle or cystic clamp.

There must be a low threshold to convert to median sternotomy. A sternotomy allows for retrograde cardioplegia and assessment of the coronary ostium to verify as to whether an obstruction is present. If there is any doubt, and the operation proceeds in a minimally invasive fashion, the valve should be removed to facilitate redosing the cardioplegia via the coronary ostium and to ensure there is no obstruction post reimplantation.

Potential questions/alternative scenarios

A 62-year-old man with severe mitral regurgitation in the setting of anterior leaflet prolapse is scheduled to undergo minimally invasive mitral valve repair with ring. What are the operative steps?

Femoral artery and vein cutdown are performed by a 2–3 cm transverse incision in the right groin. Retrograde perfusion is performed through the right femoral artery and venous cannula is placed in right femoral vein with the tip in the SVC.

A right lateral mini-thoracotomy is performed simultaneously 4 cm in length in the 4th intercostal space. A soft tissue retractor is utilized to protect the incision and spread tissue. A chitwood or cygnet aortic cross-clamp is introduced bluntly after a small incision is made in the inferior to the lateral thoracotomy. The camera port is then introduced bluntly following a similar incision and CO2 is flooded into the field via the side port. A left ventricular vent is placed in the right superior pulmonary vein. Alternatively, a drop pump sucker can be placed through the left atriotomy or the wound directly into one of the pulmonary veins.

Antegrade cardioplegia is administered directly into the aortic root following cross clamp. A left atrial retractor is used to expose the mitral valve. The valve is assessed and repaired. Annular sutures are placed using shafted instruments and the annuloplasty ring is deployed. After satisfactory valve competency testing, the left atrium is closed. Following conclusion of the procedure, deairing is performed via the left ventricle vent and cardioplegia site.

During a mitral valve repair what is the difference between a cross clamp and endoballoon?

When a crossclamp is used, antegrade cardioplegia through the aortic root is usually preferred, which introduces a potential site of bleeding and should be investigated post-procedure as you would for an open surgical procedure. If an endoballoon is used, antegrade cardioplegia is delivered through the port-access catheter and there is no cannulation of the aortic root at all.

Prior to administering protamine, a new severe aortic regurgitation is noted on transesophageal echocardiography. What is the next step in this management?
There is concern that a deep suture has involved aortic valve leaflet tissue. This suture will have to be removed. The location of this stitch is likely at the left and non-coronary cusp of the aortic valve at the aortic-mitral curtain.

The patient undergoes an uneventful mitral valve repair with use of root antegrade cardioplegia, cross clamp and femoral artery and vein cutdown however, on post-operative day one, the patient presents with a decrease in cardiac index to 1.7 from 2.2, and a slight increase in central venous pressure and remains tachycardic despite volume resuscitation. His chest tube output has substantially decreased since yesterday. What is the concerning diagnosis of this patient?
This patient has concern for cardiac tamponade. It is important to investigate further with echocardiography and return to the OR for evacuation of hemopericardium if necessary.

What if the patient undergoes an uneventful mitral valve repair with use of root antegrade cardioplegia, cross clamp and femoral artery and vein cut down however, on post-operative day zero patient presents with decrease in cardiac index 1.7 to 2.2, decrease in central venous pressure and remains tachycardic despite volume resuscitation. His chest tube output has substantially increased since yesterday. What is the concerning diagnosis of this patient?
This patient's findings are concerning for hemorrhagic shock. The patient will require return to the operating room for re-exploration of bleeding to prevent exsanguination. Given the expertise of the surgeon, the bleed can be re-explored through the minimally invasive incision, however a median sternotomy should be preferentially performed.

Pitfalls
- Aortic dissection
- Intrathoracic bleeding with post-operative exploration consider median sternotomy
- Retrograde dissection s/p femoral cannulation

69. CATHETER-BASED APPROACHES TO STRUCTURAL HEART DISEASE
Jatin Anand, MD and Adam Williams, MD
Concept
- Understand TAVR workup, procedural technique, common pitfalls, and surgical management
- Understand indications and limitations of transcatheter balloon therapies for aortic and mitral valve disease
- Understand indications for percutaneous closure of patent foramen ovale in cryptogenic stroke
- Review role for percutaneous technologies in mitral and tricuspid valve disease

Chief complaint
"An 88-year-old female with a history of severe aortic stenosis (AS) presents with worsening fatigue and shortness of breath (SOB). Other past medical history is significant for breast cancer with prior left modified mastectomy and adjuvant radiation. She is otherwise independent in her activities of daily living and wishes to pursue intervention."

Differential
Aortic stenosis, coronary artery disease, heart failure (HF), arrhythmia, primary pulmonary disease, pulmonary embolism, recurrent malignancy

History and Physical
Focused history to elicit risk factors for mortality in severe AS: angina, syncope, and HF. Additionally, evaluate for risk factors for each differential diagnosis: coronary artery disease (myocardial infarction or prior percutaneous coronary interventions (PCI), atherosclerosis,

family history); pulmonary disease (asthma, chronic obstructive pulmonary disease, smoking, occupational exposures, pneumonia); arrhythmia (history of atrial fibrillation, palpitations); and cancer history. Baseline functional status, neurological or orthopedic disorders, and other signs of frailty should be noted.

Physical exam should include focused heart and lung evaluation to elicit murmurs, arrhythmias, pulmonary abnormalities, and peripheral edema. A focused peripheral vascular examination should also be performed, noting carotid, radial, femoral, and pedal pulse characteristics.

Tests

- *Chest x-ray-* PA and lateral radiograph to evaluate cardiac contour, pulmonary lesions, pleural effusion, cardiac and vascular calcification
- *Electrocardiogram-* evaluate for baseline arrhythmia, conduction abnormality such as bundle branch block, and evidence of prior infarction
- *Labs -* complete blood count and metabolic panel to evaluate for hematologic, infectious, electrolyte and renal abnormalities, as well as brain natriuretic peptide to evaluate HF
- *Pulmonary function testing-* Severe disease is indicated if either forced expiratory volume in 1 second (FEV1) or diffusion capacity of lung for carbon monoxide (DLCO) are < 50% predicted. Oxygen dependence is another marker of severe lung disease.
- *Transthoracic echocardiogram-* Usually the first test obtained.
  - When LV function is normal, severe aortic stenosis confirmed by valve area <1cm^2, peak velocity >4m/s, or mean gradient >40mmHg.
  - If LV function is severely reduced, obtain dobutamine stress echo with severe AS confirmed if maximum jet velocity rises >4m/s while AVA remains <1 cm^2.
  - Note aortic regurgitation, other valvular pathology, ventricular systolic and diastolic function, and estimate right-sided pulmonary pressures.
- *Three-dimensional transesophageal echo-* can be used to further evaluate possible cardiac pathology as well as accurately assess aortic annulus.
- *Heart catheterization-*
  - Right heart catheterization evaluates filling pressures, cardiac index, and degree of pulmonary hypertension.
  - Left heart catheterization is recommended in all patients undergoing transcatheter valve replacement workup as coronary artery disease is common in this patient population. Coronary angiography should be performed with possible percutaneous coronary intervention (PCI) performed when indicated. Crossing the aortic valve is not routinely performed unless there are discrepancies between the echocardiographic findings and the patient's clinical presentation. If performed, aortic and left ventricular pressures are simultaneously obtained.
- *Multidetector Computed Tomography (MDCT)-* "CT TAVR Protocol," essential to plan vascular access, transcatheter heart valve (THV) sizing, and assessing the aortic root. MDCT allows assessment of tortuosity, diameter, and degree of calcification of the peripheral vasculature.

Index scenario (additional information)

Chest xray reveals enlarged cardiac silhouette and diffuse calcification of the ascending aorta. EKG shows normal sinus rhythm. PFTs reveal FEV1 25% and DLCO 30%. Echocardiogram shows severe calcific AS (mean gradient 70 mmHg and AVA 0.6cm^2), no other valvular abnormalities and reduced ventricular function (EF 30%). LHC shows no significant coronary disease. MDCT reveals diffuse calcifications of the aortic valve and ascending aorta. The descending aorta appears normal with minor calcific disease. Iliofemoral vessels are patent with minimal tortuosity or calcification, lacking aneurysmal segments, and are at least 6mm bilaterally.

Treatment/management

Given this patient's pulmonary disease, prior chest radiation, ascending aortic calcification, reduced ventricular function, and advanced age, she has significant surgical risk and would be best managed with a percutaneous intervention.

Indications for TAVR (2017 AHA/ACC Focused Update of Valvular Heart Disease):

- Symptomatic patients with severe AS and a prohibitive risk for surgical AVR (SAVR) who have a predicted post-TAVR survival greater than 12 months. (Class Ia)
- Symptomatic patients with severe AS and high risk for SAVR, depending on patient-specific procedural risks, values, and preferences. (Class Ia)
- Reasonable alternative to SAVR for symptomatic patients with severe AS and an intermediate surgical risk, depending on patient-specific procedural risks, values, and preferences. (Class IIa)
- Note: The FDA has recently approved TAVR for low risk patients. It is important to assess patient anatomy (bicuspid morphology, degree of valve calcification) when considering TAVR in low risk patients.

Additionally, all patients must be evaluated by a Heart Valve Team:

- For patients being considered for TAVR or SAVR, a heart valve team consisting of an integrated, multidisciplinary group of healthcare professionals with expertise in valvular heart disease, cardiac imaging, interventional cardiology, cardiac anesthesia, and cardiac surgery should collaborate to provide optimal patient care. (Class Ic)

This patient was evaluated by the heart valve team and determined to be at high risk for SAVR.

Operative risk assessment may be performed using the Society of Thoracic Surgeons (STS) and/or the TransVascular Therapeutics (TVT) risk scores. It is also important to evaluate for frailty and to consider other comorbidities that may not be represented in the risk profiling tools, such as liver failure and pulmonary hypertension. Mortality risk is generally used to classify patients into risk categories. These categories and the major US clinical trials are noted below:

- Inoperable or Extreme Risk: >15% (PARTNER 1B, CoreValve Extreme Risk)
- High Risk: >8% (PARTNER 1A, CoreValve High Risk)
- Intermediate Risk: 4-8% (PARTNER 2, SURTAVI)
- Low Risk: <4% (PARTNER 3, Evolut Low Risk)

Preoperative planning

Once deemed an appropriate candidate, the heart valve team plans transcatheter heart valve (THV) type and size as well as optimal route for vascular access.

- *THV type* is broadly categorized as balloon expandable or self-expanding. Currently approved balloon expandable valves include the Edwards SAPIEN 3 and SAPIEN Ultra. Currently approved self-expanding valves have supra-annular leaflet position and include the Medtronic Evolut and Evolut PRO.
- *Annular size* is determined using multiple imaging modalities, with MDCT and 3D-TEE being the most accurate in assessing annular diameter. The virtual aortic annular plane, which extends from the lowest attachment sites of each of the three aortic cusps, is measured in mid-systole.
- *Vascular access* options include peripheral (femoral, subclavian/axillary, carotid), direct aortic, transcaval, and transapical. Femoral access for TAVR is preferred, as subgroup analyses of clinical trials and meta analyses have demonstrated better outcomes than alternative (nontransfemoral) access. Smaller delivery devices have increased the rate of transfemoral access from approximately 50% to 95%. Vessel sizes greater than 5mm without extreme tortuosity or extensive calcium burden are typically feasible for transfemoral approach.

Pros/Cons in Aortic THV Choices

432

Balloon Expandable Valve

Pros:
- o Catheter delivery system can be flexed, allowing for better alignment of valve in patients with steep annular angle
- o Lower profile of stent frame, allowing for easier access to coronary arteries if possible future PCI may be needed

Cons:
- o Cannot be recaptured or repositioned after deployment

Self-Expandable Valve

Pros:
- o Valve can be recaptured and redeployed
- o Does not require rapid pacing for deployment
- o Has an in-line sheath

Cons:
- o Large stent frame may make future access to coronary arteries difficult
- o Delivery system is not flexible, therefore, not optimal valve choice for patients with steep annular angle

TAVR Operative steps

- Confirm heart valve size and vascular access sites based on imaging
- Obtain vascular access for delivery of the valve
- Place transvenous right ventricular pacing catheter
- Insert THV delivery sheath
- Place diagnostic pigtail catheter at the non-coronary cusp (for self-expanding valves) or right coronary cusp (for balloon expanding valves)
- Using coplanar view, cross the aortic valve and obtain hemodynamics
- Advance and properly position the transcatheter valve
- For the self-expanding Corevalve Evolut, assess placement at 2/3 deployment, at which point it may still be recaptured and repositioned
- Deploy valve using rapid pacing to reduce cardiac output
- Assess post-deployment hemodynamics, evaluate TEE and obtain arteriogram
- Remove device and sheath, and perform vascular closure

Potential questions/ alternative scenarios

During workup, the patient is found to have bicuspid aortic valve disease. How is this best managed?

Bicuspid aortic disease is an area of ongoing investigation and requires meticulous planning if TAVR is being considered. No randomized data exists but a number of case series demonstrate safe use of TAVR in bicuspid disease. Challenges include appropriate sizing due to a more elliptical shaped annulus, higher risk of paravalvular leak, and higher rate of permanent pacemaker requirement. Recent data also suggests higher incidence of stroke in patients undergoing TAVR for bicuspid valve disease. The gold standard remains SAVR +/- aortic root replacement.

The patient is found to have mixed severe aortic stenosis and 3+ aortic regurgitation. How does this affect management?

Isolated aortic insufficiency (AI) is a contraindication to current TAVR technology. The primary reason is that the lack of calcification may not support the valve as the calcium allows anchoring of the valve in the aortic root. This patient may still be able to have TAVR in setting of mixed AS/AI as long as there is calcium deposition on the valve.

What intraoperative complications should surgeons be prepared for during TAVR and how are they managed?

It is important to note that most intraoperative complications can be prevented by meticulous preoperative planning and excellent communication between team members, particularly with pre-procedural "huddle." Surgeons should always be prepared for catastrophic situations.

Vascular injury, coronary obstruction, paravalvular leak, annular rupture, and ventricular perforation are some of catastrophic complications one should prepare for.

- *Vascular complications* can often be predicted by careful evaluation of arterial calcification, tortuosity, and dimensions on preoperative imaging. Intraoperative angiography is the ideal test to confirm vascular injury (perforation, dissection or stenosis). Management of iatrogenic aortic dissection is discussed elsewhere. For femoral access complications, the pigtail catheter at the aortic root can be repositioned just above the aortic bifurcation, or an Omni catheter can be placed into the contralateral femoral artery. Management may include endovascular techniques (angioplasty, stenting) or open cutdown for repair.

- *Coronary obstruction* can usually be predicted with careful evaluation of MDCT. Low coronary or sinus height (<10mm), small sinotubular junction, narrow sinus of Valsalva (<30mm), and valve-in-valve procedures are risk factors that should prompt careful planning and preparedness. Avoiding oversized valves, considering recapturable self-expanding valves, and wire placement into coronary ostia prior to valve deployment can mitigate risk. Coronary obstruction can cause hypotension, arrhythmia, ST segment elevation, or cardiac arrest and immediate intraoperative angiography remains the diagnostic modality of choice. Coronary stents may be deployed if a wire is already in place, but in the face of hemodynamic compromise mechanical support may be the most prudent first step. If coronary stenting is not possible, perform sternotomy and attempt resection of obstructing calcium at the coronary ostium or proceed with coronary artery bypass grafting.

- *Paravalvular leak* (PVL) has become less frequent with newer THVs. Risk factors include severe calcification of the LVOT, annulus or leaflets as well as bicuspid aortic valves. PVL is assessed after valve deployment and if significant PVL is present, the first step is balloon post dilatation. If this fails, a valve-in-valve procedure may help. Ultimately, surgery may be necessary if the patient is a reasonable candidate.

- *Annular rupture* is a rare complication that is associated with the use of oversized or balloon expandable valves, aggressive post-dilatation, previous mitral valve prosthesis, and severe calcification of the LVOT, annulus, or leaflet bases. Acute hypotension is usually encountered. TEE may demonstrate a new pericardial effusion, aortic dissection, or aortic root hematoma (which may compress a coronary artery). Emergent surgical intervention is indicated if the patient is a candidate. Occasionally placement of a second balloon expandable THV in a more ventricular position may seal off the LVOT annular junction.

- *Ventricular perforation* is rare, mostly iatrogenic, and commonly caused by wire or catheter handling in the left ventricle and temporary pacing wire handling in the right ventricle. Immunosuppression and connective tissue disorders place patients at higher risk. Typically, hypotension with new pericardial effusion will point to the diagnosis, and pericardiocentesis demonstrating blood confirms it. Mechanical support should be used if the patient is unstable. If the perforation is on the right side, conservative management with drainage, reversal of anticoagulation and monitoring may be all that is required. For left sided perforations, primary surgical repair is usually necessary.

After successful TAVR, the patient is noted to have atrial and ventricular dyssynchrony. How is this best managed? Are other arrhythmias common?

Conduction abnormalities are an area of ongoing concern as some data suggests decreased long term survival in those requiring a permanent pacemaker (PPM). New left bundle branch block is the most common conduction abnormality, although complete heart block can also occur immediately after valve deployment. Self-expandable valves, prolonged PR interval, and preexisting right bundle branch block (RBBB) are risk factors for PPM implantation. It is our practice to schedule a temp-perm pacemaker prior to TAVR in patients with RBBB or prolonged PR interval, which can be converted to a PPM postoperatively, if necessary.

434

New onset atrial fibrillation is another relatively common arrhythmia which increases the risk of stroke and systemic embolism. Risk factors include age, heart failure, nontransfemoral access, and balloon post dilation.

The patient awakens from their procedure with facial droop and hemiparesis.
Clinically apparent stroke complicates TAVR in about 2% of cases (TVT registry), although subclinical lesions are seen far more frequently by diffusion-weighted MRI in both TAVR and SAVR patients. Early stroke accounts for about half of cases and are due to procedural complications, while late strokes are due to atrial fibrillation or subclinical valve thrombosis. Cerebral protection devices and improved anticoagulation protocols are being studied.

A patient with prior bioprosthetic aortic valve replacement presents with severe recurrent symptomatic stenosis. The patient is a poor operative candidate for SAVR. What options are available and what considerations are important?
Valve-in-valve (ViV) TAVR is well described. Although no data is available from randomized trials, the Valve-in-valve International Data registry (VIVID) demonstrates 1-year survival up to 90% depending on indication. The vast majority of ViV TAVR has been performed in the setting of prior surgical heart valve (SHV) implant. SHV leaflets dictate the true internal diameter (TID), while the outer stent diameter dictates the reported nominal size. The TID of two valves by the same manufacturer may be different despite the same nominal size. Therefore, meticulous planning is necessary prior to selecting a ViV THV and to maximize the possibility for procedural success. A ViV smartphone app has been developed that offers fluoroscopic still frames and ex-vivo images for all SHVs and is useful in preprocedural planning. Common pitfalls during ViV implantation include coronary obstruction, THV under-expansion resulting in high gradients, and malposition of the deployed THV.

Alternative Scenarios:
A 92-year-old female presents in cardiogenic shock requiring intubation. It is determined that she has critical AS and she is deemed to be inoperable. What options exist?
TAVR in emergent settings is possible, but due to the need for complex imaging to plan an appropriate procedure, a potentially more reasonable option is percutaneous balloon aortic valvotomy (BAV) as a bridge to future intervention. BAV does not substitute for valve replacement in patients with symptomatic AS because restenosis will occur within 6 to 12 months in most cases. The natural history and long-term outcome are not improved by BAV, although short term survival and early symptomatic improvement is reported. Because there is significant risk (10-20%) for major complications, BAV is utilized rarely and SAVR or TAVR are the treatments of choice for symptomatic calcific AS.

A 40-year-old patient with a history of rheumatic fever presents with worsening dyspnea and is found to have isolated severe mitral stenosis. What considerations are important and what percutaneous options exist?
The 2017 ACC/AHA guidelines state that percutaneous mitral balloon valvuloplasty (PMBV) is preferred over surgery in symptomatic patients with severe MS (valve area ≤ 1.5 cm^2) if the valve morphology is favorable, there is no left atrial thrombus, and no moderate to severe MR (Class I). In asymptomatic patients, PMBV is indicated in severe MS with new onset atrial fibrillation (Class IIb) or very severe MS (≤ 1 cm^2, Class IIa) if the previously stated echocardiographic criteria are met.
The likelihood of successful PMBV is assessed using the Wilkins score, which is the sum of four echocardiographic factors each graded 0 to 4 (leaflet rigidity, leaflet thickening, leaflet calcification, subvalvular thickening) with a maximum score of 16. A score ≤ 8 predicts favorable outcome, while higher scores indicate increasing severity of disease and lower likelihood of successful valvotomy.

An 82-year-old man with Class IV HF is found to have severe primary mitral regurgitation and is deemed a poor surgical candidate. What percutaneous options exist? What about in secondary mitral regurgitation?

Transcatheter mitral valve repair (TMVr) is currently performed using the approved MitraClip (MC) device (Abbott), which is based on surgical edge-to-edge Alfieri valvuloplasty technique. The MC device is delivered transseptally and has two grasping arms, one for each leaflet. Application of a single MC device results in a double orifice valve with reduction of MR. Multiple clips are often necessary.

Indication for MC use in chronic primary MR is for those with prohibitive surgical risk and severe symptoms (NYHA Class III to IV) despite optimal medical therapy (Class IIb). This indication is based on the EVEREST II trial, which randomized patients to MC or surgery for both primary and secondary MR. Although MC showed significant reduction in MR, the primary composite endpoint was inferior to surgery. However, subgroup analysis revealed that high risk patients (STS mortality >12%) who received MC had an observed 30-day mortality rate of <5%. Furthermore, 1-year survival was >77%, freedom from mitral valve surgery was 98%, and an overall improvement was seen in readmission rates for HF, NYHA functional class scores, and echocardiographic characteristics of ventricular function.

Subsequent COAPT and MITRA-FR trials evaluated MC versus medical management alone in patients with moderate to severe MR and HF. The COAPT trial demonstrated significantly reduced mortality and fewer rehospitalizations at 2 years, as well as improved quality of life. The MITRA-FR trial showed no significant difference in mortality or rehospitalization at 1 year. The COAPT trial was larger, had longer follow up, and enrolled patients with more significant disease, which may account for the disparate findings. The MC device was approved for *secondary* MR based on the positive trial results.

Other notable devices currently under investigation include the repositionable and recapturable edge-to-edge PASCAL device (Edwards), the Cardioband (Edwards) and Millipede (Boston Scientific) annuloplasty devices, and the NeoChord DS 1000 (NeoChord) and Harpoon TDS-5 (Edwards) chordal repair devices.

What are the current roles and challenges in transcatheter mitral valve replacement (TMVR)?

Unlike TAVR for calcific aortic valve stenosis, TMVR has advanced slowly due to the complexity of the mitral valve apparatus (annulus, leaflets, chordae, papillary muscles, and ventricle) and limitations in patient eligibility. Patients with degenerative mitral valve disease are often younger, have very low surgical mortality rates, and experience excellent long-term outcomes after surgical repair, making immature percutaneous therapies harder to advance. Additionally, biologic mitral prostheses have poorer durability and are not ideal for many younger patients. Finally, many patients with MR have associated tricuspid valve disease and atrial fibrillation, which are better addressed using surgical techniques. For these reasons, most TMVR devices are currently focused on treating functional MR in patients with poor surgical candidacy.

There are unique challenges with TMVR compared to TAVR. The larger mitral annulus requires sizeable prostheses and therefore larger delivery systems, which are currently designed for transapical access. Transfemoral iterations using transseptal delivery, often requiring subsequent ASD closure, are under development. There is higher risk for paravalvular leak due to a D-shaped annulus and less calcification than is typically seen with calcific AS (other than in cases of severe mitral annular calcification). Finally, there is substantial risk for new left ventricular outflow tract obstruction (LVOTO), which can be predicted by a small aortomitral angle, long anterior MV leaflet, or thick interventricular septum. LVOTO has been one of the main reasons for patient exclusion in ongoing clinical trials. Notable mitral THVs currently under investigation include the Tendyne (Abbott), Intrepid (Medtronic), CardiAQ (Edwards), and Caisson (Caisson) valves.

What is the current role for transcatheter interventions in tricuspid valve disease?

Most tricuspid regurgitation (TR) is functional, and repair or replacement is often performed at the time of left-sided cardiac surgery. An independent association between severe TR and mortality has been demonstrated in those with HF, and yet it remains unclear if correction of severe TR may have prognostic benefit. Current experience with transcatheter tricuspid valve

436

interventions (TTVI) has therefore evolved around patients with advanced HF who are poor surgical candidates.

To better understand TTVI, an international, multicenter TriValve registry was developed to record interventions with all devices. Most cases have involved off-label use of the MitraClip (Abbott) device in the tricuspid position. Other technologies include annuloplasty devices, such as Trialign (Mitralign Inc), TriCinch (4Tech Cardio Ltd), and Cardioband (Edwardd), as well as the FORMA spacer (Edwards), an implantable transvalvular prosthetic that improves leaflet coaptation. Transcatheter tricuspid valve replacement (TTVR) has been performed in the setting of prior surgical tricuspid valve replacement (valve-in-valve) or repair (valve-in-ring). Caval implants of THVs, including the Sapien 3 (Edwards), have been performed in order to reduce hepatic, abdominal and peripheral venous congestion. Further data is necessary to delineate future roles for TTVI.

A 55-year-old man suffered an ischemic stroke. An extensive workup revealed large right cortical brain infarct and absence of arrhythmias, potential cardioembolic sources, or large vessel disease. A large patent foramen ovale (PFO) was noted on TTE with positive bubble-study and right-to-left shunting. What considerations are important for percutaneous PFO device closure?

Cryptogenic stroke or transient ischemic attack (TIA) is a diagnosis of exclusion, considered after ruling out lacunar (small, non-cortical) infarct, non-ischemic brain lesion, large vessel stenosis or occlusion in the infarct territory, proximal aortic vasculopathy, atrial fibrillation, and other potential cardioembolic sources. Paradoxical embolism through a PFO with evidence of right to left shunt (positive "bubble study") may be considered as the etiology when no other explanation is found.

Early randomized data failed to show benefit for percutaneous device closure over anticoagulation alone in patients with cryptogenic stroke and PFO. However, subsequent meta-analysis and more stringent randomized trials showed fewer recurrent strokes after PFO closure. This led to approval of the Amplatzer PFO occluder device in 2016 in patients aged 18-60 years after cryptogenic stroke with a PFO.

TTE is often the first test but TEE should be obtained in patients considered for percutaneous device closure. Atrial septal anatomy should be carefully evaluated, including thickness of rims around the PFO, presence of atrial septal aneurysm, and whether concomitant atrial septal defect(s) are present. Rarely, surgical closure is necessary when anatomy is prohibitive or if another indication for cardiac surgery is present.

PFO device closure is performed in the cath lab under fluoroscopic and echocardiographic guidance. A transfemoral venous approach is used. After administration of unfractionated heparin, a wire is advanced to the right atrium, across the PFO into the left atrium. A stiff guidewire is exchanged and advanced into a pulmonary vein. A balloon may be used to size the PFO, typically selecting a device twice the diameter of the balloon. The device is advanced and the left-sided occluder is deployed first, followed by the right. The device is released, and TEE is used to evaluate for residual shunting. Complications are rare, with new onset atrial fibrillation being the most common adverse effect. The patient is typically treated with dual antiplatelet therapy.

Pearls/Pitfalls

- A Heart Team approach is vital to ensure optimal outcomes in transcatheter therapies for structural heart disease.
- Careful preoperative planning can prevent most mishaps. Be prepared for common and potentially catastrophic surgical emergencies.
- Transfemoral TAVR is preferred to alternative access due to better outcomes.
- Percutaneous balloon aortic valvotomy (BAV) is infrequently performed due to high risk of complications. When utilized, it is typically as a bridge to future intervention.
- Percutaneous mitral balloon valvuloplasty (PMBV) is more likely to be successful with Wilkins score ≤8

- Transcatheter mitral valve repair (TMVr) using the MitraClip device has shown survival benefit in patients with severe secondary MR, advanced HF, and failure of optimal HF medical therapy
- Other devices for TMVr as well as all current transcatheter mitral valve replacement (TMVR) and transcatheter tricuspid valve intervention (TTVI) technologies are currently investigational.
- Select patients with cryptogenic stroke and PFO have lower rates of recurrent stroke after percutaneous closure with the Amplatzer occluder device.
- Surgeons would be wise to remain current with rapidly advancing transcatheter structural heart technologies.

Suggested readings

- Transcatheter Heart Valve Handbook: A Surgeons' and Interventional Council Review - American College of Cardiology. Available at https://www.acc.org/membership/features/transcatheter-heart-valve-handbook-a-surgeons-and-interventional-council-review
- Nishimura RA, Otto CM, Bonow RO, et al. 2017 AHA/ACC Focused Update of the 2014 AHA/ACC Guideline for the Management of Patients with Valvular Heart Disease: A Report of the American College of Cardiology/American Heart Association Task Force on Clinical Practice Guidelines. Circulation. 2017;135(25):e1159-e1195.

III. Congenital Cardiothoracic Surgery

70. PATENT DUCTUS ARTERIOSUS

Trung Tran, MD and Michiaki Imamura, MD

This chapter is a revision and update of that included in the previous edition of the TSRA Clinical Scenarios written by Kristopher B. Deatrick, MD, and Richard G. Ohye, MD.

Concept

- Diagnosis
- Medical and surgical treatment options
- Current surgical vs percutaneous/catheter- based therapies
- Indications for surgery, Operative steps
- Surgical complications
- Pearls and pitfalls

Chief complaint

"An infant born at 28 1/7 weeks estimated gestational age with a weight of 1100g is admitted to the neonatal intensive care unit for treatment of respiratory distress syndrome with mechanical ventilation and multiple doses of surfactant. Her ventilator course has been characterized by persistent inability to wean. She is noted to have a continuous murmur."

Diagnosis

PDA is usually suspicious in a premature neonate with low birth weight and associated with the presence of a classic "machine-like" holosystolic murmur with respiratory failure. Infants presenting with PDA may also have signs of over-circulation, congestive heart failure, tachypnea, recurrent respiratory infections, failure to thrive, or steal phenomenon from systemic circulation resulting in end organ ischemia such as renal insufficiency or necrotizing enterocolitis. Adults may be asymptomatic if having small restrictive PDA or present with CHF or Eisenmenger's syndrome; rarely, they can present with infective endocarditis, ductal aneurysm, aortic or pulmonary aneurysm, or aortic dissection.

Supportive clinical findings include wide pulse pressure, hyperactive precordium and continuous murmur. Differential diagnoses are aortopulmonary window, truncus arteriosus, atrial septal defect, ventricular septal defect, Tetralogy of Fallot, pulmonary stenosis.

The diagnosis of PDA is typically confirmed by echocardiography. TTE is the most useful tool to assess the presence and size of PDA, direction of flow, degree of shunting, size and function of chambers, and presence of associated intracardiac defects. Exclusion of other lesions is essential so as not to close a physiologically necessary left-to-right or right-to-left shunt.

CXR and EKG may be helpful but are not sensitive nor specific. Cardiac catheterization is usually needed when considering percutaneous therapy or in combination with other congenital heart diseases.

Index scenario (continued)

"On cardiac exam, she has RRR, continuous murmur at the left upper sternal border, radiating towards midclavicular line. Her CXR shows bilateral hazy opacities, Echocardiogram shows a large PDA with left-to-right flow in both systole and diastole, and a mildly dilated left atrium. There is normal left ventricular size and hyperdynamic systolic function. No other intracardiac defects are noted."

Treatment/management

Indication for closure:

- Moderate or large PDA with symptoms of left-to-right shunt, clinical evidence of volume overload or reversible PAH.

- Prior episode of endocarditis regardless of the size of PDA and in the absence of severe PAH.
- Small but audible PDAs even in the absence of a significant left-to-right shunt: the long-term benefit of closure (e.g., prevention of endocarditis) outweighs the risk of intervention. An alternative approach is routine follow up.
- Small silent PDAs: indication for closure is controversial.
- Closure is not recommended for severe irreversible PAH and/or right-to-left shunting

Observation:
Patients need follow ups regularly to monitor for signs of increased cardiac workload and/or pulmonary vascular changes. Antibiotic prophylaxis for medical or dental procedures is not necessary.

PDA closure:
In the present scenario, the failure of respiratory improvement and failure to wean from mechanical ventilation are due to a clinically significant PDA and surgical closure should be undertaken.
PDA may be closed medically, via percutaneous catheter-based intervention, or by open or minimally invasive surgical ligation.

1. Medical closure: is the first line of treatment in preterm infants. This usually is accomplished with indomethacin (0.2 mg/kg infused over 20 minutes and repeated at 12 and 24 hours) or ibuprofen (10 to 20 mg/kg PO or IV followed by two additional doses of 7.5 to 10 mg/kg administered every 12 to 24 hours). They act by blocking the action of endogenous prostaglandins and are usually given in combination with diuresis and fluid restriction if there are symptoms of heart failure and volume overload. Up to 80% of premature infants will have successful closure of the PDA with medical treatment. Indomethacin is ineffective in term infants and older patients with a PDA. Side effects of indomethacin include impaired renal function, impaired platelet aggregation and impaired host defenses. Contraindications to treatment with indomethacin include sepsis, renal failure, and known bleeding disorders.

2. Percutaneous closure:
If medication fails or is contraindicated, surgical or percutaneous closure is considered. In the past, catheter-based closure could only be considered for >5 kg patients. Recently, with the advancement of techniques and availability of closure devices, the patient size and age limitations are lower than previously. Percutaneous catheter-based therapies can be done even for patients smaller than 5 kg. Decision of interventions is generally dependent upon patient weight, the size and morphology of the PDA, and availability of experienced clinicians to perform the procedure.

Femoral artery or vein are generally used for access. Coils or occlusion devices are the two most common catheter-based therapies. Coils are highly efficacious and cost-effective for occluding small PDAs, but have a higher rate of complications (e.g., residual PDA, coil embolization) with larger ducts. Occlusion devices have been developed with improving safety and efficacy. Amplatzer ductal occluder II was approved by the FDA in 2013 for use in children ≥6 months and ≥6 kg. PFM Nit-Occlud device was approved by FDA in 2013 for use in children ≥5 kg. Amplatzer vascular plug II, approved by the FDA in 2007, has shown to be effective in closing all PDA shapes. The percutaneous approach is occasionally impractical on very sick premature infants due to inability to transport from NICU to the catheterization laboratory.

3. Surgical closure:

PDA can be exposed through median sternotomy, left anterior thoracotomy, left posterolateral thoracotomy or VATS. VATS for PDA ligation is safe, effective and less invasive, however, it is not recommended for >9mm PDAs, previous thoracotomy, ductal calcifications, active infection, and ductal aneurysm. For premature neonates, open ligation is the standard technique. They are often unstable with very high risks for transport and the procedure can be done bedside in the NICU.

Operative steps
PDA ligation in premature infants with left sided arch
- General endotracheal anesthesia through a single lumen endotracheal tube.
- Left posterolateral thoracotomy at third or fourth interspace.
- Retract lung anteriorly.
- Open the mediastinal pleura and reflect it anteriorly and posteriorly.
- Division of the left superior intercostal vein may aid the exposure.
- Identify the ductus just opposite to the left subclavian artery (LSCA). Knowledge of the location of the left pulmonary artery, descending aorta, aortic arch, LSCA, and recurrent laryngeal nerve is a critical part of the operation since most misadventures result from inadvertent ligation of structures other than the PDA.
- Avoid cautery near the recurrent laryngeal nerve and take great care to ensure that recurrent laryngeal nerve is not clamped.
- Avoid unnecessary dissection around the ductus. Life-threatening hemorrhage may result from tearing a friable ductus.
- Prior to ligating the duct, temporarily occlude it with forceps. This should be followed by an augmentation of the diastolic pressure, with continued pulsatility in the aorta.
- Ultimately, the duct is ligated either with a simple clip (< 10 mm duct) or silk ligature.

Surgical complications:

- Recurrent laryngeal, phrenic nerve paralysis
- Respiratory compromise, pleural effusion/chylothorax, pneumothorax
- Bleeding, infection
- Aortic obstruction, pulmonary obstruction
- Scoliosis (more likely after thoracotomy)
- Residual ductal flow

Potential questions/alternative scenarios
"The patient is noted to have a calcified ductus. How should surgical closure be approached?"
This can be hazardous and is the type of case that may have been best served with transcatheter occlusion. In the operating room, it is safest to approach the PDA via median sternotomy using CPB. After CPB is initiated, ductal flow can be controlled initially by inverting the anterior wall of the main pulmonary artery against the ductus while cooling to 28-32° C. Low-flow CPB can then be instituted and the MPA opened. The opening of the ductus is then patched closed with PTFE. Care must be taken to prevent the entrainment of air into the systemic circulation. A brief period of deep hypothermic circulatory arrest may be necessary.

"The test occlusion is performed, and the patient becomes hypotensive, bradycardic, and the SpO2 begins to fall. What is the likely cause and what is your strategy?"
First ensure that you have not clamped the aorta or the left main PA. Release the clamp and resuscitate as needed. Make sure you clearly see the LSCA, ductus, aortic arch, descending aorta and left PA. If you confirm that you have clamped the ductus, then this patient may have a ductal dependent systemic circulation and further diagnosis is required.

442

"A PDA is identified in a previously asymptomatic adult. Is closure indicated? How will you proceed?"

A PDA in an adult should be closed. There is a risk of endocarditis even in clinically insignificant PDAs. Any PDA that becomes symptomatic should be closed. Transcatheter closure is ideal if feasible.

"An aneurysmal PDA is detected in a patient with a history of endocarditis on preoperative imaging."

Plan for a median sternotomy, CPB, and resection of the aneurysmal ductus. In the absence of dense left pleural adhesions, a left thoracotomy with left heart bypass would be an acceptable alternative.

"As you clamp and divide the PDA through a left thoracotomy a tear develops in the left PA with severe hemorrhage."

This is an uncommon event, but you should anticipate this if the duct is wide and friable. Obtain local hemostasis with direct digital pressure. Heparinize and cannulate the descending aorta and left atrium. Once on CPB the hemorrhage should significantly decrease allowing you to close the defect in the PA.

"The patient has persistent milky white chest tube output after 5 days of conservative management."

Chylothorax is a risk of PDA ligation due to lymphatic channels near the aortic arch and around the PDA. It is rare for the actual thoracic duct to be ligated or injured. A conservative trial of observation is not unreasonable, as many will stop spontaneously. A low-fat diet, a trial of NPO, or octreotide infusion may be attempted. Some would return to the OR sooner as the culprit lesions may be easier to identify earlier rather than later in the postoperative period. Most often you will enter the same left thoracotomy site. An alternative would be a right thoracotomy with supradiaphragmatic mass ligation of the thoracic duct.

Pearls/pitfalls

- PDA is common, affecting between 1 in 1200 and 1 in 5000 births.
- Physiologic closure may fail in neonates due to lack of normal O2 tension, decreased sensitivity to signals for closure, and increased sensitivity to vasodilators.
- Medical closure is highly successful and is first-line therapy for most neonates.
- Decision for surgical closure in a neonate is based on symptoms and hemodynamic significance.
- Closure can be accomplished via a limited thoracotomy and often at the bedside in the neonatal intensive care unit.
- Attempted medical closure (Indomethacin, 0.2 mg/kg, 3 doses) is indicated for all *neonatal* PDA unless there is a contraindication.
- Elective closure of even small PDAs should be undertaken due to the late risk of bacterial endocarditis.
- Before attempting any closure, the presence of ductal dependent circulation must be excluded.
- Complications usually result from injury to surrounding structures during dissection including: left recurrent laryngeal nerve, lymphatics, phrenic nerve, transverse aortic arch, descending thoracic aorta, left main pulmonary artery.
- Knowledge of surrounding structures is critical, as the PDA may be larger than the aortic arch in some cases.

Suggested readings

- Ardehali, A, Chen, J.M., Patent Ductus Arteriosus. Ardehali, A, Chen, J.M.,(eds). *Khonsari's Cardiac Surgery: Safeguards and Pitfalls in Operative Technique.* 5th ed. Philadelphia, PA: Lippincott Williams and Wilkins, 2017: 205-212.

- DeCampli, W.M. Patent Ductus Arteriosus. Kaiser, L.R, Kron, I.L, Spray, T.L. (eds) *Mastery of Cardiothoracic Surgery.* 3rd ed., Philadelphia, PA: Lippincott Williams and Wilkins, 2014: 788-796.

- Jonas, R.A., Patent Ductus Arteriosus, Aortopulmonary Window, Sinus of Valsalva Fistula, And Aortoventricular Tunnel. Jonas, R.A., (ed). *Comprehensive Surgical Management of Congenital Heart Disease.* 2nd ed. Boca Raton, FL: Taylor and Francis Group, LLC, 2014: 267-288.

71. ATRIAL SEPTAL DEFECTS

Reilly D. Hobbs, MD, MBS and Ming-Sing Si, MD

This chapter is a revision and update of that included in the previous edition of the TSRA Clinical Scenarios written by William Stein, MD and Brian Kogon, MD

Concept
- Presentation
- History and Physical
- Tests
- Treatment/Management
- Operative Steps
- Alternate Scenarios
- Surgical management of secundum and sinus venosus atrial septal defects (ASD)

Chief Complaint
"A 4-year-old girl with a history of a fixed split S2 heart sound and a systolic murmur is referred to you by a pediatric cardiologist for evaluation of an ASD that was found on transthoracic echocardiogram"

Differential
Although the diagnosis of an ASD has already been made in this case, the differential of exertional dyspnea in a 4-year-old is broad and all extra-cardiac and cardiac causes should be investigated including asthma, bronchiolitis, airway disorders, other pulmonary or CNS conditions, ASD, VSD, PAPVR, and PDA among others.

History and Physical
A complete history and physical examination should be performed. The majority of uncomplicated ASDs are asymptomatic and the presence of symptoms should raise suspicion of other contributing illness or concomitant cardiac lesions. Once extra-cardiac causes of dyspnea have been eliminated, it is likely that the child's symptoms are the result of pulmonary over-circulation. Other symptoms of pulmonary over-circulation include respiratory infection, failure to thrive, and exertional dyspnea.

Physical exam findings typically demonstrate a fixed split S2 heart sound and a systolic murmur from the increased blood flow across the pulmonary valve. It is also possible to note a diastolic murmur from the increased blood flow across the tricuspid valve as well.

Atrial septal defects are grouped into categories; 1) ostium primum defects, 2) ostium secundum defects, 3) sinus venosus defects, 4) coronary sinus septal defect. Ostium primum defects involve the endocardial cushion where the atrial septum meets the ventricular septum. Typically, there are both atrial and ventricular components of these defects which are commonly termed atrioventricular septal defects. Ostium secundum defects result from inadequate growth of the septum secundum and are found in the foramen ovale. Sinus venosus defects are located adjacent to either the superior vena cava or inferior vena cava and are associated with partial anomalous pulmonary venous drainage. Coronary sinus septal defects (also known as unroofed coronary sinus) result from developmental failure of the coronary sinus wall which results in communication between the right and left atrium.

Tests
- *EKG*: Will demonstrate varying degrees of right ventricular hypertrophy along with right axis deviation. The presence of left axis deviation should raise suspicion of an atrioventrical septal type defect.
- *CXR*: Varying degrees of cardiomegaly will be present depending on the degree of shunting and age of the patient.

- *Transthoracic echocardiogram (TTE)*: The gold standard for diagnosis of ASD. TTE has the ability to visualize the direction of flow across the lesion along with its location and size. It is also important to visualize the location of the pulmonary veins and coronary sinus along with the right and left heart function. In cases where the presence of an ASD is not obvious, a bubble study may be helpful.
- *Cardiac catheterization*: Although not typically needed for uncomplicated ASDs, three situations in which a cardiac catheterization may be necessary are, 1) concern for severe heart failure, 2) concern for pulmonary hypertension, or 3) inability to adequately delineate the anatomy with echocardiography.
- *Cardiac MRI or CT*: Typically, not necessary in the management of uncomplicated ASDs. In the presence of suspected anomalous pulmonary venous drainage specialized cross-sectional imaging can be extremely helpful.

Index scenario (additional information)
"Further history reveals the child has difficulty keeping up with her siblings and has a chronic cough. She also has an iodine allergy. Physical exam reveals a well appearing child in the 35th percentile for height and weight. There is a fixed split S2. Review of TTE imaging reveals a 22 mm secundum ASD with a Qp:Qs of 2:1. There is a nearly absent inferior rim"

Treatment/management
Surgical closure is the treatment of choice for this child. Observation of asymptomatic ASDs is appropriate for patients between 3-5 years of age when the ASD is small (< 8 mm) and the Qp:Qs is less than 1.5:1. If the ASD fails to close spontaneously by 5 years of age and the Qp:Qs ratio is > 1.2:1, an intervention should be pursued. The patient in this case scenario meets criteria for repair based on symptoms, size, and a high Qp:Qs.

Once the decision to intervene on an ASD has been made, clinicians can choose between transcatheter and surgical closure. Transcatheter closure is the treatment of choice for ostium secundum ASDs with over 90% of lesions being amenable to transcatheter repair. Despite the popularity of transcatheter ASD closure, it is important to understand which defects are amenable to transcatheter closure. Currently, septum secundum type defects are the only type of ASD commonly closed with transcatheter techniques.

Transcatheter Closure Contraindications/Cautions
- Size: Maximum defect size approved for transcatheter closure is 38 mm. It is important to remember that most defects are elliptical and should be measured in their maximum diameter during end ventricular systole.
- Adequate Rims: In general, there needs to be at least 5 mm rim circumferentially around the defect in order for the device to form and adequate seal. A deficient superior-anterior rim will lead to impingent on the aorta and possible erosion either acutely or over time, a deficient superior-posterior rim may lead to obstruction on the superior vena cava, a deficient posterior rim can lead to obstruction of the right upper pulmonary vein, a deficient inferior-posterior rim can obstruct the inferior vena cava, a deficient inferior-anterior rim can impinge on the AV valves.
- Difficult anatomy: most notably fenestrated or multiple defects
- Pulmonary hypertension: closure of a defect with right to left shunting secondary to pulmonary hypertension may precipitate right ventricular failure.

Operative steps
- Exposure through a partial or full median sternotomy.
- Aortic arterial and bicaval venous cannulation with caval snares.
- Antegrade cardioplegia
- Atriotomy performed. Identify the coronary sinus, orifice of the inferior vena cava, mitral valve, and the tricuspid valves and the pulmonary veins.

- Patch closure is performed with either autologous pericardium or Gore-Tex® with either running or interrupted polypropylene suture. The left atrium is deaired prior to tying the final suture.
- Cross-clamp is removed and the cardioplegia catheter converted to an aortic vent.
- The right atrium is closed and caval snares are removed.
- The patient is weaned from cardiopulmonary bypass and the heart examined with TEE prior to closure.

Potential questions/alternative scenarios

"After weaning the patient from cardiopulmonary bypass, the saturations are 88% on 100% FiO2. The child was saturating 99% on room air when he was brought to the operating room. The endotracheal tube is suctioned, the pleural spaces are examined for pneumothorax, and the ventilator settings are unremarkable. How would you proceed?"

This scenario is concerning for a right to left shunt with resulting hypoxemia. It is possible to inadvertently baffle the inferior vena cava to the left side of the heart if the surgeon is not meticulous in the identification critical structures. If the child has venous access in the lower extremity, a bubble study can be performed which will show bubbles present in the left atrium only if the inferior vena cava has been baffled to the left atrium. The surgeon can also baffle the coronary sinus to the left side of the heart, however, the differences in saturations in this instance would likely be more subtle. In either scenario, the solution is to confirm the diagnosis with TEE and redo the ASD patch.

"Preoperative TTE reveals that the ASD is located at the superior aspect of the septum near the SVC. How would you proceed?"

This situation is concerning for a superior sinus venosus ASD and the pulmonary vein anatomy must be completely evaluated to rule out partial anomalous pulmonary venous return that could interfere with ASD closure. If the TTE is not diagnostic, either a TEE or MRI can be obtained preoperatively. Patients with sinus venosus ASD and PAPVR tend to have higher Qp:Qs and are symptomatic at an earlier stage than secundum ASDs. Closure of sinus venosus ASDs require creating a baffle to direct blood flow from the pulmonary veins into the left atrium. In the event of pulmonary vein drainage high on to the superior vena cava, a Warden procedure can be performed. This entails ligating and dividing the superior vena cava just above the pulmonary vein orifice, baffling the pulmonary vein into the left atrium during closure of the defect, and attaching the cephalad portion of the superior vena cava to the right atrial appendage.

"A 4-year-old boy is referred after a TTE revealed a 2 mm patent foramen ovale with left to right shunting. The Qp:Qs is calculated to be 1.2. The echo is otherwise normal. He is asymptomatic. How would you proceed?"

The echo is diagnostic of a patent foramen ovale. This occurs due to failure of the septum primum and secundum to fuse after birth. In the absence of symptoms there are currently no indications for closure. The presence of a right to left shunt, cryptogenic stroke, or the need for other cardiac surgery are the current scenarios in which closure should be considered.

Pearls/pitfalls

- The preferred diagnostic modality is a transthoracic echo, not catheterization or other cross-sectional imaging. Alternative modalities are only necessary if there is a need to further delineate anatomy.
- The vast majority of secundum type ASDs are closed percutaneously. The most common contraindication to percutaneous closure is the lack of adequate rim on the defect.
- Uncomplicated ASDs should be repaired if they fail to close by 5 years old and have a Qp:Qs greater than 1.2:1.
- Sinus venosus ASDs are frequently associated with partial anomalous pulmonary veins. When repairing these defects, pulmonary venous flow must be redirected into

447

the left atrium and the SVC should be augmented as needed to prevent development of a SVC syndrome.

Suggested readings

- Akagi, Teiji. Current Concept of Transcatheter Closure of Atrial Septal Defects in Adults. *Journal of Cardiology*. 65 (2015), 17-25

- Bichell D and Christian K. Atrial septal defect and cor triatrium. Del Nido PJ, and Swanson SJ (eds) Sabiston and Spencer - *Surgery of the Chest*. 2010; 1797-1816.

- Troise D et al. Atrial septal defects and partial anomalous pulmonary venous connections. Yuh D, Vricella LA, and Baumgartner WA (eds). *Johns Hopkins Manual of Cardiothoracic Surgery*. 2007; 1057-1076.

- Turbendian H and Chen H. Atrial septal defects. Franco K and Thourani V (eds.) *Cardiothoracic Surgery Review*. 2011.

72. VENTRICULAR SEPTAL DEFECTS

Sasha Still, MD, and Robert Dabal, MD

This chapter is a revision and update of that included in the previous edition of the TSRA Clinical Scenarios written by George Dimeling, MD, and Olaf Reinhartz, MD.

Concept

- Presentation and natural history
- Diagnostic workup
- Morphology and pathophysiology
- Indications for surgical closure
- Surgical procedure

Chief complaint

"A 4-month-old boy presents with poor feeding and growth failure. On physical exam he has a precordial pansystolic murmur. Cardiomegaly is evident on CXR."

Differential

VSD of any variety (Perimembranous, Muscular, Outlet, Inlet, or Malalignment), VSD associated with any cardiac anomaly (i.e., TOF, TGA), ASD, PDA.

History and physical

Isolated VSD is the most common congenital heart lesion and is present in approximately half of all children with CHD. Clinical presentation is related to defect size and therefore the severity of hemodynamic shunting. Small VSDs are usually asymptomatic and detected by the presence of a holosystolic murmur. Larger, hemodynamically significant VSDs result in left ventricular overload and may progress to congestive heart failure (CHF). Symptoms of CHF include tachypnea, diaphoresis with feeding, poor feeding, growth failure and, when severe, failure to thrive, respiratory distress, and cyanosis (Eisenmenger's complex).

Tests

CXR. May show increased pulmonary vascular markings with an enlarged heart.

EKG: Normal in approximately half of patients with VSD. Large shunts may demonstrate LVH, right bundle branch block, or ventricular hypertrophy.

Echocardiography (ECHO). Gold standard for diagnosis. Color Doppler TTE can detect up to 95% of VSDs. Sensitivity approaches 100% for inlet and outlet defects, 80-90% for perimembranous defects, and 50% for muscular lesions. Muscular defects can be missed on exam due to differences in contractility, equalization of ventricular pressure gradient, and obfuscation of defect due to overlying trabecular muscle. An estimation of ventricular function and filling pressures can also be obtained.

Cardiac catheterization: Indicated when ECHO and clinical findings suggest advanced pulmonary vascular disease. Catheterization allows calculation of Qp:Qs, PA pressures, PVR, response of high PVR to vasodilators, and delineation of unclear anatomy.

Index scenario (additional information)

"Echo reveals a 10 mm perimembranous VSD and left to right shunt."

Treatment/management

Therapeutic approach is based upon defect size and symptom severity. Most VSDs are small and asymptomatic. These tend to close spontaneously and can be managed with regular outpatient follow up. Moderate or large VSD tend to become symptomatic within the first 2 months of life as pulmonary vascular resistance (PVR) decreases and left to right shunt increases leading to increased left atrial pressure and subsequent left ventricular overload. When symptoms of heart failure are mild to moderate (i.e. no respiratory distress or FTT), volume overload and left-to-right shunting are managed with diuretics and nutritional optimization. If symptoms persist or worsen despite optimal medical management then referral for surgical repair is warranted. When severe symptoms are present, the patient is stabilized with aggressive medical therapies (diuretics, inotropes, supplemental nutrition) and referred for surgical closure. Transcatheter closure is an option for an isolated VSD remote from tricuspid or aortic valves, typically within the muscular septum.

Indications for surgical closure:
- Persistent symptoms despite maximal medical therapy
- Moderate to large VSD with PAH (PVR 4-8 or PAP >50% systemic arterial pressure)
- Asymptomatic VSD with Qp:Qs >2:1
- VSD with a history of endocarditis
- VSD associated with aortic valve prolapse and regurgitation
- Moderate or large VSD with LV dilation
- All inlet and outlet VSDs

Operative steps
Right atrial approach
- Supine, standard lines, shoulder roll, TEE.
- Median sternotomy.
- Resect or retract thymus, open pericardium +/- harvest pericardium for fixation and possible patch, suspend pericardium.
- Dissect between aorta and PA, evaluate for patent ductus arteriosus.
- Heparinize, aortic and bicaval cannulation. LV vent.
- Check ACT. Commence CPB. Dissect and ligate PDA if present.
- Place SVC and IVC occlusion tapes and snare.
- Place antegrade cardioplegia stitch and cannulate. Cross clamp and arrest.
- Oblique right atriotomy parallel to the AV groove.
- Place stay stitches in the atrium and tricuspid valve septal and anterior leaflets.
- Identify and measure the VSD. Trim patch material to desired size (Dacron, PTFE, bovine pericardium). If perimembranous, consider taking down of the tricuspid valve to aid in visualization.
- Perform a running or interrupted patch repair. Re-suspend tricuspid valve.
- De-air prior to closing the defect (LV vent off to allow it to fill). Test tricuspid for competence and repair if necessary.
- Remove cross clamp. LV vent back on. Root vent on.
- Close atriotomy in running fashion.
- Check TEE for residual or other undetected VSDs, aortic insufficiency, tricuspid valve regurgitation, and function.

Potential questions/alternative scenarios
"A 6 mo old child is found to have multiple defects along the muscular septum. The Qp:Qs is > 2:1 and the shunt is left to right. How would you repair this defect?"
An uncommon but extreme example of multiple muscular VSDs is referred to as "Swiss Cheese Septum" which is best approached initially by pulmonary artery banding. Many of these defects will close over time.

"A 6 mo child has an outlet (conal/supracristal/infundibular) defect. How will you approach it for closure?"
A transpulmonary approach is most often used. Exposure is via a longitudinal incision in the main pulmonary artery, extending nearly to the annulus. Patch closure is recommended to prevent injury to or distortion of the aortic valve. The PA is closed primarily.

450

"A 1-year-old child has an outlet VSD with AI."

Outlet VSD can cause the right aortic cusp to prolapse into the defect causing aortic insufficiency. In this setting, surgery is indicated before permanent damage is sustained to the valve cusp or ventricular function. Closure of VSD is sufficient to prevent progression of AI. The aortic valve generally does not require repair.

"A 2-year-old child presents with a large VSD and cyanosis."

Patients with cyanosis or right to left shunting on ECHO require a catheterization to obtain an accurate measure of PAP, PVR, and Qp:Qs. If PVR is > 8 U/m^2 and Qp:Qs is < 1.3 then check for reversibility with supplemental oxygen or inhaled nitric oxide (iNO). Reversibility is suggested if the Qp:Qs rises above 1.5:1 and PVR drops below 8 U/m^2. Lack thereof, or fixed pulmonary hypertension, is a contraindication to VSD closure.

"Describe flow patterns across the VSD and how they affect Qp:Qs."

Shunt (Qp:Qs) occurs in systole and is determined by the defect size, difference in resistance between pulmonary and systemic circulations, and the difference in pressure between the right and left ventricle. Restrictive VSDs (Qp:Qs <1.5) are small with a high pressure gradient across the defect. In this situation, shunt is determined by the size of defect. On the other hand, non-restrictive VSDs are large and characterized by an equalization of pressures in the right and left ventricle. Here, shunt is determined by pressure gradients among ventricles and between the pulmonary and systemic vascular resistance. For example, if RVp < LVp, then L to R shunt occurs. If RVp = LVp, then shunt occurs only if PVR < SVR.

"Describe the different types of VSD"

The classification of VSDs is based on their location within the intraventricular septum. The septum is composed of four parts: membranous, inlet, outlet, and muscular. The most common surgical defects are perimembranous (80%) which lie beneath aortic valve and behind the septal leaflet of the tricuspid valve. Muscular defects (10%) occur within the muscular septum and are further delineated by their location relative to the right ventricle (anterior, posterior, apical, mid-ventricular). Both may close spontaneously, however the mechanism differs. Perimembranous defects close by way of duplicated tricuspid valve tissue or adherence of septal leaflet of tricuspid tissue to the defect's margins, whereas closure of muscular VSDs is assisted by growth/hypertrophy of septal tissue and trabeculae.

Outlet/subpulmonic/supracristal/conal/ doubly committed subatrial defects (5%) are located below the semilunar valves and above the crista supraventricularis. They are associated with prolapse of right coronary cusp of the aortic valve. Inlet defects/AV cushion defects (5%) lie beneath the septal leaflet of the tricuspid valve with tricuspid annulus forming posterior border. Perimembranous and inlet defects are closely related to the conduction system which usually penetrates through the posteroinferior border. Muscular and outlet VSDs are far from the conduction system. Malalignment VSDs are a separate category which result from malalignment of the conal septum relative to the muscular septum. Anterior malalignment defects are associated with Tetrology of Fallot and posterior malalignment defects with interrupted aortic arch.

Pearls/pitfalls

- The most common type of VSD encountered at surgery is perimembranous.
- The approach for outlet VSD is transpulmonary. Outlet and perimembranous VSD typically require patch repair.
- Medical management attempts to attenuate left to right shunting by using diuretics, inotropes, and afterload reducing agents.
- Knowledge of the expected location of the conduction system is critical.

Suggested readings

- Ventricular Septal Defect. Kouchoukos NT, Blackstone EH, Hanley FL, and Kirklin JK (eds). *Kirklin/Barratt-Boyes Cardiac Surgery, 4th ed.* 1274-1325.

- Ventricular Septal Defect. Jonas RA. (ed). *Comprehensive Surgical Management of Congenital Heart Disease*: 242-255.
- Ventricular Septal Defects, Mavroudis C and Backer CL. *Pediatric Cardiac Surgery.* 298-320.

73. COARCTATION OF THE AORTA/INTERRUPTED AORTIC ARCH

W. Clinton Erwin, MD and Damien LaPar, MD, MS

This chapter is a revision and update of that included in the previous edition of the TSRA Clinical Scenarios written by Bryan Barrus, MD and George Alfieris, MD

Concept
- Indications for repair of coarctation of the aorta
- Preoperative considerations
- Steps of coarctation repair
- Pitfalls and alternative solutions

Chief complaint
"A 2-day-old girl with a normal birth history is noted to be increasingly tachypneic, increasingly pale, and less active. A CXR shows congested lung fields and mildly enlarged heart silhouette. ABG shows a pH of 7.3, Right arm SBP is 70mmHg, right leg SBP is 40mmHg. A TTE reveals descending aortic narrowing distal to the left subclavian, there is no PDA flow."

Differential
Although the diagnosis has been made in this case, differentials included with coarctation of the aorta may include peripheral arterial disease, aortic dissection, supravalvular aortic stenosis, and other conditions causing heart failure depending on clinical presentation and patient age.

History and physical
Symptoms may occur abruptly with closure of the ductus arteriosus in neonates with severe or critical coarctation but may be more gradual in older children as collaterals often develop. Evaluate vitals, focus on pulse exam of all 4 extremities, heart, and lung exam. Classic physical exam findings include brachiofemoral pulse delay, diminished or absent femoral pulses, and blood pressure gradient between upper and lower extremities. However, significant blood pressure gradients are not always present in older children with many well-developed collaterals. Diminished pulses in all extremities may signify heart failure. Listen for murmurs along left sternal border radiating to the back. Look for differential cyanosis.

Tests
- *Labs.* Arterial blood gas, serum lactate, BUN, creatinine, electrolytes, septic workup in patients presenting in shock (blood, urine, CSF cultures).
- *CXR.* May show pulmonary congestion in neonates with critical coarctation but may be normal in older children unless heart failure present (cardiac enlargement, pulmonary congestion); > 5 years old look for rib notching by intercostal vessels. The "reverse 3" sign may be evident on barium swallow.
- *Echocardiography.* Diagnostic, test of choice. Obtain Z-score of transverse arch, isthmus, and descending aorta. Score ≤ -2 is usually an indication for intervention. Doppler flow may show a diminished pressure wave in the descending aorta, which is characteristic of coarctation. 30% of patients have simple coarctation, 30% have an associated VSD, and 40% have complex coarctation. A prominent PFO or secundum ASD may be present due to increased left heart pressures, keeping the PFO open. A Bicuspid aortic valve may be present in 50% of patients. Distal arch narrowing, other valvular anomalies, and ventricular hypoplasia must be ruled out (80% of HLHS have some degree of coarctation).
- *EKG.* normal; may have left ventricular hypertrophy (LVH) in late presentations.
- *MRI.* Useful in neonates and infants whose anatomy is not completely defined by echo

- *CTA*. helpful in older patients and adults.

Index scenario (additional information)
"The patient is increasingly tachypneic, tachycardic, and has absent femoral pulses with weak brachial pulses. The lower half of the body is cyanotic. The blood pressure in the right brachial artery is 70/40 and undetectable in the legs. In addition to coarctation of the aorta, echocardiography shows a left aortic arch with normal head vessels, closed ductus arteriosus, and no intracardiac defects. The pH is 7.2 and the lactate is 5. How would you proceed?"

Treatment/management
The patient is in cardiogenic shock with a metabolic acidosis and must be medically optimized prior to surgery. Ensure reliable IV access and infuse prostaglandin E1 to open the ductus arteriosus and improve blood flow into the descending aorta. Support heart failure with mechanical ventilation, inotropes, and diuretics. Monitor ventricular dysfunction and ductus arteriosus patency with serial echos. Monitor hepatic and renal function. Keep NPO as feeding may worsen effects of transient bowel ischemia.

Operative Steps
Goals – relieve obstruction while avoiding inadvertent injury to adjacent structures and avoiding prolonged spinal malperfusion.
For simple coarctation end-to-end anastomosis repair
- *Positioning/monitoring*. Right lateral decubitus position with axillary roll, and padding, right radial arterial line, rectal and nasopharyngeal temperature probe, BP cuff and pulse oximetry on legs, foley. Allow proximal hypertension during aortic cross-clamp. For older patients or adults, a femoral arterial line may be warranted to monitor distal perfusion during cross clamp.
- Allow patient to passively cool to ~34-35° C by dropping the ambient temperature and using cooling blankets as needed.
- Left posterolateral thoracotomy via the 3rd or 4th intercostal space. Retract the lung medially. Incise mediastinal pleura overlying descending thoracic aorta and left subclavian artery (SCA).
- Important structures to identify are the descending aorta, distal arch and left subclavian, ductus arteriosus, as well as the phrenic, vagus, and recurrent laryngeal nerves to avoid injury.
- Mobilize the distal arch and left subclavian (transverse arch as necessary) first, allowing room for the proximal vascular clamp.
- Mobilize the ductus arteriosus. Special care must be taken to avoid nerve injury, as well as avoid lymphatic duct injury.
- Next mobilize the descending aorta and necessary intercostal branches, diving as few as possible, to provide sufficient cranial mobility of the descending aorta.
- Give heparin 100 u/Kg (although some surgeons/centers may not heparinize, as non-atherosclerotic arteries are less likely to clot).
- Ligate and divide the ductus arteriosus
- Place a vascular C-clamp proximally across the transverse arch. The clamp is positioned in such a way as to partially occlude the LSCA, and LCCA. A distal straight vascular clamp is placed on the mid descending thoracic aorta.
- Divide the aorta just distal to the left SCA and just distal to coarctation segment. The coarctation segment and ductus are removed en bloc.
- Use the vascular clamps on the distal arch and descending aorta to manually approximate the 2 ends and ensure that there will not be excessive tension on the anastomosis

454

- Begin the anastomosis on backwall with a running 6-0 or 7-0 polypropylene suture. Use small bites and meticulous spacing to avoid unnecessary tension on each loop of suture, or purse string effects. Complete the anastomosis.
- Prior to tying the suture, removed the distal clamp briefly to blackbleed and deair the aorta. Make sure the anastomosis is tension free. Try to limit the anastomotic time to less than 20-30 minutes to reduce the risk of paraplegia from prolonged spinal ischemia. If a long clamp time is anticipated, consider instituting a distal perfusion strategy.
- Check for pedal pulse at the end of the procedure. Assure hemostasis prior to closure. Close pleura over the aorta.
- Place a single chest tube and close the chest.

Catheter based interventions for coarctation

- Multiple studies demonstrate that surgical repair of coarctation of the aorta is superior to balloon dilation and/or stenting. While balloon dilation may offer short term relief of the coarctation gradient, there is a high rate of re-coarctation.
- There is almost no role for balloon angioplasty or stenting for coarctation in the neonatal and infant period
- However, for patients who have been repaired surgically in childhood and present with late re-coarctation, balloon dilation is the mainstay of treatment.
- Patients who present during or after adolescence may be treated with angioplasty or stenting as a first line treatment
- Achieving a gradient of <20mmHg with balloon dilation of the re-coarctation area is possible in up to 89% of patients, and up to 99% of patients when stents are deployed across the coarctation
- However, there is an appreciable risk to balloon dilating and/or stenting the aorta. With balloon dilation, the medial muscle fibers of the aorta must be torn to achieve dilation. This may pre-dispose patients to future aneurysm formation requiring further endovascular or open repair
- Stents left in the descending aorta can injure or erode through the aortic wall, leading to endoleaks and pseudoaneurysm formation

Potential questions/alternative scenarios

"Same patient as above but now with a severely hypoplastic aortic arch. How will you proceed?"

Radical extended end to end anastomosis

- Position the patient and perform left thoracotomy, dissect out structures as above. Importantly, proximal dissection must be carried out to the level of the distal ascending aorta, exposing the innominate artery takeoff.
- Wide head vessel dissection may be required to sufficiently mobilize the entire arch
- Ensure that head vessel anatomy is as expected based on pre-operative imaging (is there a bovine arch? Aberrant right subclavian?)
- Once again, the descending aorta is extensively mobilized, and the PDA is mobilized and ligated.
- The vascular C-clamp is now placed just distal to the innominate artery, clamping the arch, the LCCA, and LSCA, ensuring that the innominate is not obstructed (as all cerebral perfusion now depends on the innominate).
- The aortotomy is now extended across the lesser curvature of the aorta, and the descending aorta is brought up to meet the lesser curvature of the aorta. The anastomosis is completed in a running fashion, as described in the simple repair.

Other variations to account for arch hypoplasia

455

- Left subclavian patch aortoplasty – the subclavian is sacrificed, opened along its lateral border, and flapped downward onto the descending aorta
- Reverse subclavian flap aortoplasty – the subclavian is sacrificed, opened along its medial border, and flapped onto the aortic arch and left carotid
- Modified left subclavian patch aortoplasty – the subclavian is transected, opened at its origin, and advanced down the distal arch as a patch

These techniques may have a significant chance of re-coarctation, as the ductal tissue is often not able to be resected.

"On echo, the patient is noted to have a large perimembranous ventricular septal defect (VSD) in addition to the coarctation. How will you proceed?"

Restrictive VSDs in the muscular septum are likely to close spontaneously and can be monitored alone. Unrestrictive VSDs can be repaired in either a one-stage or two-stage approach. The one-stage approach is preferred in cases where the VSD is unlikely to close spontaneously (perimembranous, large, inlet, outlet, malaligned). In a single incision approach, perform a median sternotomy. Repair the arch as described above. During rewarming, repair the VSD through a right atriotomy.

A two-stage approach in which the coarctation is repaired first +/- pulmonary artery banding followed by VSD closure in 2-3 months can also be employed. If preoperative congestive heart failure (CHF) does not resolve, a second operation is required to close the VSD or if the VSD does spontaneously close a de-banding procedure is performed. This approach is falling out of favor.

"The patient has a bicuspid aortic valve in addition to the coarctation of the aorta."
Usually does not need to be addressed at time of coarctation surgery.

"A 14-year-old boy presents to his pediatrician with headaches and dyspnea on exertion. His blood pressure is 140/75 in his right arm but 100/70 in his right leg. His femoral pulses are diminished with a delayed upstroke. Rib notching is noted on a chest X-ray. How would you repair this anomaly?"

Obtain an echo and CT angiography to determine anatomy. Large collaterals may impede mobilization of the aorta. Perform a left thoracotomy. The initial dissection is the same as the end-to-end anastomosis described in the initial scenario.

"A 10-year-old female presents with headaches, epistaxis and is found by her primary care physician to have a right brachial blood pressure of 160/90. Her mother reports she had repair of coarctation of the aorta as an infant. Echo shows a recoarctation. How would you approach treatment?"

Balloon angioplasty +/- stent placement is 90% successful. Mortality rate is 2.5%. The risk of recurrent coarctation following surgery is 5-10%. Angioplasty +/- stenting for native coarctation has recurrence rate of 11-15%.

"A 20-year-old immigrant with discrete coarctation not previously diagnosed presents to your office. What is the treatment of choice?"

Balloon dilatation and stenting is a reasonable first approach for discrete coarctation of the descending aorta although recurrence is likely to be higher when compared with open surgery.

"After arrival to the intensive care unit, an infant's blood pressure is noted to be severely elevated. Why does this occur? If left untreated, what may occur?"

Early phase (first 24 hours) caused by increased sensitivity of the aortic and carotid baroreceptors. Late phase (48-72 hours) increased levels of renin and angiotensin. Untreated hypertension following surgery is associated with mesenteric arteritis which may require laparotomy.

"You notice a white, milky substance coming out of the chest tube when the child begins to feed. What is your management strategy for the finding?"

Most often chyle leaks are injuries to tributaries of the thoracic duct, not the duct itself. An initial attempt at conservative measures include NPO, somatostatin, and hyperalimentation. If the patient fails to improve, operative thoracic duct ligation, or ligation of lymphatic tributaries, may be attempted.

"How can you limit the chances of paraplegia during repair of coarctation of the aorta?"

Paraplegia occurs 0.5% of the time. This can be prevented by limiting cross clamp time, passive cooling, and avoid hypotension during the clamp period.

"A 1-day old boy with a normal birth history is noted to be increasingly fussy and tachypneic, with cool lower extremities and left arm. A CXR shows congested lung fields and mildly enlarged heart silhouette. ABG shows a pH of 7.2, Right arm SBP is 70mmHg, left arm SBP is undetectable. A TTE reveals an interruption in the distal aortic arch, after the takeoff of the left carotid. There is no PDA flow."

The successful management of IAA that is not prenatally diagnosed relies heavily on early detection in the post-natal period. As the PDA closes, vasculature distal to the PDA becomes nearly completely ischemic. Symptoms usually occur abruptly with closure of the ductus arteriosus in neonates with previously undiagnosed IAA.

IAA Classification

- The most common classification of IAA is that devised by Celoria and Patton, as types A, B, and C.
- Type A interruption occurs at the isthmus of the aorta, after the left subclavian artery
- Type B interruption occurs in the distal arch, between the left carotid and left subclavian. This is the most common type. An aberrant right subclavian artery from the descending aorta is often present
- Type C interruption occurs in the proximal arch, between the innominate artery and left carotid
- Interrupted aortic arch almost always presents with associated anomalies, most commonly a single VSD. However, patients

TTE is diagnostic in IAA as in coarctation of the aorta. Genetic testing is warranted, as approximately 50% of IAA patients have DiGeorge syndrome – the presence or absence of a thymus at the time of operation may give insight into this but does not change operative management. The goal of medical management is to maintain ductal patency and correct metabolic derangements in preparation for surgery.

Operative steps

Goals – provide flow to the descending aorta via the aortic arch, remove all ductal tissue if possible, close the VSD (if present).

- *Positioning/monitoring.* supine, right radial arterial line, and umbilical arterial line (preferred for pre- and post-anastomosis pressure monitoring), rectal and nasopharyngeal temperature probe, BP cuff and pulse oximetry on legs, foley.
- Median sternotomy
- *Cannulation:* Critical to repair. Flow must be established to the head vessels as well as the descending aorta; therefore, usual cannulation includes an ascending aortic cannula and a main PA cannula connected with a Y-connector. The left and right PA must be snared so that flow is preferential down the ductus and descending aorta. If there is concern for space for cannulation on the ascending aorta, a graft can be sewn onto the innominate artery in lieu of direct aortic cannulation. Cardioplegia can be administered down a sidearm of the aortic cannula, or a standard cardioplegia needle can be placed if there is space on the ascending aorta. Venous cannulation will usually be bicaval if VSD repair is planned.

- Once cardiopulmonary bypass is instituted, the patient is cooled. 18C is the often-quoted desired temperature, 20 or 24C may be acceptable if a long circulatory arrest time is not expected.
- During cooling, mobilize the innominate, LCCA, LSCA. The descending aorta should be mobilized, along with any aberrant subclavian arteries. In mobilization of the descending aorta, intercostal artery branches should be preserved whenever possible
- Next mobilize the descending aorta and necessary intercostal branches, dividing as few as possible, to provide sufficient cranial mobility of the descending aorta.
- Once cooling is complete, circulation is arrested. At this time the innominate artery, LCCA, and LSCA are snared, the arterial cannulas are removed, and repair is begun. In some instances, if the innominate artery has been cannulated, antegrade cerebral perfusion may be possible.
- Ligate the ductus at the junction with the descending aorta, Excess ductal tissue remaining on the descending aorta is resected. A C clamp is placed on the descending aorta to provide traction up to the aortic arch
- Place a vascular C-clamp proximally across the transverse arch. The clamp is positioned in such a way as to partially occlude the LSCA, and LCCA. A distal straight vascular clamp is placed on the mid descending thoracic aorta.
- Make an aortotomy on the terminal aortic arch and bring the descending aorta cranially to meet the aortotomy site. Depending on the anatomy, the anastomosis may incorporate the LCCA into the suture line
- Begin the anastomosis on backwall with a running 6-0 or 7-0 polypropylene suture. Use small bites and meticulous spacing to avoid unnecessary tension on each loop of suture, or purse string effects. Complete the anastomosis.
- The aorta and head vessels are then de-aired with saline, the ascending aorta re-cannulated (if the innominate artery has not been cannulated), and the PA bands are released, the ascending aorta crossclamped, and bypass is reinstituted.
- During the rewarming period, the VSD can be addressed through a number of approaches, either through the RA or PA/RVOT.
- After reaching a core temperature of 35C, the patient can be separated from bypass, suture lines inspected for hemostasis
- Place chest tubes and close the chest.
-

Pearls/pitfalls
- Echocardiography is the mainstay of diagnosis.
- Open the ductus arteriosus with a prostaglandin E1 infusion in infants with heart failure.
- Extended end-to-end anastomosis shows the lowest rates of recurrence.
- Angioplasty/stenting is the preferred treatment for recurrent coarctation.
- Extensive mobilization of the entire aorta and its branches is required to avoid tension
- Particularly for IAA, the full anatomy should be thoroughly understood pre-operatively, as many complex lesions are often associated with this abnormality

Suggested readings
- Jonas, R., & DiNardo, J. (2004). *Comprehensive surgical management of congenital heart disease* (pp. 207-224). London: Arnold.
- Jonas, R., & DiNardo, J. (2004). *Comprehensive surgical management of congenital heart disease* (pp. 470-482). London: Arnold.
- Backer CL, et al. Repair of coarctation with resection and extended end-to-end anastomosis. *Ann Thor Surg.* 1998;66:1365-1370.

- Fiore AC, et al. Comparison of angioplasty and surgery for neonatal aortic coarctation. *Ann Thor Surg.* 2005;80(5):1659-1665.
- Husain SA, Mokadam NA, Permut LC, and Rodefeld MD, Coarctation of the aorta and interrupted aortic arch. Yuh D, Vricella LA, and Baumgartner WA (eds). *Johns Hopkins Manual of Cardiothoracic Surgery.* 2007.

74. TETRALOGY OF FALLOT

Heidi Reich, MD, and Richard Kim, MD

This chapter is a revision and update of that included in the previous edition of the TSRA Clinical Scenarios written by Asad A. Shah, MD, and Andrew J. Lodge, MD

Concept

- Diagnosis and management of Tetralogy of Fallot
- Operative techniques and pitfalls
- Timing of intervention
- Postoperative complications and long-term outcomes
- Pearls/pitfalls

Chief complaint

"A 6-month-old infant presents to outpatient clinic with recurrent cyanotic episodes."

Differential

Although a commonly asked question, it would be virtually unheard of today for an undiagnosed infant with Tetralogy of Fallot (TOF) to present in this manner. Almost all children with TOF variants will have been previously diagnosed either prenatally or in the early neonatal period. As the physiologic manifestations of the most common form of TOF are due to the presence of a large ventricular septal defect (VSD) with some degree of pulmonary stenosis, differential diagnosis would include other cyanotic cardiac lesions with predominant right to left shunting including transposition of the great vessels, truncus arteriosus, total anomalous pulmonary venous return, and tricuspid atresia. Less frequent causes include Ebstein's anomaly or pulmonary atresia malformations. Non-cardiac causes of cyanosis in infancy include severe lung disease, hypoventilation, or hemoglobin disorders with decreased oxygen affinity, such as methemoglobinemia.

History and physical

Prenatal and birth history, prior illnesses, known medical conditions, feeding history, and events associated with cyanosis are assessed. Depending on the age of presentation, central cyanosis may be present, but more commonly only a history of occasional perioral duskiness or cyanosis is obtained, particularly in the stable patient. A more profound history of a cyanotic event requiring some form of resuscitative measure are rarely seen in the outpatient setting, as these patients undergo hospitalization for more urgent palliation or repair. Classic findings include a systolic ejection murmur at the left upper sternal border, a single second heart sound, and a prominent parasternal right ventricular (RV) impulse. The continuous murmur of a patent ductus arteriosus may also be present. Note whether syndromic features are apparent.

Tests

- *CXR*: boot shaped heart, clear lungs, or diminished pulmonary vascular markings.
- *EKG*: rightward QRS axis and RV hypertrophy.
- *Echocardiography*: large, nonrestrictive anterior malalignment-type ventricular septal defect, overriding aorta, right ventricular outflow tract (RVOT) obstruction, RV hypertrophy. Presence of right-sided aortic arch (25%), coronary anomalies or prominent conal branches, patent foramen ovale (PFO) or atrial septal defect (ASD), and multiple VSDs are assessed. Main and branch pulmonary artery (PA) sizes are measured.
- *Cardiac catheterization*: rarely necessary, unless large aortopulmonary collaterals or small PAs not adequately characterized on echo.
- *MR imaging and CT angiography*: rarely necessary, require sedation/anesthesia, selective use when PA anatomy is unclear.
- Consider referral for genetic testing (22q11 deletion, Trisomy 21).

460

"The patient is diagnosed with TOF. His cyanotic spell resolves and his room air oxygen saturation is 75%. How do you counsel his parents regarding the timing of intervention?"

Management

Treatment of hypercyanotic episodes (TET spells)

- Oxygen.
- Intravenous fluids.
- Morphine/sedation.
- Squat: knee-chest position to increase systemic vascular resistance and increase pulmonary blood flow.
- Intravenous beta blocker
- Alpha agonists, such as phenylephrine.

Timing of surgery

- Severe cyanosis is an indication for operation or palliation. A 6-month-old infant with a history of a cyanotic episode should undergo complete repair.
- A neonate with who can maintain oxygen saturation of ≥80% can be followed in the outpatient setting for elective palliation or repair at a later date.
- Elective repair in minimally symptomatic patients, prior to one year of age. Complete repair at 4-6 months of age is preferable.
- The question of neonatal complete repair of TOF is heavily institutionally dependent. Although certainly possible, initial palliation with a systemic to pulmonary artery shunt or ductal stent can be an excellent option and is still preferred by many surgeons.

Operative steps

The goals are to close intracardiac shunts, relieve obstruction to pulmonary blood flow, maintain normal function of the right ventricle and tricuspid valve, and avoid injury to the atrioventricular conduction tissue. There has been a recent paradigm shift toward preserving the pulmonic valve, even at the expense of moderate residual obstruction. Many surgeons also advocate for a transatrial-transpulmonary repair to avoid the potential short- and long-term complications associated with right ventriculotomy. However, with the modern emphasis on a limited ventriculotomy, at least the short-term advantages of avoiding an incision on the right ventricle seem difficult to prove conclusively. Many surgeons still prefer to approach all forms of TOF primarily through the ventricle.

- Median sternotomy, aortic cannulation, bicaval cannulation, cardiopulmonary bypass with moderate hypothermia (25-28° C).
- Divide systemic to pulmonary shunts (if present), ligate the ductus arteriosus.
- Identify any major coronary artery branches crossing the RVOT.
- Place a vent via right superior pulmonary vein.
- Oblique right atriotomy with gentle retraction of the tricuspid valve leaflets.
- Identify tricuspid chordae and papillary musculature, as well as the pathway between the tricuspid valve and pulmonary outflow. Resect or incise intervening and obstructing muscle bundles.
- VSD is closed using glutaraldehyde-treated autologous pericardium, bovine pericardium, PTFE, or Dacron patch. In most cases, the conduction system is protected by the inferior muscle bar found in TOF-associated anterior malalignment VSDs. However, extension of the VSD to the perimembranous location is fairly common and, in these circumstances, the conduction system at the posterior/inferior location of the VSD is more exposed.

- Close ASD/PFO, if present. A PFO may be left to allow some right-to-left shunting to when significant postoperative RV dysfunction or pulmonary hypertension is anticipated.

- The pulmonary valve can be visualized from either direction and both blunt and sharp approaches to commissurotomy are utilized. The pulmonic valve is commonly bicuspid, has a small annulus and thickened, dysplastic leaflets.

- Depending on the valve orientation, it occasionally is possible to divide the annulus through an anterior commissure, however in most cases, the anterior leaflet will need to be divided. A standard transannular patch will be fashioned to augment both the main pulmonary artery as well as the pulmonary infundibulum. Given the recent enthusiasm for valve sparing approaches, many surgeons limit the size of the transannular patch and the size of the reconstructed annulus. The amount of residual stenosis that is reasonable to leave behind remains highly debated, but RV systolic pressures $\leq 2/3$ systemic are generally well tolerated.

Potential questions/alternative scenarios

"After dividing obstructive fibers in the RVOT and performing a longitudinal pulmonary arteriotomy, the annulus appears inadequate for the patient's age and size. You decide to make a transannular incision but are impeded by an anomalous LAD originating from the RCA. How would you proceed?"

Anterior descending coronary artery arising from right coronary artery and crossing the RVOT is found in 3-5% of patients with Tetralogy. Alternatively, a large conal branch of the right coronary artery that also limits the transannular incision may be present. These anomalies are often apparent on preoperative imaging and should be assessed for by visual inspection early in the operation. A few options in this scenario include a transatrial approach, a transventricular incision above or below the coronary artery, or construction of a double barrel outflow tract consisting of the native outflow tract combined with an RV-PA conduit using homograft or bovine jugular vein originating below the observed coronary artery.

"What is the operative and late survival after repair of TOF?"

Operative mortality should be <2%; late survival exceeds 90% at 25-35 years. Most patients will eventually require reoperation, most commonly pulmonic valve replacement. Pulmonary insufficiency is recognized as a leading cause of progressive exercise intolerance, RV failure, ventricular arrhythmias, and sudden death for patients with repaired TOF.

"What are some perioperative complications?"

- RV dysfunction – Postoperative low cardiac output syndrome with preserved biventricular systolic function is described following TOF repair. Restrictive physiology is noted by echo, with tachycardia, an underfilled left ventricle, and elevated right sided filling pressures. Treatment is supportive, with inotropes and diuretics. Will usually resolve within 72 hours.

- Arrhythmias - Ensure properly functioning pacing wires prior to chest closure. Junctional ectopic tachycardia (JET) is a common malignant arrhythmia. Treatment of JET entails core cooling to 35° C, electrolyte correction, pain control and/or sedation, and amiodarone. Overdrive pacing to restore AV synchrony may be helpful. Dexmedetomidine may reduce the incidence of postoperative JET

"You come off bypass and TEE shows a residual VSD."

Typically, small residual defects are well tolerated and defects <2 mm in size are commonly not addressed. However, larger defects should be considered for closure and most surgeons will address VSDs >2 mm in size. The need for closure needs to be weighed against the adverse consequences of reinstitution of cardiopulmonary bypass and aortic cross-clamping. Residual VSDs in the setting of TOF repair, RV dysfunction and pulmonary insufficiency may not be as well tolerated as those following repairs of isolated VSD. A shunt fraction could be calculated but may be relatively low compared to size of the hole. In general, surgeons will address residual VSDs > 3mm. TEE may be useful to differentiate a peripatch leak from a muscular VSD. Muscular VSDs that were not seen previously or appeared small may be more visible once RV pressure is subsystemic following repair. Although TEE can also be helpful to localize the defect, most commonly they are found in the posterior/inferior location in VSDs with perimembranous extension, around large chordae, or the anterior transition from ventricular septum to the overriding aspect of the aortic valve.

"You come off bypass and TEE shows severe tricuspid regurgitation."

Most cases of tricuspid regurgitation are identified prior to atrial closure on static testing of the tricuspid valve and are associated with either trapping of tricuspid chordae during patch placement or distortion of the anteroseptal commissure following annular detachment of the tricuspid leaflet. Many times, simple closure of the commissure with interrupted suture can be highly effective. Severe tricuspid regurgitation under these circumstances most likely should be addressed.

"A 2-week-old boy presents with severe cyanosis and is diagnosed with TOF. Additional comorbidities include liver dysfunction due to biliary atresia. How would you manage this patient?"

TOF and biliary atresia can be found together in patients with Alagille syndrome with either a JAG1 or NOTCH2 gene mutation. Severe cyanosis under these circumstances should undergo more durable palliation via systemic to pulmonary shunt or ductal stenting if the ductus can be reopened. In some institutions, surgeons may elect to perform a complete repair. Patients with Alagille syndrome may require multiple interventions on their pulmonary arteries. Management of the biliary atresia including the timing and need for a Kasai portoenterostomy or liver transplantation is obviously highly individualized.

"A newborn with a prenatal diagnosis of TOF with absent pulmonary valve demonstrates respiratory distress immediately upon delivery. A respiratory acidosis is present on arterial blood gas. Transthoracic echo shows enormous dilation of the main, right, and left PAs. The child is intubated and stabilizes with positive pressure ventilation. CT scan shows severe main PA dilation with tracheal and bronchial compression. What is your surgical plan?"

TOF with absent pulmonary valve is characterized by the presence of an absent or dysplastic pulmonic valve, free pulmonic insufficiency, annular stenosis and aneurysmal PAs causing tracheal and bronchial compression. Patients can present with respiratory, rather than cardiac, symptoms with a wide spectrum of severity, ranging from infants or neonates with severe respiratory compromise to older children presenting with less severe symptoms. Tachypnea, air-trapping, cyanosis, and wheezing may be present. The above scenario suggests significant tracheal/bronchial involvement. It is also possible for cardiac symptoms to predominate over respiratory symptoms and can include both cyanosis as well as heart failure. In a minimally symptomatic child, elective repair should be undertaken, usually in the 3 to 6-month age range.

Operation

Unlike more common forms of TOF, the absent pulmonary valve defect is characterized by grossly dilated central branch PAs with aberrant proximal arborization. Within the limited confines of the aortopulmonary window, significant compression of the central bronchial structures can occur. Most surgical approaches are thus aimed at reducing this compression, including anterior plication of the branch PAs and translocation of the branches anterior to the ascending aorta (LeCompte maneuver). Insertion of a competent pulmonary valve is a common adjunct. Residual tracheobronchomalacia may be expected and careful postoperative ventilatory management is required.

Pearls/pitfalls

- Tetralogy of Fallot is the most common cyanotic congenital heart defect.

- Recurrent cyanotic spells and room air oxygen saturation of less than 80% are indications for urgent operation. Otherwise, "complete repair" is electively performed between 4-6 months of age.
- The key steps of repair include closure of the ventricular septal defect, division of muscle bundles to relieve the right ventricular outflow tract obstruction, and pulmonary valvotomy or transannular patch.
- Pulmonary regurgitation resulting in right ventricular dilation is a late complication, particularly after transannular patch, and is treated with pulmonic valve replacement (detailed in Adult Congenital Heart Disease Chapter).

Suggested readings

- Jonas RA. Tetralogy of Fallot with Pulmonic Stenosis. In: Jonas RA (Ed). Comprehensive Surgical Management of Congenital Heart Disease, 2nd ed. Boca Raton, FL: CRC Press, 2014:347-68.
- Fraser CD and Khan MS. Contemporary Surgical Therapy for Tetralogy of Fallot. In: Kaiser LR, Kron IL, Spray TL (Eds). Mastery of Cardiothoracic Surgery, 3rd ed. Philadelphia, PA: Lippincott Williams & Wilkins, 2014:990-1005.
- Elliot MJ. Absent Pulmonary Valve Syndrome. In: Stark JF, de Leval MR, and Tsang VT (Eds). Surgery for Congenital Heart Defects, 3rd ed. Chichester, West Sussex: John Wiley & Sons, 2006:425-33.

75. MAJOR AORTOPULMONARY COLLATERAL ARTERIES (MAPCAs)

David Blitzer, MD and Damien LaPar, MD

Concept

- Presentation
- Differential
- Diagnostic evaluation
- Surgical repair
- Pitfalls

Chief complaint

"A 6-month-old, full term 5 kg boy is transferred to you after experiencing multiple respiratory tract infections and failure to thrive. He was born by normal vaginal delivery and was asymptomatic until 2 months of age. His first hospitalization was 1 month ago when he developed pneumonia and respiratory failure which responded to diuretics. On exam in your office, he is tachypneic and dyspneic without clear evidence of congestive heart failure. A loud P2 murmur is appreciated as is a continuous heart murmur."

Differential

The differential diagnosis of cyanotic congenital heart disease with right ventricular (RV) outflow tract obstruction includes:

- Tricuspid atresia
- Pulmonary atresia with intact ventricular septum
- Double-outlet RV with pulmonary atresia
- Double inlet left ventricle (LV) with pulmonary atresia
- Congenitally corrected transposition of the great arteries (L-TGA) with ventricular septal defect (VSD) and pulmonary atresia

History and physical

Pulmonary atresia with ventricular septal defect (PA-VSD) is an extreme subset of tetralogy of Fallot (ToF) characterized by heterogeneity in the source of pulmonary blood flow. PA-VSD accounts for 1-2% of congenital heart defects, and in 35-70% the pulmonary flow is provided entirely by a patent ductus arteriosus via the pulmonary arteries, and in the remaining 30-65%, pulmonary blood flow is derived from major aortopulmonary collateral arteries (MAPCAs).

Extracardiac anomalies are frequently associated with PA-VSD, with common associations including 22q deletion syndromes, DiGeorge syndrome, VATER syndrome, and Alagille syndrome. Associated cardiac anomalies include atrial septal defects, coronary artery anomalies, persistent left superior vena cava, and retroaortic innominate vein.

Given the variable source of pulmonary blood flow, the clinical presentation for PA-VSD is equally variable. Patients with duct dependent circulation often present with cyanosis as the duct closes. These patients may also present with evidence of pulmonary overcirculation and congestive heart failure. Patients with the most severe form of the disease may initially be asymptomatic until progressive stenosis or pulmonary vascular disease distorts their physiologic equilibrium. This contrasts with those patients with the least severe form of the disease who present early with cyanosis as the ductus arteriosus closes in early life.

Tests

- *Chest X-ray:* The appearance of the chest x-ray will vary depending on the stage of disease and the state of pulmonary blood flow. In the case of excessive flow, the heart may be enlarged, and the lung fields will appear congested. In cases of low pulmonary flow, the heart will be of normal size and the lungs may appear dark as a mark of underperfusion. Due to the intraindividual variability of pulmonary circulation, different lung fields may have signs of over- and under-circulation within the same patient.

- *Transthoracic echocardiography (TTE)*: Echocardiography is a useful modality in that it can accurately diagnose PA-VSD in utero. It cannot, however, accurately assess for the source of pulmonary blood flow. The absence of a PDA raises the likelihood of MAPCAs being the source of pulmonary flow. Echocardiography can also be used to diagnose associated cardiac anomalies as listed above.

- *Cardiac catheterization*: A key evaluative measure in the work up of MAPCAs. Catheterization is used to assess the pressure in each collateral vessel and the blood flow to each lung segment. Pulmonary venous angiography may be used to define the true pulmonary arteries, which may be absent in 10-30% of patients. Catheterization can also be used to estimate the neopulmonary artery index, a sum of the indexed cross-sectional areas of the unifocalized vessels, which is helpful in determining if a patient will tolerate VSD closure at the time of unifocalization. An index greater than 200mm2/m2 is considered adequate for VSD closure. In the case of a lung segment receiving dual blood supply, the anatomy must be diligently investigated and understood. Catheterization is also key for the work-up of patients that have undergone previous palliation.

- Computed tomographic angiography (CTA): This modality is becoming an increasingly useful tool in the preoperative work-up, particularly as a guide to future catheterization and in surgical planning. Magnetic resonance imaging (MRI) can be utilized in a similar fashion.

Index scenario (additional information)
"Chest X-ray demonstrated cardiomegaly. Echocardiography showed severe dilation of the right atrium, ventricle, and pulmonary arteries. Pulmonary artery pressure, derived by tricuspid regurgitation jet velocity, was suprasystemic (111 mmHg). No other structural abnormality was seen. Multiple MAPCAs were visualized on CT."

Treatment/management
Medical management
Initial medical management for these patients should focus on maintaining adequate pulmonary blood flow and systemic oxygenation. For patients with duct dependent pulmonary flow, prostaglandin E1 should be used to maintain ductal patency. In the case of stenotic MAPCAs, vasopressors can be initiated to increase the systemic afterload and increase shunting to the pulmonary vascular bed. Unrestricted MAPCAs can result in excess pulmonary blood flow and subsequent pulmonary congestion and heart failure. These patients should be managed as typical heart failure patients, with the initiation of digoxin and diuretics.

Transcatheter Management
Transcatheter interventions are an increasingly important component of the management of MAPCAs. These interventions include coil embolization of collateral vessels providing bronchopulmonary segments with duplicate blood supply, and balloon dilation to dilate stenoses in the pulmonary arteries or collateral vessels. Balloon dilation may also be implemented for stenosis at anastomotic sites after unifocalization. These strategies are particularly important in patients at the more severe end of the spectrum with MAPCAs and severe stenoses of the true pulmonary arteries that results in excessive pulmonary flow.

Surgical management
Regarding surgical strategies, patients with PA-VSD can generally be divided into subgroups. The first group is comprised of those with large pulmonary arteries that feed all lung segments and duct dependent circulation. These patients can generally be treated similarly to patients with ToF and their management will not be the focus of this chapter. A second group consists of patients with pulmonary arteries of diminished size which connect to most lung

466

segments and MAPCAs that supply lung segments that would otherwise be supplied by the atretic vessels. A last group consists of patients with no native pulmonary arteries who are entirely dependent on MAPCAs for pulmonary blood flow. For these last two groups, surgical management has been evolving as understanding of the pathophysiology continues to improve. Increasingly data supports the ability of the true pulmonary arteries to enlarge and alveolar development to improve when antegrade pulmonary blood flow is established earlier in life.

The overarching goal of surgical intervention is circulatory normalization, with minimization of right ventricular afterload being the clinical marker of that normalization. Right ventricular afterload is a function of pulmonary arterial resistance, which can be decreased operatively by unifocalization, which increases the total cross-sectional area of the pulmonary vascular bed. The current preferred strategy is early, single staged, unifocalization which has several distinct advantages. Early repair has protective benefits against right ventricular hypertrophy and the negative consequences of cyanotic spells.

Surgical strategy can also be subdivided into 4 groups based on preoperative workup and intraoperative considerations:

1. One stage unifocalization with intracardiac repair: The appropriate strategy for patients with adequately sized MAPCAs, a healthy distal bed, and stenotic segments that can be approached through a median sternotomy.
2. One stage unifocalization with systemic to pulmonary shunt: Even if approachable through a median sternotomy, intracardiac repair should not be attempted in patients with hypoplastic MAPCAs and hypoplastic distal vascular bed. A systemic to pulmonary artery shunt is created. Alternatively, some groups advocate for a fenestrated VSD repair.
3. Aortopulmonary window creation: This strategy should be used for patients with hypoplastic pulmonary arteries that supply a majority of the lung segments. For these patients the collateral vessels feeding the true pulmonary arteries are ligated.
4. Staged unifocalization: When MAPCAs have distal stenotic segments that cannot be reached through a sternotomy, this strategy can be utilized and performed via a thoracotomy.

Operative steps

1. One stage unifocalization with intracardiac repair:
    a. Median sternotomy is performed
    b. All collateral vessels are identified and controlled
        i.   Collaterals from the aorta are controlled by opening both pleural spaces anterior to the phrenic nerve
        ii. Collaterals originating from the upper descending thoracic aorta are identified by dissecting between the superior vena cava and the aorta.
        iii. The pericardial reflection in the transverse sinus is opened to expose the aorta and any MAPCAs in this area.
    c. Collaterals are ligated and unifocalized, with as much of this work being done off bypass as possible. Following the ligation of each collateral, the arterial oxygen saturation is checked. When the level of cyanosis is no longer tolerable, partial cardiopulmonary bypass is started and the patient is cooled to 25C.
    d. A valved aortic allograft right ventricle to pulmonary artery (RV-PA) conduit is used. The distal anastomosis is performed first.
    e. Intracardiac repair is performed. The cross-clamp is applied and cardioplegia is administered. Intracardiac repair is performed as necessary.
        i.   Intraoperatively, a pulmonary flow study can be performed if there is concern about the patient's ability to tolerate

intracardiac repair. A pulmonary artery catheter and perfusion cannula are placed into the neo-pulmonary

artery. Using the perfusion cannula, flow to the lungs is increased to at least one cardiac index as a means of predicting mean pulmonary artery pressure once the VSD is closed. A pressure </=25mmHg is considered viable for closure in infants.

    f.   The cross clamp is removed, and the proximal anastomosis of the RV-PA conduit is completed.

    g.   Cardiopulmonary bypass is weaned.

    h.   Aortic, pulmonary artery, and atrial pressures are measured continuously

2.   One stage unifocalization with systemic to pulmonary shunt

    a.   The procedure is performed as outlined above.

    b.   A Gore-tex tube graft from the ascending aorta to the neopulmonary artery is used as a shunt. One should err on the size of a larger diameter tube to allow for growth of the pulmonary bed while simultaneously being weary of excessive pulmonary flow through the shunt.

3.   Aortopulmonary window creation:

    a.   Median sternotomy is performed

    b.   The central and branch pulmonary arteries are dissected.

    c.   The branch pulmonary arteries are temporarily clamped.

    d.   The main pulmonary artery is divided as near the infundibular origin as possible.

    e.   The pulmonary artery is anastomosed to the ascending aorta with a partially occluding clamp. The optimal location is dictated by the patient's anatomy. Care should be given to ensuring that the right branch pulmonary artery is not kinked or stretched at the selected anastomosis site.

    f.   Diastolic pressure and systemic arterial saturations are closely monitored upon removal of all clamps.

4.   Staged unifocalization:

    a.   A posterolateral thoracotomy is performed in the 4th or 5th intercostal space.

        i.   The first staged procedure is performed on the most highly affected side to preserve the patient's oxygenation.

    b.   MAPCAs are dissected and controlled.

    c.   Unifocalization is performed.

    d.   The neopulmonary artery is anastomosed to the aorta or the subclavian artery using a PTFE shunt.

    e.   The neopulmonary artery is placed as centrally as possible to facilitate midline completion.

Potential questions/alternative scenarios

"What are the embryological and genetic origins of MAPCAs?"

Normal development of the aorta and pulmonary arteries begins with the fusion of the right and left sixth dorsal aortic arch to the systemic arterial plexus of the lung buds. MAPCAs are a result of failed fusion which results in pulmonary atresia and the persistence of collaterals from the aorta. The variability in the extent of pulmonary atresia is a result of variability in the point of gestation at which the failure of fusion occurs.

There is newer evidence demonstrating an association between 22q11.2 deletion and tetralogy of Fallot, and more specifically with a higher prevalence of MAPCAs within that population.

468

"What are some of the unique features of postoperative care for patients with MAPCAs?"

Patients are prone to pulmonary reperfusion injury and bronchospasm. This can generally be managed with permissive hypercapnia, though in some cases prolonged mechanical ventilation or even veno-venous ECMO may be necessary, but elevated peak pressures should be avoided due to the risk of exacerbation of pulmonary injury. There is also risk of pulmonary parenchymal hemorrhage as a result of reperfusion injury. This can generally be managed expectantly or with bronchoscopy in the setting of hemorrhage into the bronchial tree.

"What are the key elements in the follow-up care of these patients?"

These patients must be actively monitored for signs of elevated right ventricular pressure, right ventricular dilation or failure. All patients should have a lung perfusion scan prior to discharge after the index operation. Echocardiograms and subsequent lung perfusion scans should be performed to assess the state of the right ventricle. Repeat catheterization should generally performed within 3-6 months of unifocalization, with the eventual timing dependent on the patient's status. Many patients will require further pulmonary arterioplasty or balloon dilation after the index operation.

If the VSD was left open after the index procedure, post-operative catheterization should be used to assess for possible repair. If the Qp:Qs ratio is greater than 2:1 than the patient should tolerate a repair. If the Qp:Qs is inadequate, further investigation should be performed to identify previously unaddressed site of stenosis in the pulmonary artery system.

Pearls/pitfalls

- PA-VSD is a clinical spectrum of disease. The mild end of the spectrum includes ductal dependent pulmonary circulation and minimal pulmonary artery stenosis. The extreme end of the spectrum consists of severe proximal pulmonary artery stenosis and MAPCA dependent pulmonary artery circulation.

- Cardiac catheterization is a critical component of the preoperative workup. It is used to assess the pressures in the collateral vessels as well as the blood flow to each broncho-pulmonary segment. Neopulmonary artery index can also be assessed and indicates if a patient will tolerate VSD closure at the time of unifocalization.

- The management of MAPCAs requires a multidisciplinary team. Medical management should be employed for ductal dependent circulation and in the management of congestive heart failure. Transcatheter interventions can be used to coil embolize collateral vessels and balloon dilate the pulmonary arteries. Balloon dilation may be employed in the pre- and post-operative setting.

- The surgical strategies for management of PA-VSD vary in accordance with anatomic variability. Depending on the pre-operative assessment, surgical interventions include single stage unifocalization with intracardiac repair, single stage unifocalization with systemic to pulmonary artery shunt, aortopulmonary window, and staged unifocalization.

- Postoperative management should include repeat catheterizations and many patients will at the very least require repeat balloon dilation of pulmonary artery stenosis or stenoses of the anastomotic sites.

Suggested readings

- Surgical Treatment of Pulmonary Atresia with Ventricular Septal Defect. Mavroudis C. and Backer CL (eds). *Pediatric Cardiac Surgery*, 4e West Sussex, UK: Wiley-Blackwell; 2013.

- Tetralogy of Fallot with Pulmonary Atresia. Jonas R. (ed). *Comprehensive Surgical Management of Congenital Heart Disease*. 2e Boca Raton, FL: CRC Press. 2014.

76. CONGENITAL AORTIC STENOSIS/ROSS

Reilly D. Hobbs MD, MBS and Ming-Sing Si, MD

This chapter is a revision and update of that included in the previous edition of the TSRA Clinical Scenarios written by Ashok Muralidaran, MD and Katsuhide Maeda, MD, PhD

Concept

- Presentation
- Background
- Diagnosis
- Medical/Interventional Treatment Strategies
- Surgical Treatment Strategies
- Ross-Konno Technique
- Pearls/Pitfalls

Chief complaint

"A newborn infant is transferred to your center due to the presence of a systolic murmur and a screening transthoracic echocardiogram suggestive of aortic stenosis. Physical exam reveals a systolic murmur radiating to the carotid arteries and palpable thrill in the second intercostal space. Complete cardiac echocardiogram reveals a thickened unicuspid valve, severe stenosis, and mild regurgitation. The pulmonary valve is normal"

Differential

Differential for a systolic murmur in an infant can be extensive depending on symptomatology. A few considerations include: Left ventricular outflow tract obstruction (LVOTO) with either valvular, subvalvular or supravalvar obstruction. Others include: Ventricular septal defect (VSD), Atrial Septal Defect (ASD), AV canal defect, Coarctation of aorta, Ebstein's anomaly. Several of these can have either very benign initial presentations all the way to severe decompensating CHF symptoms.

History and physical

Congenital aortic stenosis accounts for approximately 3-6% of patients with congenital heart defects. Valvar aortic stenosis is more common in males and is associated with a number of other congenital heart lesions including patent ductus arteriosus (PDA), hypoplastic left ventricle, VSD, mitral stenosis, and coarctation of the aorta. Congenital aortic stenosis can present from infancy to adulthood with a broad spectrum of anatomic and clinical variations. In the neonatal period, patients may have severely hypoplastic aortic valves and depend on reverse PDA flow for survival, conversely, adults with bicuspid or unicuspid aortic valves may present in later years with progressive stenosis or regurgitation requiring valve replacement. Optimal management of congenital aortic stenosis requires complete understanding of the many transcatheter and surgical options for palliation in both infants and adults. The presentation depends on the severity of aortic stenosis. Mild aortic stenosis may be clinically silent but slowly worsen over weeks to decades. Presenting symptoms depend on the age of the patient, severity of the stenosis, and the degree of heart failure present. Older patients may report dyspnea, chest pain, syncope, or chronic fatigue. Children may have a history of failure to thrive, feeding difficulty, delayed milestones, and irritability. Infants with critical aortic stenosis at birth will typically show overt signs of heart failure.

Physical exam findings may include cool extremities, reduced pulses throughout, a systolic ejection murmur that radiates to the carotids, a prominent apical impulse, and a precordial thrill. In infants with critical aortic stenosis, these exam findings are typically overshadowed by circulatory collapse and overt heart failure.

Tests

- *EKG*: Left ventricular hypertrophy or biventricular hypertrophy, ventricular strain patterns, or may be normal.
- *CXR*: Typically, normal but may show signs of pulmonary congestion or an enlarged cardiac silhouette.
- *Cardiac Catheterization*: Provides peak-to-peak gradient measurements, LV and RV direct pressure measurements, valve gradients, and cardiac function
- *Echocardiography and Doppler Flow Studies*: Typically, the most informative test, which has the ability to assess aortic valve morphology (unicuspid, bicuspid, tricuspid, etc.), LVOT and annular size, leaflet mobility and thickening, ventricular function, severity of hypertrophy, and to as evaluate for synchronous lesions. Additionally, doppler flow studies can estimate gradients, visualize valvular insufficiency, and define valvar morphology.

Index scenario (additional information)
"The child developed tachycardia, hypotension, inability to feed, tachypnea and diaphoresis. He underwent a cardiac catheterization and balloon valvuloplasty that resulted in severe AI with residual moderate AS. How would you proceed?"

Treatment/management
In the neonatal period, aortic stenosis with signs and symptoms of congestive heart failure or ductal dependent systemic blood flow are indications for urgent intervention. Past the neonatal period, indications for treatment are symptoms of congestive heart failure and elevated aortic valve gradients (catheter measured peak-to-peak gradient > 20-30 mmHg or a peak doppler derived gradient > 30-40 mmHg). It is important to carefully consider the patient age, likelihood for medication compliance (if considering a mechanical valve), need for future reintervention, and lifestyle prior to counseling the patient and/or their parents.

Balloon valvuloplasty is the treatment of choice for infants with critical aortic valve stenosis. Significant contraindications are aortic insufficiency or a prohibitively small aortic annulus. In comparison to surgical aortic valvotomy, balloon valvuloplasty typically leaves lower residual gradients and a higher incidence of aortic insufficiency. Surgical and balloon valvuloplasty have similar rates of survival and need for reintervention. As demonstrated in our case example, a notable risk of balloon valvuloplasty is significant aortic insufficiency which is reported in 18% of cases. For this reason, it is important for surgical backup to be available. Commonly utilized surgical techniques for children with growth potential include 1) surgical valvotomy (relatively contraindicated in the presence of significant aortic insufficiency); 2) The Ozaki procedure (aortic valve reconstruction with pericardium); 3) root replacement with aortic homograft; and 4) the Ross procedure.

In additional to the above, alternatives for older children and adults include 1) aortic valve replacement with/without annular enlargement techniques; 2) aortic root replacement; and 3) aortic valve repair with/without annular stabilization techniques.

In the above case scenario, the most appropriate surgical technique is the Ross-Konno procedure, whose steps are listed below.

Operative Steps
Ross-Konno procedure
- Median sternotomy, bicaval cannulation and hypothermia to 25° C.
- After aortic cross clamping, a transverse aortotomy is performed, aortic leaflets are excised, and coronary buttons mobilized.
- Branch pulmonary arteries are snared and the pulmonary artery (PA) is transected proximal to the bifurcation.
- The pulmonary autograft is harvested with a cuff of infundibular muscle.
- An anterior aortic root enlargement incision (Konno) is now performed. The incision is made just to the left of the right coronary artery (RCA) ostium site, extending on to the ventricular septum thus enlarging the subaortic area.

471

- If significant LV endocardial fibroelastosis (EFE) is observed, it is stripped.
- The pulmonary autograft is now implanted into the aortic annulus and the ventricular septal incision.
- The left coronary button is reimplanted followed by the right button.
- The distal autograft to ascending aortic anastomosis is now performed.
- The crossclamp is removed after deairing maneuvers.
- A pulmonary homograft is anastomosed to the PA bifurcation.
- The proximal pulmonary homograft is then anastomosed to the infundibulum taking care at the leftward aspect to not compromise the left anterior descending coronary artery.
- The patient is fully rewarmed, ventilated and weaned off cardiopulmonary bypass.
- A post-operative transesophageal echocardiogram is performed.

Potential Questions and Alternative Scenarios

"What other preoperative echocardiographic findings are important before a Ross-Konno procedure?"

It is important to identify the pulmonary valve morphology and rule out significant incompetence or stenosis. Additionally, it is important to assess for the presence of other associated lesions associated with aortic stenosis (mitral stenosis, coarctation, ascending and transverse aortic arch anomalies).

"What intra-operative echocardiographic features are assessed post-repair?"

It is important to evaluate biventricular function, look for any residual VSD, neoaortic valve structure and function, homograft function, and assess coronary flow.

"A 10-day-old neonate is diagnosed with critical aortic stenosis. He has pulmonary congestion, dyspnea, cold and clammy extremities. The NICU has asked for your opinion and evaluation."

This is a surgical emergency. Initial medical stabilization with intubation, mechanical ventilation, and inotropic support is required. If there is ductal dependent systemic perfusion, prostaglandin infusion will help maintain a patent ductus and improve systemic perfusion. Percutaneous transcatheter balloon aortic valvotomy is the procedure of choice. Nearly 50% of patients will require a repeat procedure within 5 years.

"A 14-year-old girl presents with severe symptomatic aortic stenosis. She is 8 years s/p balloon valvuloplasty. What are her surgical options?"

The management of adolescents can be challenging. Her size and growth potential should be assessed. In female patients, the inability to conceive a pregnancy while on systemic anticoagulation is important to consider. Moreover, many young adults will have difficulty maintaining therapeutic INR levels or may engage in hobbies that are exceedingly dangerous while on systemic anticoagulation. This patient and her parents should be counselled on the risks and benefits of 1) mechanical/tissue aortic valve replacement; 2) Ross procedure; 3) Ozaki procedure; and 4) Aortic valve repair

"An echocardiogram is performed on a 6-year-old child with chest pain and syncope. A diagnosis of subaortic stenosis is made. How would you proceed?"

Subaortic stenosis is classified as either discrete or diffuse with most cases having a discrete stenosis. The discrete form typically involved a membranous web that connects the anterior leaflet of the mitral valve and the aortic valve annulus. In the diffuse form, there is a fibromuscular ridge the extends from the aortic annuls towards the apex of the left ventricle, which may be difficult to distinguish from hypertrophic cardiomyopathy. In patients with discrete subaortic stenosis, surgical excision through the aortic valve is the treatment of choice. In cases of diffuse subaortic stenosis, a modified Konno-Rastan procedure is performed.

- The primary intervention for critical neonatal aortic stenosis is balloon valvuloplasty with surgical backup available. In comparison to surgical valvotomy, balloon valvuloplasty results in higher rates of aortic insufficiency but lower mean gradients. Survival and reintervention rates are similar between groups.
- Depending on the type of LVOTO and the institution, indications for surgery vary. Generally accepted indications for surgery are:
  - *Discrete subaortic membrane*: symptoms, peak Doppler gradient 40-50 mmHg, or new onset AI.
  - *Diffuse subaortic stenosis*: generally, a slightly higher peak Doppler gradient (50-60 mmHg) used as a guideline for surgery due to complexity of procedure, or symptoms.
  - *Hypertrophic obstructive cardiomyopathy*: symptoms rather than gradient typically dictate need for surgical intervention. Surgery for HOCM in children is rare.
- In the Ross-Konno procedure, the autograft harvest should include a generous anterior free-wall lip to fill the ventricular septal incision.
- Any septal perforator injury should be repaired immediately to prevent coronary steal.
- The Konno incision on the ventricular septum should be made leftward and not directed toward the LV apex, to avoid the conduction system.
- The pulmonary autograft to ventricular septal anastomosis should be adequately reinforced to prevent any residual septal defects.
- *Posterior root enlargement maneuvers (see Aortic Stenosis Chapter for more details).*
  - *Nicks*. The aortotomy is extended down the middle of the non-coronary cusp just across the aortic annulus. A Dacron patch is sewn from the apex of the incision. Interrupted valve sutures are placed from the outside-in along the width of the patch.
  - *Manouguian*. The aortotomy is initiated as in the Nicks maneuver but extended beyond the aortic annulus onto the anterior mitral leaflet. The left atrium is hence incised and should be closed along with a patch repair of the Mitral leaflet onto the aortic annulus.

Suggested readings

- Long-Term Survival and Reintervention After the Ross Procedure Across the Pediatric Age Spectrum. Nelson JS, Pasquali SK, Pratt CN, Yu S, Donohue JE, Loccoh E, Ohye RG, Bove EL, Hirsch-Romano JC. Ann Thorac Surg. 2015 Jun;99(6):2086-94; discussion 2094-5. doi: 10.1016/j.athoracsur.2015.02.068. Epub 2015 Apr 25
- Douglas J. Schneider, John W. Moore. Aortic Stenosis. Allen, Hugh D.; Driscoll, David J.; Shaddy, Robert E.; Feltes, Timothy F.(eds). *Moss and Adams' Heart Disease in Infants, Children and Adolescents: Including the Fetus and Young Adults.* 2008;968-986.
- Richard A. Jonas. Left Ventricular outflow tract obstruction: aortic valve stenosis, subaortic stenosis, supravalvar aortic stenosis. Richard A. Jonas (ed). *Comprehensive surgical management of congenital heart disease.* 2004;320-340.
- Katsuhide Maeda, Rachel E. Rizal, Michael Lavrsen, et al. Midterm results of the Modified Ross/Konno procedure in neonates and infants. *Annals of Thoracic Surgery* 2012;94:156-63.
- Shigeyuki Ozaki, Isamu Kawase, Hiromasa Yamashita, Shin Uchida, Yukinari Nozawa, Mikio Takatoh, So Hagiwara. A total of 404 cases of aortic valve reconstruction with glutaraldehyde-treated autologous pericardium. *The Journal of Thoracic and Cardiovascular Surgery* 2014; 147: 301-306

77. ANOMALOUS PULMONARY VENOUS CONNECTION

Trung Tran, MD and Michiaki Imamura, MD

This chapter is a revision and update of that included in the previous edition of the TSRA Clinical Scenarios written by Eric Griffiths, MD and James Gangemi, MD

Concept

- Diagnosis modalities
- Initial management and timing for TAPVC repair
- Operative steps
- PAPVR: diagnosis and management
- Pearls and pitfalls

Chief complaint

"A 4-day old baby boy with cyanosis, hypoxemia and respiratory distress is found on echocardiogram to have total anomalous pulmonary venous connection."

Differential

Differential diagnoses include cyanotic heart diseases: Transposition of the great arteries, Tetralogy of Fallot, Truncus arteriosus, TAPVC, and other causes such as double outlet right ventricle, pulmonary atresia, multiple variations of single ventricle, hypoplastic left heart syndrome, complex conditions associated with heterotaxy syndromes, or anomalous systemic venous connection (left SVC connect to LA).

Although the diagnosis has been established in this case, important information regarding the defect is required. In the suspicion of mixed type TAPVC, CT might be helpful to clarify the venous anatomy.

History and physical

TAPVC is a cyanotic congenital defect in which all pulmonary veins are not connecting to the left atrium, but instead draining to the systemic venous circulation. Patients without significant obstruction usually present in infancy or childhood with symptoms of heart failure, failure to thrive, feeding intolerance or hepatomegaly. Patients with complete pulmonary venous obstruction present in extremis with pulmonary congestion, poor oxygenation and life-threatening cyanosis. Physical exam should focus on vitals, degree of cyanosis and evidence of CHF, or other physical abnormalities.

Tests

Generally, TAPVC is diagnosed by Echocardiography. CXR is nonspecific, lung fields may be normal in non-obstructive TAPVC or show evidence of pulmonary edema, pulmonary vein congestion.

Angiography was formerly the gold standard for diagnosis of TAPVC, but it is now rarely done. It may be indicated in cases that require more hemodynamic information or plan for palliative intervention procedures such as atrial septostomy or stenting of the obstructed vertical vein.

CTA and MRA are helpful to evaluate pulmonary pathways and connections in detail. CT provides better anatomical features, while MRI provides information regarding flow and velocity which can reveal differential lung perfusion and venous stenoses. They may rarely be needed since most information can be obtained by echo and they both require IV contrast to evaluate the vascular anatomy.

Echocardiography: TAPVC is diagnosed based on the following findings:

- No normal pulmonary venous connections to the left atrium
- Ascending collecting vein with dilated SVC and innominate vein (in case of supracardiac lesions)

- Descending collecting vein with connection to hepatic or portal vein, and a dilated IVC (in case of infracardiac lesions)
- Direct connection between the pulmonary venous system and the right atrium or coronary sinus (in case of intracardiac TAPVC)
- Dilated right atrium and ventricle, evidence of right heart overload.
- Right-to-left shunting PFO/ASD, VSD or PDA
- Doppler imaging can estimate PA pressures, and measure the blood flow rates through the ascending or descending vertical veins, evidence of obstruction on Doppler with turbulent flow in venous pathway
- Aortic arch and left heart size are needed to be evaluated because occasionally hypoplastic left heart syndrome is accompanied with TAPVC.

Index scenario (additional information)
"The baby has a supracardiac confluence of veins with evidence of obstruction."
Treatment/management
Surgical repair is indicated when the diagnosis is made, and the patient is stabilized for all TAPVC regardless of the degree of obstruction. However, initial management and timing for TAPVC repair depends on the degree of obstruction:

- **Obstructed TAPVC:** stabilize prior to surgery with supplemental oxygen, mechanical ventilation, inotropic support, and PGE as needed (to maintain the PDA). Some patients may require ECMO to correct severe hypoxemia, acidosis, and hemodynamic instability. Palliative cardiac catheterization may be helpful to stabilize patients prior to surgical correction, such as atrial septostomy for patients with restrictive interatrial blood flow, or stent placements into severely obstructed pulmonary and common vertical veins.
- **Unobstructed TAPVC:** diuretics for newborn with pulmonary over-circulation

Surgical repair: the goal is to identify the anomalous connection and re-establish the connection of pulmonary veins and left atrium, avoiding obstruction of pulmonary venous drainage flow, and close the interatrial connection (PFO/ASD).

Operative steps
- Cardiopulmonary bypass often with DHCA.
    - Single arterial and venous cannula (bicaval cannulation optional)
    - Ligate PDA if present
- *Supra and infracardiac venous confluence*: direct anastomosis to left atrium, ligate and divide vertical vein.
- *Cardiac venous confluence*: unroof of the coronary sinus, connect ASD and coronary sinus ostia, then place a patch over the defect so that both pulmonary vein and coronary vein flow returns to the left atrium.
- Pulmonary veins drain directly into SVC: intracardiac baffle to create a channel for blood from the RA across the atrial septum into the LA.
- *Sutureless repair*: Anastomotic stricture is a serious concern for TAPVC procedures. Sutureless repair is used for small veins or obstruction at venous confluence:
    - LA is incised as well as the pulmonary veins including areas of obstruction or narrowing.
    - LA sutured to the pericardium adjacent to the pulmonary veins with continuous suture line.
    - Creates a "controlled bleed" into the LA.

Potential questions/alternative scenarios
"Postoperatively, the baby has difficulty weaning from ventilator, CXR shows right pleural effusion and congestion."

This patient likely has an obstruction at the anastomosis of the right veins. Obtain an echo (transthoracic) to evaluate the right sided pulmonary venous return. Consider contrast enhanced MRI, CTA of the heart, or possibly catheterization to look for obstruction. May need surgical revision with sutureless technique (see above).

"A 4-month-old baby boy with no other symptoms, found to have a heart murmur. Echocardiography revealed drainage of the right upper pulmonary vein into the superior vena cava with an associated atrial septal defect."
PAPVR is the abnormal return of one or more but not all the pulmonary veins to the right side of the heart. It can present isolated or in combination with other cardiac abnormalities, mostly with a sinus venosus ASD. The most common form of PAPVR is the left upper pulmonary vein connects to the left innominate vein, which drains into the SVC. Most patients with this form of PAPVR are asymptomatic throughout childhood, then eventually develop symptoms usually in 3rd or 4th decade of life with fatigue and exercise intolerance. Younger patients may be found to have heart murmur, abnormal CXR or recurrent pulmonary infections.
Other forms of PAPVR include PAPVR to SVC without ASD and Scimitar syndrome. Scimitar syndrome consists of right pulmonary veins draining into the IVC, anomalous arterial supply from the abdominal aorta, and often pulmonary sequestration. For these patients, the history and physical should focus on evidence of CHF, arrhythmias, failure to thrive, and paradoxical embolus.

Management
Surgical goal is to separate the systemic and pulmonary venous systems and avoid stenosis of SVC or pulmonary venous flows.
If there is no pulmonary hypertension then proceed with repair. Cardiac catheterization is indicated to evaluate pulmonary vascular resistance if there are signs of pulmonary hypertension.

- PVR normal → surgical repair
- Increased PVR but responsive to 100% O2 and/or inhaled nitric oxide → surgical repair
- Increased PVR and not responsive → may require ASD closure and lung transplant, or possible heart/lung transplant.

Operative steps for PAPVR with sinus venosus ASD
- Median sternotomy, bicaval cannulation, caval tapes, superior right atriotomy.
- Intra atrial patch (bovine pericardium or autologous pericardium) to baffle venous opening into left atrium.
- Second patch often used to close the opening over the superior cavoatrial junction.

"The venous confluence is too high on the SVC to baffle to left atrium."
Warden procedure: transect the SVC at the cavoatrial junction and relocate it to right atrial appendage, the pulmonary venous return is then baffled to left atrium through the ASD.

Pearls/pitfalls
- Obstructed TAPVC represents a surgical emergency.
- Limited role for medical management in TAPVC beyond intubation and inotropes. Prostaglandins and pulmonary vasodilators should be avoided in non-obstructive cases.
- *Approach*: bicaval cannulation, DHCA may be used for better intraatrial visualization.
- Repair depends on site of confluence: supracardiac, cardiac, or infracardiac.
- Consider sutureless repair for small veins or obstruction at confluence.
- PAPVR requires evaluation for pulm HTN.
    - If pulmonary hypertension is suspected, proceed to cardiac catheterization to determine PVR (normal or reversible, may proceed with repair).

- Fixed pulm HTN requires ASD closure and lung transplant, or possible heart/lung transplant.

Suggested readings

- Ardehali, A, Chen, J.M., Total Anomalous Pulmonary Venous Connection. Ardehali, A, Chen, J.M.,(eds). *Khonsari's Cardiac Surgery: Safeguards and Pitfalls in Operative Technique.* 5th ed. Philadelphia, PA: Lippincott Williams and Wilkins, 2017: 253-261.
- Calderone CA. (2013, Mar 21) "Sutureless" pulmonary vein stenosis repair. Retrieved Aug 26, 2019 from https://www.ctsnet.org/article/sutureless-pulmonary-vein-stenosis-repair.
- Jonas, R.A., Total Anomalous Pulmonary Venous Connection and Other Anomalies of the Pulmonary Veins. Jonas, R.A., (ed). *Comprehensive Surgical Management of Congenital Heart Disease.* 2nd ed. Boca Raton, FL: Taylor and Francis Group, LLC, 2014: 535-548.
- Mery, C.M., Gangemi, J.J., Kron, I., Anomalies of Pulmonary Venous Return. Kaiser, L.R, Kron, I.L, Spray, T.L. (eds) *Mastery of Cardiothoracic Surgery.* 3rd ed., Philadelphia, PA: Lippincott Williams and Wilkins, 2014: 1041-1054.

78. Palliative operations in congenital heart surgery

William Chancellor, MD and Mark Roeser, MD

Chief complaint
"A five-week-old girl born at 38 weeks gestation with prenatally-diagnosed multiple muscular ventricular septal defects was transferred to your center due to hypoxia, increased work of breathing, and poor feeding. She weighed 3kg at birth but is now only 2.7kg. On physical exam she is tachypneic, cachectic, her liver is 2 cm below the costal margin, and she has a holosystolic murmur. She is on 1 mg/kg of Lasix PO TID and on NG feeds. What are the next steps in the work-up of this infant with hypoxia and failure to thrive?"

Differential
The differential diagnosis for congestive heart failure in an infant includes:
- Patient ductus arteriosus
- Ventricular septal defect (VSD)
- Common atrioventricular canal (AV canal)
- Truncus arteriosus
- Aortic stenosis
- Coarctation of the aorta
- Endocarditis
- Arrhythmias

History and physical
Pulmonary over circulation can be observed in patients with multiple or large VSDs or single ventricle defects with unrestricted pulmonary blood flow. Such lesions may be well compensated until after the pulmonary vascular resistance decreases, which is often delayed in these patients. Left untreated, pulmonary over circulation can cause congestive heart failure, failure to thrive, and irreversible changes in pulmonary vasculature. Definitive repair of the causative anatomic lesion may not be possible due to small size or inability to tolerate cardiopulmonary bypass or may be postponed in hopes of achieving biventricular repair once the patient grows. However, if the patient exhibits signs and symptoms of heart failure or is not gaining weight a palliative operation may be indicated.

Tests
CXR – When symptomatic pulmonary over circulation is present, chest X-ray findings include prominent pulmonary vasculature with active congestion or interstitial pulmonary edema.

EKG – Electrocardiogram demonstrates normal rate and rhythm. Biventricular hypertrophy left atrial enlargement, and right axis deviation may be seen in advanced disease.

Echocardiography – Two-dimensional echocardiography allows identification of lesions responsible for left to right shunting, including atrial septal defect, ventricular septal defects, and patent ductus arteriosus. Additionally, AV valve regurgitation and dilated chamber sizes, especially the right ventricle and left atrium, may be evident in symptomatic patients. Finally, the aorta should be evaluated for the presence and severity of coarctation and the pulmonary arteries should be evaluated for dilatation.

Cardiac catheterization – Although not routinely indicated for ventricular septal defects, catheterization may be obtained to diagnose the degree of left to right shunt in symptomatic patients and to ensure that the pulmonary vascular bed is responsive to 100% oxygen or nitric oxide.

Index scenario (additional information)
"Cardiac catheterization was consistent with significant left to right shunt, no coarctation, and pulmonary artery pressure that decreased with 100% oxygen. Echocardiography demonstrated multiple muscular ventricular septal defects with left to right shunting and normal ventricular size and systolic function."

Treatment/management
Medical management
The mainstay of medical treatment for congestive heart failure is aggressive diuresis with loop diuretics. Depending on volume status and the degree of shunting, inotropes, such as milrinone or epinephrine may also be indicated to maintain systemic perfusing pressures. Supplemental oxygen is often required but should be used sparingly because of its pulmonary vasodilatory effects. Finally, infants that are failing to thrive should receive nutritional supplementation with continuous nasogastric feedings.

Surgical management
Given our patient's degree of over circulation, her current weight, and her inability to gain weight despite NG feeding, she will undergo pulmonary artery band placement until she is a better candidate for VSD repair. Ideally, in addition to decreasing pulmonary blood flow, restricting the main pulmonary artery will also cause RV hypertrophy, leading to spontaneous closure of the smaller ventricular septal defects. Then the larger defects can be closed surgically or via catheter depending on their location.

Operative steps
- Place patient in supine position with radial arterial line.
- Insert a transesophageal echo probe to measure the band gradient and to assess for new tricuspid regurgitation.
- Perform median sternotomy and total thymectomy.
- Open and suspend the superior portion of the pericardium overlying the great vessels.
- Use electrocautery to dissect out the aorta and main pulmonary artery.
- Place a tonsil or large right angle in the transverse sinus under the aorta and pulmonary artery. Then pass the banding material (Mersilene, Ethibond, or Goretex) through the transverse sinus.
- Reach between the aorta and pulmonary artery with the tonsil or right-angle clamp and grasp the end of the banding material on the aorta side of the transverse sinus. Then bring the banding material under the aorta proximal to the takeoff of the right pulmonary artery. This technique is known as the subtraction method and ensures that the left main coronary artery will never be compressed by your instrument. Neonates with heart failure do not tolerate compression of the left main, which may lead to fatal arrhythmias.
- Place a DLP catheter in the distal pulmonary artery for pressure monitoring.
- Begin by securing the band at a circumference calculated using Trusler's Rule (20mm plus 1mm for each kg of bodyweight). Place serial hemoclips to tighten the band so that the pulmonary artery pressure falls to ½ of the systemic pressure. As the band is tightened the systemic pressure will increase and the PA will end up smaller in diameter than the aorta.
- Place an interrupted suture through the band above or below the hemoclips so the band will not loosen over time.
- Secure the band to the main PA with 6-0 prolene sutures. This is an important step as it keeps the band form migrating distally onto the branch PA's.

- Place a 15F Blake drain in mediastinum.
- Close the chest in the standard fashion.

"What are the indications for PA banding?"
There are three general categories of congenital defects that can benefit from palliation by pulmonary artery banding:

1) Lesions allowing for significant left to right shunting that are not amenable to definitive repair until the neonate has grown (e.g. so-called "swiss cheese" VSD, premature AV canal, VSD with coarctation, or tricuspid atresia types Ic and IIc)

2) Single ventricle lesions with unrestricted pulmonary blood flow (e.g. tricuspid atresia and variants of hypoplastic left heart syndrome)

3) Lesions that could potentially be repaired to allow for biventricular physiology, but the left ventricle needs to be "trained" (most commonly transposition of the great arteries)

"How do you determine the initial size of the PA band and how much to tighten it?"
Trusler's rule states that the circumference of the PA band should be 20mm plus 1mm for each kg of bodyweight unless the patient's primary lesion allows for intracardiac bidirectional mixing, in which case the band should start at 24mm plus 1mm per kg. Single ventricles have tighter bands placed than biventricular repairs as they will undergo a Glenn procedure at 4-6 months of life, while biventricular repairs may wait longer. These children will all double in size before their next operation. The band is sequentially tightened using hemoclips then secured using an interrupted 6-0 prolene suture when the pulmonary artery pressure is approximately ½ of the systemic arterial pressure. Arterial oxygen saturation will be 75-90%.

"What are the advantages of sternotomy over thoracotomy for PA band placement?"
Median sternotomy allows for excellent exposure of the great vessels without compression or collapse of a lung, which provides more accurate intraoperative physiologic monitoring to guide the degree of pulmonary artery narrowing.

"What are the risks of PA band placement?"
The operative risks of pulmonary artery banding include distortion of the pulmonary valve, compression of coronary arteries, and kinking or stenosis of branch pulmonary arteries, particularly the right pulmonary artery. Post operatively these patients may be difficult to manage because the pulmonary vascular bed can be reactive, and the patient may have episodic desaturations. If this occurs 100% FiO2 and/or nitric oxide may be needed. Alternatively, raising the systemic vascular resistance with vasopressin or epinephrine will shunt more blood into the pulmonary circulation and raise oxygen saturations. Longer-term risks include main and branch pulmonary artery stenosis and theoretical ventricular hypertrophy that can increase a subaortic obstruction.

"Describe the technique for the removal of a PA band?"
The band should be removed at the time of surgical correction of the primary lesion. The inflamed, thin-walled segment of the main PA that has been compressed by the band should be excised back to normal tissue. Every effort should be made to sew native tissue to native tissue at the back of the PA to ensure future growth, while placing a patch of gortex, bovine pericardium, or autologous pericardium anteriorly to ensure there is no stenosis. If the thin, inflamed tissue extends to the commissure of the pulmonary valve, then cut into each pulmonary sinus and patch this area to relive any residual stenosis.

"What are the palliative options for cyanosis?"
Congenital cardiac defects that limit pulmonary artery blood flow may lead to cyanosis that requires palliation prior to definitive repair. The classic operation to augment pulmonary artery blood flow and relieve cyanosis, known as the Modified Blalock-Taussig shunt,

involves placement of a 3.5-mm PTFE interposition graft between the right subclavian artery and right branch pulmonary artery. In the case of a right-sided aortic arch the shunt can be placement between the left subclavian and pulmonary arteries. The use of a PTFE interposition graft, rather than ligation of the subclavian artery and primary anastomosis to the branch PA as in the "original" BT shunt, avoids the potential for stunted growth of the ipsilateral arm and kinking of the PA due to upward traction. PTFE is also easily ligated and transected at the time of the full repair. Patients are typically maintained on Aspirin for graft patency as long as the shunt is in place. A central shunt can be used if the anatomy is not amenable to a modified BT shunt.

"What are the indications for performing a palliative modified BT shunt?"
Cyanotic lesions such as Tetralogy of Fallot and Truncus Arteriosus types Ia and IIa that are causing severe hypoxemia in a neonate less than 4kg can be palliated with a BT shunt prior to definitive repair once the child has grown. Typically, patients that require surgical palliation are those who continue to desaturate despite maximum medical therapy, including inhaled prostacyclin.

"Is cardiopulmonary bypass necessary for BT shunt placement?"
If the patient is on prostacyclin, likely it can be performed off bypass. If the patient is having desaturations, they will likely not tolerate having the right pulmonary artery temporarily clamped and may require pump assist. If this is a concern, cannulation stitches should be placed to make crashing onto bypass less time consuming. Systemically heparinize with 300 units/kg and check an ACT prior to starting the first anastomosis in order to safely initiate bypass if needed.

"Describe the operation for BT shunt placement."
- Place patient supine and insert transesophageal echocardiography probe
- Insert peripheral arterial line in an extremity not receiving the BT shunt
- Perform median sternotomy and total thymectomy
- Fully open and suspend the pericardium
- Dissect out the aorta, AP window, the right pulmonary artery, and the innominate artery as well as the right carotid and subclavian arteries
- Place a partial occluding clamp at the junction of the innominate and subclavian arteries proximal the recurrent laryngeal nerve.
- Bevel the proximal end of a 3.5mm PTFE shunt.
- Perform the arteriotomy and extend with Potts scissors
- Sew proximal anastomosis with 8-0 prolene
- Remove clamp and flash the shunt to make sure it is widely patent
- Then let the shunt lay over the PA and mark on the shunt where it will be transected
- Place a clip or temporary ligature on the proximal shunt and trim it to length
- Place a partial occluding clamp on the right PA and pause to ensure the patient tolerates clamping
- Perform an arteriotomy and extend with Potts scissors
- Sew the shunt to the PA using 8-0 prolene
- Remove the clamp and the ligature from the shunt
- Close the chest in the standard fashion

Pearls/pitfalls
- PA bands should be tightened until the pulmonary artery pressure is ½ of the systemic artery pressure. This can be determined using a radial arterial line and cannula placed in the distal PA.
- Use hemoclips rather than interrupted sutures to tighten the PA band because clips can easily be removed if the patient becomes hypoxic or hemodynamically unstable.
- If the patient is unstable or the band size is difficult to get correct, leave the chest open and see if the band needs readjustment over the next 48 hours.

481

- Almost all patients undergoing BT shunt will require blood transfusion, ask anesthesia to maintain the hematocrit over 40% to optimize oxygen delivery
- While performing the distal anastomosis of a BT shunt remember that the PA will stretch but can easily tear. This is not a timed anastomosis, so take 2 bites and be safe.
- If the diastolic pressure starts to rise after BT shunt placement, the shunt is likely becoming occluded and may require revision
- Goal SaO2 at BT shunt is 75-85%. If hypoxemic, raising the systolic pressure will increase flow through the shunt and increase oxygen saturation.

Suggested readings

- Albus RA, Trusler GA, Izakawa T, Williams W. Pulmonary artery banding. J Thorac Cardiovasc Surg 1984;88:645–53.
- Franco KL, Thorani VH (editors). *Cardiothoracic Surgery Review*. 1st ed. Philadelphia, PA: Lippincott Williams & Wilkins; 2012: 315-327.
- Mavroudis K, Backer CL (editors). *Pediatric Cardiac Surgery*. 4th ed. Hoboken, N: Blackwell Publishing Ltd; 2012: 155-168.

79. HYPOPLASTIC LEFT HEART SYNDROME

Garrett Coyan, MD, MS and Victor Morell, MD

Concept
- Presentation
- Differential for HLHS
- Diagnostic Evaluation
- Staged Surgical Repair
- Additional Questions and Alternative Scenarios
- Pearls/Pitfalls

Chief complaint
"A 3kg male infant who initially appeared healthy develops sudden shock and cyanosis 48 hours following delivery. He was born to a G2P1 mother at 37 weeks gestational age following an uncomplicated pregnancy; no pre-natal testing or ultrasonography was conducted due to the patient being born in a small rural town. He was started on PGE1 and the patient was transferred to your facility for further evaluation and management. What is your differential and diagnostic plan?"

Differential
The differential for cyanotic heart disease includes hypoplastic left heart syndrome (HLHS), transposition of the great arteries, Ebstein's anomaly, Tetralogy of Fallot, truncus arteriosus, pulmonary or tricuspid atresia, total anomalous pulmonary venous return, and more complex congenital heart pathologies with right to left shunt. Lesions with ductal-dependent circulation can present in a delayed fashion with circulatory collapse and new cyanosis when the duct begins to close, necessitating PGE1 initiation and aggressive resuscitation.

History and physical
HLHS accounts for approximately 3-4% of congenital heart defects in infants, with a prevalence of 2.5 per 10,000 live births in the US. It is associated with over 25% of neonatal cardiac mortalities despite the low incidence. HLHS is a spectrum of disease characterized by inadequate sized and underdeveloped left-sided heart structures that are unable to support systemic circulation. Hypoplasia occurs in the left ventricle, left-sided heart valves, and the ascending aorta/arch; because of the inability for the left heart to support systemic circulation, HLHS is by necessity a ductal-dependent circulation and also requires an ASD for adequate mixing of oxygenated blood in the right ventricle. HLHS is universally fatal if left untreated; advances in early medical and surgical palliation have significantly improved outcomes over time with a 5-year survival approaching 65%.

Though many cases of HLHS are currently diagnosed on pre-natal ultrasonography, this technology is not uniformly used in all expectant mothers and post-natal presentation does still occur. Many children are born apparently healthy with a period of stability while the neo-natal circulation continues to support the child. When the PDA begins to close and PVR falls in the first several days following birth, patients will become symptomatic presenting with cyanosis, respiratory distress, failure of oral intake, and diminished pulses/systemic perfusion. This rapidly deteriorates into cardiogenic shock and heart failure. In 10% of cases, a restrictive or absent PDA/ASD will be present, and these patients present with cardiogenic shock and severe cyanosis immediately after birth; this will progress to death quickly without emergent intervention. Physical exam of HLHS infants can identify cyanosis, tachypnea, no murmur but a single pronounced S2 reflecting aortic valve absence, hepatomegaly, and cool extremities. Although usually absent in HLHS, a history of other genetic conditions or congenital abnormalities can be identified in 10-20% of patients.

Tests

483

- *Transthoracic echocardiography (TTE)*: serves as the primary modality for diagnosing HLHS. Characteristic factors include hypoplastic left ventricle, stenotic or atretic mitral and aortic valves, diminutive ascending aorta, and bidirectional flow through a PDA. In most cases there will be an ASD with left to right flow. Typically, the ventricular septum is intact.
- *CXR*: demonstrates increased pulmonary vascular markings and cardiomegaly, possible pulmonary white out in cases of restricted atrial septum
- *EKG*: right ventricular hypertrophy and right axis deviation are commonly observed on post-natal EKG
- *Pulse Oximetry*: will be characteristically low secondary to obligate right to left shunting and can be used as a screening test in post-natal screening for cyanotic heart disease
- *Cardiac catheterization*. Not routinely performed. In HLHS, balloon atrial septostomy may be required in the 10% of cases presenting with restrictive or absent ASD.

Index scenario (additional information)
"TTE demonstrates hypoplastic left ventricle with mitral and aortic valve atresia, atretic ascending aorta, large ASD and an open PDA. The infant has stabilized following transfer, resuscitation, and administration of PGE1. What is your next course of action?"

Treatment/management
Medical Management
Historically comfort care was the sole option for infants born with HLHS, and the condition was uniformly fatal. In some cases, with multiple congenital abnormalities, genetic syndromes, or extreme prematurity comfort measures may still be elected. However, in the modern era, surgical palliation or primary heart transplantation have taken over as the mainstay of treatment. In order to prepare a patient for either of these strategies, aggressive early management and referral to a tertiary care facility are required. The goal of initial management is to ensure adequate mixing of deoxygenated and oxygenated blood and allow for adequate systemic cardiac output. PGE1 (0.01 to 0.05 mcg/kg/min) is initiated to maintain ductal patency. In the 10% of patients with a restrictive or absent ASD, emergent balloon atrial septostomy is undertaken to ensure adequate mixing across the septum; if this procedure fails emergent surgical septectomy may be warranted. In cases of cardiogenic shock/ventricular dysfunction, aggressive management in the intensive care unit may include inotropic support, diuretics, and mechanical ventilation. Management of acidosis is paramount to stabilizing patients in extremis. Maneuvers to balance to systemic and pulmonary circulation by adjusting PVR (using the addition/subtraction of oxygen and carbon dioxide) and SVR (using α agonists/antagonists) can be required to stabilize patients prior to undergoing surgical correction.

Surgical Management
Patients electing to undergo treatment either enter a staged surgical palliation pathway or undergo primary heart transplantation. Because of the scarcity of neonatal organ donors and the increasing success of palliative surgery, most centers will recommend a surgical palliation strategy for infants presenting with HLHS.
Staged palliation consists of 3 sequential procedures for a single ventricle repair strategy:
Stage 1: The Norwood procedure is performed during the first weeks of life
Stage 2: The Bidirectional Glenn procedure or Hemi-Fontan is performed at 3-6 months
Stage 3: The Fontan procedure is performed between 2-4 years of age
This staged sequence is required to allow for the high PVR at birth, which then declines over time allowing for the passive pulmonary circulation required in the Stage 2 and Stage 3 operations.
For patients who present with anatomical or cardiac functional abnormalities that would prevent a staged palliation sequence, primary cardiac transplantation may be offered. It is important to realize that over 20% of infants listed for transplant will experience mortality

prior to being offered a transplant, but near-term post-operative survival following transplant is good. The long-term immunosuppression risks, along with graft failure/rejection make delaying transplant for as long as possible in those who can undergo staged palliation desirable. For this reason, staged palliation has become the standard of care for nearly all centers treating patients born with HLHS.

Operative Steps
Stage 1 (Norwood)
The goals of the Norwood operation include (1) ensuring unobstructed pulmonary venous blood flow to the RV (2) providing flow from the RV to the systemic circulation and (3) establishing a balanced source of pulmonary blood flow. There are several reported modifications to the Norwood procedure, and important modifications will be discussed in the alternative scenarios section.

- Median Sternotomy
- The pulmonary artery just inferior to the main PA/PDA junction (arterial) and right atrial appendage (venous) are cannulated and cardiopulmonary bypass is instituted
- The right and left pulmonary arteries can be snared to provide adequate systemic circulation
- Cooling for deep hypothermic circulatory arrest is commenced to 18°C
- Mobilization of the hypoplastic aorta and arch, branch vessels, main and branch PAs is completed during cooling; snares are placed around head vessels and a silk ligature around the PDA and left loose at this point
- The MPA is transected just proximal to the bifurcation, and the branch PA confluence is closed with a patch of PTFE or pulmonary homograft
- Once cooled, a clamp is placed on the descending thoracic aorta, head vessels snared, and cardioplegia delivered through the aortic cannula
- The PDA is then ligated proximally with the encircled suture and oversewn; the venous and arterial cannulas are removed
- Atrial septectomy is performed through the cannulation site or a separate inferior incision
- An aortotomy is made proceeding distal from the PDA insertion (with the PDA insertion being resected) to normal caliber descending aorta, then proximally along the lesser curve of the arch down the left side of the ascending aorta to the level of the distal open MPA
- The MPA is anastomosed to the ascending aorta with interrupted proline sutures being careful not to distort the coronary anatomy
- A crafted pulmonary allograft patch is then used to reconstruct the remainder of the ascending aorta/aortic arch sewn distal to proximal; care is taken when anastomosing near the aortic/PA anastomosis because this area is prone to bleeding
- The neoarota is re-cannulated through the pulmonary allograft, and the venous cannula re-inserted with re-warming instituted (head vessels are opened)
- During re-warming, a 3.5mm modified BT shunt is fashioned using a PTFE graft
- The patient is weaned from cardiopulmonary bypass
- The chest may be closed immediately or in a delayed fashion, depending on hemodynamic stability and bleeding/coagulopathy

Stage 2 (Bi-Directional Glenn Shunt)
The goal of the second stage is to begin to establish a pathway for systemic venous return to passively fill the pulmonary circulation now that post-natal PVR has decreased to a point where this is feasible. A Bi-Directional Glenn Shunt (described here) is used to shunt the SVC return to the pulmonary circulation. The Hemi-Fontan modification is a well-described alternative stage II discussed as an alternative scenario.

- Median sternotomy is performed

485

- Cardiopulmonary bypass is instituted with neoarotic cannulation for systemic arterial flow and right atrial appendage cannulation + proximal SVC cannulation for venous drainage
- The modified BT shunt is ligated, as is the azygous vein
- After circumferential mobilization, the SVC cannulas is snared and a vascular clamped applied just above the SVC/RA junction
- The SVC is transected, and the SVC/RA junction is oversewn
- The SVC is anastomosed to the right pulmonary artery using a running proline suture
- Patient is weaned from CPB and the sternum is closed in the usual manner

Stage 3 (Fontan Operation)
The third stage completes the routing of systemic venous return to the pulmonary system by shunting the IVC to the RPA. Described here is the extra-cardiac Fontan which goes smoothly with the previously described Glenn shunt. An alternative is the intracardiac lateral tunnel Fontan which involves a baffle and pairs well with the Hemi-Fontan (both described in the alternative scenarios below).
- Median sternotomy is performed
- Ascending aortic cannulation (arterial) with SVC and IVC (low on the IVC) bi-caval cannulation is carried out and cardiopulmonary bypass is initiated
- The lateral right atrium, IVC and right PA are mobilized, and a clamp is applied 2 cm above the IVC/atrial junction
- The IVC is divided just on the atrial side of the IVC/atrial junction, and the atrial stump is oversewn
- An 18-22 mm PTFE tube graft is anastomosed end to end with the IVC stump
- The opposite end of the graft is measured, cut, and anastomosed to the right pulmonary artery offset from the previous SVC anastomosis performed during the Bidirectional Glenn
- A 4 mm fenestration is created between the new IVC-PA conduit and the right atrium to serve as a "pop-off" valve should high pulmonary resistance be encountered in the post-operative period
- Weaning from bypass, decannulation, and sternotomy closure are performed as usual

Potential Questions and Alternative Scenarios
"What are the different morphologies of HLHS?"
HLHS is typically characterized by the degree of stenosis/atresia to the left-sided heart valves. The four classifications include:
1. Aortic Atresia/Mitral Atresia: most common presentation ($\approx$40% of cases)
2. Aortic Atresia/Mitral Stenosis: $\approx$30% of cases
3. Aortic Stenosis/Mitral Stenosis: $\approx$25% of cases, depending on degree of valvular stenosis and LV development, may be able to be taken down a biventricular repair pathway, otherwise staged palliation for repair
4. Aortic Stenosis/Mitral Atresia: $\approx$5% of cases (rare), highest risk cohort

"What can be expected post-operatively following operative staged palliation in HLHS patients?"
Following Stage I operations, patients with HLHS can have extremely labile hemodynamic profiles given the parallel nature of their circulation. Balancing pulmonary and systemic blood flow is the primary concern in the immediate post-operative period. PVR is managed by manipulating $FIO2$ levels and $CO2$ levels on the ventilator circuit, while SVR is manipulated using α-adrenergic agents. After several days the patient's hemodynamics typically reach a baseline with the new physiology, and support can be de-escalated. Oxygen saturation following a Stage I repair should typically be in the low to mid 80% range. Oral intake is begun and usually is the factor extending the length of stay in many circumstances

(avg of approximately 21 days). Patients are usually put on aspirin therapy for shunt thrombosis prophylaxis.

Inter-stage morbidity/mortality following Stage I can be significant, which is why close at home and in clinic monitoring is typically conducted on these patients tracking SPO2, weight, vital signs, and development. When an HLHS patient post Stage I repair is dehydrated, ill, or even simply fussy/upset, changes in the SVR/PRV balance can drastically affect oxygenation and cause cyanosis. Administering oxygen to obtain a saturation above the normal Stage I range may cause PVR to decrease making the patient decline further. Close coordination with the patient's cardiologist/surgeon is needed to manage any illnesses/issues in the inter-stage period.

For Stage II and Stage III repairs, the length of stay is around 7 days, and the post-operative courses are much more benign. There is significantly less inter-stage morbidity and mortality following Stage II repair, but patients are still closely monitored as discussed above.

"Discuss the shunt options for the Stage I Norwood procedure, and the pros and cons to the use of each."
In the operative description above, a modified Blalock-Taussig shunt was described (3.5 mm shunt from the innominate artery to the right pulmonary artery). A popular alternative is the RV-PA shunt (Sano shunt) consisting of a PTFE graft tunneled through a small incision in the infundibulum of the RV to the main PA. The Single Ventricle Reconstruction trial was the first multi-center randomized trial in congenital heart surgery, and compared outcomes following mBT shunt vs RV-PA shunt placement in HLHS. The early follow-up data suggested an early mortality benefit to the RV-PA shunt, but longer-term follow up over several years demonstrated no significant differences in mortality, and a higher re-intervention rate for RV-PA shunts compared to mBT shunts. This was mostly related to pulmonary artery stenosis requiring reconstruction or catheter-based interventions. There remains no consensus on which of the 2 shunts is preferred, with many centers of excellence utilizing both shunts with excellent outcomes throughout the world.

"Are there any alternatives to using deep hypothermic circulatory arrest for Stage I repair?"
Over the last several years, some centers have transitioned to utilizing antegrade cerebral perfusion (ACP) at 40cc/kg/minute with moderate (26-28°C) systemic cooling during the circulatory arrest period of the Stage I procedure for arch reconstruction. This method has been shown in observational studies to be safe with good post-operative neurocognitive outcomes. As with many other modifications to the Stage I Norwood palliation, no prospective randomized data exists on this subject, and both deep hypothermia and moderate hypothermia w/ ACP are used with excellent outcomes at many centers.

"Describe the Hemi-Fontan modification for Stage II and the Lateral Tunnel Fontan modification for Stage III."
Some centers prefer a Hemi-Fontan operation for Stage II in lieu of the Bi-directional Glenn shunt. The Hemi-Fontan consists of opening the superior portion of the RA onto the SVC/RA junction, anastomosis of the SVC to the RPA, and patch closure connecting the RPA to the SVC opening, while simultaneously excluding the SVC circulation from the RA. There is no data demonstrating a difference in mortality between Bi-directional Glenn and the Hemi-Fontan. However, there is a higher rate of atrial dysrhythmias associated with the Hemi-Fontan in some reports, likely due to the atrial suture lines. The Hemi-Fontan is also a more technically demanding operation, yet it allows for RPA augmentation in patients with stenosis and some proponents site improved hydrodynamics of the Hemi-Fontan circulation.

The Hemi-Fontan lends itself to the Lateral Tunnel Fontan modification of the Stage III operation. Instead of an extra-cardiac IVC-PA shunt, the lateral tunnel provides for an intra-atrial baffle between the IVC and the RPA. This is typically created with a PTFE patch through a right atriotomy. Compared to the extracardiac Fontan, the lateral tunnel tends to have higher rates of atrial arrhythmias and heart block/nodal dysfunction in several observational cohorts. There are no reported differences in mortality or other post-operative metrics between the two alternatives.

"A 2 kg infant born at 32 weeks gestational age is transferred to your facility after having undergone successful cardiopulmonary resuscitation after developing cyanosis 24 hours after birth. His lactate is 7, he is acidotic, and a TTE performed in the NICU demonstrates HLHS with AA/MA subtype, moderate tricuspid regurgitation, and a RV EF of approximately 40%. Are there alternatives to a traditional Stage I approach, and is this patient a candidate for palliation?"

In this scenario, the patient presents with several features that would classify them as a "high risk" candidate to undergo a traditional Stage I Norwood repair. Although low-moderate risk patients undergoing Stage I are quoted 90% survival at many specialty centers, patients presenting with high risk features (such as prematurity, low birth weight <2.5 kg, impaired RV function, moderate or severe tricuspid regurgitation, refractory cardiogenic shock, and co-existing genetic/extra-cardiac abnormalities) are at a much greater risk of mortality with a Norwood procedure.

Over the last several years, a "hybrid" approach to Stage I palliation has been shown to not only be safe in high risk patients but allows patients with these risk factors to clinically improve prior to undergoing a more comprehensive Stage II repair. The hybrid procedure consists of stenting of the PDA, bilateral PA banding, and balloon atrial septostomy (if required for a restrictive atrial septum). This eliminates the risk of cardiopulmonary bypass/deep hypothermic circulatory arrest in these higher risk patients. A comprehensive Stage II repair is them performed consisting of creation of the Bi-directional Glenn Shunt in addition to reconstruction of the hypoplastic aortic arch that would have been completed in the traditional Stage I repair. There has been a higher rate of PA stenosis requiring reconstruction at Stage II due to the pulmonary banding, but outcomes at centers utilizing this strategy have been promising. There have been no randomized studies adequately powered to demonstrate differences in long-term outcomes between a traditional and hybrid approach to Stage I palliation.

"What are the outcomes following surgical palliation of HLHS? Are there any long-term complications?"

Those undergoing stage palliation for HLHS have seen improved outcomes over the years. Currently, post-operative mortality following Stage I palliation in standard risk patients approaches 90%, with >80% reaching Stage II repair following the interstage period. Stage II boasts a 95% survival, with >98% survival post-operatively following Stage III Fontan completion. Ten-year survival is now >65-70% in the HLHS population.

Following staged palliation and Fontan completion, patients remain at risk for pleural effusions, atrial arrhythmias, exercise intolerance, atrioventricular valve dysfunction ventricular failure, and sudden cardiac death. Protein losing enteropathy can present following Fontan procedure in a limited number of cases but can be notoriously difficult to manage. This is thought to arise from altered lymphatic drainage patterns associated with the low-flow state during periods following Fontan completion. Patients present with progressive malnourishment that can be refractory to nutritional optimization and supplementation. Another rare but potentially deadly complication from dysregulation of the lymphatic system following Fontan completion is plastic bronchitis. Treatment of these disorders resolves around optimizing Fontan performance/hemodynamic status by addressing any shunt obstructions, valvular abnormalities, or volume status issues affecting cardiac performance. Supportive therapy including nutrition optimization is also required. Some specialized centers have experience with lymphangiography and embolization of abnormal lymphatic tracts in the treatment of refractory cases.

For patients presenting with failure of their Fontan physiology due to the above complications, either revision of the Fontan or heart transplantation may be the only intervention capable of improving their condition.

- HLHS is responsible for over 25% of neonatal cardiac deaths, but accounts for only 5% of congenital heart disease
- Infants with HLHS can present in a delayed fashion following birth when the ductus arteriosus closes; however, prenatal diagnosis has been increasing due to the ability to see the under-developed left heart structures on routine prenatal ultrasonography; post-natal TTE remains the gold standard for confirming the diagnosis
- PGE1 is the cornerstone of stabilization after HLHS is recognized; atrial septostomy is emergent in cases with a restrictive or non-existent ASD to provide adequate mixing
- Stage surgical palliation (consisting of the Stage I Norwood, the Stage II Bi-Directional Glenn or Hemi-Fontan, and the Stage III Fontan procedure) is the standard of care at most specialized centers dealing with HLHS patients
- Cardiac transplantation is typically reserved for circumstances where cardiac anatomy and dysfunction would prohibit a palliative repair, or for failure of patients who have undergone the palliative repair sequence
- Careful monitoring of patients in the interstage period between Stage I and Stage II is critical to minimize mortality given the continued hemodynamic lability of the Norwood circulation and need for balancing pulmonary and systemic blood flow
- RV-PA conduits during a Stage I repair may provide improved survival in the early post-operative period, but at the cost of increased re-interventions due to PA stenosis and RV dysfunction longer-term. There is no difference in longer-term survival between the 2 shunts demonstrated in the Single Ventricle Reconstruction trial studying this issue.
- Care should be taken during creation shunts to the PA to avoid narrowing and cause stenosis/narrowing in these regions; reconstruction of the PA prior to proceeding to the next Stage may be required to optimize the passive flow into the pulmonary circulation

Suggested readings

- Hirsch J., Devaney, E., Ohye R., and Bove E.; Chapter 31: Hypoplastic Left Heart Syndrome. Mavroudis C. and Backer CL (eds). *Pediatric Cardiac Surgery*, 4e Philadelphia, PA: Mosby; 2013.
- Chapter 31: The Norwood Principle. Khonsari S, Sintek CF(eds). *Cardiac Surgery: Safeguards and Pitfalls in Operative Technique*. 4th ed. Philadelphia, PA: Lippincott Williams & Wilkins; 2008.
- Gruber P., Spray T.; Chapter 96: Hypoplastic Left Heart Syndrome. Kaiser, LR, Kron, IL, and Spray, TL (eds). *Mastery of Cardiothoracic Surgery*, 3e Philadelphia, PA: Lippincott Williams & Wilkins; 2014.

80. TRANSPOSITION OF THE GREAT ARTERIES

Mallory Hunt, MD and J. William Gaynor, MD

This chapter is a revision and update of that included in the previous edition of the TSRA Clinical Scenarios written by Muhammad Aftab, MD, Elizabeth Pocock, MD, and Charles D. Fraser, Jr., MD

Concept

- Presentation
- Differential for TGA
- Diagnostic evaluation
- Surgical repair
- Pitfalls and Alternative Scenarios

Chief complaint

"A full-term 3.2kg male is found to be severely cyanotic at birth. His mother is a 17-year-old G1P0 who received no prenatal care. At his birth hospital, he was started on PGE1. Due to lack of advanced cardiac intervention capability, he is transferred to your hospital for further evaluation. What is your differential diagnosis for cyanotic heart disease and how would you proceed?"

Differential

The differential diagnosis of cyanotic congenital heart disease at birth includes:
1. Transposition of the great arteries (TGA)
2. Tetralogy of Fallot (TOF)
3. Truncus arteriosus (TA)
4. Ebstein's anomaly
5. Total anomalous pulmonary venous connection (TAPVC)
6. Single ventricle anomalies, including (but not limited to):
   a. Hypoplastic left heart syndrome (HLHS)
   b. Tricuspid atresia
7. Double outlet right ventricle (DORV)
8. Pulmonary atresia or pulmonary stenosis (PA/PS)

History and physical

Transposition of the great arteries (TGA) comprises 9.9% of all congenital cardiac defects and is characterized by reversal of the anatomic relationship of the great arteries (ventriculoarterial discordance), with the aorta arising from the right ventricle and the pulmonary artery arising completely, or mostly, from the left ventricle. The resulting physiologic abnormality, i.e. systemic and pulmonary circulations that are arranged in parallel, is incompatible with life unless surgically corrected. TGA may coexist with other congenital lesions, including coarctation of the aorta and patent ductus arteriosus.

TGA is associated with IVS in approximately 50% of cases; the remainder present with VSD (25%) or VSD with left ventricular outflow tract obstruction (pulmonary stenosis) (25%). The degree of cyanosis present at birth is determined by the extent of intracardiac mixing of pulmonary and systemic blood flow. Neonates with TGA and intact ventricular septum (IVS) have the most severe cyanosis, which is discernible at birth after removal of ductal-dependent flow. By contrast, patients with TGA and non-restrictive ventricular septal defect (VSD) may exhibit mild cyanosis at birth, which can be clinically underappreciated. With the gradual fall in pulmonary vascular resistance (PVR) in the neonatal period, these patients will develop pulmonary overcirculation and congestive heart failure, symptoms of which commonly appear by 1 month of age. Systolic murmurs are audible in almost 50% of patients.

490

Tests

- *Transthoracic echocardiography (TTE)*: postnatally, TTE is the mainstay of diagnosis. Diagnosis is confirmed by the presence of a posterior vessel that branches into right and left pulmonary arteries arising from the left ventricle; with an anterior aorta arising from the right ventricle. The classic echocardiographic findings are: great vessels seen parallel to each other instead of classic wrapping pattern (on the long axis view), two semilunar valves (mitral-pulmonary contiguity) visible within the same slice (on the short axis view) and an early branching pattern of the great artery associated with the left ventricle (pulmonary artery). Subsequent views can delineate the size and location of VSDs, and Doppler ultrasound can clarify the extent of intracardiac shunting. The echocardiogram should also be able to define the relative position and size of great vessels, the relative size of aortic and pulmonary valves, and the location of coronary ostia.

- *CXR*. Classically demonstrates the "egg on a string" sign suggestive of a narrow superior mediastinum. Initial CXRs may reveal unremarkable lung fields, with increasing pulmonary edema as PVR falls and pulmonary overcirculation develops.

- *EKG*. Usually normal for age at birth. In neonates with TGA/IVS, EKG may later demonstrate RV hypertrophy with right axis deviation. In patients with TGA/VSD, EKG typically shows biventricular hypertrophy with a normal axis.

- *Cardiac catheterization*. No longer routinely performed. Cardiac catheterization is indicated in the presence of inadequate intracardiac mixing, or if other intra- or extracardiac lesions are present that require intervention. In patients with TGA/IVS, therapeutic cardiac catheterization to perform balloon atrial septostomy may be warranted in cases of clinical or hemodynamic instability pre-operatively.

Index scenario (additional information)

"Two-dimensional echocardiogram reveals a posterior vessel that branches into right and left pulmonary arteries arising from the left ventricle; with an anterior aorta arising from the right ventricle, with a patent ductus arteriosus (PDA), a small restrictive atrial septal defect (ASD) and an intact ventricular septum (IVS). How would you proceed?"

Treatment/management
Medical management
The goal of medical management of a neonate with TGA is stabilization of the patient, adequate systemic (including cerebral) perfusion, acceptable oxygen delivery, and correction of metabolic derangements caused by cyanosis. PGE1 is immediately initiated to restore ductal patency and increase pulmonary blood flow. Balloon atrial septostomy should be performed within hours of diagnosis of TGA in the absence of sufficient shunting at the atrial (ASD), ventricular (VSD), and/or arterial (PDA) level. If a prenatal diagnosis has already been established, the child should be delivered in a center where balloon atrial septostomy can be performed expeditiously.

Due to the risk of severe CHF resulting from increased pulmonary blood flow in the setting of declining PVR, early repair is typically advocated in neonates with favorable anatomy. Typically, the neonate is stabilized and resuscitated in the ICU for several days prior to surgical intervention.

Surgical management
The diagnosis of TGA in a neonate is an indication for surgery.
TGA/IVS. An arterial switch operation (ASO) is indicated in patients with TGA/IVS early in the neonatal period. In infants with uncomplicated TGA who present beyond 4-6 weeks after birth, LV deconditioning is a matter of concern. In these patients if the LV muscle mass is adequate and the LV posterior wall thickness is normal for the age, a single stage ASO can be performed. For patients with a marginal LV, a two-stage approach can be used. This approach consists of placement of a pulmonary artery band (PAB) for LV retraining, with or without modified Blalock-Taussing shunt (BTS) followed by an ASO. However, two-stage

491

approaches are less common in the current era, when ASO followed by perioperative mechanical circulatory support (i.e. ECMO or VAD) is utilized increasingly more frequently. *TGA/VSD.* An arterial switch operation with VSD closure is indicated for TGA/VSD diagnosed at any age, if there is a non-restrictive VSD and the patient has not developed fixed pulmonary vascular obstructive disease (PVOD). While TGA/VSD repair used to be postponed until about 2-3 months of age, most centers now repair these patients as neonates due to data suggesting that delayed repair is detrimental.

TGA/VSD/PS (LVOTO). The surgical options for patients with TGA/VSD/PS include ASO, Bex-Nikaidoh, Réparation à l'Etage Ventriculaire (REV) and the Rastelli operation. The choice of operative procedure varies based on the size of pulmonary valve annulus, degree and etiology of pulmonary stenosis and the resectability of LVOT obstruction. For patients with an isolated pulmonary valve abnormality (i.e., focal area of pulmonary stenosis), it is possible to resect the obstruction and perform a primary ASO.

For the subset of patients having TGA/VSD with moderate pulmonary valve hypoplasia and septal malalignment, an anatomical repair can be performed using the Bex-Nikaidoh operation. These patients usually have a VSD non-committed to the great arteries (inlet or trabecular type), so construction of an LV to aorta tunnel is not possible.

Patients with TGA/VSD and pulmonary atresia, significant valvular pulmonary stenosis or hypoplasia can undergo anatomic repair using the REV procedure or the Rastelli operation. These procedures can be performed safely only after the neonatal period, so it is crucial to carefully monitor these patients for any worsening cyanosis. A ductal stent may be necessary for these patients prior to any definitive repair.

TGA/VSD/Aortic Arch Obstruction. When arch obstruction is present (i.e. coarctation or interrupted aortic arch), arch repair should be performed at the time of the definitive TGA operative procedure.

Operative Steps
The Arterial Switch Operation
The goal of the arterial switch operation (ASO) is to correct ventriculoarterial discordance by transecting and replacing the great vessels. Concurrently, the coronary arteries are re-implanted to the aorta following repositioning. The ASO is performed through a median sternotomy with cardiopulmonary bypass under mild or moderate hypothermia, +/- a period of circulatory arrest, and proceeds generally as outlined below:

- Following sternotomy, the great vessels and coronary arteries are closely examined. The presence of anomalous coronary relationships must be thoroughly investigated, in order to plan for the most appropriate repair. While normal coronary anatomy is most common, the next most common relationship is an aberrant left circumflex artery originating from the right coronary artery.

- The pericardium is opened, and a portion is harvested for reconstruction of the defects created by excision of coronary buttons from the native aortic root (pulmonary artery).

- Cardiopulmonary bypass is established using bicaval cannulation. The aorta is cannulated as far distally as possible to allow for manipulation of the aorta during reconstruction.

- If the operation is to be performed under hypothermia, cooling will begin. However, most centers use mild or no hypothermia. The repair of TGA/IVS and TGA/VSD usually do not require deep hypothermic circulatory arrest.

- The PDA is dissected out, doubly ligated and divided.

- A left atrial vent is placed via the right superior pulmonary vein or directly through a right atriotomy across the PFO.

- Extensive mobilization of pulmonary arterial branches is performed, to the hilum bilaterally. Adequate mobilization of the branch pulmonary arteries is essential for safe relocation of the pulmonary artery during the Lecompte maneuver.

- The ascending aorta is cross clamped, and the heart is arrested with antegrade cardioplegia.

492

- If a VSD is present, it can be repaired through the tricuspid valve via a right atriotomy. Occasionally, a VSD may be repaired through the anterior great vessel or pulmonary artery; however, doing so greatly increases the risk of neoaortic insufficiency and so this approach is typically avoided. Generally, the VSD is repaired with a pericardial or Gore-Tex patch. The ASD is usually closed partially to allow for mixing in the early post-operative period, either primarily or by patch closure.

- Following VSD repair, additional cardioplegia is administered as needed. The aorta and the main pulmonary artery are then transected above the semilunar valves.

- After repositioning of the aortic cross clamp, the pulmonary artery confluence is relocated in front of the aorta (Lecompte maneuver).

- At this point, the coronary ostia are inspected, and coronary buttons are excised from the native aortic root and re-implanted into the native pulmonary root (neoaortic root) taking great care to avoid twisting, kinking, and excess tension. (Coronary reimplantation may also be accomplished after anastomosis of the neoaortic root. A "closed technique" uses marking stitches on the outside of the neoaortic root to identify the commissures so that a safe location for button reimplantation can be found after the anastomosis is complete when the root is temporarily filled).

- Aortic continuity is established by anastomosing the native pulmonary root (neoaortic root) to the ascending aorta.

- The defects of coronary buttons in the native aortic root (neopulmonary root) are patched using autologous pericardium. Pulmonary arterial continuity is then reestablished by anastomosing the neopulmonary root to the pulmonary artery bifurcation. Pulmonary anastomoses may be completed following clamp removal, allowing for adequate inspection of hemostasis.

- Rewarming is started, the aortic cross clamp is removed, and deairing is accomplished under TEE guidance.

- The patient is separated from the cardiopulmonary bypass, protamine is administered to reverse heparin, and the heart is decannulated.

- Hemostasis is secured. Chest tube(s) are placed. The sternum is closed in the standard fashion.

Potential Questions and Alternative Scenarios

"What is the morphology of TGA and what are the clinical subtypes and most common coronary patterns?"

Morphology of TGA

TGA is characterized by ventriculoarterial discordance. The aorta arises from the right ventricle and the pulmonary artery from left the ventricle. The looping of ventricles is normal (i.e. d-looping; the right atrium is related to the right ventricle and left atrium to left ventricle). TGA is further classified into:

- *Simple TGA* (50%). These patients have an Intact Ventricular Septum (IVS) and no other cardiac anomaly except a patent ductus arteriosus (PDA) and patent foramen ovale (PFO).

- *Complex TGA with ventricular septal defect-VSD* (50%). VSDs associated with TGA are more commonly of conoventricular (perimembranous) or outlet morphology. Approximately 25% of the patients with TGA and VSD have pulmonary stenosis resulting in LVOTO. TGA with an anterior malalignment VSD is also frequently associated with Interrupted Aortic Arch (IAA) or marked hypoplasia of aortic arch with coarctation.

Although the coronary anatomy is variable among patients with TGA, the most common (60%) distribution consists of the left main coronary artery originating from the leftward and posterior facing sinus and the right coronary artery arising from the rightward and posterior facing sinus. In almost 1/3 of patients with TGA, the coronary arteries are found looping either anterior or posterior to the great arteries. Other coronary variations include all arteries

493

arising from a single sinus and intramural coronary arteries. The coronary branching pattern is variable and contributes to increasing technical complexity of treatment.

Clinical variations of TGA and physiologic implications
The common resulting physiologic abnormality in TGA is the presence of parallel systemic and pulmonary circulations. As mentioned previously, the degree of cyanosis presents at birth, and the neonate's prognosis, depends upon the communication between these two circulations. Communication can occur at several levels, including at the atria (ASD), ventricles (VSD), and/or ductus arteriosus (PDA).
Several clinical forms of TGA exist, as described below.
1.   Transposition of the Great Arteries with Intact Ventricular Septum (TGA/IVS)
In patients with TGA/IVS, there is no intracardiac mixing; therefore, a patent ductus arteriosus must be maintained by a PGE1 infusion for survival. Closure of the PDA will result in loss of mixing, severe cyanosis, and hemodynamic compromise. If warranted, balloon atrial septostomy should be performed early in this situation. Occasionally, patients with TGA/IVS may survive without diagnosis due to adequate atrial level shunting. In these patients, the LV becomes deconditioned and loses its ability to support the systemic circulation in the setting of decreasing pulmonary vascular resistance. These patients will need LV reconditioning by pulmonary artery banding (PAB) prior to ASO.
2.   Transposition of the Great Arteries with Ventricular Septal Defect (TGA/VSD)
Patients TGA and a nonrestrictive VSD typically have more effective mixing between both pulmonary and systemic circuits, resulting in pulmonary overcirculation. Moreover, because of the equalization of pressure between both ventricles, the LV maintains its ability to support the systemic circulation. These patients are at significant risk of early onset pulmonary vascular obstructive disease (PVOD). As such, early repair is advocated.
3.   Transposition of the Great Arteries with Ventricular Septal Defect and Left Ventricular Outflow Tract Obstruction (TGA/VSD/LVOTO)
Neonates with TGA/VSD and LV outflow tract obstruction (LVOTO) exhibit physiologic abnormalities similar to those seen in Tetralogy of Fallot. Mild PS protects the lungs from the development of pulmonary vascular obstructive disease. Usually, these patients have adequate intracardiac mixing. Moreover, the LV pressure load from PS and the VSD prevents deconditioning of the LV. Patients with significant pulmonary stenosis may require a PGE1 infusion to maintain ductal patency and provide adequate pulmonary blood flow.
4.   Transposition of the Great Arteries with Ventricular Septal Defect and Aortic Arch Obstruction (IAA/Arch Hypoplasia/Coarctation)

Patients with TGA/VSD and aortic arch obstruction (e.g. interrupted aortic arch, arch hypoplasia or coarctation) are at risk of lower extremity malperfusion following ductal closure. These patients exhibit reverse differential cyanosis; i.e., *blue fingers and pink toes*. This results from a supply of fully saturated blood reaching the lower body through the LV and PDA, while the upper body is desaturated.

"What is the REV procedure and how does it compare with the Rastelli operation?"
The Rastelli operation is the classic corrective procedure for patients with TGA/VSD/LVOTO (PS). In this procedure, left ventricular blood flow is diverted by an intraventricular baffle across the VSD to the aorta. The right ventricle to pulmonary artery continuity is then established using an extracardiac valved conduit. The reported mortality from this procedure ranges from 10-29% with acceptable long-term results. Long-term survival is usually affected by the presence and degree of LV dysfunction as well as conduit stenosis/subaortic stenosis which may require multiple reoperations.

The Réparation à l'Etage Ventriculaire (REV procedure), which consists of reconstructing the RVOT without a prosthetic conduit, was introduced by Lecompte to decrease the number of reoperations from conduit replacement. This procedure consists of extensive resection of the conal septum for VSD enlargement, creating a short and straight LV-to-aortic tunnel without reducing the size of the RV cavity. An intraventricular baffle is created to divert LV blood flow to the aorta, and the great vessels are transected and repositioned as in the ASO.

494

The operative mortality of the REV procedure is less than 5%. The advantage of the REV procedure over the Rastelli operation is that the LV function remains preserved among most survivors with a very low risk of subaortic stenosis.

"What is the Bex-Nikaidoh operation?"
The Bex-Nikaidoh procedure consists of harvesting the aortic root, as in the Ross procedure, and reconstructing the LVOT by the translocated the aortic root. LVOT obstruction is relieved by dividing the outlet septum and/or enlarging the outflow tract with a patch if necessary. Coronary arteries are individually re-implanted after translocation or transferred en bloc with the root. The RVOT is reconstructed by anterior translocation of the pulmonary artery (or using pulmonary homograft) and direct anastomosis to the right ventricle. The major advantage of this approach is that it is an anatomic repair in which the LVOT and RVOT are normally aligned.

"What are the outcomes of an Arterial Switch Operation and how would you follow your patient after ASO?"
The reported 30-day mortality rate following an ASO is 1.6%, with expected long term survival of > 95% with a normal lifestyle and LV function. Close long-term follow-up is necessary to monitor for the development of conditions that may require surgical intervention, such as proximal coronary artery stenosis, supravalvular pulmonary stenosis, and dilation of the neoaortic root and resulting aortic insufficiency.

"What is the relevance of left ventricular outflow tract obstruction in TGA?"
Isolated LVOTO sometimes occurs in patients with TGA and IVS. This is a functional obstruction, usually caused by the leftward bulging of the septum due to higher RV (systemic) pressure compared to the lower pressure LVOT. The functional LVOTO usually resolves with anatomic correction resulting in a rightward shift of the septum. However, sometimes this can progress into fixed LVOTO.

Hemodynamically significant valvular and sub-valvular stenosis causing LVOTO is more common in patients with TGA/VSD. Organic LVOTO results in reduced pulmonary blood flow which, in combination with TGA physiology, causes a profound cyanosis which may affect surgical decision making.

"After coming off pump following an ASO, significant ST changes are noted on EKG with hemodynamic instability. LV function is severely depressed on TEE. What would you do next?"
The scenario describes myocardial ischemia due to coronary insufficiency. Poor myocardial preservation or an intraoperative complication of coronary transfer must be considered. Assuming myocardial protection was adequate, coronary insufficiency may be due to proximal occlusion, stenosis, or dissection. Proximal occlusion or stenosis can be caused by twisting of the artery during coronary artery button rotation prior to reimplantation, tension on the coronary artery, or by other distortion. Coronary artery dissection is possible during manipulation of the artery before, during, and after harvesting the buttons, or may be due to a retraction injury.
The most important treatment is prevention of these conditions before they occur. Reimplantation of a coronary button with repositioning and patching can be attempted but is very difficult and usually requires taking down the pulmonary anastomosis and re-arresting the heart. The most common management strategies include proximal patch (autologous pericardium) coronary arterioplasty, coronary artery bypass grafting (usually with the internal thoracic artery), or a combination of both techniques. Stenting has been successfully used to treat coronary artery dissection following a Ross procedure and may be an option in larger patients after ASO. Management decisions should be based on patient characteristics, surgeon comfort level and institutional practice, as well as the availability of a catheterization lab and a skilled interventionalist.

- Most cases of TGA are diagnosed prenatally. When a child presents with a new diagnosis of TGA at birth, transthoracic echocardiogram is diagnostic, and will show two great vessels running parallel to each other in the long-axis view, or the "double-barrel" appearance of the great vessels in the short-axis view. Cardiac catheterization is indicated only if concurrent intervention is needed.

- The degree of cyanosis and hemodynamic compromise present at birth are determined by the level of intracardiac mixing. Mixing occurs at several levels: atrial (ASD), ventricular (VSD), and/or ductal (PDA). Usually, two levels are needed for adequate mixing.

- PGE1 should be initiated immediately after birth to maintain ductal patency.

- The diagnosis of TGA in a neonate is an indication for surgery.

- While patients with TGA/IVS present with severe cyanosis at birth, those with TGA/VSD may be less symptomatic in the neonatal period. However, these patients risk severe symptomatic CHF resulting from decreased pulmonary vascular resistance. As such, early repair is warranted.

- The arterial switch operation (ASO) is the definitive procedure of choice for TGA/IVS, and TGA/VSD. Surgical options for patients with TGA/VSD/LVOTO include the Rastelli, Bex-Nikaidoh, and REV procedures in addition to the ASO.

- When an arch abnormality (e.g. IAA, hypoplasia, or coarctation) is present, it should be addressed at the time of definitive repair.

- In infants with simple TGA who present beyond 4-6 weeks after birth, LV deconditioning is a matter of concern. For patients with an unprepared or marginal LV, a two-stage approach consisting of LV retraining by placement of pulmonary artery band (PAB) with or without modified Blalock-Taussing shunt (BTS) followed by an ASO is undertaken.

- Avoiding coronary complications is critical, as surgical correction can be very difficult.

Suggested readings

- Transposition of the Great Arteries. Kaiser, LR, Kron, IL, and Spray, TL (eds). *Mastery of Cardiothoracic Surgery*, 3e Philadelphia, PA: Lippincott Williams & Wilkins; 2014.

- Coronary artery anomalies. Mavroudis C. and Backer CL (eds). *Pediatric Cardiac Surgery*, 3e Philadelphia, PA: Mosby; 2003.

- Transposition of the Great Arteries. Jonas R. (ed). *Comprehensive Surgical Management of Congenital Heart Disease*. Hodder Arnold Publication. 2004.

- Khonsari S, Sintek CF. *Cardiac Surgery: Safeguards and Pitfalls in Operative Technique*. 4th ed.Philadelphia, PA: Lippincott Williams & Wilkins; 2008.

- Franco KL, Thorani VH (editors). *Cardiothoracic Surgery Review*. 1st ed. Philadelphia, PA: Lippincott Williams & Wilkins; 2012: 315-327.

81. EBSTEIN'S ANOMALY

Stephanie Nguyen, MD and Damien J. LaPar, MD, MSc

This chapter is a revision and update of that included in the previous edition of the TSRA Clinical Scenarios written by Dr. Damien J. LaPar, MD, MSc and Dr. Pedro J. del Nido, MD.

Concept

- Diagnosis and classification of Ebstein's anomaly
- Indications for surgical repair
- Critical steps of tricuspid valve repair (cone procedure)
- Alternative surgical techniques
- Pitfalls and alternative solutions

Chief complaint

"A 10-year-old boy with a neonatal diagnosis of Ebstein's anomaly presents with worsening cyanosis, new onset palpitations, and fainting spells.

Differential

The diagnosis has been established and the patient was medically managed throughout infancy and childhood. It is likely that the degree of tricuspid valve malformation and regurgitation at birth were not severe enough to warrant repair; however, the new heart failure symptoms and palpitations are most likely related to a progression of his Ebstein's. If cyanosis is present in the neonatal period one should also consider other causes of cyanotic congenital heart disease including: Tetralogy of Fallot, total anomalous pulmonary venous return, hypoplastic left heart syndrome, d-transposition of the great arteries, truncus arteriosus (persistent), tricuspid atresia, pulmonary atresia, and critical pulmonary stenosis.

History and physical

Focused history for presence of cyanosis, palpitations, fatigability, reduced exercise tolerance, dyspnea on exertion, or other manifestations of reduced cardiac functional status. Most patients with Ebstein's anomaly have an atrial shunt (PFO or secundum ASD) which accounts for the cyanosis. The presence of symptoms or cyanosis suggest a malformation severe enough to warrant surgery. A focused physical exam should clarify the presence of cyanosis, a systolic murmur of tricuspid regurgitation, a prominent jugular venous "v" wave, liver enlargement, as well as evidence of irregular cardiac rhythm and tachyarrhythmia.

Tests

- *Laboratory analysis*: may reveal polycythemia.
- *EKG*: right bundle branch block with right axis deviation and atrial arrhythmias (15% Wolff-Parkinson-White [WPW] syndrome; 1-2% atrioventricular node reentrant tachycardia [AVNRT]))
- *Imaging:*
  - *CXR*: significant cardiomegaly (cardiothoracic ratio > 0.65), decreased pulmonary vascular markings.
  - *Echocardiography*: diagnostic test of choice; provides essential preoperative information.
    - LV function, RA and RV size and function, TV annulus size, extent of RV atrialization.
    - Doppler - estimate severity of TR and RV outflow obstruction.
    - Atrial shunt type and direction (ASD, PFO).
    - TV leaflet anatomy – degree of tethering/lamination, apical displacement of the septal leaflet, mobility of the anterior leaflet, presence of fenestrations

- Carpentier classification of Ebstein's anomaly (helps determine severity of malformation and depicts important components of the echo and gross inspection):
  - *Type A*
    - small atrialized RV (adequate-sized functional RV)
    - moderate displacement of septal/posterior leaflets
    - normal anterior leaflet
  - *Type B*
    - large atrialized RV (small functional RV)
    - marked displacement of septal/posterior leaflets
    - hypoplastic, adherent septal leaflet
    - normal anterior leaflet
  - *Type C*
    - large atrialized RV (very small functional RV)
    - marked displacement of septal/posterior leaflets
    - hypoplastic, adherent septal and posterior leaflet
    - restricted anterior leaflet (may cause obstruction)
  - *Type D*
    - almost completely noncontractile atrialized RV
    - marked displacement of septal/posterior leaflets
    - hypoplastic, adherent septal and posterior leaflet
    - adherent anterior leaflet (severe RVOTO)
- *Great Ormond Street Score (GOSE)*: ratio of combined RA area and atrialized RV to the combined areas of the functional RV and left heart chambers in diastole on 4 chamber view (Score 1-4).
  - Score 1: ratio < 0.50
  - Score 2: ratio 0.50-0.99
  - Score 3: ratio 1.00-1.49
  - Score 4: ratio > 1.50
  - Studies demonstrating Scores 3-4 (ratio > 1.00) predict high mortality (44-100%).
- *Cardiac catheterization*: rarely necessary and may precipitate arrhythmias. Only useful if ruling out severe pulmonary vascular resistance.
- *MRI:* quantitative assessment of ventricular size and function. Although not routinely used, may be useful in planning more complex or re-operative repairs.
- *Associated anomalies*: rare; bicuspid AV, mitral valve prolapse, and ASD are the most common considerations.

Index scenario (additional information)
"EKG demonstrates a WPW pre-excitation pattern and CXR with severe cardiomegaly. Echocardiography shows a large atrialized RV, severe TR, apical displacement of the TV with an elongated anterior leaflet, rudimentary septal leaflet, and a secundum ASD."

Treatment/management
Treatment is dictated by age of presentation, constellation of clinical features, and anatomy. Most symptomatic children will undergo surgical correction before medical therapy is required; however, those with overt heart failure will require medical stabilization prior to surgery. Indications for surgery include the presence of the following:
1) Symptomatic NYHA functional class III or IV
2) Progressive RV dilation with severe TR by echocardiography or cardiomegaly on CXR (cardiothoracic ratio ≥ 0.65)
3) Cyanosis
4) Paradoxical embolism
5) Atrial or ventricular arrhythmias

Early surgical intervention is encouraged prior to deterioration of right and/or left ventricular function. Mortality for late-stage operations increases significantly.

The fundamental goals for surgical correction of Ebstein's anomaly:

- Preoperative electrophysiologic mapping of accessory conduction pathways in patients with ventricular preexcitation
- If present, closure of ASD (+/- fenestration)
- Ligation of prior shunts and correction of associated cardiac anomalies
- Performance of any indicated anti-arrhythmia procedure (such as cryoablation of AV nodal reentrant tachycardia, right/biatrial maze, etc).
- Tricuspid valve repair (versus replacement with bioprosthetic) whenever a good to excellent result can be expected
- Possible plication of the atrialized right ventricle
- Reduction right atrioplasty
- Avoiding the major pitfalls - injury to the coronary sinus, right coronary artery or conduction.

Biventricular TV repair: the cone reconstruction

- Place TEE probe
- Access via median sternotomy
- Aortic and bicaval venous cannulation and initiation of cardiopulmonary bypass (CPB)
- Mild systemic hypothermia (32-34° C), aorta cross clamped with antegrade cardioplegia, snare IVC and SVC
- Oblique right atriotomy parallel to AV groove
- Left heart vent (often placed through PFO/ASD if present)
- Investigate presence of ASD
- Inspection of TV leaflets and annulus; assessment of size and extent of atrialized RV (see Carpentier's classification above)
- Incise anterior leaflet at 12:00 (surgeon's view), a few millimeters from the true annulus and extend in a rightward/clockwise fashion using scissors. Detach ("delaminate") the body of the anterior and posterior leaflets from the underlying RV myocardium, leaving all attachments and chordae to the leading edge intact
- Examine edge of leading leaflet for direct attachment to myocardium ("linear attachment"). If present, create fenestrations in distal leaflet to allow blood flow into RV cavity
- Mobilize the septal leaflet off of the true annulus and underlying myocardium in a similar fashion if sufficient tissue is present. Leave all apical attachments intact. The septal leaflet is typically diminutive and displaced toward the apex more so than the other leaflets
- Rotate the free edge of the anterior/posterior leaflet complex clockwise and suture its septal edge (interrupted 5-0 or 6-0 monofilament) to the septal leaflet, thus increasing the height of the septal leaflet. If too little septal leaflet tissue, suture free edge of posterior leaflet to the septal edge of the anterior leaflet
- Internal plication of atrialized RV with running 5-0 monofilament with caution as to avoid compromising branches of the RCA externally
- Annuloplasty (usually partial/posterior +/- prosthetic ring)
- Suture the 360° cone-shaped valve to true tricuspid annulus with interrupted 5-0 or 6-0 monofilament
  - Superficial bites near AV node to avoid heart block

499

- Test valve while occluding PA
- Fenestrated closure of ASD
- +/- ablation or right or biatrial maze
- Right reduction atrioplasty. Close RA, remove cross clamp
- Patient rewarmed and weaned from CPB
- PRN inotropic support and RV afterload reduction (dopamine, milrinone, iNO)

Potential questions/alternative scenarios

"Immediately after birth, a neonate with prenatal diagnosis of Ebstein's anomaly presents with severe right heart failure and cyanosis. CXR shows cardiothoracic ratio > 0.80. Describe the approach to management in the neonatal period."

This unstable patient requires intubation and paralysis, inotropic support, and PGE infusion to decrease metabolic demands, improve cardiac output, and increase pulmonary blood flow. Other efforts to decrease RV afterload include hyperventilation, alkalosis, and nitric oxide. As native PVR falls, PGE can be weaned off and surgery may be delayed beyond the neonatal period. However, surgery should be performed if there is evidence of ventricular deterioration, or pulmonary atresia (anatomic and functional) in the acute period.

"What are the other indications for surgery in the neonate/infant?
- Congestive heart failure refractory to medical therapy
- Severe cyanosis
- GOSE score of 3 or 4 with mild cyanosis
- Cardiothoracic ratio > 0.80
- Severe TR with persistent right heart failure

"Describe alternative options for patients that are not candidates for biventricular repair alone."

For most patients, a biventricular repair alone is possible, and the cone procedure is the repair of choice. However, those with significant RV dysfunction, TR, or anatomic/functional pulmonary atresia require alternative surgical management. Some patients may benefit from a 1.5-ventricle repair (addition of bidirectional superior cavopulmonary shunt) to reduce RV hemodynamic stress or flow across a small effective orifice area following TVr. In neonates, other surgical options include a univentricular approach using the Starnes palliation (fenestrated patch exclusion of the RV, inter-atrial connection enlargement, and placement of a systemic-to-pulmonary artery shunt) or a modified BT shunt, both leading to a Fontan circulation. In severe cases of biventricular failure, heart transplantation is an option but limited due to donor shortage for this patient population and improved early results of biventricular and univentricular repair.

"If initial TV repair proves inadequate, what other surgical options are available?"

Re-repair of residual anatomic defect is performed. Usually in children, a repair with even moderate TR is preferred over valve replacement. If unable to repair the valve, replacement with a bioprosthesis is preferred over a mechanical valve due to lack of lifetime anticoagulation requirement and good durability in the tricuspid position. However, young patients will inevitably require future upsizing of valve prosthesis due to annular growth and valve degeneration. In order to avoid damage to the conduction system, the coronary sinus may be left to drain into the RV if there is not enough room between it and the AV node during valve implantation. To protect the RCA, the valve suture line may need to deviate above the tricuspid annulus posterolaterally where tissues are typically thin.

"What is the role of concomitant arrhythmia ablation?"

Concomitant surgical ablation or cryoablation at the time of surgical repair should be added for all patients with supraventricular tachycardia, accessary pathway-mediated tachycardia, and atrioventricular nodal reentrant tachycardia not amenable to percutaneous intervention. Patients with atrial fibrillation or flutter can undergo a right-sided or biatrial maze procedure.

The latter is preferable to catheter ablation for those with persistent or permanent A fib/flutter.

Pearls/pitfalls

- *Common clinical presentation includes*: cyanosis, palpitations, arrhythmia
- *Classic CXR finding*: cardiomegaly (cardiothoracic ratio > 0.65)
- Wolff-Parkinson-White syndrome is commonly associated with Ebstein's anomaly and may predispose to tachyarrhythmia presenting as fainting spells. Use preoperative EP mapping for localization/ablation of accessory conduction pathways and consider concomitant surgical ablation
- Aggressive medical management required in early neonatal period to support RV dysfunction until reduction of native PVR
- Early surgical repair encouraged to avoid ventricular deterioration (associated with increased mortality)
- Surgical management largely guided by TV leaflet morphology, degree of RVOTO, and degree of RV atrialization
- Cone reconstruction is the preferred biventricular TV repair technique
- Single ventricle palliation and heart transplantation reserved for severe cases

Suggested readings

- Dearani JA, Bacha E, and Da Silva JP. Cone Reconstruction of the Tricuspid Valve for Ebstein's Anomaly: Anatomic Repair. *Oper Tech Thorac Cardiovasc Surg* 2008;13(2):109-125.
- Da Silva JP and Da Silva Lda F. Ebstein's Anomaly of the Tricuspid Valve: The Cone Repair. *Semin Thorac Cardiovasc Surg Pediatr Card Surg Annu.* 2012;15(1):38-45.
- Da Silva JP et al, Baumgratz JF, Fonseca L, et al. The cone reconstruction of the tricuspid valve in Ebstein's anomaly. The operation: early and midterm results. *J Thorac Cardiovasc Surg*; 133: 215-23.
- Knott-Craig CJ, Goldberg SP. Management of Neonatal Ebstein's Anomaly. *Semin Thorac Cardiovasc Surg Pediatr Card Surg Ann.* 2007;10(1):112-116.
- Stulak JM et al, Schaff HV, Dearani JA. Optimal Surgical Ablation of Atrial Tachyarrhythmias During Correction of Ebstein Anomaly. *Ann Thorac Surg.* 2015;99(5):1700-1705.
- http://www.ctsnet.org/sections/videosection/videos/vg2012_CaputoM_coneReconstruct.html

82. DOUBLE OUTLET RIGHT VENTRICLE

Aditya Sengupta, MD and Raghav A. Murthy, MD, DABS, FACS

Concept
- Presentation and natural history
- Diagnostic workup
- Morphology and pathophysiology
- Surgical repair
- Potential questions and alternative scenarios
- Technical pearls/pitfalls

Chief complaint

"A 3-kg female was born at 36 weeks to a G2P1 mother via Cesarean-section; the pregnancy was complicated by preterm premature rupture of membranes. Immediately after birth, she was cyanotic with O2 saturations in the low 80s. Echocardiography confirmed the prenatal diagnosis of double-outlet right ventricle-Tetralogy of Fallot type (subaortic ventricular septal defect with pulmonary stenosis). How would you proceed?"

Differential

Double-outlet right ventricle (DORV) represents a complex array of congenital heart disease and presents with multiple phenotypes with varying anatomical and physiological properties. Ventricular septal defect (VSD) with overriding aorta (tetralogy of Fallot type) lies at one end of this spectrum, and transposition of the great arteries (TGA) with VSD lies at the other. Thus, the differential diagnosis includes:

- TGA
- Tetralogy of Fallot (TOF)
- VSD with overriding aorta with or without pulmonary stenosis
- Truncus arteriosus
- Pulmonary atresia/stenosis (PA/PS)

History and physical

Tachypnea and failure to thrive can be present in those with CHF, while cyanosis is seen in DORV patients with reduced pulmonary blood flow. DORV is a type of ventriculoarterial connection whereby both the aorta and pulmonary artery (PA) arise predominantly or entirely from the right ventricle (RV). Thus, DORV is not a specific congenital malformation, but rather a descriptive term. Discontinuity of the arterial and atrioventricular valves is a prominent feature of this condition. ~85-90% of patients have concordant atrioventricular connections, and hearts with DORV have a variable number of coni (bilateral coni with a single conus beneath each of the semilunar valves, a unilateral conus, or no conus). In most cases, the aorta is situated posteriorly and to the right of the pulmonary trunk, and the two arteries spiral around each other in the usual fashion. However, the relationship of the great arteries to each other, along with the size and orientation of the infundibular septum, can be highly variable. The coronary artery pattern is typically normal in DORV patients with a right-sided and anterior aorta, but the left anterior descending artery (LAD) may anomalously originate from the right coronary artery (RCA) in ~5-25% of patients. The clinical presentation depends on the relationship of the VSD to the great arteries and the presence or absence of RVOTO:

- DORV-VSD & DORV-remote VSD types: These patients have unrestricted pulmonary blood flow and present with congestive heart failure (CHF). They are not clinically cyanotic since the high pulmonary blood flow results in well saturated blood in the RV (due to mixing with left ventricular blood through the VSD).

- DORV-TOF type: Such patients are cyanotic given the reduced pulmonary blood flow, and present similar to TOF patients. The degree of cyanosis depends on the severity of the pulmonary stenosis.

- DORV-TGA type: Patients with the Taussig-Bing malformation preferentially direct well saturated left ventricular blood to the pulmonary artery due to the sagittal orientation of the infundibular septum. They mimic patients with TGA and VSD, and present early in infancy with cyanosis and CHF since relatively desaturated right ventricular blood is directed into the aorta (phenomenon of "streaming").

Electrocardiogram (EKG): Right axis deviation, right ventricular/biventricular hypertrophy.
Chest radiography (CXR): Evidence of pulmonary overcirculation or clear lung fields in those with RVOTO.

Transthoracic echocardiography (TTE): 2-D TTE is crucial in characterizing the following:
- Diameter, location, number, and commitment of the VSDs
- Origins of the aorta and pulmonary trunk, and their relationship to each other
- Semilunar-atrioventricular valve continuity, along with atrioventricular valve abnormalities
- Absence of the normal left ventricular outflow tract (LVOT)
- Presence of associated cardiac anomalies

Cardiac catheterization: This can be performed to define associated cardiac anomalies that have not been clearly identified by TTE, including coronary artery anomalies, peripheral pulmonary artery stenosis, and irreversible pulmonary vascular disease.

Index scenario (additional information)
"The patient required prostaglandin therapy for two weeks of post-natal life with appropriate weight gain and subsequent discharge home. Surgical consultation was obtained at five months of age, at which point she weighed 4.3 kg. TTE revealed DORV-TOF type with side-by-side great vessels and a large subaortic anteriorly malaligned VSD. There was significant anterior deviation of the conal septum leading to sub-pulmonary obstruction. In addition, multi-level RVOTO was noted, and the pulmonary annulus was ~0.5 cm (Z-score -2.9). The pathway from the left ventricle to the aorta appeared to be unobstructed. How would you proceed?"

Treatment/management
Classification of DORV
A VSD (unrestrictive in ~90% of patients) is typically necessary for survival in DORV. Most are conoventricular in location, lying between the anterior and posterior limbs of the trabeculoseptomarginalis (TSM), and are usually described in relation to the great arteries.

- Subaortic VSDs are the most prevalent, occurring in approximately half of all DORV patients. ~77% of patients with DORV and subaortic VSDs have bilateral coni and 23% have just a subpulmonary conus. When the subaortic conus is absent and aortic-mitral continuity is present, the posterosuperior margin of the VSD is formed by the left coronary cusp/base of the anterior leaflet of the mitral valve. Furthermore, the VSD is usually subaortic when L-malposition of the aorta is present. Variable amounts of right ventricular outflow tract obstruction (RVOTO) may be present (e.g., infundibular, valvar with or without a small pulmonary valve annulus, or central PA hypoplasia).

- Subpulmonary VSDs (Taussig-Bing malformation) are present in 30% of DORV patients. ~55% of such patients have bilateral coni. When the subpulmonary conus is absent (and there is pulmonary-mitral continuity), the pulmonary valve overrides the

VSD and forms its superior boundary. Furthermore, the orientation of the infundibular septum commits the VSD to the pulmonary artery, which generally arises biventricularly. The great arteries lay side-by-side and do not spiral around each other. There is usually a variable amount of subaortic obstruction, and coarctation of the aorta occurs in ~80% of patients.

- Doubly-committed VSDs occur in ~10% of patients. Here, the infundibular septum is usually deficient or absent, and thus the semilunar valves are contiguous. RVOTO may be present.

- Non-committed VSDs occur in 10-20% of cases. These are not sandwiched between the limbs of the TSM and are generally located within the inlet septum/trabecular interventricular septum.

The current Society of Thoracic Surgeons-European Association of Cardiothoracic Surgery (STS-EACTS) classification is as follows:

- DORV-VSD type (subaortic and doubly-committed VSDs without RVOTO)
- DORV-TOF type (subaortic and doubly-committed VSDs with RVOTO)
- DORV-TGA type (subpulmonary VSDs/Taussig-Bing malformation)
- DORV-remote VSD type (uncommitted VSDs with/without RVOTO)
- DORV-AVSD type (complete atrioventricular septal defect)

Surgical Management
The diagnosis of DORV is an indication for complete anatomic repair. The timing of surgery and the corrective approach to be used depend on the patient's anatomy (especially of other cardiac anomalies associated with the DORV) and the symptomatic state of the patient. Initial palliative procedures may be needed, but complete repair is advocated at as early an age as possible. Repairs are usually performed through the tricuspid valve and/or a right ventriculotomy.

Contraindications to anatomic repair include:

- Surgically important ventricular hypoplasia (this requires single ventricle palliation)
- Severe abnormalities of either atrioventricular valve
- Very remote or multiple VSDs
- Irreversible pulmonary vascular disease
- Severe straddling and/or overriding of either atrioventricular valve

Operative steps
DORV-VSD Type
Complete repair is advocated in early infancy before the onset of pulmonary vascular disease. An intraventricular tunnel repair is used for these patients, and is performed as follows:

- The VSD is exposed through a longitudinal right ventriculotomy, and its size and location relative to the aorta are noted. If it appears restrictive, it is enlarged by making an incision anterosuperiorly or by resecting a wedge of the interventricular septum (IVS).

- Obstructive right ventricular muscle bundles are resected, and a portion of the IVS may be resected to facilitate construction of the straight tunnel between the VSD and aorta.

- The intracardiac tunnel is created with an appropriately trimmed flat Gore-Tex patch/tailored Dacron or Gore-Tex tube graft secured with running or interrupted sutures.

504

- The patch should be 2/3 of the aortic circumference and the width should extent from the inferior edge of the VSD to the superior margin of the aortic annulus. Posteriorly, the patch should be secured to the base of the septal leaflet of the tricuspid valve (thus completely avoiding the posteroinferior margin of the VSD and the conduction tissue).

- The right ventriculotomy is then closed with a patch to avoid RVOTO created by the intraventricular tunnel.

Complications include complete heart block, tunnel or pathway obstruction, residual VSD (patch dehiscence), localized subaortic stenosis, and RVOTO.

DORV-TOF Type
Repair is advised by 6 months of age, but a palliative systemic-to-pulmonary artery shunt may be required (depending on the degree of cyanosis after birth) prior to definitive repair. The principles of repair are like those described for TOF, except that the VSD is closed with the intraventricular tunnel technique (usually requires a ventriculotomy):

- The VSD is exposed through the tricuspid valve, and when necessary, a right ventriculotomy is performed.

- The infundibular os is resected to enlarge the RVOT. When a transannular patch is necessary for pulmonary annular hypoplasia and/or pulmonary valve stenosis, transatrial and transpulmonary endocardial resection of hypertrophied/obstructive muscle is performed.

- If the pulmonary annulus and arterial tree are normal, and only pure valvar pulmonary stenosis exists, then pulmonary valvotomy is adequate.

- A valved, extracardiac conduit is necessary in cases where an anomalous coronary artery crosses the RVOT immediately beneath the pulmonary valve annulus (especially when endocardial resection and pulmonary valvotomy alone will not relieve the RVOTO).

- The VSD is closed using the tunnel technique as previously described, and as with DORV-VSD type, the right ventriculotomy is then closed with a patch to avoid RVOTO.

DORV-TGA Type (Subpulmonary VSD with/without Pulmonary Stenosis)
In patients with the Taussig-Bing malformation with no RVOTO, the arterial switch operation (ASO) with tunnel closure of the VSD to the pulmonary artery is the procedure of choice. Intraventricular tunnel repairs can also be performed, and these are discussed in greater detail later (see "Potential Questions & Controversies"). With the ASO, single-stage repair is preferred and usually carried out in the first week of life.

For Taussig-Bing patients *without* aortic arch obstruction, the ASO is performed as follows:

- Through a standard median sternotomy, the ascending aorta, main pulmonary artery (MPA), and patent ductus arteriosus (PDA) are circumferentially dissected. The PDA is snared during the initial cooling phase of cardiopulmonary bypass (CPB) and is thereafter suture ligated and divided.

- The VSD is closed transatrially or transventricularly.

- The sites for coronary artery transfer to the pulmonary trunk (neoaorta) are marked with sutures.

505

- If the Lecompte maneuver is to be carried out, a relatively high aortic transection and low transection of the MPA are performed.

- The great arteries are transected, and the coronary artery orifices are excised with a button of native aortic wall. Ovals of the neoartic root are then removed at the previously marked sites.

- The defects in the aortic wall (neopulmonary root) are repaired with autologous pericardium/pantaloon patch, and the mobilized coronary arteries are transferred to the neoartic root and sutured.

- Finally, the neoartic root is sutured to the distal transected ascending aorta and the neopulmonary root is sutured to the distal transected MPA.

For Taussig-Bing patients *with* aortic arch obstruction (~80% incidence), the repair is similar to that described above, but with a few modifications. The PDA is first divided, and the pulmonary end is oversewn. The ascending aorta and aortic isthmus are divided. The descending thoracic aorta is mobilized, and all coarctation/ductal tissues are excised, following which partial direct anastomosis of the proximal descending thoracic aorta to the transected aortic isthmus is performed (along with augmentation of this anastomosis, the transverse aortic arch, and the ascending aorta with a homograft patch).

DORV-Remote VSD Type
Two-ventricle repair is necessary for patients with DORV-remote VSD type. Here, an intracardiac tunnel is constructed between the VSD and either the aorta or PA. This is best performed in early infancy (rather than the neonatal period) and initial palliation may be necessary.

- For those *without* RVOTO, the intraventricular tunnel can be directed either to the aorta or PA. The former can be performed if there is adequate distance between the tricuspid and pulmonary valves. If this is not anatomically feasible, an ASO with tunneling of the VSD to the PA is necessary. This often results in a shorter tunnel with relative sparing of the tricuspid subvalvular apparatus.

- For those *with* RVOTO, the repair strategy depends on the level of obstruction:

    o Subvalvular RVOTO is treated in a similar manner to that described above with the addition of a right ventricular infundibular patch augmentation.

    o With valvar obstruction, the VSD can be tunneled to the aorta and the pulmonary outflow tract can be closed. This is then followed by a Rastelli- or REV-type procedure (see below).

Single ventricle repair may be necessary when there is significant ventricular hypoplasia and/or severe atrioventricular valve straddling/overriding. Here, an initial systemic-to-PA shunt or PA band is followed by a bi-directional cavopulmonary anastomosis at 6 months. This is completed with a total cavopulmonary connection by 3-4 years of age.

Potential questions/alternative scenarios
"What are the long-term outcomes of DORV repair?"
Intraventricular tunnel repair for DORV-VSD type is associated with very favorable in-hospital and short-term outcomes, and 15-year actuarial survival is ~95%. Increasing pulmonary vascular disease with older age may be a risk factor for death after repair. Similarly, the functional status of DORV-TOF type patients after repair is excellent. Early- and late-survival are improved if the repair did not necessitate placement of an extracardiac conduit/transannular patch for pulmonary stenosis. Not surprisingly, the 10-year time-related

506

actuarial freedom from reoperation after placement of a RV-PA heterograft valved conduit is ~50%. The hospital mortality of the ASO for DORV-TGA type ranges from 3-15%, with higher mortality reported for patients with concomitant aortic arch anomalies. Actuarial 10-year survival is ~85% with a 10% rate of reoperation (for RVOTO, aortic regurgitation, arch/coronary obstruction). Finally, hospital mortality rates have been reported to be as low as ~6-7% for two-ventricle repair of DORV-remote VSD type.

"What options are available for patients with DORV-TGA type and pulmonary stenosis, and what are the long-term outcomes?"

The ASO with VSD closure to the neoaorta is contraindicated in patients with the Taussig-Bing malformation and pulmonary stenosis as this could create stenosis of the neoartic valve. A number of procedures have evolved over the years to combat this rare anatomical situation, including the Rastelli procedure, the REV (*reparation a letage ventriculaire*) procedure by Lecompte, and the Nikaidoh procedure. The Rastelli procedure involves VSD closure to the aorta with placement of a right ventricular-to-pulmonary artery (RV-PA) conduit. However, 20-year survival is only ~50-60% (likely related to the long-term liabilities of the conduit). In 1982, the REV procedure was introduced to mitigate several of these unfavorable long-term outcomes. Here, the pulmonary outflow tract is reconstructed without using a RV-PA conduit: the LV outflow is directed to the aorta, the pulmonary trunk is transected, and the distal segment is directly anastomosed to the right ventricle. Numerous others have modified the original REV operation, and some even advocate harvesting the intact pulmonary root rather than simply transecting the MPA (thus improving the competency of the neopulmonary root). Hospital mortality of the REV procedure has been reported at 18% with normal right ventricular size and contractility in 83% of patients at greater than one-year follow-up. Finally, the Nikaidoh procedure involves a complex aortic translocation and biventricular outflow tract reconstruction which results in an anatomically aligned LVOT and RVOT. Hospital mortality ranges from ~0-10% in reported series. Among the three, the Rastelli procedure is the most familiar and technically feasible operation, while the Nikaidoh procedure is the most complex. The latter might be advocated in cases where coronary artery anomalies interfere with a vertical right ventriculotomy, an inlet VSD is present, or there exists atrioventricular valve straddling/RV hypoplasia. However, the ideal procedure for this rare anatomical variant of DORV is unknown as long term data are scarce.

"What is the Kawashima operation and when can it be used?"

The Kawashima operation is an alternative repair strategy for patients with side-by-side great vessels (with the aorta to the right of the PA) and a subpulmonic VSD. This procedure avoids the need for the ASO/use of an extracardiac conduit. It is an intraventricular tunnel repair that connects the LV directly to the aorta with a tunnel that runs posterior to the PA between the tricuspid and pulmonary valves. When the great arteries have an oblique/anterior-posterior relationship, there may not be adequate separation of the tricuspid and pulmonary valves, thus making tunnel creation difficult. The ASO should be used in such situations.

Pearls/pitfalls

- During closure of the VSD in patients with DORV, it is very important to follow and stay close to the suture line at the aortic annulus. DORV patients may have several hypertrophied muscle bands and suturing the patch to these bands will result in a residual VSD.

- Complex tunnel repairs, especially in DORV patients with AVSD and heterotaxy patients, may require use of multiple patches for creation of the pathway.

- There should be a low threshold to perform a ventriculotomy. The malaligned VSD repair is often hard to perform transatrially.

- 3-D printing and segmentation, if available, may be utilized in the surgical planning of complex, biventricular repairs.

- In patients with DORV-TGA type, care has to be taken with coronary artery translocation when employing the ASO. Coronary artery anomalies are frequent, and the RCA button often gives rise to the LAD or circumflex coronary artery. In these situations, the RCA button should be placed superiorly by creating a relatively high defect in the pulmonary artery (neoaorta) and by interdigitating as much of the button into the aortic suture line. The left coronary button should be placed just high enough to prevent kinking.

Suggested readings
- Walters HL & Mavroudis C. Chapter 25: Double-Outlet Ventricles. In: Mavroudis C, Backer CL, Idriss RF, eds. Pediatric Cardiac Surgery, 4th ed. Blackwell Publishing Ltd; 2013.
- Thompson J & Dearani JA. Chapter 71: Double Outlet Right Ventricle. In: Yuh DD, Vricella LA, Yang SC, Doty JR, eds. Johns Hopkins Textbook of Cardiothoracic Surgery, 2nd ed. McGraw-Hill Education; 2014.
- Mavroudis C. Chapter 14: Double-Outlet Ventricles (with Two Adequate Ventricles). In: Mavroudis C, Backer CL, eds. Atlas of Pediatric Cardiac Surgery, 1st ed. Springer; 2015.

83. ANOMALOUS ORIGIN OF THE LEFT CORONARY ARTERY FROM THE PULMONARY ARTERY

Syed Faaz Ashraf, MD, and Mario Castro-Medina, MD
This chapter is a revision and update of that included in the previous edition of the TSRA Clinical Scenarios written by Michael C. Monge, MD and Hyde M. Russell, MD

Concept

- Presentation
- Differential for ALCAPA
- Diagnostic Evaluation
- Surgical Repair
- Pearls and pitfalls

Chief complaint

"A two-month-old infant presents with diaphoresis, tachypnea, and failure to thrive."

Differential

The differential for new heart failure in the infant includes dilated cardiomyopathy, myocarditis, Kawasaki disease, Ebstein's anomaly, large ventricular septal defect, ostium primum atrial septal defect, coarctation of the aorta, patent ductus arteriosus, atrioventricular canal, congenital aortic stenosis, left ventricular outflow tract obstruction, aortic or mitral regurgitation, and Anomalous Origin of the Left Coronary Artery from the Pulmonary Artery (ALCAPA).

History and physical

After birth but before duct closure the pulmonary artery retains an adequately high pressure for perfusion of the anomalous coronary artery. After ductal closure, and as the pulmonary vascular resistance drops, there is increasing coronary artery steal with gradual myocardial ischemia. Feeding, the most strenuous activity in which an infant engages, may be poor due to angina, resulting in failure to thrive. Most infants with ALPACA present between 4-6 weeks of age. Worsening ischemia leads to heart failure heralded by diaphoresis, tachypnea, and tachycardia. As with cardiomyopathy, a precordial lift from cardiomegaly is frequently appreciated. In addition, a systolic murmur from mitral regurgitation may be auscultated at the apex, in association with a gallop rhythm. Lung auscultation will reveal rales due to interstitial pulmonary edema and hepatomegaly can be palpated.

Tests

- *CXR*: severe cardiomegaly, pulmonary edema.

- *EKG.* Q-waves and ST segment elevation from anterolateral ischemia are frequently present. Evidence of left ventricular hypertrophy may be apparent.

- *Echocardiography.* Dilated left ventricle with markedly reduced function. Dilated right coronary artery (RCA) may be evident. Color Doppler echocardiography can detect retrograde flow from the anomalous coronary artery into the pulmonary artery. Mitral regurgitation is often present. The hyper-echogenicity of endocardial fibroelastosis may be observed.
  Although echocardiography can establish ALCAPA, it is not adequate to rule-out the diagnosis. Only cardiac catheterization can rule-out ALCAPA in patients presenting with classic symptoms.

- *Cardiac catheterization.* Single, dilated right coronary artery arising from the aorta. Characteristic blush in the pulmonary artery from retrograde filling of the left coronary artery. Prominent collaterals are observed in adult-type ALCAPA. An oxygen step-up in the pulmonary artery will be present from left-to-right shunting through the anomalous coronary artery and collateral vessels. Care should be taken in the already compromised patients undergoing invasive diagnostic testing.

- *Magnetic resonance angiography (MRA)*: similar sensitivity and specificity to coronary angiography in diagnosis of ALCAPA.
- *Computed tomographic angiography (CTA)*: assessment of coronary anatomy may be difficult because of tachycardia.

Index scenario (additional information)

"An apical pansystolic murmur was auscultated. Left-axis deviation was noted on EKG with Q-waves and ST elevation in I, aVL, and V4-V6. CXR demonstrated cardiomegaly. A dilated left ventricle with markedly reduced function is evident with echocardiography. Severe mitral valve regurgitation with calcification of the papillary muscles is observed. The coronary arteries are not well-visualized. What additional studies, if any, would you like to perform?"

Treatment/management

Although an anomalous coronary artery from the pulmonary artery was not seen on echocardiography, further diagnostic testing is mandatory to rule-out ALCAPA. Cardiac catheterization, demonstrating retrograde flow through from the coronary artery into the pulmonary artery should be performed. Alternatively, CTA may be used, although the quality may be limited by tachycardia. Identification of ALCAPA is an indication for surgical intervention, which should be performed within days of the diagnosis to promote rapid left ventricular recovery.

The accepted optimal surgical treatment is restoration of a two-coronary system via the direct re-implantation method.

Operative steps
Aortic re-implantation of ALCAPA

- *Place transesophageal echocardiography (TEE) probe*: used to assess postoperative patency of re-implanted coronary artery, assess postoperative ventricular function, assess degree of mitral valve regurgitation.
- Median sternotomy.
- Harvest pericardial patch.
- Ischemic myocardium with poor ventricular function is prone to ventricular fibrillation. Myocardial contact should be minimized prior to initiation of cardiopulmonary bypass.
- *Cannulation.* Cannulate ascending aorta near innominate artery to provide enough length for aortic implantation of anomalous coronary artery. Bicaval cannulation is utilized to protect myocardium from warm blood entering heart. Cardioplegia is delivered via an angiocatheter in aortic root. A left ventricular vent is placed via the right superior pulmonary vein to decompress the left ventricle.
- Bilateral pulmonary arteries should be mobilized and the ligamentum arteriosum divided. The branch pulmonary arteries are encircled with Rumel tourniquets, which are snared once bypass is initiated to increase pressure in the left coronary artery system by preventing run-off.
- The aorta is cross-clamped and cardioplegia is delivered into the aortic root.
- The main pulmonary artery is transected after fully mobilizing the branch pulmonary arteries.
- A large coronary artery ostial button is developed. The left main coronary artery is mobilized off the epicardium.
- With care taken to prevent injury to the aortic valve, an opening is created in the left posterolateral wall of the ascending aorta, approximately 30-40% smaller than the coronary button. By excising a large ostial button, the pulmonary wall can be used to extend the coronary artery to create a tension-free repair. A flap of aortic wall can be created to augment the anastomosis as needed to prevent tension at the coronary button anastomosis.

510

- The left coronary artery-to-aorta anastomosis is performed with 7-0 prolene suture.
- After completion of the anastomosis, the aortic root is de-aired via the angiocatheter. The aortic cross-clamp is removed.
- The sinus of the pulmonary artery, in which the ostial button was harvested, is reconstructed with a fresh autologous pericardial patch using 6-0 prolene suture.
- The pulmonary artery is re-anastomosed at the site of transection with 6-0 prolene suture.
- Left atrial pressure is monitored with a catheter placed through the vent site in the right superior pulmonary vein.
- The patient is weaned from cardiopulmonary bypass by allowing venous return to fill the left side of the heart.
- TEE will demonstrate poor ventricular function unimproved from the preoperative study; and therefore, careful monitoring of blood pressure and left atrial pressure is required.

Potential questions/alternative scenarios

"The preoperative echocardiogram demonstrates severe mitral regurgitation with severely reduced left ventricular dysfunction."
Most patients present with some degree of mitral regurgitation related to annular dilatation from left ventricular enlargement or to ischemic papillary muscle dysfunction. Left ventricular function has been shown to recover to normal or near-normal levels within one to two years following repair. With the improvement in left ventricular function, the mitral regurgitation improves in most patients, and secondary mitral valve operations are rarely necessary. The increased cross-clamp time required to repair the mitral valve can be detrimental to the already compromised myocardium.

"Upon weaning from cardiopulmonary bypass, the patient is hypotensive with an elevated atrial pressure."
The left ventricular function may remain markedly depressed in the early postoperative period. Because significant improvement in function is expected, an aggressive approach to supporting the damaged myocardium with mechanical assistance should be used. If significant hypotension or supraventricular or ventricular arrhythmias persist, total cardiopulmonary support with ECMO should be instituted. Most patients demonstrate myocardial recovery in 48 to 72 hours. Need for post-operative support with signs of ischemia should prompt cardiac catheterization.

"Upon transection of the pulmonary artery, the origin of the anomalous coronary artery is observed to be from the non-facing sinus."
In ALCAPA the left coronary artery commonly originates from the posterior facing sinus of the pulmonary artery. Even anomalous coronary arteries that arise from the non-facing sinus of the pulmonary artery can be successfully re-implanted. A large segment of the pulmonary artery wall is excised and fashioned into a tube, lengthening the proximal end of the coronary artery. The Takeuchi operation provides an alternate approach in this scenario. It involves the creation of an aortopulmonary window along with an intrapulmonary tunnel from the aorta to the anomalous coronary artery ostium. This approach, however, has been associated with supravalvular pulmonary artery stenosis and baffle leaks.

"A 30 y/o asymptomatic woman is incidentally found to have an anomalous origin of the left coronary artery from the pulmonary artery on CT imaging."
A small subset of patients, often with pronounced right coronary dominance and/or a restrictive ostium of the anomalous coronary, survive to adulthood. Significant intercoronary collateral vessels develop. These patients may be asymptomatic or present with exertional angina, dyspnea, pre-syncope, or syncope. Mitral regurgitation from ischemic papillary muscle dysfunction can exist, despite left ventricular function being relatively well preserved.

511

Because of the risk of sudden death, these patients should undergo operation on an elective basis.

Pearls/pitfalls

- In patients presenting with classic symptoms, in whom echocardiography has not confirmed ALCAPA, a cardiac catheterization must be performed to rule-out the diagnosis.
- Mild-to-moderate or greater mitral valve insufficiency is often present preoperatively. The mitral insufficiency improves over time, in most patients. Mitral valve repair/replacement is rarely indicated at the initial operation.
- Rapid initiation of mechanical assistance with ECMO support should be performed if the patient is unable to be weaned from cardiopulmonary bypass.

Suggested readings

- Dodge-Khatami A, Mavroudis C, Backer CL. Anomalous origin of the left coronary artery from the pulmonary artery: collective review of surgical therapy. *Ann Thorac Surg* 2002; 74:946-955.
- Ben Ali W, Metton O, Roubertie F et al. Anomalous origin of the left coronary artery from the pulmonary artery: late results with special attention to the mitral valve. *Eur J Cardiothorac Surg.* 2009; 36(2):244-8, discussion 248-9.
- Schwartz ML, Jonas RA, Colan SD. Anomalous origin of the left coronary artery from pulmonary artery: Recovery of the left ventricular function after dual coronary repair. *J Am Coll Cardiol.* 1997; 30:547-553.
- Turley K, Szarnicki RJ, Flachsbart KD et al. Aortic implantation is possible in all cases of anomalous origin of the left coronary artery from the pulmonary artery. *Ann Thorac Surg.* 1995. 60:84-89.

84. CORONARY ARTERY ANOMALIES

Syed Faaz Ashraf, MD and Mario Castro-Medina, MD

Concept

- Presentation
- Differential for AAOCA and Coronary artery fistula
- Diagnostic Evaluation
- Surgical Repair
- Pearls and pitfalls

Chief complaint

"A 10-year-old boy presents with chest discomfort and dizziness just after exercise. These symptoms resolve after resting for 1 minute."

Differentials

Hypertrophic obstructive cardiomyopathy (HOCM), Aortic stenosis, left ventricular outflow tract obstruction, Anomalous aortic origin of a coronary artery (AAOCA).

History and physical

AAOCA is the second most common cause of sudden cardiac death (SCD) in young athletes and represents one third of all coronary artery anomalies. Anomalous right coronary artery (ARCA) is 3-6 times more common than anomalous left coronary artery (ALCA), however the latter carries a higher risk of SCD. The cause of SCD is hypothesized to be due to decreased anomalous coronary blood flow resulting in myocardial infarction and/or ventricular arrhythmias. Unlike ALCAPA, AAOCA can be difficult to diagnose as most of these patients are asymptomatic. Those who are will commonly present with chest pain, dizziness, palpitations, pre-syncope or syncope during/just after exertion. For many patients their only presenting complaint is SCD. Physical examination is almost always normal.

Tests

- *CXR*: Most often normal

- *EKG*: Often normal, should be used to evaluate arrhythmias, ventricular hypertrophy and signs of previous MI's – indicative of ischemia.

- *Echocardiography*: Can be used to diagnose the majority of AAOCA. Echo with color flow mapping of the proximal coronary arteries is mandatory to diagnose the extramural and/or intramural course of an AAOCA. AAOCA with an intramural course is characterized by an acute angulation of the coronary origin with diastolic color flow in its proximal course within the aortic wall. The AAOCA can be posterior, anterior or even course in between the great vessels. Finally, echo may also show areas of abnormal wall motion which would signify history of ischemia.

- *MRI or CT angiography*: Can be used to confirm the diagnosis of AAOCA where TTE does not provide an answer.

- *Cardiac catheterization*: Still considered the gold standard test for elucidating coronary artery anatomy. Used in adult patients to evaluate for other coronary disease before undergoing surgery. Invasive, not the first choice in children with the advances seen in TTE and its techniques.

- *Exercise stress test with ECHO/ECG, nuclear perfusion study*: Used to evaluate signs of ischemia during stress. For the AAOCA population, seen as unreliable due to high rate of false negatives.

Index scenario (additional information)
"The patient's EKG and CXR are normal. His transthoracic echocardiogram shows a single right coronary artery that originates from the right aortic sinus. It also shows a single left coronary artery that originates from the right aortic sinus and courses in between the aorta and pulmonary artery. Color flow mapping shows diastolic color flow in the left coronary's proximal course within the aortic wall. The patients exercise stress EKG is negative for signs of ischemia."

Treatment/management
The presentation and anatomy of AAOCA is variable and therefore its management strategy differs. The decision to operate for certain AAOCA anatomy is controversial. The aim of surgical repair for AAOCA is to reduce or eliminate the future risk of SCD. It is widely accepted that patient's with AAOCA whom are symptomatic or have signs of myocardial ischemia, regardless of ALCA vs ARCA, should undergo surgical intervention. Some surgical teams recommend patients with AAOCA with high risk anatomy – long intramural course, abnormal ostium or coronary compression, have an undue risk of SCD. Therefore, they should undergo surgical repair even if asymptomatic with no signs of ischemia. The management of asymptomatic patients with ARCA, with no signs of ischemia, has not been universally agreed upon.

The aim of surgery is to restore a normal anatomic position of the left or right coronary ostium. The surgical procedure of choice for AAOCA with an inter-arterial and intramural course is the unroofing procedure. For AAOCA without an intramural course but an inter-arterial one the pulmonary artery (PA) translocation procedure can be performed. The distal main PA is transected at the branched PA confluence. The PA is repaired with a pericardial patch, the left PA is incised longitudinally, and the main PA is re-anastomosed here towards the left hilum. This increases the gap between the PA and aorta reducing the risk of the inter-arterial coronary from obstructing.

Operative steps
Unroofing procedure
- *Place transesophageal echocardiography (TEE) probe*: used to assess postoperative patency of re-implanted coronary artery, assess postoperative ventricular function,
- Median sternotomy.
- *Cannulation.* Cannulate ascending aorta near innominate artery to provide sufficient length for aortic re-implantation of anomalous coronary artery. Insert two stage venous cannula into the right atrial appendage. Cardiopulmonary bypass is initiated with moderate hypothermia. A left ventricular vent is placed via the right superior pulmonary vein to decompress the left ventricle.
- The aorta is cross-clamped and cardioplegia is delivered via an angiocatheter into the aortic root.
- Once adequate cardiac arrest is achieved a transverse aortotomy is performed and the two coronary ostia are identified
- The 'slit like' ostium of the ALCA is identified. A coronary dilator is inserted into the anomalous ostium and advanced into the intramural tunnel to the correct cusp and measured. The ostium is opened longitudinally from the ostium along the length of the intramural course to the correct aortic sinus until the exit point of the coronary artery is reached.
- The common wall between the aorta and the coronary is excised and the intimal layers are approximated with 8-0 Prolene tacking sutures thereby preventing dissection and thrombosis.
- The aortotomy is then repaired and the cross clamp removed after de-airing.

514

- The patient is rewarmed, and the EKG closely monitored to evaluate for signs of myocardial ischemia.
- The patient is then weaned and separated from cardiopulmonary bypass

Potential questions/alternative scenarios

"Intraoperatively the 'slit like' ostium of the left coronary is seen to be in close proximity to the aortic valve commissure."
When the abnormal ostium is located close to a commissure, the commissure should be taken down. This will allow space to enlarge the ostium and to make the longitudinal incision along the coronary's intramural course. Once the intimal layers between the coronary and aorta and approximated, the aortic valve commissure will need to be re-suspended with a pledgeted suture. Take down and re-suspension of the aortic valve commissure runs the risk of causing iatrogenic aortic insufficiency. An alternative technique, for an intramural segment of the anomalous coronary that passes below the aortic valve commissure, is the creation of a neo-ostium. A probe is passed through the original ostia of the anomalous coronary, through its intramural segment and into its correct sinus. At the point where the coronary exits the aorta, a neo-ostium is created. 8-0 Prolene sutures are used to re-approximate the intimal layers in the neo-ostium. This technique avoids the longitudinal incision and therefore the takedown and re-suspension of the commissure.

"Intraoperatively there are two separate coronary ostia in the right aortic sinus. There is a single right coronary artery that originates from the right aortic sinus. A single left coronary artery also originates from the right aortic sinus and courses in between the aorta and pulmonary artery. The left coronary has no intramural course."
When there are two separate ostia and the anomalous artery has an interarterial course but not an intramural course, the coronary artery translocation procedure with reimplantation can be used. This is similar to the repair described for the ALCAPA procedure. The left coronary artery is excised with a button. The left coronary with its button is then re-located to its correct sinus above its commissure.

"A 23-year-old otherwise healthy male presents with a 2-month history of shortness of breath and chest tightness when walking up hills. On auscultation there was a continuous murmur heard best at the left upper sternal border. The patient's EKG showed sinus rhythm and chest x-ray showed mild cardiomegaly. The transthoracic echocardiogram demonstrated an enlarged right coronary artery along with right ventricle hypertrophy. The patient underwent cardiac catheterization which again confirmed a dilated and tortuous proximal right coronary artery along with contrast entering directly into the right ventricle from the right coronary artery from a single point."
Coronary artery fistulas can arise from either the left or right coronary artery. They can terminate in any of the 4 cardiac chambers or other cardiac structures such as the coronary sinus, pulmonary artery and the SVC. The most common site of termination is the right ventricle. Various surgical series have shown the RCA and LAD to be the most common sources of the fistula. Fistulas terminating in a right sided chamber will result in a left-to-right shunt. Whereas fistulas terminating into a left cardiac chamber will have a left-to-left shunt with physiology like aortic regurgitation. The signs and symptoms of coronary artery fistulas depend on the size of the fistula and its location. Patients with coronary artery fistulas are usually asymptomatic with most starting to present after the second decade of life. Over time the fistula gradually increases in size with common symptoms being shortness of breath on exertion along with fatigue. Others may suffer from angina due to coronary steal, palpitations, dizziness and in older adults' symptoms of congestive heart failure. On auscultation often a continuous machinery like murmur can be heard, similar to a PDA, however it is heard lower on the left sternal border. It is widely regarded that patients with symptomatic coronary artery fistulas should undergo closure. Similarly, all large coronary fistulas regardless of symptoms should be closed due to their natural tendency to enlarge and become symptomatic over time. Consensus has not yet been reached for indications and timing of closure for small to medium sized asymptomatic coronary artery fistulas.

515

Operative Steps:

Internal cameral closure on cardiopulmonary bypass

- *Place transesophageal echocardiography (TEE) probe*: used to assess location of coronary artery fistula along with identifying a residual shunt post repair.
- Median sternotomy.
- *Cannulation.* Cannulate ascending aorta. Bicaval cannulation is utilized for blood free access to the right side of the heart. Cardiopulmonary bypass is initiated.
- The aorta is cross-clamped and cardioplegia is delivered via an angiocatheter into the aortic root.
  This operation can be performed without the need for cross clamping or cardioplegia but on a beating heart
- Once adequate cardiac arrest is achieved a right atriotomy is performed and the coronary fistula is identified in the right ventricle whilst looking through the tricuspid valve. Using anterograde blood cardioplegia can help in locating the coronary artery fistula.
- The coronary artery fistula termination site is closed primarily via a purse string suture on the internal ventricular side.
- Further anterograde blood cardioplegia is given to check for total occlusion of the fistula and identify any missed openings.
- The atriotomy is then repaired and the cross clamp removed after de-airing.
- The EKG is closely monitored to evaluate for signs of myocardial ischemia. TEE is also monitored to look for signs of a residual shunt.
- The patient is then weaned and separated from cardiopulmonary bypass

"A similar patient presents but with a large coronary artery fistula in his distal LAD communicating to his right ventricle. How would your surgical approach change?"

Coronary artery fistulas located at the distal/terminal end of the artery, with no viable myocardium distal to the fistula, can be ligated. This procedure does not require going on cardiopulmonary bypass. A ligature (3-0 Prolene) is placed immediately proximal to the origin of the coronary fistula. This temporarily occludes the fistula. The EKG is then monitored to look for signs of ischemia. If there are no signs of ischemia and there is adequate myocardial perfusion, then the ligature can be tied. Again, TEE should be used to confirm the fistula has been closed. Cardiopulmonary bypass for midpoint fistulas is also not always necessary. If there is a lateral and easily identifiable fistula, then it may be closed by passing multiple pledgeted sutures of 3-0 Prolene placed underneath the coronary artery. This should close the fistula tract without impairing distal perfusion. Regardless this runs the risk of injuring a feeding artery e.g. septal perforator and has a higher risk of leaving residual fistulae.

"Whilst delivering anterograde cardioplegia at the start of the case, you notice you are requiring large amounts with little success in stopping the heart"

In patients with large coronary fistula/fistulas, a large amount of the anterograde cardioplegia may be shunted into the cardiac chamber. During delivery of cardioplegia it is beneficial to temporarily occlude the fistula to prevent this from occurring. If this technique still produces inadequate arrest, retrograde cardioplegia may be helpful.

Pearls/pitfalls

- It is widely accepted that patient's with AAOCA whom are symptomatic or have signs of myocardial ischemia, regardless of ALCA vs ARCA, should undergo surgical intervention.
- Coronary artery fistula: Distal fistula's can be ligated without CPB; however it is imperative to first test the ligation for signs of cardiac ischemia before tying the ligature.

516

Suggested readings

- Mery CM, De León LE, Molossi S et al. Outcomes of surgical intervention for anomalous aortic origin of a coronary artery: A large contemporary prospective cohort study. J Thorac Cardiovasc Surg. 2018;155(1):305-319.e4.

- Poynter JA, Bondarenko I, Austin EH et al. Repair of anomalous aortic origin of a coronary artery in 113 patients: a Congenital Heart Surgeons' Society report. World J Pediatr Congenit Heart Surg. 2014 Oct;5(4):507–14

- Mangukia CV. Coronary artery fistula. Ann Thorac Surg. 2012 Jun;93(6):2084–92

85. PULMONARY ARTERY SLING AND VASCULAR RINGS

Laura Seese, MD and Harma Turbendian, MD

This chapter is a revision and update of that included in the previous edition of the TSRA Clinical Scenarios written by Robroy MacIver, MD, MPH and Igor E. Konstantinov, MD. PhD.

Concept

- Differential for vascular anomalies that can cause respiratory issues
- Embryological and anatomical reason for sling
- Diagnostic options prior to surgical therapy
- Conduct of operation and pitfalls

Chief complaint

"A 7-month-old boy is referred to your clinic from his primary provider with question of tracheal stenosis. The child has had repeated episodes of stridor and respiratory tract infections since birth and was intubated for 48 hours two months ago secondary to pneumonia at an outside hospital while the family was on vacation."

Differential

- Congenital or acquired tracheal stenosis
- Complete Vascular Ring
- Incomplete Vascular Rings
- Tumor
- Foreign Body

Table 1. Common Vascular Rings

Complete Vascular Ring	Description	Presenting Symptoms
Double Aortic Arch - **Right Arch Dominant** - **Left Arch Dominant** - **Balanced Arch**	Two arches arise from the ascending aorta and pass on both sides of the trachea and esophagus, joining the descending aorta. The right (posterior) arch typically gives origin to the right carotid and right subclavian arteries. The left (anterior) arch usually gives rise to the left carotid and the left subclavian. In most infants, the right arch is the dominant arch.	Compression of both the esophagus and trachea leads to symptoms of respiratory distress, recurrent respiratory infections, stridor, apnea or cyanosis, dysphagia, slow feeding and "brassy" cough.
Incomplete Vascular Rings	Description	Presenting Symptoms
Pulmonary Artery Sling	The left pulmonary artery originates from the right pulmonary artery, instead of the main pulmonary artery. The left pulmonary artery passes around the right mainstem bronchus and courses between the trachea and the esophagus.	Compression on the tracheobronchial tree or "ring-sling" complex from absence of a portion of the membranous tracheal usually leads to airway symptoms such as cough, stridor, cyanosis, frequent respiratory infections, and dyspnea.

Left Aortic Arch with Aberrant Right Subclavian	Occurs when the right fourth arch between the subclavian and carotid artery regresses. The right subclavian originates from the left-sided distal aortic arch, passing posterior to the esophagus.	Usually asymptomatic (90%). May cause dysphagia lusoria due to esophageal compression.
Innominate Artery Compression	Results from anterior compression of the trachea by the innominate artery, which originates more posterior and leftward on the arch. Considered significant when 70% of the tracheal lumen is compressed.	Symptoms result from tracheal compression including apneic spells, cyanosis, "brassy" cough, recurrent infections due to inability to clear secretions, and respiratory distress with feeding.

History and physical

The focus should be to elucidate the quality and timing of symptoms. Typically, patients with PA slings primarily demonstrate airway symptoms only, such as cough, stridor, frequent infections, and dyspnea. Patients born with PA sling and complete tracheal rings may rarely present with life threatening respiratory distress in infancy. In contrast, vascular rings will potentially present with both respiratory and feeding symptoms. Physical exam should identify any murmurs suggestive of coexisting cardiac malformations. History and physical exam should also encompass associated systemic congenital anomalies.

Tests

- *CXR.* It is important to review prior CXRs. Although either lung may appear hyperinflated secondary to varying location of tracheal stenosis, traditionally unilateral hyperinflation of the right lung may suggest a pulmonary artery sling. On a lateral film the left pulmonary artery on end will appear as a mass anterior to the esophagus and posterior to the trachea.

- *Echocardiography.* There is up to a 50% incidence of congenital heart defects with PA sling. These include atrial septal defects, left superior vena cava, ventricular septal defect, and patent ductus arteriosus. The anomalous take-off of the left pulmonary artery can usually be diagnosed by echocardiography.

- *Contrast esophagram.* In PA sling, unlike other vascular rings, the indentation on the esophagus will occur on the anterior margin rather than the posterior aspect. The esophagus may appear deviated slightly to the right. Alternative studies include computer tomography and magnetic resonance imaging.

- *Computed tomography/magnetic resonance imaging (CT/MRI).* Useful to delineate both airway and vascular anatomy. On these imaging modalities, the left pulmonary artery will be seen originating from the right pulmonary artery, encircling the trachea and extending to the left hilum posterior to the trachea and anterior to the esophagus and aorta. Similarly, MRI can provide similar information without the use of ionizing radiation. Both CT and MRI imaging can be useful in identifying areas of tracheal narrowing or the presence of complete tracheal rings. A notable disadvantage of MRI is the length of time required and the potential need for sedation, which may be unsafe in those in respiratory distress.

- *Bronchoscopy.* Complete tracheal rings occur when the membranous portion of the posterior tracheal is absent resulting in fully cartilaginous stenotic rings. Complete tracheal rings or "ring-sling complex" occurs in 50-65% of patients with PA slings. Bronchoscopy is utilized to assess for areas of tracheal stenosis, complete tracheal rings, and other unanticipated tracheal anomalies. Importantly, care must be taken after bronchoscopy as the already narrowed tracheal lumen may become edematous following manipulation.

Table 2. Key Diagnostic Findings for Differentiating Common Vascular Rings

Complete Vascular Ring	Key Diagnostic Findings
Double Aortic Arch	**Contrast Esophagram:** Indentation on the posterior esophagus in lateral view. Bilateral indentation on the esophagus from anteroposterior view. **CT/MRI:** With a balanced double aortic arch, the key findings are a 4-vessel sign and completely encircled trachea and esophagus. If not balanced, the most common dominant arch is right-sided (posterior) and usually appears higher and larger than the nondominant arch. **CXR:** Tracheal narrowing at the level of the aortic arch. **Bronchoscopy:** External, pulsatile compression just above the carina.
Incomplete Vascular Rings	**Key Diagnostic Findings**
Pulmonary Artery Sling	**Contrast Esophagram:** Indentation on the anterior esophagus in lateral view. **CT/MRI:** Left pulmonary artery can be appreciated originating from the right pulmonary artery and passing between the trachea and esophagus. **CXR:** Unilateral hyperinflation of the right lung. **Bronchoscopy:** May demonstrate complete tracheal rings in 50-65% of patients. Pulsatile indentations can be seen posteriorly on the trachea or at the level of the right mainstem.
Left Aortic Arch with Aberrant Right Subclavian	**Contrast Esophagram:** A high, posterior, oblique indentation (directed towards the right shoulder) on the posterior esophagus. This is known as a bayonet deformity. **CT/MRI:** Demonstrates the aberrant right subclavian artery arising from the distal left aortic arch and coursing rightward posterior to the esophagus. May be associated with a Kommerell's diverticulum at the origin of the aberrant right subclavian artery.
Innominate Artery Compression	**CT/MRI:** Innominate artery arises to the left of the trachea and causes appreciably tracheal compression as it courses anteriorly. **CXR:** tracheal compression and deviation may be appreciated. **Bronchoscopy:** Pulsatile anterior compression of the cervical trachea.

Index scenario (additional information)

"The patient's history and physical exam reveal symptoms of recurrent stridorous breathing, respiratory infections and shortness of breath. The child has no problems with either liquid or solid feeds. He has no other associated congenital anomalies. A CT scan reveals a left pulmonary artery originating from the posterior aspect of the right pulmonary artery and coursing behind the trachea contributing to tracheal compression."

Treatment/management

Patients diagnosed with PA slings should undergo surgical repair via median sternotomy. The key step in the operation is reimplantation of the left pulmonary artery. Subsequently, tracheal stenosis or complete tracheal rings may be addressed. If the stenosis is less than 30%

the length of the total tracheal length or less than 4 tracheal rings, an end-to-end anastomosis can be conducted. Otherwise, a slide tracheoplasty should be pursued and is the recommended approach at most institutions. Postoperatively, care may be complicated if there is residual trachea stenosis, which can tend to worsen due to tissue edema. Unfortunately, this edema usually occurs at the level of the bifurcation, distal to the end of the endotracheal tube, which can make respiratory support challenging.

Embryology and Anatomy

Normally, the primitive lung buds connect to their ipsilateral sixth arch, which will develop into the pulmonary arteries. A pulmonary sling occurs when the primitive left lung bud connects to derivatives of the right sixth arch through capillaries that are caudal rather than cephalad to the tracheobronchial tree. The left pulmonary artery then develops off the right pulmonary artery, rather than the main pulmonary artery. The left pulmonary artery passes around the right main bronchus and then runs posteriorly to the trachea and anterior to the esophagus. The ductus arteriosus / ligamentum arteriosum usually arises from the main PA and travels anterior and superior to the left main bronchus before inserting into the descending thoracic aorta. This creates a vascular sling that compresses the tracheobronchial tree (17).

Operative steps

- Median Sternotomy and if necessary, a collar neck incision can be added for visualization of the cervical trachea.

- Pericardial sac is opened and the aorta, right and left pulmonary arteries are mobilized extensively and isolated. Care is taken while mobilizing the LPA posterior to the trachea, especially in the absence of complete tracheal rings as it may be intimately associated with the membranous trachea.

- Cardiopulmonary bypass is established with an aortic and single venous cannula. Alternatively, bicaval cannulation may be used, especially if there are associated intracardiac lesions that will be repaired as well.

- If there is no tracheal reconstruction required, divide the left pulmonary artery at its origin on the right pulmonary artery and repair the defect in the right pulmonary artery. Carefully remove the left pulmonary artery from between the trachea and esophagus. Correct the vascular anomaly by anastomosing the left pulmonary artery to a longitudinal incision in the main pulmonary artery. This anastomosis is performed using running 6-0 polypropylene suture. Most often it is best to place the left pulmonary artery slightly posterior on the proximal main pulmonary artery just above the pulmonary valve. Some groups use the origin of the ligamentum arteriosum as a reference point.

- If tracheal reconstruction is required, the trachea is dissected out in the plane between the aorta and the superior vena cava.

  - Disruption of the lateral tracheal blood supply should be avoided.
  - Care should be taken to avoid injury to the recurrent laryngeal nerve that passes in the tracheoesophageal groove.

- The trachea is transected at the midportion of the stenosis. The left pulmonary artery is divided at its origin on the right pulmonary artery and the defect in the right pulmonary artery is repaired. The left pulmonary artery is retracted while the tracheal anastomosis is performed.

- For short segment stenosis, the proximal and distal ends of the trachea are resected until a satisfactory luminal size is identified. The anastomosis is performed with 5-0 or 6-0 polydiaxone or Maxon suture.

- For long segment stenosis, a slide tracheoplasty is performed. The proximal tracheal segment is incised longitudinally on the posterior side. The distal segment is incised longitudinally on the anterior side. The ends of the trachea are beveled. The anastomosis is performed with a running 5.0 or 6.0 PDS or Maxon suture (parachute technique) beginning at the superior border.

- A pedicled pericardial flap can be harvested to separate the tracheal anastomosis from the mediastinum. More specifically, this helps to prevent erosion of the reconstructed trachea into the vessels and also ensures that the tracheal anastomosis is well sealed.

- The left pulmonary artery is then reimplanted into the main pulmonary artery.

  - Any associated intra-cardiac anomalies can be repair at this time.

- Bronchoscopy should be performed to inspect the anastomosis and clear any residual secretions. The anastomosis is then tested with a peak airway pressure of 35 cm H_2O.

Potential questions/alternative scenarios

"After inspection of the trachea by bronchoscopy in the operating room, you realize the child has complete tracheal rings of 3 mm diameter and extending the length of 5 tracheal rings. What is your operative approach?
Complete tracheal rings do not necessarily need resection or tracheoplasty. The normal size of the trachea for an infant is 5-6 mm, so a 3 mm sized trachea is approximately 50% of normal lumen size. Good results have been obtained with pulmonary artery reimplantation alone. Many groups feel that the presence of complete tracheal rings with diameter < 50% of expected size warrants operation. The decision to perform a slide tracheoplasty versus resection depends on the length of the stenosis. Considering that this child has a long segment (≥5 tracheal rings), the tracheal repair should be done using the slide tracheoplasty technique.

"After the operation the patient develops dense granulation tissue at the anastomosis causing airway compromise. What are the treatment options?"
Stenting is the most commonly used method, but not the first choice. Balloon dilatations with rigid bronchoscopy must be tried first followed by stenting if needed. Laser therapy can be used if available. Aggressive nebulizer treatments with humidified air and mucolytic therapy must be used while the stent is in place. The majority of patient deaths in series of PA sling with tracheal stenosis are due to repeated airway collapse and inability to clear secretions leading to infectious complications.

"The child is 14-year-old and presents after a CT scan performed for blunt trauma incidentally shows a PA sling. The child is asymptomatic."
Although most pulmonary artery slings are symptomatic when found, the natural history is unknown. Most institutions offer surgery even in the absence of symptoms. An echocardiogram should be performed as well to rule out coexisting cardiac anomalies.

Pearls/pitfalls

- Use caution during the dissection of the pulmonary artery and posterior trachea/bronchus.
- Rule out coexisting cardiac malformations.

- The left pulmonary artery should be implanted slightly posteriorly on the proximal main pulmonary artery. Care must be taken to avoid kinking at its origin as it arises more distally than normal.
- Extensive tracheoplasty can cause carinal collapse requiring tracheal stenting.
- Early extubation to limit positive pressure ventilation on the tracheal repair is essential in stable patients.

Suggested readings

- Backer CL, Russell HM, Kaushal K, et al. Pulmonary artery sling: Current results with cardiopulmonary bypass. *Journal of Thoracic and Cardiovascular Surgery* 2012; 143:144–151.
- Huang SC, Chen YS, Chang CI, et al. Surgical management of pulmonary artery sling: Trachea diameter and outcomes with or without tracheoplasty. *Pediatric Pulmonology* 2012; 47:903-908.
- Stephens EH, Eltayeb O, Mongé MC, Forbess JM, Rastatter JC, Rigsby CK, Backer CL. Pediatric Tracheal Surgery: A 25-year Review of Slide Tracheoplasty and Tracheal Resection. *Ann Thoracic Surgery*. 2019 Aug 7.
- Yong MS, Zhu MZL, Bell D, Alphonso N, Brink J, d'Udekem Y, Konstantinov IE. Long-term outcomes of surgery for pulmonary artery sling in children. *European Journal of Cardiothoracic Surgery*. 2019 Jan 31.
- Yong MS, d'Udekem Y, Brizard CP, et al. Surgical management of pulmonary artery sling in children. *The Journal of Thoracic and Cardiovascular Surgery* 2012. Epub June 12.

86. PEDIATRIC MECHANICAL CIRCULATORY SUPPORT

Aditya Sengupta, MD and Raghav A. Murthy, MD, DABS, FACS

Concept
- Case
- Extracorporeal Membrane Oxygenation
- Short- & Mid-Term Mechanical Circulatory Support
- Durable Support
- NHLBI Pediatric Circulatory Support Program & PumpKIN Trial
- Technical Pearls/Pitfalls
- Potential Questions & Alternative Scenarios

Chief complaint
"A 4-year-old boy at 19-kg with Kawasaki disease and giant coronary aneurysms (on prophylactic enoxaparin and aspirin) suffered acute coronary ischemia (STEMI) secondary to thrombosis of the aneurysm. He was initially rescued in the catheterization laboratory with recanalization of the left coronary system, and then maintained in the ICU on anticoagulation and antiplatelet therapy. After an initial improvement of cardiac function and reduction of inotropic requirements, the aneurysm re-thrombosed, leading to severe left heart failure (EF 20%) and ventricular arrhythmias (unresponsive to amiodarone). How would you stabilize this patient?"

Differential
In this case, the differential shock in this patient is hypovolemic, cardiogenic, distributive/septic shock, or mixed. The exact cause in this case appears to be related to the patient's underlying cardiac condition, bringing cardiogenic shock higher in the differential. In any event, rapid stabilization and resuscitation are required.

History and physical
The patient in this scenario requires emergent cardiovascular and pulmonary support given the profound state of shock. Patients in shock will demonstrate tachycardia, tachypnea, hypoxia, and cool extremities (except in distributive shock where extremities may be warm). Patient may be undergoing active CPR, mechanical ventilation, or resuscitation with high-dose inotropic and vasopressor agents. For emergent situations such as this, extracorporeal membrane oxygenation (ECMO) is the primary means of provided support. Venoarterial extracorporeal membrane oxygenation (VA-ECMO) is the most prevalent form of pediatric mechanical circulatory support (MCS) used given its versatility and ability to be used in patients of any size. It is especially useful in the acute setting given the ease of cannulation either via sternotomy or via peripheral sites, and it remains the only resuscitative measure when significant hypoxemia and respiratory failure contribute to the underlying physiology. However, ECMO can only be used for short-term support. Furthermore, it limits attempts at ambulation and effective physical rehabilitation, and bleeding and thromboembolic complications are frequent. Survival to discharge for pediatric cardiac patients requiring ECMO has been ~40-50%, and long-term survival (if successfully supported by ECMO in the short-term) is ~90% after discharge.

Indications:

- Preoperative stabilization (e.g., prior to implantation of a durable device)
- Postcardiotomy shock or cardiac arrest
- Bridge-to-transplant (BTT)
- Cardiopulmonary arrest (extracorporeal cardiopulmonary resuscitation, or ECPR)
- Acute myocarditis
- Cardiomyopathy (dilated, hypertrophic, or restrictive)

- Pulmonary hypertension
- Intractable arrhythmias
- Heart failure after repair of congenital heart disease or single ventricle palliation
- Respiratory failure refractory to venovenous ECMO (VV-ECMO)

Although limited in scope compared to VA-ECMO, VV-ECMO can be particularly useful in cases where pulmonary hypertension and elevated pulmonary vascular resistance lead to right ventricular dysfunction in the perioperative period.

Left heart decompression can be enhanced if there is an adequate atrial septal defect (or one can be created in the catheterization laboratory), or by the placement of a transseptal/left atrial drainage cannula. Allowing the patient to be "pulsatile" also allows for left heart decompression.

Complications:

- Bleeding (e.g., at the cannulation site, cerebral)
- Infection
- Thrombosis
- Pulmonary edema (inadequate left heart decompression)
- Hemolysis
- Cannula malposition

Tests
Echocardiography: Used to assess cardiac function and subsequent recovery following initial stabilization on ECMO or other support. Used to determine if heart is decompressed on full circulatory support and need for further venting. With more durable support, can be used to help position support devices in the heart.
Laboratory Evaluations: Complete blood count is important to obtain to determine need for blood/platelet transfusion on mechanical support. Metabolic profile assists in determining renal function for titration of support and need for renal replacement therapy. Blood gas analysis is used to titrate level of ECMO support (oxygen concentration, gas sweep levels, ect.).

Index scenario (additional information)
"The patient underwent femoral veno-arterial ECMO placement with direct cannulation of the femoral vein and cannulation of the femoral artery with a "chimney graft". Hemodynamic stability was achieved, inotropes were weaned, and minimal ventilatory settings were required. End-organ function improved. Given that this patient currently has good right ventricular function, what are the options for continued left ventricular support?"

Treatment/management
Short- & Mid-Term Mechanical Circulatory Support
Short-term MCS devices are typically used for weeks, but support can be extended to months. Examples of such devices include the PediMag (for patients <10 kg; provides 0.4-1.7 L/min of cardiac output), CentriMag (provides 2-10 L/min of cardiac output), Rotaflow (for patients with BSA <1.3 m²), Impella 2.5 (for those with BSA 0.6-1.3 m²), Impella 5.0 (used for patients with BSA >1.2 m²), and TandemHeart (BSA >1.3 m²; provides up to 5 L/min of output). Right ventricular support can be achieved with ECMO, the Impella RP, or with the TandemHeart.

Indications:
- Inability to wean from cardiopulmonary bypass (CPB).

- Persistent heart failure, along with evidence of end-organ dysfunction in at least one other system, following maximal inotropic support. Examples of end-organ dysfunction include:

The decision to discontinue MCS or transition to another type of support depends on the clinical situation and institutional availability of devices. A short-term ventricular assist device (VAD) allows for better ventricular decompression, and thus, recovery. This increases the odds of VAD explantation and allows the patient to be a better candidate for long-term VAD support/BTT. Use of ECMO beyond two weeks increases the risk of complications. When used as a bridge-to-transplant, ECMO results in a higher wait-list mortality and lower survival post-transplantation. Use of a VAD as BTT results in lower complication rates, presumably due to a simpler circuit and a smaller incidence of thrombosis. The associated wait-list mortality and post-transplantation survival are much improved as well.

Use of a short-term VAD also allows for "down-categorization" of a child's PEDIMACS category (see below), which in turn allows for durable VAD implantation at a lower category with better results post-implantation.

PEDIMACS Profile (At Time of Implant):

- PEDIMACS 1: Critical Cardiogenic Shock
- PEDIMACS 2: Progressive Decline
- PEDIMACS 3: Stable but Inotrope-Dependent
- PEDIMACS 4: Resting Symptoms
- PEDIMACS 5: Exertion Intolerant
- PEDIMACS 6: Exertion Limited
- PEDIMACS 7: Advanced NYHA Class 3

Durable (Long-Term) Mechanical Circulatory Support
Durable VAD implantation is preferred when a patient with PEDIMACS profile <3 is in chronic heart failure. Here, patient size is the most important determinant of the eventual device to be implanted. In small patients, the Berlin Heart EXCOR is the only durable VAD with regulatory approval. For larger patients, options include the Berlin Heart EXCOR, Thoratec's HeartMate II and III, the HeartWare HVAD, and the SynCardia Total Artificial Heart. "Size", however, is a moving target. While the EXCOR can be used in pediatric patients of all sizes, implantation of the other durable devices may require CT imaging and "fit-testing". HeartWare's HVAD has been used in children with body-surface-areas as small as 0.6 m^2.

Operative steps
- ECMO cannulation strategies, when peripheral, involve either the neck (carotid artery and internal jugular vein) or groin (femoral artery and vein). Groin cannulation is usually reserved for children >15 kg. Here, limb ischemia is an obvious concern. This can be minimized by sewing in a graft in an end-to-side manner to the artery and then cannulating the graft, or with the use of an antegrade or retrograde perfusion catheter. Central cannulation requires a sternotomy and temporary sternal closure.

- Impella: The Abiomed Impella 2.5/5.0/RP can be used for left or right heart support. The support duration is limited to days. The device can be inserted by direct puncture of the femoral or axillary artery or by indirect cannulation via a chimney graft, is placed in a retrograde fashion, and sits across the aortic valve (guided in place by the use of fluoroscopy and echocardiography). It is usually used in patients with acute myocarditis or allograft rejection during recovery. Complications include dislodgement, hemolysis, bleeding, and thrombosis.

- TandemHeart: This device has been shown to provide better ventricular decompression than the Impella. Here, the inflow cannula is positioned across the atrial septum through the femoral vein and the outflow is to the femoral artery.

- PediMag, CentriMag, & Rotaflow: These devices can provide either univentricular or biventricular support for days to weeks. For isolated LVAD support, inflow cannulas can be placed across the left ventricular apex or the left atrium. The outflow cannula can be placed in the aorta or its branches (either directly or with a graft sewn to the vessel). RVAD inflow cannulas are usually placed directly into the right atrium with the outflow into the pulmonary artery. An oxygenator can also be added to the RVAD circuit.

- Berlin Heart EXCOR: This pulsatile, paracorporeal VAD can be used in patients of any size. It harbors pneumatically driven, thin membrane pumps that come in a variety of sizes (10-80 mL). This system allows for extubation and ambulation and can provide uni- and bi-ventricular support. It is superior to ECMO in providing moderate- to long-term support and has previously been used for BTT or bridge-to-recovery indications. The EXCOR system includes cannulas that are specifically designed for left- and right-sided support, and the extracorporeal pump can serve in either configuration. The inflow cannula for left heart support can be placed by cannulation of either the apex of the left ventricle or the left atrium. The outflow cannula can be directly sutured to the ascending aorta or sewn to a graft. This is often performed under cardiopulmonary bypass, and most surgeons prefer myocardial arrest. The cannulae are brought out through skin puncture sites to allow for sternal closure. Right heart support can be achieved via cannulation of the right atrium and pulmonary artery. Some centers prefer to initially connect these cannulae to a PediMag or CentriMag device. This allows for lower levels of anticoagulation in the initial post-operative period, and also enables one to determine the actual flows required for an adequate cardiac index. After a few days of stable anticoagulation and cessation of post-operative bleeding, these pumps can be exchanged for the continuous-flow pumps.

- HeartWare HVAD & HeartMate II/III: Implantation of these devices are similar. Most surgeons prefer performing a sternotomy, but other minimally invasive approaches are also possible. After initiation of cardiopulmonary bypass, the left ventricular apex is cannulated with the inflow cannula. This requires suturing a ring and coring the apex. The device is then connected to the ring and secured. The outflow graft is then sutured to the ascending aorta in an end-to-side fashion. After de-airing the device and graft, cardiopulmonary bypass is weaned as device flows are ramped up. If needed, right heart support can be provided by placing an additional HeartWare or HeartMate device. However, this comes with an increased risk of thrombosis. Thus, most centers prefer to provide additional right heart support with a paracorporeal device.

Potential questions/alternative scenarios
"Can ventricular assist devices be used for patients who have undergone single ventricle palliation?"
One of the greatest advances in pediatric cardiac surgery has been the development of single ventricle palliation. An initial palliative procedure results in a parallel circulation with the single ventricle pumping blood to both the systemic and pulmonary circuits. This is converted, in a staged fashion, to an in-series circulation with the Glenn operation and the Fontan completion. Heart failure can result during any stage requiring mechanical assistance for BTT. For patients that have undergone Fontan completion, this includes ventricular failure (left-sided failure) or "Fontan-concept" failure (right-sided failure). These patients are also the likeliest (among all single ventricle patients) to be candidates for VAD implantation. Numerous innovative techniques have been developed to allow for mechanical circulatory support during all stages of single ventricle palliation.

527

"What are the various anticoagulation strategies following institution of mechanical circulatory support?"
Heparin remains the mainstay of therapy. The timing of initiation and level of anticoagulation depend on the patient's clinical status. Heparin, or alternatively bivalirudin, has been the choice for patients supported on ECMO, the PediMag, CentriMag, and Rotaflow. The Berlin Heart EXCOR requires a higher level of anticoagulation, and two or more antiplatelet medications are generally employed. Heparin can be substituted with bivalirudin, enoxaparin, or warfarin. The HeartMate and HeartWare devices require warfarin in addition to an antiplatelet agent.

"What are some of the complications of MCS?"
Some of the commonly encountered complications include bleeding (e.g., post-operative, at the cannula insertion sites, gastrointestinal, and cerebral), thrombosis of the device or cannulae, stroke, and infection of the cannulae, driveline, or device.

"Is there a role for destination therapy in the pediatric population?"
Adults who are not deemed to be transplant candidates but receive long-term VAD support are termed to have destination therapy. This concept has been extended to the pediatric population. Destination therapy is being increasingly considered in children with certain forms of muscular dystrophy where skeletal myopathy far exceeds the cardiomyopathy, patients with malignancies where cure is unlikely or unproven, and certain patients with graft failure (to minimize immunosuppressive therapy or when compliance is an issue).

"What pediatric specific devices have been evaluated for durable mechanical circulatory assist in smaller children?"
The National Heart, Lung and Blood Institute (NHLBI) Pediatric Circulatory Support Program was established in 2004 to support development of innovative MCS devices for use in children. Devices supported by this program that were originally under active investigation include:

- PediaFlow VAD (University of Pittsburgh, Pittsburgh, PA)
- PediPump (Cleveland Clinic, Cleveland, OH)
- Pediatric Cardiopulmonary Assist System or pCAS (Ension Inc., Pittsburgh, PA)
- Pediatric Jarvik 2000 (Jarvik Heart Inc., New York, NY)
- Penn State Pediatric VAD or PVAD (Pennsylvania State University, Hershey, PA)

The Infant Jarvik 2015, one of the original devices investigated under the Pediatric Circulatory Support Program, has become the first continuous-flow VAD specifically designed for small children that obtained the Investigational Device Exemption from the U.S. Food and Drug Administration (FDA). This approval is a prerequisite to initiate a clinical trial (i.e., the PumpKIN trial). The PumpKIN trial was originally designed as a prospective, two-arm randomized study to compare the Infant Jarvik 2015 to the standard (and only) pediatric device, the Berlin Heart EXCOR. The study design, however, is now being reevaluated, and the trial may be transitioned to a single-arm pivotal study. The discussion regarding study design modification is currently underway among the trial executive committee, participating centers, the NHLBI, and FDA.

Pearls/pitfalls
- Proper cannula selection for carotid cannulation is of utmost importance and is based on the size of the carotid artery and the projected amount of blood flow through the cannula. Oversizing of the cannula can lead to injury to the carotid endothelium and catastrophic vascular disruption.

- Advancing the arterial cannula too far into the aorta can lead to partial occlusion of the aortic arch, injury to the facing aortic wall, or retrograde orientation of the cannula into the ascending aorta (thus placing undue mechanical stress on the aortic valve, leading to injury to the leaflets and valvar insufficiency).

- Femoral artery cannulation can be useful in larger patients and in those with compromised carotid blood flow. In patients with small femoral vessels, a side graft can be sewn onto the femoral artery, followed by placement of the cannula into the side graft. Alternatively, antegrade or retrograde cannulas can be used to perfuse the extremities.

- After LVAD implantation, right ventricular dysfunction and failure must be prevented and aggressively managed. Empiric use of inhaled nitric oxide and inotropic support, careful fluid management to prevent RV dilatation, and early implantation of an RVAD can tremendously improve outcomes.

- Implantation of the Heartware HVAD, HeartMate III, and SynCardia TAH in small patients requires pre-operative "fit-testing".

- Directing the inflow cannula away from the septum during positioning at the left ventricular apex can help prevent "suction" events in the post-operative period.

Suggested readings

- Duncan BW. Chapter 45: Pediatric Mechanical Circulatory Support. In: Mavroudis C, Backer CL, Idriss RF, eds. Pediatric Cardiac Surgery, 4th ed. Blackwell Publishing Ltd; 2013.
- Karamlou T, McMullan D, Baden HP, Jeffries H, & Cohen GA. Chapter 87: Extracorporeal Membrane Oxygenation in Pediatric Cardiac Care. In: Yuh DD, Vricella LA, Yang SC, Doty JR, eds. Johns Hopkins Textbook of Cardiothoracic Surgery, 2nd ed. McGraw-Hill Education; 2014.
- Nelson K & Vricella LA. Chapter 88: Ventricular Assist Devices in Children. In: Yuh DD, Vricella LA, Yang SC, Doty JR, eds. Johns Hopkins Textbook of Cardiothoracic Surgery, 2nd ed. McGraw-Hill Education; 2014.
- Adachi I. Current status and future perspectives of the PumpKIN trial. Transl Pediatr 2018;7(2):162-168.
- McMillan KN & Jaquiss R. Chapter 40: Ventricular Assist Device Therapy. In: Ungerleider R, Meliones JN, McMillan KN, Cooper DS, Jacobs JP, eds. Critical Heart Disease in Infants and Children, 3rd ed. Elsevier; 2019.

87. Adult Congenital Heart Disease: Pulmonary Valve Replacement

Michael Kasten, MD and Jeremy Herrmann, MD

Concept
Preoperative Workup of Adult Congenital Heart Disease
- Operative Conduct
- Alternative Choices
- Pearls/Pitfalls

Chief complaint
"A 36-year-old male presents to his cardiologist with general fatigue and worsening dyspnea on exertion. He underwent a modified Blalock-Taussig shunt as a neonate and a full repair of his tetralogy of Fallot as a four-month-old. He does not recall specific details about the procedures, which were performed in another state. He is a nonsmoker and is otherwise healthy, though is stamina limits his work and personal life. What is the differential and how would you proceed?"

Differential
1. Pulmonary insufficiency
2. Residual VSD
3. Right ventricular outflow tract obstruction
4. Arrhythmia

History and Physical
The natural history of patients with repaired tetralogy is emerging. Overall survival is 87% at 20 years, though by 30 years, 50% of repaired patients will require a reintervention. Late pulmonary valve insufficiency is most common, particularly in patients in whom the native pulmonary valve was not present (e.g., transannular patch repair, Right Ventricular to Pulmonary Artery (RVPA) conduit). Right ventricular aneurysms occur uncommonly following infundibular patching, but most commonly relate to distal pulmonary arterial stenosis. Supraventricular arrhythmias may occur late and are more likely to cause sudden death.

Patients should be evaluated by examining for scars, especially examining the lateral chest for thoracotomy scars that would indicate previous B-T shunting. A systolic murmur loudest at the left upper sternal border is most common and correlates with pulmonary stenosis. A diastolic murmur may be heard at the left second intercostal space and the S_2 may be split, indicating pulmonary insufficiency. Peripheral edema or ascites may be present in the setting of severe, chronic right heart failure.

2018 AHA/ACC Guidelines for Adult Congenital Heart Disesase:

Pulmonic Stenosis – Classified by gradients of <36 (mild), 36-64 (moderate), >64 mmHg (severe). Treatment: Moderate or severe and symptomatic: Balloon valvuloplasty 1ˢᵗ line, Surgical replacement 2ⁿᵈ line (COR I, Level B-NR). Severe asymptomatic: surgical or percutaneous intervention (COR – IIa, Level C-EO).

Pulmonary Insufficiency after PS intervention – Surgical replacement indicated in symptomatic patients and moderate or greater insufficiency. (COR I, Level B-NR)

Pulmonary Insufficiency after ToF repair- Valve replacement (surgical or percutaneous) in symptomatic patients with moderate or greater insufficiency. (COR I, Level B-NR) Valve replacement is also indicated for asymptomatic patients with ventricular enlargement, (COR II, and Level B-NR).

Tests

Previous operative reports: May contain key information regarding previous technical details and descriptions of coronary anomalies.

Chest X-ray: Should be ordered on all patients. Film may show cardiomegaly. Pleural effusions ae uncommon with PI.
ECG: May demonstrate a right bundle branch block or prolonged QRS interval.
A QRS interval greater than 180 msec increases the risk for ventricular tachycardia and sudden cardiac death. If any other history of arrhythmia, Holter event monitoring should be considered to determine whether ablation before or during surgery will be necessary.

Echocardiogram: Transthoracic Echocardiograms should be ordered on all patients with adult congenital heart disease. Comparison to previous is essential in determining timing of surgery. In this case, likely will demonstrate a dilated right ventricle, dilated right atrium, severe pulmonary regurgitation, and diminished right ventricular function, without stenosis and moderate tricuspid regurgitation. Left ventricular function is usually normal or mildly diminished. Tricuspid regurgitation may also be present. Also may demonstrate any intracardiac shunts (ASD, VSD).

Cardiac MRI: If no contraindication (ICD, pacemaker, etc), cardiac MRI will provide more information about ventricular function, valve function and morphology, pulmonary artery anatomy, and presence of myocardial fibrosis. A Right Ventricular End Diastolic Volume index (RVEDVi) >150 ml/m^2 and a RVEDV: LVEDV >2 are common indications for PVR. RVOT size can be evaluated for consideration of transcatheter PVR. Will visualize the relationship of the great vessels to the sternum in consideration for reentry.
Cardiac catheterization: Generally, not necessary in patients under 40 years unless there are specific concerns for coronary atherosclerosis, myocardial ischemia or previously documented coronary abnormalities. Can be beneficial for transcatheter PVR planning.
Chest Computed Tomography: Will demonstrate superior anatomic detail though without physiologic information, when compared to cardiac MRI. Useful for planning sternal reentry.

Index scenario (additional information)
Previous operative reports indicate the patient initially received a right modified BT shunt as in infant then underwent tetralogy of Fallot repair with a PTFE transannular patch. No coronary branches were seen crossing the RVOT. His echocardiogram demonstrates severe pulmonary insufficiency and no residual ASD or VSD. A bubble study was negative for atrial communication. Cardiac MRI demonstrated a RVEDV: LVEDV ratio of 2.6:1 and his anatomy was not suitable for percutaneous replacement.

Treatment/Management
2018 AHA/ACC Guidelines for Adult Congenital Heart Disease:
Pulmonic Stenosis: Classified by gradients of <36 (mild), 36-64 (moderate), >64 mmHg (severe). Treatment: Moderate or severe and symptomatic: Balloon valvuloplasty 1st line, Surgical replacement 2nd line (COR I, Level B-NR). Severe asymptomatic: surgical or percutaneous intervention (COR – IIa, Level C-EO).
Pulmonary Insufficiency after PS intervention: Surgical replacement indicated in symptomatic patients and moderate or greater insufficiency. (COR I, Level B-NR)
Pulmonary Insufficiency after ToF repair: Valve replacement (surgical or percutaneous) in symptomatic patients with moderate or greater insufficiency. (COR I, Level B-NR) Valve replacement is also indicated for asymptomatic patients with ventricular enlargement, (COR II, and Level B-NR).

Operative Steps
Redo sternotomy, right ventricular outflow tract reconstruction/pulmonary valve replacement

Setup:

Arterial lines should be placed on the opposite side of B-T shunt. Central access should be obtained but a pulmonary artery catheter is unnecessary. Groins should be prepped in the field in case urgent femoral cannulation is needed during reentry. Care should be taken during reentry to avoid injuring the RV free wall, RVPA conduit or RVOT patch, which can be densely adherent to the sternum.

Bypass Strategy:
If no atrial communication is present, the operation can be performed on bypass without arresting the heart. Bicaval venous cannulation may offer better venous drainage. If the TEE shows atrial communication (or a VSD repair is planned), the heart should be arrested with antegrade cardioplegia to facilitate. Additionally, if the patient has a history of atrial fibrillation or flutter and a right atrial MAZE procedure is planned, bicaval cannulation with snaring will be necessary. Retrograde cardioplegia is not necessary. Mild hypothermia (32-34°C) can be used.

Conduct of Repair
The RVOT should be opened through the existing patch after evaluating the branch pulmonary arteries. The infundibulum should be inspected for muscle bundles or RVOTO. Native valve leaflets are excised. Pulmonary valve replacement is performed using stented or stentless prosthesis. Occasionally a hood of bovine pericardium or other patch material is needed to augment the proximal anastomosis to avoid conduit compression. If the main PA or RVOT is significantly dilated and a stented bioprosthesis is chosen, the valve may be placed within the RVOT without the need for additional patch material. Any branch PA stenosis should be patched during the procedure. Separate from bypass in normal fashion. Pacing wires are not placed routinely unless a concomitant arrhythmia procedure is performed.

Potential questions/alternative scenarios
What conduits are available and are they placed in orthotopic or heterotopic position?
For patients less than 18 years, conduit options include bovine jugular vein (placed in a heterotopic position) or homograft. For patients older than 18 years, options included stented bioprostheses, stentless porcine aortic root, and homografts. During placement of stentless conduits, avoid narrowing the distal anastomosis with pursestringing and excise the main PA to shorten the length between the native pulmonary annulus and PA bifurcation. The key is to maximize laminar flow. Currently, there do not appear to be any differences in long-term durability and need for reintervention between these valve options. Mechanical valves are rarely used in the pulmonary position.

Bright red blood is encountered upon dissecting the posterolateral pulmonary root
Evaluate the left atrial appendage for bleeding; if not arrested, this could introduce left sided air. Repair with suture and continue dissection.

Your patient has moderate TR on preoperative echo, would this change your operative plan? Severe TR?
Moderate TR should improve with a competent pulmonary valve, so can be observed. However, severe TR should be addressed with annuloplasty (de Vega and/or annuloplasty ring) at the time of PVR.

Is there a role for percutaneous valve placement in the RVOT? What risks with placement
Patients are increasingly being evaluated for transcatheter pulmonary valve replacement as a first-line option. In appropriately selected patients (e.g., those with RVOT <28 mm), transcatheter pulmonary valve replacement can be safe and effective. However, no long-term data exist for transcatheter pulmonary valve replacements. A multidisciplinary discussion should be had for each patient, though criteria for this are not as strict as with transcatheter aortic valve replacement.

Pearls/pitfalls

- Adult congenital heart disease is becoming much more common as neonatal/infant repairs have improved over time
- Late pulmonary valve insufficiency is the most common presentation of adults who had congenital heart surgery for tetralogy of Fallot earlier in life
- Care should be taken during re-do sternotomy as RV-PA conduits and RVOT repairs can be densely adherent to the sternum
- Annular patch should be used as needed during pulmonary valve replacement
- Patching of branch PAs may be necessary depending on degree of stenosis
- Percutaneous valves may be considered for those with acceptable anatomy though long-term data is scarce

Suggested Readings

- Bhagara CJ, Hickey EJ, Van De Bruane et al. Pulmonary valve procedures late after repair of tetralogy of Fallot: current perspectives and contemporary approaches to management. *Can J Cardiol* 2017;33:1138-1149.
- Stout KK, Daniels CJ, Aboulhosn JA, et al., 2018 AHA/ACC Guideline for the Management of Adults with Congenital Heart Disease, *Journal of the American College of Cardiology* (2018) doi 10.1016

88. CONGENITAL DIAPHRAGMATIC HERNIA

Amir A. Sarkeshik, DO and Gary Raff, MD

Concept

- Recognition of congenital diaphragmatic hernia (CDH) in a neonate
- Early management strategies of symptomatic neonate with a CDH
- Role of concomitant congenital anomalies in prognosis
- Timing of surgical management on recognition of diagnosis
- Conduct of the operative repair

Chief Complaint

"A 2.2-kg newborn with no known antenatal history was delivered vaginally. Shortly following birth, the newborn becomes increasingly dyspneic and cyanotic. Exam reveals a scaphoid abdomen, prominent chest, and decreased breath sounds on the left. Plain films reveal lung parenchymal compression on the left with loops of bowel in the hemithorax."

Differential

The differential diagnosis of respiratory distress in a newborn can be extensive, ranging from meconium aspiration and pneumonia to cardiac defects. Evidence of lung compression on chest x-ray can result from congenital pulmonary airway malformations (CPAM), pulmonary sequestration, or teratomas.

History and physical

The constellation of dyspnea, cyanosis, scaphoid abdomen and a prominent chest should raise a high clinical suspicion for congenital diaphragmatic hernias (CDH). Diagnosis is secured with plain film which typically reveal loops of intestine in the associated hemi-thorax and mediastinal shift. Placement of a nasogastric tube often will lead to coiling in the left chest on imaging. Our attention to CDH in this chapter will be on left-sided posterolateral (Bochdalek) CDH as they (a) are more common, and (b) present an emergency.

Associated congenital anomalies involving other systems include cardiac (VSD, ASD, TOF, hypoplastic left heart), renal (ectopic kidney), central nervous system (neural tube defects) and gastrointestinal (Meckel diverticulum, anal atresia). Although prognosis is dependent on the severity of underlying pulmonary hypoplasia and pulmonary hypertension, the impact of these associated anomalies cannot be overstated. Studies have shown that 60% of non-survivors beyond the neonatal period typically have an associated anomaly. It is reported that those with an isolated CDH have a survival advantage. As such, prenatal diagnosis of CHD should prompt referral to a tertiary care center for judicious work-up, planning and multi-disciplinary management.

Tests

Pre-natal ultrasound- Diaphragm can be evaluated for defects
- Fluid-filled stomach or loops of intestine in chest
- R-Sided lesion = R Lobe of liver herniating to chest = ↓Prognosis
- L-Sided lesion = Rightward heart
- Evaluate for cardiac, renal, CNS and GI anomalies
- Diagnosis can typically be made by 2nd -trimester

Neonatal chest x-ray - Gas-filled loops of bowel in the chest
- Right-sided heart +/- mediastinal shift
- Compression of lung parenchyma on ipsilateral side
- Coiling of nasogastric tube in the chest

Neonatal echocardiogram
- Evaluate for structural cardiac anomalies
- Evaluate biventricular function

"The patient arrives with severe acidosis, dyspnea, and trouble with oxygenation on supplemental oxygenation. What is your next step, and what is the timing of definitive treatment for this patient?"

Treatment/management

Newborns with CDH often present in respiratory distress shortly after birth. This can result from the underlying pulmonary hypoplasia leads to a detrimental cycle of hypoxia, hypercarbia and acidosis. Initial goals in care should focus on the disruption of this cycle through optimization of *oxygenation* and *correction of acidosis*, in addition to *controlling the pulmonary hypertension*. While historically CDH was considered a surgical emergency, improvements in our understanding of its etiology have led to immediate medical stabilization with delayed surgical repair as the core tenants of practice. In the index scenario, the clinician should focus on rapid intubation, ventilation and neuromuscular blockade. Mask-bagging should be avoided as it will result in increased herniation and worsened respiratory status. Pre- and post-ductal monitoring is prudent and can be obtained through a right and left hand (*or lower extremity*) pulse-oximetry, respectively. A nasogastric Salem Sump tube should be advanced and placed to low-continuous suction to minimize intestinal distention within the thoracic cavity. Ventilation strategy should focus on (a) adequate post-ductal SpO2, (b) avoidance of respiratory acidosis and (c) limiting barotrauma in the hypoplastic lungs. Most cases can be managed using pressure-cycled mode with higher respiratory rates and lower peak airway pressures, while titrating FiO2 to a pre-ductal PaO2 <60-mmHg. Permissive hypercapnia can be tolerated, so long the PaCO2 remains <60-mmHg. If this is ineffective then high-frequency oscillatory ventilation (HFOV) strategies may be employed. Generally, when peak inspiratory pressure exceeds 25-cmH2O with conventional ventilation, HFOV should be considered to avoid barotrauma. In addition to resuscitative efforts and ventilation management, echocardiography must be done to (a) rule out associated cardiac anomalies and (b) assess ventricular function. Inhaled NO and sildenafil may be used to decrease pulmonary vascular resistance. Finally, judicious fluid and inotropic resuscitative efforts should not be overlooked. ECMO management may be necessary in select cases refractory to medical stabilization.

Historically, CDH was considered a surgical emergency under the pretext that decompression of the lungs through reduction of abdominal content offered the best chance for survival. As our understanding of the underlying pulmonary hypoplasia and pulmonary hypertension has evolved, CDH is now recognized as a *physiologic* emergency requiring pre-operative stabilization and delayed repair. Optimal timing of surgical intervention is unclear and institution dependent. Having said that, the criteria established by most centers mandate cardiopulmonary stabilization, resolution of acidosis and improvement in pulmonary hypertension before surgical intervention.

Operative Steps

The key principles of CDH repair are the identification of a hernia sac, reduction of involved content and repair of associated defect. The CDH is typically approached through a *subcostal incision*. Abdominal viscera are then identified and returned into the abdominal cavity. In the rare case (10%) that a hernia sac is present, it should be excised. If the associated diaphragmatic defect is small, it can be repaired with interrupted, non-absorbable sutures. For larger (and more common) defects or in the case of an absent hemidiaphragm, a polytetrafluoroethylene (PTFE) membrane is used for repair. This can be fixated to the ribs anteriorly and posteriorly with the medial edge sutured to the contralateral hemidiaphragm. There are also reports of several reconstructive techniques using latissimus dorsi, the internal oblique and transverse abdominus muscles in lieu of applying prosthetic material. Having said that, if the patient is clinically tenuous and may require ECMO post-operatively, strategies that require extensive dissection should be avoided to limit bleeding risk. Chest tubes are not routinely used unless there is a concern for active bleeding or evidence of an air-leak from preceding barotrauma.

Abdominal wall closure following CDH repair can lead to high intra-abdominal pressures with potential compromise of respiratory excursion post-operatively. This can be avoided by closing the skin over a fascial layer that is left open. In the case of more unstable patients, one may use silo closure with eventual abdominal wall re-approximation when appropriate.

Potential questions/alternative scenarios

"Despite aggressive HFOV strategies and medical efforts, the neonate remains hypoxic and hypercapnic— with an SpO_2 of 75% and $PaCO_2$ of 70 mmHg, respectively. How would you proceed?"
With improvements in the management of CDH, the past two decades have witnessed a decrease in ECMO requirement. Having said that, if ECMO is considered, the neonate should demonstrate some evidence of adequate, revivable, lung parenchyma. General criteria for ECMO use in CDH are listed below. Meeting these criteria has been associated with a significant ECMO survival benefit, resulting in survival of over 75% of eligible patients. In addition to these criteria, VV-ECMO should be considered if there is a reversable process that can be treated on recovery of lung function.

CRITERIA FOR USE OF ECMO IN CDH	
Consider ECMO...	No ECMO...
A-a gradient > 600-mm Hg for 4-hours	Weight < 2-kg – *cannula size limitation*
Oxygen Index > 40 | OI: *(MAP x FiO_2 x 100) / PaO_2*	Newborn with <34-weeks gestation
PaO_2 < 40 and/or pH < 7.15 ≥ 2-hours	Lethal associated congenital anomalies
"Failure to respond to conventional therapy"	Evidence of intracranial hemorrhage

"Describe the two main types of congenital diaphragmatic hernias."
Most commonly, CDH occurs through the posterolateral diaphragmatic defect of Bochdalek. Of these, left-sided defects are more common, constituting 90% of presentations, while right-sided defects represent the remaining 10%. As opposed to Bochdalek diaphragmatic hernias, Morgagni hernias are anterior (retrosternal) defects, representing less than 2% of all CDH. They are typically asymptomatic and if ever an issue, they present with gastrointestinal features typically later in life.

Pearls/pitfalls

- Respiratory distress in CDH is due to pulmonary hypoplasia, hypercarbia and acidosis
- CDH represents a *physiologic* emergency requiring immediate attention on diagnosis
- Gentle ventilation strategies should be employed to avoid barotrauma
- Defined algorithms in care are institutional dependent with no major consensus
- Management should focus on stabilization, evaluation for other anomalies with delayed repair
- Timing of repair depends on adequacy of pulmonary parenchyma and presence of other congenital anomalies

Suggested Readings

- J, D., Meyerson, S. L., A, P. (Ed.), & JD, C. (Ed.) (2008). *Pearson's Thoracic and Esophageal Surgery 3rd edition*. Philadelphia: Churchill Livingstone.
- Coran, A. G., & Adzick, N. S. (2012). *Pediatric surgery*. Philadelphia, PA: Elsevier MosbyFoker JE et al. Development of a true primary repair for the full spectrum of esophageal atresia. *Ann Surg* 1997, 226(4):533-41.

89. CONGENITAL TRACHEOESOPHAGEAL FISTULA
Amir A. Sarkeshik, DO and Amy L. Rahm, MD

Concept
- Pre-operative evaluation and work-up
- Risk stratification and decision making
- Role of associated anomalies in management
- Surgical conduct, pearls and potential pitfalls

Chief complaint

"A 2.5 kg newborn with an antenatal diagnosis of Tetralogy of Fallot (TOF) was born by C- section. Maternal history was significant for polyhydramnios during pregnancy. At birth, TTE confirmed TOF but no significant gradient across the right ventricle outflow tract with an SpO2 of 95%. On first feed, the child develops significant choking, coughing and cyanosis. The cyanosis improved with supplemental oxygen. Multiple attempts at nasogastric (NG) tube placement were met with failure as it did not traverse beyond 10-cm from the alveolar ridge. Plain radiograph reveals curling of the NG tube in the esophagus, as well as dense right upper lobe opacification."

Differential

The differential diagnosis of respiratory distress in a newborn is extensive. Common causes include meconium aspiration, pneumonia, transient tachypnea of the newborn, structural heart defects, and tracheoesophageal fistula.

TEF and EA are typically described using the Gross classification. Esophageal atresia with a distal tracheal fistula, or Type C, is the most common form (*Think C = Common*) seen in 85% of cases. Pure esophageal atresia, or Type A, comprises 8% of the cases (*Think A = Atresia Alone*). Other, more rare variations include an isolated fistula (Type E), an esophageal atresia with a proximal fistula (Type B) and esophageal atresia with both proximal and distal fistula (Type D).

History and physical

The triad of choking, coughing and cyanosis on first feed with an inability to pass an NG-tube beyond 10-cm is pathognomonic for esophageal atresia +/- fistula. A scaphoid abdomen and radiographic evidence of air in the stomach are indicative of a distal tracheoesophageal fistula (TEF), whereas a gasless abdomen and maternal polyhydramnios are more suggestive of isolated esophageal atresia (EA).

TEF is associated with other congenital anomalies in 50% of patients. Cardiac abnormalities, particularly VSD and TOF are common, mandating a TTE to be done as part of basic work-up. In addition, TEF is part of the VACTERL association (*v*ertebral anomalies, *a*nal atresia, *c*ardiac defects, *t*racheo-*e*sophageal fistulas, *r*enal defects and *l*imb defects) and presentation of these conditions should prompt a higher level of clinical suspicion for a TEF diagnosis.

Tests
- *Pre-natal Ultrasonography.* Polyhydramnios with a small (*or no*) stomach bubble
- *Chest X-Ray.* Most important diagnostic study. Inability to pass NGT beyond 10-cm (*resistance*). NGT tip curled in esophageal pouch
- *Abdominal X-Ray.* No air in stomach: isolated EA, no TEF. Air in stomach: EA + distal TEF.
- *Transthoracic Echocardiography.* Perform in all patients to rule out CHD. Aortic arch sidedness can affect surgical approach (*R-sided aorta = L surgical approach*).
- *Renal Ultrasound.* Rule out renal agenesis.
- *Genetic Karyotyping.* Rule out chromosomal abnormalities. Trisomy 13 or 18 = No surgical intervention.
- *Thin Barium Esophagography.* Confirms diagnosis and detects any proximal fistula.
- *Rigid Bronchoscopy.* Performed for definitive diagnosis if unclear. Identify simultaneous proximal and distal fistula(s).

"The patient develops progressive respiratory distress. Chest x-ray reveals ground glass opacification of the right upper lobe lung and a very distended stomach. How would you proceed?"

Treatment/management
Pre-operative management

- Keep neonate in semi-upright sitting position (30° - 45°)
- Place soft stump tube in atretic esophageal pouch on low-intermittent suction
- Perform frequent oropharyngeal suctioning
- Empiric antibiotics (ampicillin and gentamicin) + acid suppressors
- Endotracheal intubation in case of ↑ respiratory distress + **gentle low-pressure ventilation**
- If extremely unstable then emergent decompressive gastrostomy can be considered
- If remains unstable, may consider emergent ligation of fistula with delayed primary repair

Risk stratification and timing of repair
Decision to proceed with early vs delayed repair is dependent on the risk profile of the patient. Neonates with a low birthweight (<1500 g) +/- major cardiac anomalies are deemed to be "high-risk" and should undergo palliative gastrostomy with delayed repair. In the case of worsening respiratory status from escaped ventilatory gases, a transpleural ligation of the fistula can be performed to stabilize the patient with plans for delayed repair. Significant improvement in diagnosis, neonatal care, anesthetic care and management of associated comorbidities has evolved since the risk classification was initially proposed. Sptiz et al proposed the most recent classification based upon birth weight +/- cardiac abnormality.

Sptiz Classification	
Criteria I	Birth weight > 1500-g and no major cardiac anomaly
Criteria II	Birth weight < 1500-g or major cardiac anomaly
Criteria III	Birth weight < 1500-g and major cardiac anomaly

Currently, individualized decisions dictate operative timing and approach. Early repair is generally employed on neonates with an adequate birth weight (>1200-g) in the absence of pneumonia or other major associated anomalies.

Operative Steps
Open TEF Repair
TEF repair may be performed through an open or thoracoscopic approach. Side of entry is contralateral to the side of aortic arch, highlighting the importance of a thorough pre-operative work-up. For a left-sided aortic arch, one should enter the right chest and vise versa. Below, we highlight the major steps involved in an open approach in a patient with a left-sided aortic arch.

- General anesthesia with adequate venous access
- Left lateral decubitus position and flexible bronchoscopy to confirm ETT position
- Right posterolateral thoracotomy with entry through the 4th or 5th intercostal space
- Perform extrapleural dissection to limit any esophageal leak to retropleural space
- Identify, ligate and divide the azygos vein
- Identify and preserve the vagus nerve as it courses along the side of esophageal pouch
- Retract the mediastinal pleura anteriorly to identify the trachea and esophagus
- Identify distal esophagus and circumscribe with vessel loop to inhibit air-leak through fistula

- Identify proximal esophagus by asking anesthetist to push to proximal pouch to right
- Perform posterior and lateral (blunt) dissection of the proximal pouch
- Isolate and divide fistula, closing tracheal side in interrupted fashion with absorbable sutures
- Perform a water-bubble test to ensure air-tight closure of tracheal repair
- Perform judicious dissection of distal esophagus to ensure a tension-free repair
- Amputate tip of proximal esophageal pouch to open the lumen and reveal mucosa
- Perform a single layer anastomosis between the esophageal ends (end-to-end | 5-0 Vicryl)
- Prior to completion of the anastomosis, an NG-tube is passed beyond the site into stomach
- Place a drain anchored to the posterior chest wall (not adjacent to the suture line)
- Chest closure with gentle re-approximation of the ribs to prevent overlapping

Potential Questions and Alternative Scenarios

"You are consulted on a term 3.2-kg neonate with TEF and pulmonary atresia with ductal dependent pulmonary circulation. The patient is maintained on prostaglandins and SpO2 is in the low-90s. His hemodynamic status is stable. How would you proceed with timing and sequence of shunt and TEF surgery?"

Patients with cardiac lesions that predispose them to high pulmonary blood flow can safely proceed to esophageal repair in the immediate neonatal period. Since the pulmonary resistance is high, the consequences of high pulmonary blood flow are mitigated. As the pulmonary resistance falls and pulmonary over-circulation develops, appropriate palliative or reparative measures can be taken. In patients with ductal dependent circulation, the clinical status of the patient dictates timing of esophageal repair. If the clinical condition is appropriate and duct is patent, prostaglandin infusion is maintained, and esophageal repair can be carried out prior to cardiac surgery. If there is evidence of systemic or pulmonary hypoperfusion with hypoxemia, then a prostaglandin infusion should be initiated, and judicious resuscitation carried out. Once stable, the patient may undergo esophageal repair. If clinical stability cannot be achieved, then the definitive or a palliative cardiac procedure should be carried. In general, it is rare that cardiac surgery precedes palliative or definitive TEF repair.

"You are attempting a thoracoscopic repair and notice a right-sided aortic arch."

Aortic arch-sidedness should be confirmed with echocardiography prior to surgery. If a right-sided arch is discovered, a left thoracotomy is the side of choice. While open repair can be performed through the right chest, the aorta may limit critical exposure. In the present scenario, further attempts through the right side should be abandoned and a left approach undertaken.

"After division of fistula, you notice there is a significant gap between the esophageal ends."

Long gap atresia has traditionally been defined as greater than 3-cm or three vertebral bodies. It is a somewhat subjective term which literally means that the gap cannot be bridged together and differs from surgeon to surgeon. It is classically associated with esophageal atresia without fistula. Management of these patients is very difficult and there is no best technique. Esophageal stretching first proposed by Foker et al uses traction sutures on the esophagus that are brought out through the skin. The ends of the esophagus are marked by radio opaque metallic clips. Progressive traction is applied over the course of the subsequent days and as the esophageal ends overlap, definitive surgery is carried out. The results of this procedure have been controversial. These patients have classically been managed with gastrostomy and bouginage until overlap is seen with serial fluoroscopy and then staged repair is completed. Other methods used to lengthen the esophagus include circular myotomies (achieve 1-cm lengthening with each myotomy), proximal esophageal flap with tubularization and limited mobilization of the distal esophagus. Post-operative strictures and impaired esophageal function are common and require close monitoring and serial dilations. In addition, given that this anastomosis is under tension, the patient is kept sedated, paralyzed and managed with the neck in flexion for up to 5-7 days. If the gap cannot be bridged in patients with long gap atresia, then esophageal replacement options are entertained. These include gastric, colonic, or jejunal interposition to bridge the gap.

"You obtain an esophagram after a routine TEF repair on day five and note extravasation of contrast at the anastomosis."
Minor leaks occur in 15-20% of neonates following repair; most of these can be managed conservatively with drainage, antibiotics and parenteral or enteral jejunal nutrition. Significant disruptions are rare and present with pneumothorax and signs of sepsis. Anastomotic disruptions warrant a return to the OR for mediastinal drainage, gastrostomy, and takedown of the anastomosis with diverting esophagostomy. Minor leaks are associated with a significant rate of esophageal stricture and should be followed in a serial fashion with esophagoscopy and dilatation. Aggressive acid suppression with proton pump inhibitors should not be overlooked.

"You are seeing a patient six months after a TEF repair; parents report poor feeding and regurgitation."
The long-term complications of TEF repair include esophageal stricture, esophageal dysmotility, gastroesophageal reflux, tracheomalacia, and scoliosis. In rare cases a missed laryngopharyngeal cleft is diagnosed. Reflux and esophageal strictures predominate due to universal distal esophageal dysmotility. There is approximately a 30% incidence of stricture formation and about 40% of patients have significant gastroesophageal reflux.
Aggressive screening for stricture with esophagram is recommended and any stricture should be dilated. pH probe monitoring and manometry should be carried out. Failure of acid suppression presents a second set of challenges. Nissen fundoplication has a high early failure rate in patients with TEF. Inherent esophageal dysmotility in children with TEF and the foreshortened esophagus make the wrap difficult. One strategy is to use nasal or gastro-jejunal feeding until the child grows and then reassess the need for an anti-reflux procedure. Although prokinetic agents are recommended for esophageal dysmotility, their efficacy and treatment results have been disappointing.

Pearls/pitfalls

- TEF diagnosis mandates an aggressive evaluation of concomitant congenital abnormalities

- Staged repair for neonates <1200-g or unstable ductal dependent cardiac anomaly

- Establishing arch sidedness is essential for employing appropriate surgical approach

- A small cuff of esophageal tissue should be retained to prevent tracheal narrowing

- Limit mobilization (as possible) of the distal esophagus to prevent esophageal necrosis

- Long gap atresia encountered during surgery is best managed by a staged approach

- Feeding difficulty is common after surgery due to esophageal strictures, dysmotility and reflux; an aggressive approach to counter these is necessary

Suggested readings

- Sptiz L. Oesophageal atresia. *Orphanet J Rare Dis* 2007 May 11;2:24.

- Poenaru D et al. A new prognostic classification for esophageal atresia. *Surgery* 1993, 113(4):426-432.

- Foker JE et al. Development of a true primary repair for the full spectrum of esophageal atresia. *Ann Surg* 1997, 226(4):533-41.

90. CONGENITAL PULMONARY AIRWAY MALFORMATION (CPAM)

Stephanie N. Nguyen, MD and Jennifer C. Romano, MD, MS

This chapter is a revision and update of that included in the previous edition of the TSRA Clinical Scenario written by Immanuel Turner, MD. Jennifer C. Nelson, MD, and Jennifer C. Hirsch-Romano, MD, MS.

Concept

- Classification of congenital pulmonary airway malformation (CPAM)
- Prenatal/neonatal diagnosis and management
- Surgical indications
- Pearls and alternative scenarios

Chief complaint

"A 2-day-old 3.4 kg boy presents with acute respiratory failure and cyanosis. Prenatal ultrasound revealed multiple cystic lesions in the left lower lobe and postnatal CXR shows a gas-filled shadow and mild flattening of the left hemidiaphragm."

Differential

Congenital pulmonary airway malformation (CPAM), formerly known as congenital cystic adenomatoid malformation (CCAM), is the most common congenital lung lesion and should be suspected given the radiologic findings. Other congenital thoracic lesions to consider include pulmonary bronchogenic cysts, congenital lobar emphysema, pulmonary sequestration, cystic bronchiectasis, pneumatocele formation, foregut malformations, and congenital diaphragmatic hernia.

History and physical

The history and physical exam aids in establishing the diagnosis and yields important information about the maternal and fetal clinical course. Elicit whether hydrops fetalis or polyhydramnios were present prenatally, as these may be clinical indicators of disease severity. After birth, symptoms may include tachypnea, labored breathing, hypoxemia, hypercarbia, poor feeding, and overt respiratory failure requiring invasive or noninvasive ventilatory support. In infants and older children, a history of recurrent respiratory infections is key. Severe respiratory distress is rare, with persistent cough, dyspnea, or cyanosis being common complaints. Depending on the size of the lesion(s), exam findings include focally diminished/absent breath sounds, hyperresonance, and chest wall asymmetry. Additionally, chromosomal microarray testing may also be performed if there is concern for other congenital anomalies. The presence of other associated cardiac, gastrointestinal or renal anomalies should be noted and evaluated.

Classification of CPAM

There are 5 types of CPAM, each with distinct pathologic characteristics and prognosis:

- *Type 0 (1-3%):* Small cysts (< 0.5 cm in diameter) originating from tracheal or bronchial tissue with diffuse lung involvement. Severe and usually lethal at birth.
- *Type 1 (50-70%):* Multiple or a single dominant cyst (3-10 cm) arising from the distal bronchus or proximal bronchiole. Often unilateral lung involvement with potential for significant mass effect and malignant transformation.
- *Type 2 (15-20%):* Small cysts (0.5-2 cm) with solid components arising from terminal bronchioles. Highest incidence of associated congenital anomalies (60%), which are often the presenting feature and determinant of prognosis. These include congenital heart disease, intestinal atresia, renal agenesis, congenital diaphragmatic hernias, and pectus excavatum.

- *Type 3 (5-10%):* Solid lesions with small cysts (< 0.5 cm) arising from acinar tissue which proliferate to occupy entire lung lobes. Present with respiratory distress or neonatal death.
- *Type 4 (5-10%):* Large cysts (5-10 cm) arising from alveolar tissue. Often present with tension pneumothorax or recurrent infection. Strong association with malignancy, particularly pleuropulmonary blastoma.

Tests
Prenatal ultrasound:
CPAM is usually detected in the second trimester, appearing as a cystic intrathoracic mass(es). Cysts may be unilateral, bilateral, macrocystic (>5 mm; anechoic) or microcystic (<5 mm; hyperechoic). Depending on CPAM size and location, mediastinal shift, hydrops fetalis, pulmonary hypoplasia, and polyhydramnios may also be present. Significant mass effect suggests a poor prognosis and often occurs when the cysts occupy > 50% of the thoracic cavity. The CPAM volume ratio (CVR) is a sonographic indicator of outcome and is obtained by dividing CPAM volume by head circumference. CVR > 1.6 is highly predictive for the risk of hydrops, respiratory insufficiency, and early intervention. Though 50% of CPAMs may regress during gestation, the majority persist postnatally.
Postnatal imaging:
- *CXR:* All infants with a prenatal diagnosis of CPAM should have a CXR shortly after birth to assess for mass effect. Cysts appear as fluid-filled or solid lesions, or an ill-defined shadow.
- *CT:* Confirms the diagnosis by further delineating cyst location and characteristics. The best test for differentiating CPAM from other thoracic lesions and identifying associated congenital anomalies. CTA is particularly useful for distinguishing CPAM from bronchopulmonary sequestration (BPS), which has a systemic feeding vessel.
- *MRI:* Also helpful for confirming CPAM diagnosis and identifying associated anomalies; however, clinical utility has not been well studied.

Index scenario (additional information)
"In this symptomatic neonate, CT scan confirmed a 7cm multi-cystic lesion in the left lower lobe with no aberrant systemic vasculature. No other congenital anomalies were present. How would you proceed?"
Treatment/management
Early surgical resection is indicated and curative for symptomatic cases. Lobectomy is preferred over parenchymal-sparing resection as it is often difficult to delineate between CPAM and normal lung parenchyma and incomplete resection carries the risk of recurrent infection and malignant transformation. Overall, lobectomy is generally well-tolerated in this patient population and may lead to compensatory lung growth. Extensive multi-lobar disease can be managed by pneumonectomy or segmental resection to preserve pulmonary parenchyma. Management of asymptomatic CPAM is somewhat more controversial; however, given the risk of malignancy and/or infection that complicates further intervention, the general consensus is to resect.

Operative steps
Goals – complete resection of abnormal lung parenchyma to relieve symptoms and prevent infection and malignant transformation.
- Single lung ventilation (by selective mainstem intubation in neonates)
- Posterolateral thoracotomy and entrance into the chest cavity through the 5th or 6th interspace. Thoracoscopic approach for small peripheral lesions in experienced centers.
- Completion of major and minor fissure
- Sequential division of arterial branches, pulmonary veins, and segmental bronchus
- Lobectomy vs. pneumonectomy vs. parenchymal-sparing resection

Potential questions/alternative scenarios
542

"The previously described patient is noted to have hydrops fetalis at 22 weeks gestational age."

Development of hydrops fetalis (due to IVC compression and cardiac displacement) is associated with high mortality rate. It is usually seen when CVR > 1.6. Prenatal intervention aims to alleviate the mass effect and to prevent progression and complications of CPAM. First-line treatment is maternal betamethasone administration for stabilization or regression of lesions. Invasive approaches include thoracentesis, thoracoamniotic shunts, and fetal thoracotomy. Pre-term delivery may be indicated in severe cases and should be performed at institutions with capacity for advanced cardiorespiratory support, including extracorporeal membrane oxygenation (ECMO). Furthermore, fetal echocardiogram is important to fully assess cardiac anatomy and function.

"The patient is asymptomatic at birth."

Regression may occur in 40-60% of cases. Early surgical resection is controversial, as risk and morbidity may outweigh the benefits. Close observation with routine CT imaging is performed, delaying surgery until 6 months of age to minimize risk of operation. Nonetheless, asymptomatic patients with high-risk features (large, bilateral or multifocal cysts, recurrent infection, and pneumothorax) should undergo surgical evaluation for resection during infancy.

"A 3-year-old boy presents with progressive weight loss and sudden onset dyspnea and right-sided chest pain. CXR reveals a tension pneumothorax and CT scan demonstrates a 6cm solid mass in the right upper lobe. Lobectomy was performed and histologic analysis was positive for malignancy."

Pleuropulmonary blastoma (PPB) is a rare and aggressive childhood lung tumor, arising from the lung or pleura. There is a known association with Type 4 CPAM and oftentimes the two may be indistinguishable, as up to 30% of PPB present in a purely cystic form. Pneumothorax is a common feature of Type 4 CPAM and may be the first manifestation of PPB. A weak association also exists between Type 1 CPAM and bronchoalveolar carcinoma (adenocarcinoma in situ).

"A 10-year-old girl presents with recurrent cough and pneumonia. A CXR shows a left lower lobe consolidation and CT reveals a left lower lobe lung mass with an infra-diaphragmatic aortic blood supply."

This patient has a bronchopulmonary sequestration (BPS), which presents differently from CPAM in that patients tend to be older with more subtle respiratory symptoms. Treatment is also resection, which should be delayed for 3-4 weeks after appropriate antibiotic therapy in the setting of active infection. CT angiography is a useful diagnostic test, as BPS is characterized by aberrant systemic blood supply from the abdominal aorta, thoracic aorta or even subclavian or coronary vessels. In contrast, CPAM is supplied by the pulmonary arteries. BPS can be intralobar or extralobar depending on whether the mass lies within or outside normal lung tissue.

Pearls/pitfalls

- If symptomatic, early resection is indicated, and lobectomy is standard of care.
- If asymptomatic, elective resection after 6 months of age should be considered to minimize risk of recurrent infections and malignant transformation.
- Hydrops fetalis is associated with a poor prognosis and fetal intervention may be indicated.

- Fetal echocardiogram is important to fully assess cardiac anatomy and function in the setting of hydrops and Type 2 CPAM (commonly associated with other congenital anomalies)
- Controversy still exists regarding the malignant potential for an unresected asymptomatic CPAM.

Suggested readings

- Baird R, Puligandla PS, Laberge J-M. Congenital lung malformations: Informing best practice. *Seminars in Pediatric Surgery.* 2014;23(5):270-277.

- David M, Lamas-Pinheiro R, Henriques-Coelho T. Prenatal and Postnatal Management of Congenital Pulmonary Airway Malformation. *Neonatology.* 2016;110(2):101-115. doi:10.1159/000440894.

- Hung-Wen et al. Management of Congenital Cystic Adenomatoid Malformation and Bronchopulmonary sequestration in Newborns. *Ped Neonatol.* 2010; 51 (3):172-177.

- Kim et al Treatment of Congenital Cystic Adenomatoid Malformation: Should lobectomy always be performed? *Ann Thorac Surg.* 2008; 86:249-53.

- Nagata et al. Outcome and treatment in an anenatally diagnosed congenital cystic adenomatoid malformation of the lung. *Ped Surg Int.* 2009; 25:753-757.

91. Chest Wall Deformities

Mallory Hunt, MD and J. William Gaynor, MD

Concept

- Presentation and overview of pectus deformities
- Diagnostic workup
- Surgical technique: Ravitch and Nuss procedures
- Potential questions/alternative scenarios
- Pearls/pitfalls

Chief complaint

"A 16-year-old male with a history of asthma presents to his primary care physician with a two-week history of palpitations. He has been otherwise healthy, although he's noticed that he is more fatigued with exercise over the past several months. He denies tobacco or other drug use. His family history is notable for aortic insufficiency in his mother. He tells you that his chest "looks funny" and that it has been that way his entire life, but he has noticed it more recently. Physical exam reveals a tall, thin male with a pectus excavatum deformity, and normal cardiopulmonary exam."

Differential

The patient above presents with pectus excavatum on physical exam, the most common chest wall deformity. Other chest wall/thoracic deformities include pectus carinatum, scoliosis of the thoracic spine, and absent pectoralis muscle as found in Poland syndrome.

History and physical

Pectus excavatum, also known as sunken or "funnel chest," accounts for >90% of all chest wall deformities, occurring in up to 1 in 300 live births, with a 4:1 male predominance. It is characterized by a posterior depression of the sternum beginning below the insertion of the second costal cartilage, with posterior angulation of the costal cartilage-sternal junction. In childhood, it is generally well-tolerated, but older children and teenagers may present with a variety of symptoms, including palpitations, precordial pain during exercise, and decreased exercise tolerance. The severity of pectus excavatum depends on the degree of posterior displacement; with the most severe form being those cases in which the sternum nearly abuts the vertebral bodies, resulting in RV compression.

Pectus carinatum, also known as "keel chest," occurs with less frequency compared to pectus excavatum, and again demonstrates a male predominance. It is characterized by outward protrusion of the sternum and is typically asymptomatic.

A genetic predisposition for the pectus deformities has been suggested, as anywhere between 25-40% of patients have a family history of chest wall deformities. Some have hypothesized that abnormal connective tissue development plays a role, as these deformities have been associated with other musculoskeletal disorders such as scoliosis and Marfan Syndrome. While most patients tolerate pectus well in infancy and childhood, others may become symptomatic in their later childhood and teenage years, due to associated comorbidities or resulting cardiac compression, particularly during exercise. However, the cosmetic disfigurement associated with these deformities often remains the dominant issue, affecting self-esteem and social behavior. Thus, even asymptomatic patients may present for elective repair.

Tests

*Calculation of the **Haller Index** (CT or MRI):* the Haller Index is a measure of pectus severity and is obtained by divided the transverse thoracic diameter by the anteroposterior (AP) distance between the posterior sternum and anterior vertebral body. Haller Index <2.5 is considered normal, and values >3.1 are considered severe.

Pulmonary function testing: including spirometry. Frequently normal but may show restrictive physiology.

EKG: expected to show some changes, even in asymptomatic patients, due to displacement of the heart by the deformity. Frequent changes of note include a) S1S3 or S1Q3, b) negative p waves in V1, and c) RSR' pattern in V1. Notably, these changes frequently disappear postoperatively, with correction of cardiac malpositioning.

Echocardiogram: transthoracic imaging may be challenging due to posterior displacement of the heart, and often transesophageal echocardiogram is necessary for optimal evaluation. Many echocardiographic findings may be observed in patients with pectus, including but not limited to RV dysfunction, RV enlargement, mitral and/or tricuspid valve prolapse, aortic root enlargement, and atrial or ventricular septal defects.

Index scenario (additional information)
"MRI of the chest is performed and reveals a Haller Index of 3.2. Pulmonary function testing is normal at rest, and EKG shows frequent premature atrial contractions with RSR' pattern in V1. Given the patient's history of palpitations, a Holter monitor is ordered and the event log notes frequent PACs and PVCs, with several runs of SVT. Echocardiogram demonstrates RV compression with mildly decreased function, normal LVEF, and no valvular abnormalities."

Treatment/management
Due to worsening of pectus deformities during the axial growth spurt period, patients often present for operative evaluation currently. Careful surgical planning must involve a discussion of optimal timing, due to the potential for recurrence if the axial growth spurt has not completed at the time of repair.

The **Ravitch procedure**, originally described in 1949, has been dubbed the "ideal" surgical repair for pectus excavatum. It consists of bilateral subperichondrial resection of all deformed costal cartilages (typically from cartilages 3 through 7), in addition to an anterior wedge-shaped osteotomy to elevate the sternum which is supported by a strut for 6 months to 1 year while the perichondrium heals and ossifies.

The **Nuss Procedure**, first described in 1988, involves the insertion of a convex steel bar underneath the sternum and takes advantage of the flexibility of the anterior chest wall. Performed via a thoracoscopic/minimally invasive approach, it has gained popularity in recent years, particularly among patients.

Preoperative Considerations
- Preoperative evaluation should include a careful history, and if any family or patient history of allergy to nickel or metal is noted, allergy testing should be performed. In the event of an allergy, titanium bars may be used; however, these are significantly more expensive and should be reserved for cases of necessity.
- Bar sizing can be determined preoperatively using cross-sectional imaging by measuring the mid-axillary to mid-axillary distance across the deepest segment of pectus depression. The optimal bar is 1 inch shorter than the distance from the right-to-left mid-axillary line.
- Pre-operative discussion about pain control is crucial to recovery and may include thoracic epidural and/or patient-controlled anesthesia (PCA).

Operative steps
Ravitch Procedure
- The procedure is performed under general anesthesia, with the patient positioned supine and arms abducted.
- A transverse incision is made at the level of the inframammary crease between the nipples, and skin flaps are mobilized above the deformity.
- The pectoralis muscles are reflected off the sternum and costal cartilages, with careful attention to identify an avascular plan and avoid the intercostal neurovascular bundles. If needed, rectus abdominus insertions are divided to expose inferior cartilages.

- Subperichondrial resection begins by incising the pericondrium anteriorly and developing a plane between it and the costal cartilage. Clamps can be used to elevate the edges of the cartilage as necessary. When coming around the cartilage to the posterior aspect, it is important to avoid incising the perichondrium.
- A perichondrial elevator is placed posterior to the costal cartilage as it is divided from the sternum. The divided cartilage is grasped with a clamp, elevated anteriorly, and the costal cartilage removed from the costochondral junction.
- This process is repeated bilaterally from costal cartilages 3 through 7, or fewer levels depending on the extent of the deformity.
- Following resection of all affected costal cartilage, a wedge-shaped osteotomy is created anteriorly above the level of the deformity to correct the excavatum deformity. The base of the sternum is elevated, and the posterior aspect is fractured behind the osteotomy.
- A retrosternal strut is placed posterior to the sternum to support it in its corrected position. It is then secured to the ribs bilaterally to prevent migration. The strut is typically removed 6-12 months after repair, at which time sufficient ossification has usually occurred to fix the sternum in its new location.
- A more common modification of the Ravitch procedure involves more limited cartilage resection, with only small pieces of parasternal and costochondral cartilage removed at each level. This modification improves operative time and extent.

Nuss Procedure
- The operation is performed under general anesthesia, with the patient positioned supine and arms abducted.
- The right-to-left mid-axillary distance is confirmed in the operating room, and the bar bent to allow for sternal correction. A 2 to 4 cm region in the middle of the bar is left flat for sternal support.
- The deepest portion of the pectus deformity is identified; and once this is done, subcutaneous incisions are made in the mid-axillary line bilaterally. A trochar is introduced through a separate incision just inferior to one of these incisions, and a scope inserted for visualization and safety during bar introduction.
- Under direct visualization, the pectus introducer bar is passed through the subcutaneous tunnel to the pectoral ridge and into the thoracic cavity at the deepest point of sternal depression. Note that this point often occurs adjacent to the pericardium, and a gentle sweeping motion can be utilized to create a plane of entry with the introducer tip always under direct view. Once the introducer reaches the contralateral pectoral ridge, it is pushed out of the thorax and into the subcutaneous tunnel.
- The Nuss bar is then pushed across the mediastinum. Upward traction on the bar by the assistant may be employed for ease of entry. Some surgeons also employ a third, subxiphoid incision, in order to elevate the sternum with a towel clip or manually.
- Once the definitive Nuss bar is in place, it is rotated 180 degrees and each end is attached to the stabilizer, which is attached to the chest wall with suture around the bar and rib.
- Timing of bar removal is surgeon- and patient-specific, but bars are typically left in place for 2 to 4 years.

Potential questions/alternative scenarios

"A 17-year-old male patient presents for surgical repair of a pectus carinatum defect. He is otherwise healthy. You have discussed the surgical options with the patient and his family, and a Ravitch approach is chosen. How can this procedure be modified to treat pectus carinatum defects?"

The Ravitch procedure is easily modified for surgical treatment of pectus carinatum. Once cartilage resection accomplished, a transverse osteotomy is made across the anterior sternum, and a wedge of autologous cartilage is placed within it to depress the sternum to its proper location.

"What are the most common complications following repair of pectus deformities?"

Prior to introduction of Nuss bar stabilizers, bar migration was not uncommon, and reoperation following the Nuss procedure for bar correction was required approximately 4% of the time. Following the introduction of bar stabilizers, this complication has nearly disappeared. More common complications in the current era are pneumothorax, which occurs up to two-thirds of the time but rarely requires intervention. Wound infection (1%) and hemothorax (0.5%) are also recognized complications.

Pearls/pitfalls
- Pectus excavatum and pectus carinatum are the most common chest wall deformities, with pectus excavatum representing most cases presenting for surgical repair.
- More common in males, and frequently associated with Marfan syndrome/connective tissue disorders.
- Haller Index (transverse thoracic diameter divided by AP distance from posterior sternum to anterior vertebral bodies) >3.1 considered to be severe.
- Both the Ravitch and Nuss procedures both well-tolerated with low post-operative complication rates.

Suggested readings
- Martins de Oliveira., et al. "The electrocardiogram in pectus excavatum". British Heart Journal 20.4 (1958): 495-501.
- Silbiger, J. J., & Parikh, A. (2016). Pectus excavatum: echocardiographic, pathophysiologic, and surgical insights. Echocardiography, 33(8), 1239-1244.
- Operative Correction of Pectus Excavatum and Pectus Carinatum. Kaiser, LR, Kron, IL, and Spray, TL (eds). Mastery of Cardiothoracic Surgery, 3e Philadelphia, PA: Lippincott Williams & Wilkins; 2014.
- Davis, J. T., & Weinstein, S. (2004). Repair of the pectus deformity: results of the Ravitch approach in the current era. The Annals of thoracic surgery, 78(2), 421-426.
- Kelly, R. E., Goretsky, M. J., Obermeyer, R., Kuhn, M. A., Redlinger, R., Haney, T. S., ... & Nuss, D. (2010). Twenty-one years of experience with minimally invasive repair of pectus excavatum by the Nuss procedure in 1215 patients. Annals of surgery, 252(6), 1072-1081.

Made in the USA
Columbia, SC
07 December 2024

48679141R00328